Neurodevelopmental Disorders: Pathogenesis, Diagnosis and Management

Neurodevelopmental Disorders: Pathogenesis, Diagnosis and Management

Edited by Ella Keller

hayle
medical

New York

Hayle Medical,
750 Third Avenue, 9th Floor,
New York, NY 10017, USA

Visit us on the World Wide Web at:
www.haylemedical.com

ISBN: 978-1-63241-677-3

Cataloging-in-Publication Data

Neurodevelopmental disorders : pathogenesis, diagnosis and management / edited by Ella Keller.
    p. cm.
Includes bibliographical references and index.
ISBN 978-1-63241-677-3
1. Nervous system--Diseases--Pathogenesis. 2. Nervous system--Diseases--Diagnosis.
3. Nervous system--Diseases--Treatment. 4. Developmental neurobiology.
5. Nervous system--Growth. 6. Neurology. I. Keller, Ella.
RC346 .N48 2019
616.8--dc23

Table of Contents

Preface

Neurodevelopmental disorder is a mental disorder that affects emotion, self-control, learning ability and memory. It manifests after the individual grows. Such disorders can be genetic, such as attention deficit hyperactivity disorder, fragile-X syndrome, Down syndrome, etc., or caused due to neurotoxicants such as Minamata disease and fetal alcohol spectrum disorder. Intellectual disabilities and autism spectrum disorders also fall under neurodevelopmental disorders. The development of the nervous system is a tightly regulated genetically encoded process that is influenced by the environment. Any deviation from this process can result in such disorders and lead to potentially distinct pathologies later in life. Deprivation from emotional and social care in children, genetic influences, immune dysfunction, traumatic brain injury and nutritional deficits can cause such disorders. These can be diagnosed using chromosomal microarray analysis. Through support from therapists, counselors, families and groups, such disorders can be managed. This book covers in detail some existing theories and innovative concepts revolving around neurodevelopment disorders. The objective is to give a general view of the different aspects of their pathogenesis, diagnosis and management. It will help the readers in keeping pace with the rapid changes in this field.

After months of intensive research and writing, this book is the end result of all who devoted their time and efforts in the initiation and progress of this book. It will surely be a source of reference in enhancing the required knowledge of the new developments in the area. During the course of developing this book, certain measures such as accuracy, authenticity and research focused analytical studies were given preference in order to produce a comprehensive book in the area of study.

This book would not have been possible without the efforts of the authors and the publisher. I extend my sincere thanks to them. Secondly, I express my gratitude to my family and well-wishers. And most importantly, I thank my students for constantly expressing their willingness and curiosity in enhancing their knowledge in the field, which encourages me to take up further research projects for the advancement of the area.

Editor

Differential effects of anxiety and autism on social scene scanning in males with fragile X syndrome

Hayley Crawford[1,2]* ⓘ, Joanna Moss[2,3], Chris Oliver[2] and Deborah Riby[4]

Abstract

Background: Existing literature draws links between social attention and socio-behavioural profiles in neurodevelopmental disorders. Fragile X syndrome (FXS) is associated with a known socio-behavioural phenotype of social anxiety and social communication difficulties alongside high social motivation. However, studies investigating social attention in males with FXS are scarce. Using eye tracking, this study investigates social attention and its relationship with both anxiety and autism symptomatology in males with FXS.

Methods: We compared dwell times to the background, body, and face regions of naturalistic social scenes in 11 males with FXS ($M_{age} = 26.29$) and 11 typically developing (TD) children who were matched on gender and receptive language ability ($M_{age} = 6.28$). Using informant-report measures, we then investigated the relationships between social scene scanning and anxiety, and social scene scanning and social communicative impairments.

Results: Males with FXS did not differ to TD children on overall dwell time to the background, body, or face regions of the naturalistic social scenes. Whilst males with FXS displayed developmentally 'typical' social attention, increased looking at faces was associated with both heightened anxiety and fewer social communication impairments in this group.

Conclusions: These results offer novel insights into the mechanisms associated with social attention in FXS and provide evidence to suggest that anxiety and autism symptomatology, which are both heightened in FXS, have differential effects on social attention.

Keywords: Eye tracking, Fragile X syndrome, Autism spectrum disorder, Anxiety, Social attention

Background

Fragile X syndrome (FXS) is the most common cause of inherited intellectual disability affecting approximately 1 in 2500 males and 1 in 4000–6000 females [1]. FXS is caused by excessive cytosine-guanine-guanine (CGG) repeats on the Fragile X Mental Retardation 1 (FMR1) gene located on the Xq27.3 site. Individuals with the FXS premutation have 45–200 repeats whereas individuals with the full mutation have in excess of 200 repeats. The excessive CGG repeats cause the FMR1 gene to become methylated, resulting in reduced production of the protein FMRP. As FXS is an X-linked disorder, males are more severely affected than females. The phenotype associated with FXS encompasses mild to profound intellectual disability alongside physical, cognitive, and behavioural manifestations [2].

FXS is associated with a socio-behavioural phenotype that includes being motivated to interact with others and demonstrating interest in the social world. However, these features co-occur with heightened anxieties and social communication impairments [2, 3]. The social communication impairment associated with FXS is reflected in the heightened prevalence of autism spectrum disorders (ASD). Although prevalence figures often vary across studies, a recent meta-analysis has indicated that approximately 30% of males with FXS meet criteria for ASD [4]. This is in comparison to 1% of the

* Correspondence: hayley.crawford@coventry.ac.uk
[1]Centre for Research in Psychology, Behaviour and Achievement, Coventry University, Coventry CV1 5FB, UK
[2]Cerebra Centre for Neurodevelopmental Disorders, School of Psychology, University of Birmingham, Edgbaston B15 2TT, UK
Full list of author information is available at the end of the article

general population [5]. However, it is increasingly recognised that subtle differences exist between individuals with FXS and those with idiopathic ASD, as those with FXS often display a milder profile of autism symptomatology. A recent review of existing literature highlights several studies indicating less severe social impairments in individuals with FXS and comorbid ASD compared to individuals with idiopathic ASD, particularly on measures of social responsiveness [6].

Anxiety is also commonly reported in FXS with over 80% of males meeting criteria for one anxiety disorder and 60% meeting criteria for multiple anxiety disorders. The most common types of anxiety disorder in FXS are specific phobia, selective mutism, and social phobia. Approximately 60% of males with FXS display clinically significant features of social phobia [7]. Despite social communication impairments and social anxiety, individuals with FXS are reported to show behaviours suggestive of a willingness to interact with others; thus, they appear socially motivated [8–10].

Relevant to the features of FXS described above, existing literature within the field of developmental disorders has drawn links between socio-behavioural characteristics and social attention. Research has primarily identified atypically reduced social attention in ASD (behaviourally associated with social withdrawal) and atypically prolonged social attention in Williams syndrome (WS; behaviourally associated with hyper-sociability) [11–14]. Specifically, this research has demonstrated that people with ASD spend less time than typically developing (TD) individuals viewing people and faces in static pictures of social interaction. Attention to social stimuli in this group has also been linked to social behaviour, with reduced social attention being associated with more severe autism symptomatology and consequently more social communication difficulties [15–17]. Much research has focussed on the association between social behaviour and social attention in ASD. However, little is known about the way in which behavioural characteristics interact with social attention in males with FXS despite the known social profile associated with this group, and the heightened risk of autism.

Studies that have been conducted in FXS have identified atypical social attention, in the form of reduced looking to the eye region of static isolated faces, compared to TD individuals [18–20] and individuals with ASD [20, 21]. However, every one of these studies used isolated face images displaying different emotional expressions. Whilst this offers rich information regarding looking patterns to facial features in FXS, it is known from the literature on both typical development and ASD that such stimuli lack ecological validity as there is no 'competition' between social and non-social attention capture (e.g. see discussions by [16]). One study that has investigated social attention to more naturalistic social

scenes reported that a largely female sample of people with FXS spent a 'typical' amount of time looking at social information, but that they also looked away quicker than TD participants, indicating active social avoidance [22]. The issue that 12 out of the 14 FXS participants in that study were female is important due to the striking differences in the severity and prevalence of the FXS phenotype between males and females. Therefore, it is problematic to generalise findings from studies using largely female samples to males with FXS who are often more severely affected.

There is a need to utilise ecologically valid social scene stimuli to understand the social attention of males with FXS. Furthermore, given the socio-behavioural profile of the disorder, preliminary insight into the role of anxiety and autistic features is important to understand the potential mechanisms underlying social attention in this group. In typical development, it is known that socially anxious individuals fixate longer on the eye region of faces than those without social anxiety [23]. Anxiety has previously been related to social attention in people with WS, but in a different way, with high levels of anxiety being associated with reduced fixation on faces and eye regions of threatening facial expressions [24]. In FXS, some studies have reported that reduced fixation to the eye region of isolated emotionally expressive faces is not associated with social anxiety [20] or autism symptomatology [19, 21], whereas other studies have reported a positive correlation between self-reported social anxiety and time spent looking at the eye region of faces [25]. Studying FXS, a genetic syndrome with heightened risk of autism and anxiety, offers novel insight into the association between these behavioural characteristics and social attention, which may inform understanding of other neurodevelopmental disorders associated with a similar socio-behavioural profile, e.g. ASD and Cornelia de Lange syndrome [26].

Whilst existing eye-tracking studies in FXS have offered rich information regarding the extent of eye gaze aversion, the current study makes a significant contribution to investigating the influence of anxiety and autism symptomatology on social attention in males with FXS using naturalistic social scenes that reflect the complexities of our social world. This study aims to (1) compare and contrast social attention in males with FXS to TD children matched on gender and receptive language ability, (2) investigate the relationship between social attention and anxiety in males with FXS, and (3) investigate the relationship between social communication impairment and social attention in males with FXS.

Methods

Participants

Participants were 11 males with FXS aged between 14 and 43 years (M_{age} = 26.29; 9.06). All participants had a confirmed diagnosis from a professional (paediatrician, general practitioner, or clinical geneticist). Participants with FXS were recruited through the Cerebra Centre for Neurodevelopmental Disorders participant database at the University of Birmingham.

Participants with FXS were group-matched to 11 male TD children on receptive language ability (t (20) = −1.208, p = .242) using the raw scores from the British Picture Vocabulary Scale (BPVS; [27]). As previous literature indicates that receptive language is commensurate with nonverbal mental age in adolescents with FXS [28], receptive language was used as a proxy indicator of general intellectual ability. TD children were recruited through the Infant and Child Laboratory participant database, also at the University of Birmingham. None of the TD children scored above 15 on the Social Communication Questionnaire (SCQ; [29]), the score suggested by the authors to be indicative of ASD. All of the TD children scored within the normal range on the Spence Child Anxiety Scale—Parent version (SCAS-P; [30]), defined as the mean + 1 standard deviation, using the national normal data from TD boys aged 6–11 years [31]. The same criterion was used to rule out anxiety in children under the age of 6 years in the current study. Table 1 presents the final participant characteristics.

All participants had normal or corrected to normal vision. All participants aged 16 years and over provided informed written consent, and parents of children aged under 16 provided written consent before taking part in the study, in line with the ethical approval granted from the Science, Technology, Engineering and Mathematics Ethical Review Committee at the University of Birmingham.

Stimuli and apparatus

The stimuli used were identical to those used by Riby and Hancock [11]. Stimuli consisted of 20 colour photographs of naturalistic social scenes including human actors engaged in natural activities. Example scenes included a bride and groom on their wedding day, a woman on the phone, a group of friends talking to one another, and a teacher in a classroom. Actors in the photographs were not directing their attention towards the camera and displayed natural facial expressions. Specifically, the emotional valence of the actors in the social scenes was mostly neutral, interspersed with a few images where actors were displaying a happy facial expression. The scenery was naturalistic for the activities that actors were engaged in, e.g. classroom, restaurant. Participants also saw five filler photographs of landscapes with no actor, which were interspersed throughout the eye-tracking task so as to avoid a uniform pattern of solely social scenes being displayed. As filler trials contained no social stimuli, eye movements during these trials were not analysed. Stimuli were 640 × 480 pixels.

Stimuli were presented on a 24-in. widescreen LED monitor at a screen resolution of 1680 × 1050. Participants' eye movements were recorded using an EyeLink 1000 Tower Mount system, which runs with a spatial accuracy of .5–1 visual angle (°), a spatial resolution of .01°, and a temporal resolution of 500 Hz. The right eye of each participant was tracked. The eye-tracking camera was linked to a host PC separate to the one displaying the stimuli. EyeLink software (SR research, Ontario, Canada) was used to control the camera and collect data.

Measures

The participants' primary caregivers completed the SCQ [29] and the SCAS-P [30] to measure social communication impairments and anxiety, respectively, and for the purposes of investigating associations between these behavioural characteristics and social attention in the present study. The SCAS-P assesses the following six domains of anxiety: physical injury fears, obsessive-compulsive disorder, separation anxiety, social phobia, panic/agoraphobia, and generalised anxiety, and has been shown to differentiate those with and without an anxiety disorder. Internal consistencies of the total scale and subscales range from .83 to .92 in an anxiety-disordered group and .81 to .90 in typical controls. The SCAS-P total score correlates significantly with the Child Behavior Checklist [32] internalising subscale, indicating convergent validity [31]. Caregivers completed these measures either whilst their child was participating in the study or at home, returning it to the researchers

Table 1 Participant characteristics and alpha level for comparison between FXS and TD participants

	FXS (n = 11)	TD (n =11)	t	df	p
Chronological age (years)					
Mean (SD)	26.29 (9.06)	6.28 (1.31)	−7.256	20	<.001
Range	14.12–43.01	4.60–8.94			
Receptive language ability (raw score)					
Mean (SD)	87.00 (27.21)	74.18 (22.32)	−1.208	20	.241
Range	87–135	47–114			
Gender (% male)	100	100			

Comparison between participants on chronological age, receptive language ability as measured by the British Picture Vocabulary Scale, and gender on completion. All participants lived at home with the caregiver completing the questionnaire measures. The Autism Diagnostic Observation Schedule (ADOS; [33]) was administered to all participants with FXS for diagnostic purposes (module 2: $n = 2$; module 3: $n = 5$; module 4: $n = 4$). The BPVS [27] was administered to all participants to assess receptive language ability.

Procedure

Participants were tested individually at the University of Birmingham in a dimly lit room with windows blacked out to avoid luminance changes. Participants were seated approximately .6 m from the screen with their chin resting on a chinrest and their forehead against a headrest. The chinrest and desk height were adjusted so that eye gaze was central to the display screen. A 5-point calibration was performed prior to the experiment during which participants followed the location of an animated blue dolphin positioned at the edges of the display area. The calibration procedure was repeated until successful, and all participants included in the analysis achieved a full 5-point calibration. Following calibration, the participants were told that they would view a series of pictures and that they could look wherever they wished whilst these were displayed. Each image was then presented for 5 s. Between each trial, a fixation cross appeared at the centre of the screen for 1 s.

Data analysis

Areas of interest (AOI) were designated to the face, body, and background using the Data Viewer programme (SR Research). Face and body AOI were created using the FreeHand Interest Area Shape to select the outline of each actor's face and body. The background AOI was created using the Rectangular Interest Area Shape, to cover the entire image, and then subtracting fixation data from the face and body AOI prior to analysis. Data are presented as the total time, in milliseconds, that fixations were within each AOI. A trial was deemed invalid, and therefore excluded, if a participant did not look at the picture presented for any of the trial time. If any participant produced more than 40% invalid trials, their data were excluded from analyses. In the current study, one participant produced one invalid trial only. Therefore, no participants were excluded due to insufficient data. All data were subjected to the Shapiro-Wilk test for normality. Where data were not normally distributed, non-parametric tests were used for statistical analyses. For the between-group comparisons, where results from non-parametric tests did not differ from results from the equivalent parametric tests, the results from the parametric tests are reported. For within-group correlations, Spearman's correlations are used where data are not normally distributed and Pearson's correlations are used where data are normally distributed. The alpha level for significance was .05.

Results

There was no difference in the overall amount of time participants spent viewing stimuli, indicating comparable task engagement across the groups (FXS mean per image: 4202.46 ms; TD mean per image: 4237.88 ms; $t (20) = .148$, $p = .884$). The remaining analyses concern dwell time in milliseconds for each AOI (see Fig. 1).

A 3 (AOI: background, body, face) × 2 (group: FXS, TD) ANOVA was conducted, which revealed a significant main effect of AOI ($F (2, 40) = 38.153$, $p < .001$, $n^2 = .656$) but no significant main effect of group ($F (1, 20) = .009$, $p = .923$, $n^2 < .001$), and no significant interaction ($F (2, 40) = 1.066$, $p = .354$, $n^2 = .051$). Bonferroni post hoc tests indicated that the main effect of AOI was driven by longer dwell time on the background than the body and the face regions of the actors in the scenes (both $p < .001$). Dwell times on the face and body region of actors were statistically comparable ($p = .081$). However, Wilcoxon signed rank tests, which were conducted because body AOI data were not normally distributed, revealed longer dwell time on the face compared to the body region of actors ($Z = -2.029, p = .042$).

Correlations were conducted to assess the association between dwell time on each AOI and social communication difficulties, as measured by the SCQ, and social phobia and total anxiety scores, as measured by the SCAS-P for each participant group. Table 2 shows the descriptive statistics for these measures by group. A significant negative correlation between SCQ score and dwell time to the background was revealed for the TD group ($r_s (7) = -.792$, $p = .011$), indicating that those individuals with fewer social communication difficulties spent more time looking at the background. No other significant correlations were revealed for the TD participant group (all $p > .05$; Table 3). For participants with FXS, moderate-strong positive correlations were revealed between dwell time on the face AOI and social phobia ($r_p (8) = .687$, $p = .028$; Fig. 2), and between dwell time on the face AOI and total anxiety score ($r_p (8) = .742$, $p = .014$; Fig. 3). A significant negative correlation was revealed between dwell time on the face AOI and SCQ score ($r_p (7) = -.720$, $p = .029$; Fig. 4). This did not remain significant after controlling for receptive language ability ($r_p (5) = -.704$, $p = .077$). Taken together, this indicates that those FXS participants with higher anxiety scores, and fewer social communication difficulties, exhibited longer dwell times on faces.

As participant groups were not matched on chronological age, correlations were conducted to assess the relationship between chronological age and dwell time, especially due to the large age range of the FXS group.

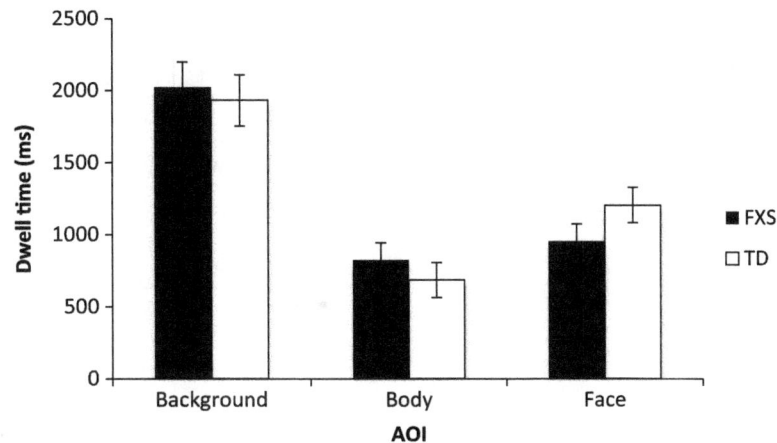

Fig. 1 Dwell time on AOIs; dwell time in milliseconds on background, body, and face AOI for the FXS and TD participant groups, when overall engagement with the stimuli did not differ across groups

These revealed no significant association between chronological age and dwell time on any AOI for either participant group (all $p > .05$). Although participant groups were matched on receptive language ability, correlations were conducted to assess the relationship between receptive language and dwell time in the event that our group-matching comparison was underpowered. These revealed no significant association between receptive language and dwell time on any AOI for either participant group (all $p > .05$).

Discussion

In the present study, we examined and compared visual attention to naturalistic social scenes in males with FXS versus TD individuals. In addition, we investigated the relationship between social attention, anxiety, and social communication difficulties. The results demonstrated statistically comparable dwell time on background, body, and face regions of the social scenes across the two participant groups. The results also demonstrated an association between increased looking at faces with

Table 2 Descriptive statistics and alpha level for the ADOS, SCQ, and SCAS-P measures

Measure	FXS	TD	t	df	p
ADOS					
Mean raw total score (SD)	8.64 (5.12)	NA			
Range	2–22				
% meeting cut-off for ASD	72.73				
% meeting cut-off for autism	18.18				
Social Communication Questionnaire[a]					
Mean raw total score (SD)	17.57 (6.27)	2.89 (2.37)	−6.569	16	<.001
Range	6–27	0–6			
% meeting cut-off for ASD	77.7	0			
% meeting cut-off for autism	22.22	0			
Spence Child Anxiety Scale[b]					
Mean raw Social Phobia score (SD)[c]	4.33 (4.53)	2.63 (2.26)	−.967	16	.348
Range	0–14.4	0–6			
Mean raw total score (SD)[d]	19.54 (16.95)	9.38 (5.32)	−1.625	16	.124
Range	1–49	1–20			

[a]SCQ was not completed for two TD participants and two FXS participants
[b]SCAS-P was not completed for three TD participants and one FXS participant
[c]The maximum Social Phobia score on the SCAS-P is 18. Normative data obtained from Nauta et al. [31] indicate a mean score of 7.3 for anxiety-disordered and a mean score of 4.3 for typically developing boys aged 6–11 years
[d]The maximum total score on the SCAS-P is 114. Normative data obtained from Nauta et al. [31] indicate a mean total score of 31.4 for anxiety-disordered and 16.0 for typically developing boys aged 6–11 years

Table 3 Correlations between behavioural characteristics and social attention, and between participant characteristics and social attention

	Fragile X syndrome			Typically developing		
	Face r_p (p)	Body r_p (p)	Background r_p (p)	Face r_p (p)	Body r_s (p)	Background r_s (p)
Social phobia	.687 (.028)	−.311 (.981)	−.161 (.657)	−.059 (.890)	−.024 (.955)	−.539 (.168)
Total anxiety score	.742 (.014)	−.153 (.673)	−.250 (.486)	−.265 (.525)	.120 (.776)	−.663 (.073)
Total SCQ score	−.720 (.029)	.077 (.845)	.099 (.800)	−.660 (.053)	.017 (.965)	−.792 (.011)
Chronological age	.593 (.055)	−.105 (.758)	.165 (.627)	.166 (.627)	−.082 (.811)	.191 (.574)
Receptive language	.383 (.246)	.073 (.831)	.422 (.196)	−.178 (.601)	.178 (.601)	.483 (.132)

Correlation matrix for correlations between dwell time on face, body, and background AOI with (1) social phobia, as measured by the SCAS-P, (2) total anxiety score on the SCAS-P, (3) social communication impairment, as measured by the SCQ, (4) chronological age, and (5) receptive language raw score, as measured by the BPVS

increased anxiety and fewer social communication difficulties in individuals with FXS. Together, these results suggest that whilst social attention to naturalistic social scenes may be developmentally 'typical' in males with FXS, anxiety and autism symptomatology are differentially related to social attention in this population.

Existing studies that have indicated atypical social attention in males with FXS have focussed on attention to the eye region of static faces. However, the current study revealed that social attention to naturalistic social scenes appears developmentally 'typical' in males with FXS. A number of important advances have indicated reduced social attention in individuals with ASD, which is associated with social withdrawal [11–14]. The milder profile of social communication difficulties, and subtle but important differences in the social impairment reported in individuals with FXS [2, 3, 6], may account

for the results presented here, documenting that these individuals do not show reduced social attention in the same way as those with ASD. Existing literature suggests that individuals with FXS demonstrate less severe impairments in social responsiveness compared to individuals with ASD, even when matched on overall autism severity [6, 34]. These different profiles go some way to explaining why reduced social attention may be expected in individuals with ASD but not in those with FXS.

Although there were no significant differences between the FXS and TD groups in relation to overall looking time, increased looking to faces was correlated with fewer social communication difficulties in individuals with FXS. This is a finding that is often reported in the ASD literature [15–17], and one that suggests autism symptomatology may play a role in the viewing of naturalistic social scenes. Interestingly, in our previous work

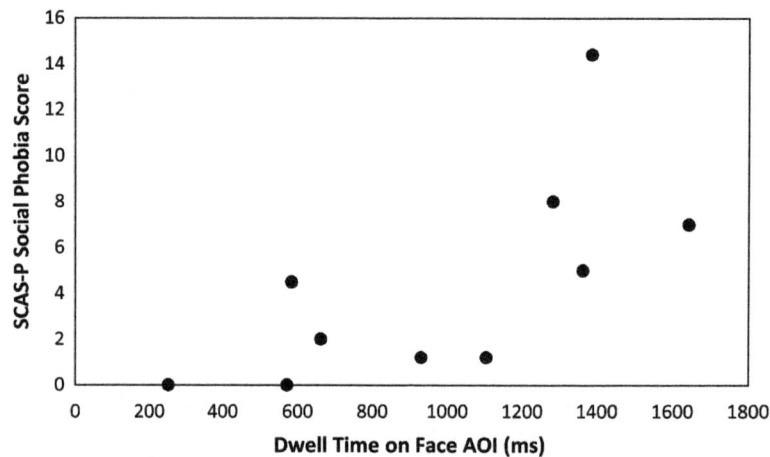

Fig. 2 Relationship between face AOI and social anxiety; a scatterplot depicting the relationship between dwell time on the face AOI in milliseconds, and the SCAS-P social phobia score for participants with FXS. The analyses indicate a significant positive correlation (r_p (8) = .687, p = .028)

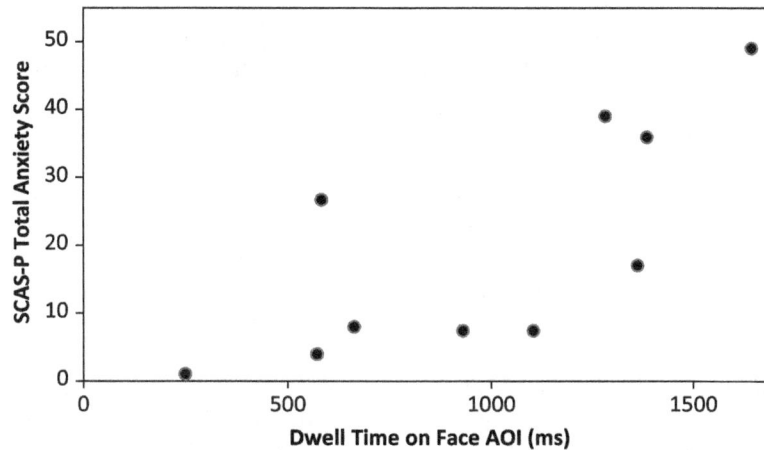

Fig. 3 Relationship between face AOI and anxiety; a scatterplot depicting the relationship between dwell time on the face AOI in milliseconds, and the SCAS-P total score for participants with FXS. The analyses indicate a significant positive correlation (r_p (8) = .742, p = .014)

directly comparing individuals with FXS and ASD, we reported that atypical eye gaze in FXS was not a product of autistic symptomatology [21]. Together, these results suggest that social attention to naturalistic scenes appears developmentally typical but may be influenced by autism symptomatology, whereas eye gaze aversion is a FXS-specific impairment that is unlikely to be a product of autism symptomatology in the same way.

The current study reported a relationship between heightened looking at faces and anxiety. A potential mechanism underlying this explanation is that individuals experiencing anxiety, and social anxiety in particular, may view faces as a more threatening aspect of a social scene. Therefore, heightened looking to threatening stimuli may reflect hyper-vigilance for threatening stimuli, supporting previous literature indicating that socially anxious TD individuals fixate longer on the eye

region of faces than those without social anxiety [23]. This potential explanation is supported by our previous eye-tracking study, which revealed a positive relationship between social dwell time on videos of actors approaching the viewer, and anxiety, in males with FXS [35]. The results of the current study are also interesting in light of existing behavioural observation research that highlighted a pattern of results in which more eye contact was associated with increased cortisol reactivity, a physiological indicator of stress, in individuals with FXS [36]. It is important to note that although the mean anxiety scores for participants with FXS did not differ from normative data from TD children, within-syndrome variability was large. Participants with FXS were therefore more likely to achieve scores on the SCAS-P indicative of more severe anxiety than children with an anxiety disorder (see [31] for normative data).

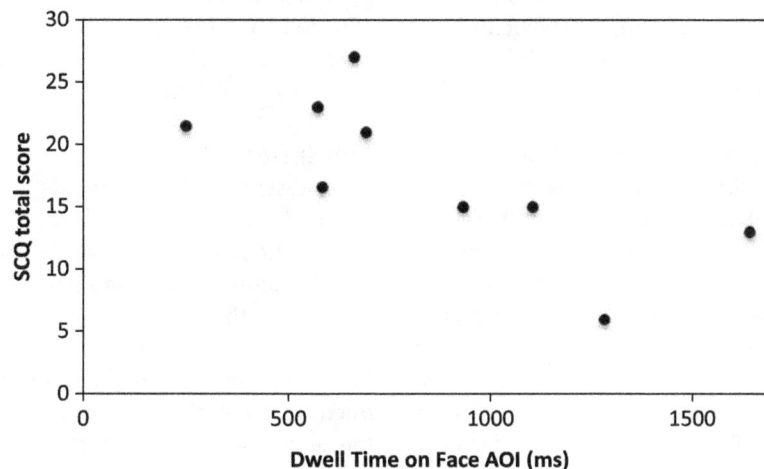

Fig. 4 Relationship between face AOI and autism symptomatology; a scatterplot depicting the relationship between dwell time on the face AOI in milliseconds and the SCQ total score for participants with FXS. The analyses indicate a significant negative correlation (r_p (7) = −.720, p = .029)

The differential relationships reported here, between social attention and both anxiety and autism symptomatology, are particularly interesting when existing literature on WS is considered. Less time spent looking at the eye region of faces has been related to higher levels of autism symptomatology in individuals with WS [37], a similar relationship to that reported in the current study where less looking at faces was associated with higher levels of autism symptomatology. Additionally, increased levels of generalised anxiety have been associated with reduced fixation on faces and eyes for individuals with WS [24], which is the opposite pattern of results to that reported in the current FXS sample where increased levels of anxiety were associated with increased dwell time on faces. One possible explanation for these cross-syndrome differences in the relationship between social attention and anxiety may be related to the different profiles of anxiety associated with these two genetic syndromes. Although both FXS and WS are associated with high levels of specific phobia, FXS is also typically associated with social anxiety [7] whilst WS is associated with generalised anxiety disorder [38]. Such cross-syndrome insights allow us to advance our understanding of syndrome-specific mechanisms that might underlie social attention patterns.

It is essential to apply caution when interpreting the results of the present study due to the small sample sizes. However, moderate to strong correlations between social attention, anxiety, and social communication impairments were revealed even with these small samples, highlighting the potential utility of further investigations in this area. The scatterplots (Figs. 2 and 3) indicate further that the significant correlations are unlikely to be driven by outliers. Whilst the between-group comparisons may have been statistically underpowered, the alpha levels are well above the significance cut-off (group × AOI interaction: $p = .354$; between-group comparisons: $p = .923$). Therefore, it seems unlikely that these results would differ with additional participants.

In addition, the wide age range of the FXS group should be considered when interpreting the results due to the possibility of age-related differences in social attention and behavioural characteristics. Group matching on chronological versus mental age is a common issue in intellectual disability research, and we, therefore, suggest our results indicate *developmentally* 'typical' social attention in FXS. The extent to which social attention in the FXS group would compare to individuals of the same chronological age is beyond the scope of this study. However, correlations to investigate the relationship between chronological age and social attention were not significant. Existing literature has reported interesting differences in social attention as a function of chronological age, with children aged 3 months looking more at eyes, and older children aged 30 months looking more flexibly at mouths (especially when talking) and hands (especially when picking up an object) [39]. The development of social attention across childhood and adolescence has focussed on specific skills such as facial expression recognition, which seems to improve with age [40, 41]. Less is known about the effect of age and social experience on social attention in a passive viewing task.

It is important to note that the sample size and age range in the current study is similar to that of other eye-tracking studies investigating social attention in FXS [18–20, 42]. However, further research in this area is required to clarify the nature of social attention to naturalistic social stimuli in males with FXS, and to disentangle the effects of developmental level and other behavioural characteristics, such as social communication impairments and anxiety, on social attention.

Furthermore, although IQ measures were not administered for the present study due to methodological impracticality of administering multiple different IQ tests to account for the wide range of ages and abilities of participants, the two participant groups were matched on receptive language. Receptive language has been reported to be commensurate with nonverbal mental age in adolescents with FXS [28]. It is possible that the statistical test to confirm that groups were matched was underpowered. To that end, receptive language ability was taken into account with our statistical tests, and correlations between receptive language and social attention were not significant. Finally, although genetic reports were not available for the current study, future research could investigate the relationship between genetic factors and social attention. Interestingly, our previous work has demonstrated a relationship between genetic variation and visual scanning of emotional faces [43]. Overall looking time indicated good levels of task engagement by both groups, highlighting the opportunities afforded by using eye tracking to investigate the mechanisms subserving clinically relevant behaviours in males with FXS.

Conclusions

The present study documents differential effects of anxiety and autism on social attention in males with FXS. To our knowledge, this is the first study to investigate visual attention to naturalistic social scenes in a sample of males with FXS. This offers insights into the potential mechanisms subserving social attention in this population and how this might differ to other genetically defined neurodevelopmental disorders. The research paves the way for future investigations of the relationship between clinically relevant, socio-behavioural phenotypes, and social attention, in theories of social attention in neurodevelopmental disorders.

Abbreviations
ADOS: Autism Diagnostic Observation Schedule; ANOVA: Analysis of variance; AOI: Area of interest; ASD: Autism spectrum disorder; BPVS: British Picture Vocabulary Scale; CGG: Cytosine-guanine-guanine; FMR1: Fragile X Mental Retardation 1 gene; FMRP: Fragile X Mental Retardation Protein; FXS: Fragile X syndrome; SCAS-P: Spence Child Anxiety Questionnaire—Parent Version; SCQ: Social Communication Questionnaire; TD: Typically developing; WS: Williams syndrome

Acknowledgements
The research reported here was supported by a grant from the Economic and Social Research Council (Grant Number: ES/I901825/1) and by Cerebra. The authors would like to thank all of the participants and their families and Professor Gaia Scerif for her contribution to the interpretation of the data.

Funding
The research reported here was supported by a grant from the Economic and Social Research Council (Grant Number: ES/I901825/1) and by Cerebra.

Authors' contributions
HC participated in the study design and coordination, performed the statistical analyses, participated in the interpretation of the data, and drafted the manuscript. JM participated in the study coordination, interpretation of the data, and helped to draft the manuscript. CO participated in the study coordination, interpretation of the data, and helped to draft the manuscript. DR conceived of the study, participated in its design and coordination, participated in the interpretation of the data, and helped to draft the manuscript. All authors read and approved the final manuscript.

Competing interests
The authors declare that they have no competing interests.

Author details
[1]Centre for Research in Psychology, Behaviour and Achievement, Coventry University, Coventry CV1 5FB, UK. [2]Cerebra Centre for Neurodevelopmental Disorders, School of Psychology, University of Birmingham, Edgbaston B15 2TT, UK. [3]Institute of Cognitive Neuroscience, University College London, 17 Queen Square, London WC1N 3AR, UK. [4]Department of Psychology, Durham University, Durham DH1 3LE, UK.

References
1. Turner G, Webb T, Wake S, Robinson H. Prevalence of fragile X syndrome. Am J Med Genet. 1996;64:196–7.
2. Cornish K, Turk J, Hagerman R. The fragile X continuum: new advances and perspectives. J Intellect Disabil Res. 2008;52:469–82.
3. Cornish K, Turk J, Levitas A. Fragile X syndrome and autism: common developmental pathways? Curr Pediatric Rev. 2007;3:61–8.
4. Richards C, Jones C, Groves L, Moss J, Oliver C. Prevalence of autism spectrum disorder phenomenology in genetic disorders: a systematic review and meta-analysis. Lancet Psychiatry. 2015;2:909–16.
5. Baird G, Simonoff E, Pickles A, Chandler S, Loucas T, Meldrum D, Charman T. Prevalence of disorders of the autism spectrum in a population cohort of children in South Thames: The Special Needs and Autism Project (SNAP). Lancet. 2006;368:210–5.
6. Abbeduto L, McDuffie A, Thurman AJ. The fragile X syndrome-autism comorbidity: what do we really know? Front Genet. 2014;5:355.
7. Cordeiro L, Ballinger E, Hagerman R, Hessl D. Clinical assessment of DSM-IV anxiety disorders in fragile X syndrome: prevalence and characterization. J Neurodev Disord. 2011;3:57–67.
8. Roberts JE, Weisenfeld LAH, Hatton DD, Heath M, Kaufmann WE. Social approach and autistic behavior in children with fragile X syndrome. J Autism Dev Disord. 2007;37:1748–60.
9. Kau ASM, Tierney E, Bukelis I, Stump MH, Kates WR, Trescher WH, Kaufmann WE. Social behavior profile in young males with fragile X syndrome: characteristics and specificity. Am J Med Genet A. 2004;126:9–17.
10. Kaufmann WE, Cortell R, Kau ASM, Bukelis I, Tierney E, Gray RM, Cox C, Capone GT, Stanard P. Autism spectrum disorder in fragile X syndrome: communication, social interaction, and specific behaviors. Am J Med Genet A. 2004;129:225–34.
11. Riby DM, Hancock PJB. Viewing it differently: social scene perception in Williams syndrome and autism. Neuropsychologia. 2008;46:2855–60.
12. Riby DM, Hancock PJB. Looking at movies and cartoons: eye-tracking evidence from Williams syndrome and autism. J Intellect Disabil Res. 2009;53:169–81.
13. Riby DM, Doherty-Sneddon G, Bruce V. Exploring face perception in disorders of development: evidence from Williams syndrome and autism. J Neuropsychol. 2008;2:47–64.
14. Riby DM, Hancock PJB. Do faces capture the attention of individuals with Williams syndrome or autism? Evidence from tracking eye movements. J Autism Dev Disord. 2009;39:421–31.
15. Klin A, Jones W, Schultz R, Volkmar F, Cohen D. Visual fixation patterns during viewing of naturalistic social situations as predictors of social competence in individuals with autism. Arch Gen Psychiatry. 2002;59:809–16.
16. Speer LL, Cook AE, McMahon WM, Clark E. Face processing in children with autism effects of stimulus contents and type. Autism. 2007;11:265–77.
17. Kliemann D, Dziobeck I, Hatri A, Steimke R, Heekeren HR. Atypical reflexive gaze patterns on emotional faces in autism spectrum disorders. J Neurosci. 2010;30:12281–7.
18. Dalton KM, Holsen L, Abbeduto L, Davidson RJ. Brain function and gaze fixation during facial-emotion processing in fragile X and autism. Autism Res. 2008;1:231–9.
19. Farzin F, Rivera SM, Hessl D. Brief report: visual processing of faces in individuals with fragile X syndrome: an eye tracking study. J Autism Dev Disord. 2009;39:946–52.
20. Holsen LM, Dalton KM, Johnstone T, Davidson RJ. Prefrontal social cognition network dysfunction underlying face encoding and social anxiety in fragile X syndrome. Neuroimage. 2008;43:592–604.
21. Crawford H, Moss J, Anderson GM, Oliver C, McCleery JP. Implicit discrimination of basic facial expressions of positive/negative emotion in fragile X syndrome and autism spectrum disorder. Am J Intellect Dev Disabil. 2015;120:328–45.
22. Williams TA, Porter MA, Langdon R. Viewing social scenes: a visual scan-path study comparing fragile X syndrome and Williams syndrome. J Autism Dev Disord. 2013;43:1880–94.
23. Weiser MJ, Pauli P, Alpers GW, Muhlberger A. Is eye to eye contact really threatening and avoided in social anxiety? An eye-tracking and psychophysiology study. J Anxiety Disord. 2009;23:93–103.
24. Kirk HE, Hocking DR, Riby DM, Cornish KM. Linking social behaviour and anxiety to attention and emotional faces in Williams syndrome. Res Dev Disabil. 2013;34:4608–16.
25. Shaw TA, Porter MA. Emotion recognition and visual-scan paths in fragile X syndrome. J Autism Dev Disord. 2013;43:1119–39.
26. Moss J, Nelson L, Powis L, Richards C, Waite J, Oliver C. A comparative study of sociability and selective mutism in autism spectrum disorder, Angelman, Cri du Chat, Cornelia de Lange, Fragile X and Rubinstein-Taybi syndromes. Am J Intellectual Dev Disabilities. in press.
27. Dunn LM, Whetton C, Burley J. The British picture vocabulary scale, second edition testbook. NFER: Windsor; 1997.
28. Abbeduto L, Murphy MM, Cawthon SW, Richmond EK, Weissman MD, Karadottir S, O'Brien A. Receptive language skills of adolescents and young adults with Down or fragile X syndrome. Am J Mental Retardation. 2003;103:149–60.
29. Rutter M, Bailey A, Lord C. The Social Communication Questionnaire. Los Angeles: Western Psychological Services; 2003.
30. Spence SH. Spence Children's Anxiety Scale (parent version). Brisbane: University of Queensland; 1999.
31. Nauta MH, Scholing A, Rapee RM, Abbott M, Spence SH, Waters A. A parent-report measure of children's anxiety: psychometric properties and comparison with child-report in a clinic and normal sample. Behav Res Ther. 2004;42:813–39.
32. Achenbach TM. Integrative guide for the 1991 CBCL/4-18, YSR, and TRF profiles. Burlington: University of Vermont, Department of Psychiatry; 1991.
33. Lord C, Rutter M, DiLavore P, Risi S. Autism Diagnostic Observation Schedule: Manual. Los Angeles: Western Psychological Services; 1999.
34. McDuffie A, Thurman AJ, Hagerman RJ, Abbeduto L. Symptoms of autism in males with fragile X syndrome: a comparison to nonsyndromic ASD using current ADI-R scores. J Autism Dev Disord. 2014;45:1925–37.

35. Crawford H, Moss J, Oliver C, Elliott N, Anderson GM, McCleery JP. Visual preference for social stimuli in individuals with autism or neurodevelopmental disorders: an eye-tracking study. Mol Autism. 2016;7:24.

36. Hessl D, Glaser B, Dyer-Friedman J, Reiss AL. Social behavior and cortisol reactivity in children with fragile X syndrome. J Child Psychol Psychiatry. 2006;47:602–10.

37. Hanley M, Riby D, Caswell S, Rooney S, Back E. Looking and thinking: how individuals with Williams syndrome make judgements about mental states. Res Dev Disabil. 2013;34:4466–76.

38. Dykens EM. Anxiety, fears, and phobias in persons with Williams syndrome. Dev Neuropsychol. 2003;23:291–316.

39. Frank MC, Vul E, Saxe R. Measuring the development of social attention using free-viewing. Infancy. 2012;17:355–75.

40. Herba C, Phillips M. Annotation: development of facial expression recognition from childhood to adolescence: behavioural and neurological perspectives. J Child Psychol Psychiatry. 2004;45:1185–98.

41. Thomas LA, De Bellis MD, Graham R, LaBar KS. Development of emotional facial recognition in late childhood and adolescence. Dev Sci. 2007;10:547–58.

42. Farzin F, Scaggs F, Hervey C, Berry-Kravis E, Hessl D. Reliability of eye tracking and pupillometry measures in individuals with fragile X syndrome. J Autism Dev Disord. 2011;41:1515–22.

43. Christou AI, Wallis Y, Bair H, Crawford H, Frisson S, Zeegers MP, McCleery JP. BDNF Val66Met and 5-HTTLPR genotype are each associated with visual scanning patterns of faces in young children. Front Behav Neurosci. 2015;9: 1–12.

2

Few individuals with Lennox-Gastaut syndrome have autism spectrum disorder: a comparison with Dravet syndrome

Na He[1,2], Bing-Mei Li[1,2], Zhao-Xia Li[1,2], Jie Wang[1,2], Xiao-Rong Liu[1,2], Heng Meng[1,2,3,4], Bin Tang[1,2], Wen-Jun Bian[1,2], Yi-Wu Shi[1,2] and Wei-Ping Liao[1,2]*

Abstract

Background: Autism spectrum disorder (ASD) in epilepsy has been a topic of increasing interest, which in general occurs in 15–35% of the patients with epilepsy, more frequently in those with intellectual disability (ID). Lennox-Gastaut syndrome (LGS) and Dravet syndrome (DS) are two typical forms of intractable epileptic encephalopathy associated with ID. We previously reported that ASD was diagnosed in 24.3% of patients with DS, higher in those with profound ID. Given the severe epilepsy and high frequency of ID in LGS, it is necessary to know whether ASD is a common psychomotor co-morbidity of LGS. This study evaluated the autistic behaviors and intelligence in patients with LGS and further compared that between LGS and DS, aiming to understand the complex pathogenesis of epilepsy-ASD-ID triad.

Methods: A total of 50 patients with LGS and 45 patients with DS were enrolled and followed up for at least 3 years. The clinical characteristics were analyzed, and evaluations of ASD and ID were performed.

Results: No patients with LGS fully met the diagnostic criteria for ASD, but three of them exhibited more or less autistic behaviors. Majority (86%) of LGS patients presented ID, among which moderate to severe ID was the most common. Early onset age and symptomatic etiology were risk predictors for ID. The prevalence of ASD in LGS was significantly lower than that in DS (0/50 vs. 10/45, $p < 0.001$), while the prevalence and severity of ID showed no significant difference between the two forms of epileptic encephalopathy.

Conclusions: This study demonstrated a significant difference in the co-morbidity of ASD between LGS and DS, although they had a similar prevalence and severity of ID, refuting the proposal that the prevalence of ASD in epilepsy is accounted for by ID. These findings suggest that the co-morbidity of ASD, ID, and epilepsy may result from multifaceted pathogenic mechanisms.

Keywords: Autism spectrum disorder, Intellectual disability, Epileptic encephalopathy, Lennox-Gastaut syndrome, Dravet syndrome

Background

Lennox-Gastaut syndrome (LGS) is a severe epileptic encephalopathy, which accounts for approximately 1–10% of childhood epilepsies [1]. The etiologies of LGS can be symptomatic with an identifiable brain disorder, or cryptogenic without known causes [2]. The clinical presentation of LGS is characterized by the following triad: multiple seizure types that are mainly tonic, specific abnormal electroencephalogram (EEG), and cognitive impairment. Majority of LGS patients typically experience cognitive regression at seizure onset, with a decreasing intelligence quotient (IQ) over time [3]. Along with cognitive problems, behavioral and psychiatric co-morbidities are commonly seen in patients with LGS, such as hyperactivity, anxiety, aggression, and depression [2]. Autism or autistic behavior has also been reported, but only in a few cases of LGS [4, 5].

Autism spectrum disorder (ASD) is a complex neurobehavioral disorder characterized by social interaction

* Correspondence: wpliao@163.net
[1]Institute of Neuroscience and Department of Neurology of the Second Affiliated Hospital of Guangzhou Medical University, Chang-gang-dong Road 250, Guangzhou 510260, China
[2]Key Laboratory of Neurogenetics and Channelopathies of Guangdong Province and the Ministry of Education of China, Guangzhou 510260, China
Full list of author information is available at the end of the article

impairments, communication deficits, and stereotyped behaviors. It has been estimated that ASD may occur in 15–35% of children with epilepsy, while epilepsy may affect 7–46% of patients with ASD [6], suggesting a strong relationship between ASD and epilepsy. Additionally, previous evidence indicates that ASD occurs more frequently in epilepsy patients with intellectual disability (ID) [7]. We previously reported that ASD was diagnosed in 24.3% of patients with Dravet syndrome (DS), which is another form of epileptic encephalopathy with ID, and ASD was more often in those with profound ID [8]. Given the severe epilepsy and high frequency of ID in LGS, it is necessary to know whether autism or autistic behavior is a common psychomotor co-morbidity of LGS. As little is known about the relative contributions of epilepsy itself, ID, or other underlying factors to the occurrence of ASD in different forms of epileptic encephalopathy, a comparison between LGS and DS will help to understand the complex pathogenesis of epilepsy-ASD-ID triad.

In this study, we evaluated the autistic behaviors and intelligence in patients with LGS and further compared that between LGS and DS, aiming to explore the prevalence of ASD and its potential risk factors.

Methods

Participants

A total of 50 patients with LGS and 45 patients with DS were recruited between 2007 and 2013 at the Epilepsy Centre of the Second Affiliated Hospital of Guangzhou Medical University. All patients were southern Han Chinese. Medical records were collected, including gender, seizure onset age, seizure types and frequency, application of antiepileptic drugs (AEDs), family history, brain MRI scans, and video-EEG records. This study adhered to the guidelines of the International Committee of Medical Journal Editors with regard to patient consent for research or participation, and study protocol was approved by the ethics committee of the hospital.

According to the criteria of Commission on Classification and Terminology of the International League Against Epilepsy [9–11], LGS was diagnosed when at least two of the following criteria were met: (1) multiple seizure types including tonic seizure, (2) generalized polyspikes or fast rhythms during sleep (required especially when daily tonic seizures are obscure), and (3) diffuse slow (≤ 2.5 Hz) spike-wave complex on EEG. Tonic seizures are essential for the diagnosis of LGS. The diagnosis of Dravet syndrome was based on the criteria (1) febrile seizures starting in the first year of life and subsequent appearance of multiple seizure types (myoclonic, atypical absence, focal); (2) prolonged seizures triggered by or sensitive to fever, which might evolve to status epilepticus; (3) generalized and focal/multifocal discharges

on EEG; and (4) normal psychomotor development before onset of seizure, but cognitive regression afterward. All EEGs were reviewed by two qualified electroencephalographers. Epileptic seizures and epilepsy syndromes were diagnosed and classified by two epileptologists in our Epilepsy Center.

Neurodevelopment assessments

ASD was diagnosed according to the Diagnostic and Statistical Manual of Mental Disorders, Fifth Edition (DSM-5), and the International Classification of Diseases, Tenth Edition (ICD-10). A diagnosis of ASD was made when patients had deficits in two core domains: (1) deficits in social communication and social interaction and (2) restricted repetitive patterns of behavior, interests, and activities. The Autism Behavior Checklist (ABC) by the parents and the Childhood Autism Rating Scale (CARS) by the same qualified psychiatrists were used as additional assessments. An ABC score of ≥ 67 and a CARS score of ≥ 30 were considered to be supporting the diagnosis. Autism Diagnostic Observation Schedule (ADOS), Autism Diagnostic Interview (ADI), and Diagnostic Interview for Social and Communication Disorders (DISCO) were occasionally used due to the lack of Chinese norms of these tools.

To assess cognitive impairment, Chinese Wechsler Intelligence Scale for Children (C-WISC), for those aged ≥ 6 years, and Gesell Developmental Scales, for those aged < 6 years, were performed by the same qualified psychiatrists in our hospital. According to IQ and developmental quotient (DQ), the cognitive outcomes were divided into five categories as in our previous study [8]: normal or borderline intelligence (IQ > 70 or DQ > 75), mild ID (IQ ranging from 55 to 70 or DQ ranging from 55 to 75), moderate ID (IQ/DQ ranging from 40 to 54), severe ID (IQ/DQ ranging from 25 to 39), and profound ID (IQ/DQ below 25).

Statistical analysis

Student t tests and χ^2 tests were performed to determine the significance of differences between groups. Two-sided p-values < 0.05 were considered statistically significant. All analysis was performed using SPSS version 19.0 (SPSS, Chicago, IL, USA).

Results

Demographic and clinical characteristics of patients with LGS

The 50 patients included 38 males and 12 females, aged from 2.2 to 33 years (mean age of 9.3 years, at cognitive evaluation), and were followed up for at least 3 years (range 3–6 years). Their clinical characteristics are summarized in Table 1.

The age at onset of seizure ranged from 10 days to 9 years, with the mean onset age of 35.3 months. Eight

Table 1 Demographic and clinical characteristics of patients with Lennox-Gastaut syndrome

	LGS (N = 50)	Cryptogenic LGS (N = 28)	Symptomatic LGS (N = 22)	p
Gender (male/female)	38/12	21/7	17/5	0.852
Age at conclusion of study (years)	12.9 ± 6.5	12.5 ± 6.1	13.5 ± 7.1	0.875
Age at evaluation (years)	9.3 ± 6.2	9.9 ± 5.6	8.4 ± 7.0	0.418
Age at seizure onset (months)	35.3 ± 29.6	49.4 ± 29.5	17.4 ± 18.1	0.007*
Seizure type				
Tonic	48 (96%)	26 (92.9%)	22 (100.0%)	0.309
GTCS/secondary GTCS	34 (68%)	18 (64.3%)	16 (72.7%)	0.525
Complex/simple partial	20 (40%)	11 (39.3%)	9 (40.9%)	0.907
Atypical absence	20 (40%)	12 (42.9%)	8 (36.4%)	0.642
Myoclonic	16 (32%)	8 (28.6%)	8 (36.4%)	0.558
Spasms	12 (24%)	1 (3.6%)	11 (50.0%)	0.001*
Drops	11 (22%)	5 (17.9%)	6 (27.3%)	0.650
Atonic	8 (16%)	5 (17.9%)	3 (13.6%)	0.988
Status epilepticus	6 (12%)	3 (10.7%)	3 (13.6%)	1.000
EEG characteristics				
Slow background activity	34 (68%)	18 (64.3%)	16 (72.7%)	0.525
Generalized polyspikes	49 (98%)	28 (100.0%)	21 (95.5%)	0.440
Diffuse SSW pattern	36 (72%)	22 (78.6%)	14 (63.6%)	0.243
Focal discharges	43 (86%)	24 (85.7%)	19 (86.4%)	1.000
Burst-suppression pattern	11 (22%)	6 (21.4%)	5 (22.7%)	1.000
Antiepileptic drugs				
2	13 (26%)	10 (35.7%)	3 (13.6%)	0.768
≥ 3	37 (74%)	18 (64.3%)	19 (86.4%)	
Seizure free	14 (28%)	13 (46.4%)	1 (4.5%)	0.001*

GTCS generalized tonic-clonic seizure, SSW slow spike-wave
* p < 0.05 (two-sided) was statistically significant

of the 50 (16%) patients evolved from infantile spasms. All patients experienced multiple seizure types, among which tonic seizure was the most common, followed by generalized tonic-clonic seizure (GTCS)/secondary GTCS. All patients were treated with 2–6 AEDs (mean 3.4). Fourteen patients (28%) were seizure-free for at least 1.5 year, and one patient has been seizure-free for more than 6 years under the combination of valproate and lamotrigine.

Based on brain MRI and medical history, 22 patients (44.0%) had known etiologies and were classified as symptomatic LGS. These etiologies included hypoxic-ischemic encephalopathy, intracranial hemorrhage, malformations of cortical development, ventriculomegaly, tuberous sclerosis, head trauma, encephalitis, hydrocephalus, and porencephaly. The other 28 patients (56.0%) had no identifiable etiology and were classified as cryptogenic LGS. Clinical characteristics of the two groups were compared (Table 1). Patients with symptomatic LGS had much earlier onset age (17.4 vs. 49.4 months in patients with cryptogenic LGS, p = 0.007). Spasms were more common in patients with symptomatic LGS than

that in cryptogenic LGS patients (11/22 vs. 1/28, p < 0.001). The patients who were seizure-free were significantly less in the symptomatic LGS group than that in the cryptogenic LGS group (4.5 vs. 46.4%, p < 0.001).

Autism and autistic behaviors in LGS

No patient with LGS could be diagnosed as ASD, and the average scores of ABC and CARS were 22.1 and 20.7, respectively.

However, three patients exhibited more or less autistic behaviors. The three patients showed speech delay and repetitive stereotypic movements. One of them had social interaction reduction, or narrow interests, or narrow interests and short temper each. Their etiologies were intracranial hemorrhage, encephalitis, and hypoxic-ischemic encephalopathy, respectively. One of them was evolved from infantile spasms. They also had a very early onset age, which were 2, 4, and 6 months, respectively. Their cognitive outcomes were poor, one patient was complicated with severe ID, and the other two had profound ID.

Intellectual disability in LGS and the potential risk factors
C-WISC was performed on 44 patients, and Gesell Developmental Scale was performed on the other 6 patients. According to the IQ or DQ values, 7 patients (14%) had normal or borderline intelligence, and the majority (86%) presented different levels of ID, including 10 patients (20%) with mild ID, 4 (8%) with moderate ID, 19 (38%) with severe ID, and 10 (20%) with profound ID.

To explore the potential risk factors for ID in patients with LGS, clinical characteristics in patients with and without ID were compared (Table 2). The patients with ID had a much earlier onset age than those without ID (26.2 vs. 50.6 months, $p = 0.009$), suggesting that seizure onset age was potentially a significant predictor for ID. Half of the patients with ID had a symptomatic etiology, significantly more often than those without ID (22/43 vs. 0/7, $p = 0.014$), implying that symptomatic etiology was potentially another risk predictor.

Furthermore, the ID severity was compared between patients with cryptogenic LGS and those with symptomatic LGS (Fig. 1). Significant difference was found between the two groups ($p = 0.027$), which showed that moderate to severe ID was more common in the symptomatic group than that in the cryptogenic group.

Comparison of ASD and ID between LGS and DS
To explore the relationships among epilepsy, ASD, and ID, we compared psychomotor development abnormalities between patients with LGS and those with DS. The demographic and clinical characteristics of the 45 patients with DS are summarized in Table 3, among whom 37 cases had been reported previously [8]. These patients aged between 2 to 16 years (mean age 8.2 years) at the neurodevelopment evaluation. There was no significant difference in age at the evaluation between the DS

Table 2 Comparison of clinical features among LGS patients with and without intellectual disability

	Without ID (N = 7)	With ID (N = 43)	p
Gender (male)	5 (71.4%)	33 (76.7%)	1.000
Age at seizure onset (month)	50.6 ± 35.6	26.2 ± 20.0	0.009*
Age at evaluation (years)	11.9 ± 8.6	8.9 ± 5.8	0.400
History of infantile spasms	0 (0.0%)	8 (18.6%)	0.580
Seizure types			
Tonic	6 (85.7%)	42 (97.7%)	0.263
GTCS/secondary GTCS	5 (71.4%)	29 (67.4%)	1.000
Complex partial seizure	2 (28.6%)	18 (41.9%)	0.687
Atypical absence	4 (57.1%)	16 (37.2%)	0.416
Myoclonic	2 (28.6%)	14 (32.6%)	1.000
Spasms	0 (0.0%)	12 (27.9%)	0.174
Drops	1 (14.3%)	10 (23.3%)	1.000
Atonic	1 (14.3%)	7 (16.3%)	1.000
Status epilepticus	1 (14.3%)	5 (11.6%)	1.000
EEG characteristics			
Slow background activity	4 (57.1%)	30 (69.8%)	0.666
Generalized polyspikes	7 (100.0%)	42 (97.7%)	1.000
Diffuse SSW pattern	6 (85.7%)	30 (69.8%)	0.657
Focal discharges	5 (71.4%)	38 (88.4%)	0.250
Burst-suppression pattern	0 (0.0%)	11 (25.6%)	0.324
Antiepileptic drugs			
2	3 (42.9%)	10 (23.3%)	0.357
≥ 3	4 (57.1%)	33 (76.7%)	
Etiology			
Symptomatic	0 (0.0%)	22 (51.2%)	0.014*
Cryptogenic	7 (100.0%)	21 (48.8%)	
Seizure free	4 (57.1%)	10 (23.3%)	0.085

GTCS generalized tonic-clonic seizure, SSW slow spike-wave
* $p < 0.05$ (two-sided) was statistically significant

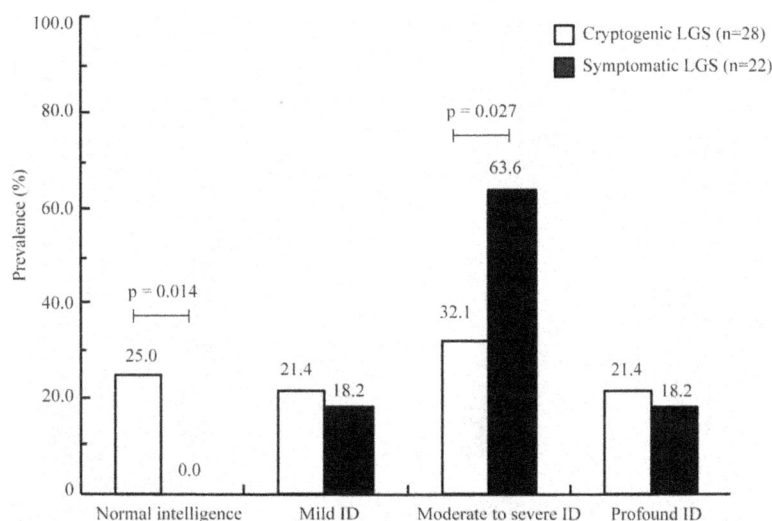

Fig. 1 Comparison of ID in patients with cryptogenic LGS and those with symptomatic LGS. The cognitive outcome in patients with cryptogenic LGS was significantly better than that in patients with symptomatic LGS ($p = 0.040$). In the cryptogenic LGS group, the patients with normal intelligence (7/28) were significantly more than that in symptomatic LGS group (0/22), while the patients with moderate to severe ID (9/28) were significantly less than in the symptomatic LGS group (14/22)

Table 3 Demographic and clinical features of patients with Dravet syndrome ($n = 45$)

Gender (male)	32 (71.1%)
Age at conclusion of study (years)	11.3 ± 5.1
Age at evaluation (years)	8.2 ± 3.7
Age at seizure onset (months)	6.2 ± 3.7
Family history of febrile seizures or epilepsy	16 (35.6%)
Antecedent febrile seizures	35 (77.8%)
Seizure type	
GTCS/secondary GTCS	40 (88.9%)
Complex partial	29 (64.4%)
Myoclonic	18 (40.0%)
Atypical absence	15 (33.3%)
Simple partial	9 (20.0%)
Atonic	4 (8.9%)
Tonic	1 (2.2%)
Status epilepticus	28 (62.2%)
EEG characteristics	
Normal	1 (2.2%)
Slow background activity	25 (55.6%)
Only focal discharge	14 (31.1%)
Only generalized discharge	5 (11.1%)
Focal and generalized discharge	25 (55.6%)
MRI abnormality	13 (28.9%)
Treatment with ≥ 3 AEDs	36 (80.0%)
Seizure free	0 (0%)

Value was expressed as n (%) or means ± SD
AEDs antiepileptic drugs, GTCS generalized tonic-clonic seizure

group and LGS group (8.2 ± 3.7 vs. 9.3 ± 6.2, mean ± SD, $p > 0.05$). The seizure onset age of patients with DS ranged from 3 days to 18 months, significantly earlier than that of patients with LGS (6.2 ± 3.7 vs. 35.3 ± 29.6, mean ± SD, $p < 0.05$). The most common seizure types were GTCS/secondary GTCS, complex partial seizures (CPS), and myoclonic seizures.

ASD was diagnosed in 22.2% (10/45) of patients with DS, significantly higher than that (0/50) in patients with LGS (Fig. 2, $p < 0.001$). The average ABC scores in the DS patients were 46.8, significantly higher than that in LGS patients (46.8 ± 25.7 vs. 22.1 ± 19.9, mean ± SD, $p < 0.001$). The average CARS scores in DS patients were also significantly higher than that in LGS patients (23.8 ± 7.8 vs. 20.7 ± 6.2, mean ± SD, $p = 0.036$). Among the ten DS patients with ASD, they all had speech delay, narrow interests, and lack of emotional reciprocity; nine of them showed stereotypic behavior; seven of them had short temper; and four of them displayed language regression.

C-WISC and Gesell Developmental Scale were performed on 36 and 9 patients with DS, respectively. According to the IQ or DQ values, 41 patients (91.1%) had ID, including 5 patients (11.1%) with mild ID, 30 (66.7%) with moderate to severe ID, and 6 (13.3%) with profound ID. There was no significant difference in the severity of ID between patients with DS and those with LGS (Fig. 2, $p = 0.245$). Nine of the ten patients with ASD showed ID, among which moderate, severe, and profound ID were found in two, three, and four patients, respectively.

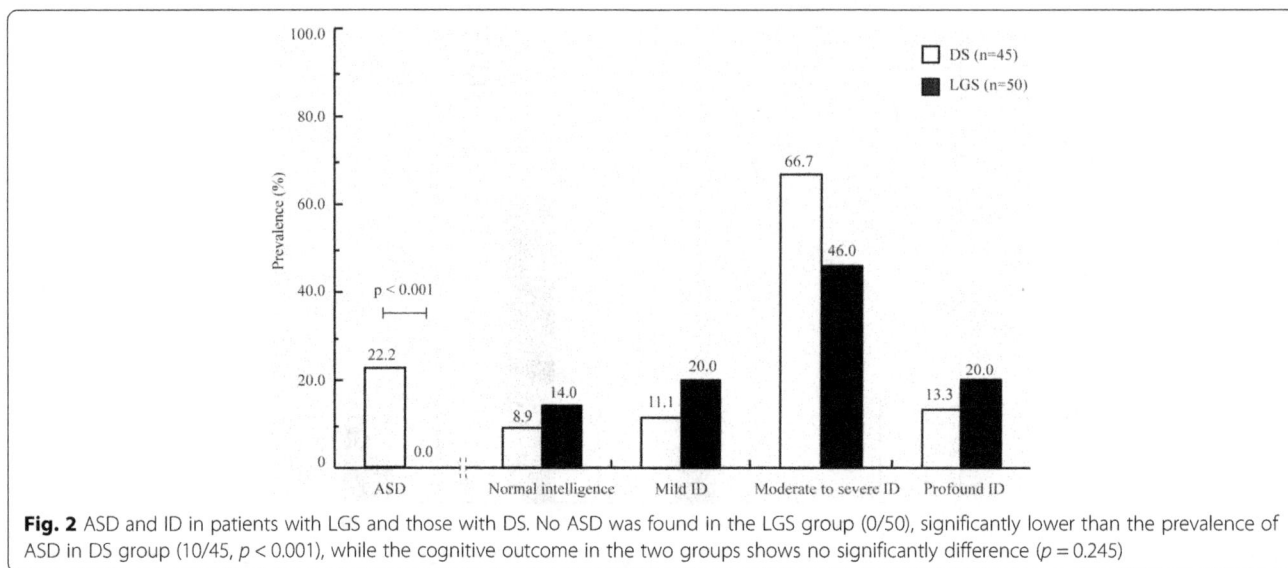

Fig. 2 ASD and ID in patients with LGS and those with DS. No ASD was found in the LGS group (0/50), significantly lower than the prevalence of ASD in DS group (10/45, $p < 0.001$), while the cognitive outcome in the two groups shows no significantly difference ($p = 0.245$)

Discussion

In the present study, no ASD was diagnosed in the 50 patients with LGS, although majority (86%) of them presented ID. The co-morbid prevalence of ASD in LGS was significantly lower than that in DS, but the ID severity did not differ significantly between LGS and DS. These findings suggest that the prevalence of ASD in epilepsy might not be accounted for by the ID. Besides ID, which has been hypothesized as a critical determinant of the co-morbid of epilepsy-ASD-ID triad previously [7, 12], other factors should be considered.

Lennox-Gastaut syndrome is a typical severe epileptic encephalopathy associated with psychomotor developmental abnormalities. Intellectual disability is a prominent feature of LGS. About 20–60% of LGS patients have apparent ID at the onset of seizures, and the proportion of patients with serious ID may increase to 75–95% 5 years after the seizure onset [2, 13]. In this study, majority (86%) of patients with LGS demonstrated ID, among which moderate and severe ID was common.

Previous studies have suggested several risk factors for ID in patients with LGS, such as nonconvulsive status epilepticus, previous diagnosis of infantile spasms, symptomatic etiology, and early seizure onset age [3, 14]. The present study confirmed symptomatic etiology and early seizure onset age as predictors of ID. After follow-up for more than 3 years, 25% of patients with cryptogenic LGS in this cohort still had normal intelligence, whereas all patients with symptomatic LGS showed ID of varying severity. Similar phenomenon was observed in a previous study, 33% of cryptogenic LGS patients had normal or borderline intelligence after a 3-year follow-up, as compared with only 3% of normal intelligence in patients with symptomatic LGS [13]. Previous study has suggested that cortical or cortical-subcortical connection intact is crucial in the cognition development [15]. It is unknown whether the severe ID in patients with symptomatic LGS was due to impaired cortical or cortical-subcortical connection. The seizure onset age is also suggested to be one of the risk factors for intellectual impairment. The seven patients with favorable cognitive outcome had a mean onset age of 50.6 months, while those with ID had a mean onset age of 26.2 months, consistent with a previous study that revealed seizure onset before age 3 years being a significant risk factor for ID in LGS [14].

ASD varies greatly in different epilepsies. The prevalence of ASD was reported to range from 17 to 63% in tuberous sclerosis [16], 24 to 61% in DS [8, 17], and be 35% in infantile spasms [18]. However, the prevalence of co-morbid ASD in LGS remains unclear, although several cases with autism or autistic behavior have been reported [4, 5]. In this study, none of the patients with LGS met the diagnostic criteria of ASD, although three of them exhibited more or less autistic behaviors.

Several variables, such as seizure onset age [19], seizure type [20], ID, and gender [21, 22], were suggested to be risk factors for ASD in epilepsy. ID is one of the factors that should be considered. Patients with epilepsy and ID had an increased risk of ASD (13.8%) relative to those with epilepsy but without ID (2.2%) [23]. A previous study proposed that the prevalence of ASD in epilepsy was accounted for by the degree of ID [7]. The proposal was not supported by the evidence in the present study. The prevalence of ASD in DS was significantly higher than that in LGS, albeit the prevalence and severity of ID were similar in the two forms of epileptic encephalopathy. Factors other than ID should be considered.

Seizure onset age was suggested to be one of the risk predictors for the ASD in the present study. Generally, seizure in DS occurs before the first year of life, while seizure in LGS happens between 1 and 8 years old [9–11]. In this study, the mean onset age in the patients with DS was 6.2 months, whereas that in patients with LGS was 35.3 months. We noticed that the three LGS patients with autistic behaviors suffered their first seizure before 1 year old, which were at 2, 4, and 6 months, respectively. Previous studies have shown that the prevalence of ASD was highest among children whose seizures started before age 2 years [24]. Generally, the stage before age 2 is critical for brain development [25]. Early onset seizure during this stage is possibly an indicator of neurodevelopmental abnormalities, which may account for ASD. However, the seizures are more visible relatively to autistic behaviors, which are often ignored by parents in daily care. It is therefore undetermined when the ASD began in the present LGS and DS cohorts, which is one of the limitations of this study.

Seizure types differed between LGS and DS in this study (Tables 1 and 3), which has been suggested to be one of the possible risk factors for ASD [20, 26]. However, it is unknown whether the seizure type itself or the underlying pathogenesis contributes to ASD.

Current data suggests that genetic etiology plays a critical role in the pathogenesis of epilepsy as well as the co-morbidity. DS is typically a genetic epileptic encephalopathy caused by *SCN1A* mutations in the majority [27]. Our recent study demonstrated 50% of DS patients had *SCN1A* mutations [28]. In contrast, LGS remains elusive in genetic etiology in the majority, although mutations in genes such as *GABRB3* and *ALG13* were occasionally detected [29]. Only a few patients with LGS were found to have causative mutations [28, 30]. Previous studies have suggested a possible involvement of several genes in ASD, such as *SCN1A*, *SCN2A*, *GABRA1*, and *GABRB1* [31]. Additionally, some genetic epilepsies are at high risk of ASD, such as tuberous sclerosis/*TSC2* gene [16] and Fragile X syndrome/*FMR1* gene [32]. However, little is known about the relative contribution of genetic factors in ASD and the underlying mechanisms. Due to the incompleteness of genetic information in the patients in this study, the relationships among genetic risk factors, ASD, and epilepsy warrant further investigation.

Conclusion

This study showed that the co-morbidity of ASD was significantly lower in LGS than in DS, although these two epileptic encephalopathies had a similar prevalence and severity of ID. It is suggested that other factors, besides ID, would be involved in the pathogenesis of ASD in epilepsy. Further studies with large sample size and basic researches are required to unveil the underlying mechanisms and interaction among epilepsy, ASD, and ID.

Abbreviations

ABC: Autism Behavior Checklist; AEDs: Antiepileptic drugs; ASD: Autism spectrum disorders; CARS: Childhood Autism Rating Scale; CPS: Complex partial seizures; C-WISC: Chinese Wechsler Intelligence Scale for Children; DQ: Developmental quotient; DS: Dravet syndrome; DSM-5: Diagnostic and Statistical Manual of Mental Disorders, Fifth Edition; EEG: Electroencephalogram; GTCS: Generalized tonic-clonic seizure; ICD-10: International Classification of Diseases, Tenth Edition; ID: Intellectual disability; IQ: Intelligence quotient; LGS: Lennox-Gastaut syndrome

Acknowledgements

We thank the family and physicians for their participation in our study. We are grateful to the He Shanheng Charity Foundation for contributing to the development of this institute.

Funding

This work was supported by the National Natural Science Foundation of China (Grant Nos. 81571273, 81571274, and 81501125), Omics-based precision medicine of epilepsy being entrusted by Key Research Project of the Ministry of Science and Technology of China (Grant No. 2016YFC0904400), the Natural Science Foundation of Guangdong Province (Grant No. 2014A030313489), and Medical Scientific Research Foundation of Guangdong Province (Grant No. A2013268). The funders had no role in the study design, data collection and analysis, decision to publish, or preparation of the manuscript.

Authors' contributions

LWP and HN conceived and designed the study, analyzed the data, and wrote the paper. LWP was the principal investigator of this study. HN, LBM, and WJ collected and analyzed the data and performed the statistical analysis. LBM, LXR, LZX, MH, and TB recruited and provided samples and data for these analyses. SYW and BWJ performed the data analysis and interpretation. All authors read and approved the final manuscript.

Competing interests

The authors declare that they have no competing interests.

Author details

[1]Institute of Neuroscience and Department of Neurology of the Second Affiliated Hospital of Guangzhou Medical University, Chang-gang-dong Road 250, Guangzhou 510260, China. [2]Key Laboratory of Neurogenetics and Channelopathies of Guangdong Province and the Ministry of Education of China, Guangzhou 510260, China. [3]Department of Neurology, The First Affiliated Hospital of Jinan University, Guangdong 510630, China. [4]Clinical Neuroscience Institute of Jinan University, Guangdong 510630, China.

References

1. Hancock EC, Cross JH. Treatment of Lennox-Gastaut syndrome. Cochrane Database Syst Rev. 2013;2:CD003277.
2. Arzimanoglou A, French J, Blume WT, Cross JH, Ernst JP, Feucht M, et al. Lennox-Gastaut syndrome: a consensus approach on diagnosis, assessment, management, and trial methodology. Lancet Neurol. 2009;8(1):82–93.
3. Bourgeois BF, Douglass LM, Sankar R. Lennox-Gastaut syndrome: a consensus approach to differential diagnosis. Epilepsia. 2014;55(Suppl 4):4–9.
4. Ferlazzo E, Nikanorova M, Italiano D, Bureau M, Dravet C, Calarese T, et al. Lennox-Gastaut syndrome in adulthood: clinical and EEG features. Epilepsy Res. 2010;89(2–3):271–7.
5. Orrico A, Zollino M, Galli L, Buoni S, Marangi G, Sorrentino V. Late-onset Lennox-Gastaut syndrome in a patient with 15q11.2-q13.1 duplication. Am J Med Genet A. 2009;149A(5):1033–5.
6. Lo-Castro A, Curatolo P. Epilepsy associated with autism and attention deficit hyperactivity disorder: is there a genetic link? Brain and Development. 2014;36(3):185–93.
7. Tuchman R, Hirtz D, Mamounas LA. NINDS epilepsy and autism spectrum disorders workshop report. Neurology. 2013;81(18):1630–6.

8.   Li BM, Liu XR, Yi YH, Deng YH, Su T, Zou X, et al. Autism in Dravet syndrome: prevalence, features, and relationship to the clinical characteristics of epilepsy and mental retardation. Epilepsy Behav. 2011; 21(3):291–5.

9.   Commission. Proposal for revised clinical and electroencephalographic classification of epileptic seizures. From the Commission on Classification and Terminology of the International League Against Epilepsy. Epilepsia. 1981;22(4):489–501.

10. Commission. Proposal for revised classification of epilepsies and epileptic syndromes. Commission on Classification and Terminology of the International League Against Epilepsy. Epilepsia. 1989;30(4):389–99.

11. Berg AT, Berkovic SF, Brodie MJ, Buchhalter J, Cross JH, van Emde Boas W, et al. Revised terminology and concepts for organization of seizures and epilepsies: report of the ILAE Commission on Classification and Terminology, 2005–2009. Epilepsia. 2010;51(4):676–85.

12. Berg AT, Plioplys S. Epilepsy and autism: is there a special relationship? Epilepsy Behav. 2012;23(3):193–8.

13. Goldsmith IL, Zupanc ML, Buchhalter JR. Long-term seizure outcome in 74 patients with Lennox-Gastaut syndrome: effects of incorporating MRI head imaging in defining the cryptogenic subgroup. Epilepsia. 2000;41(4):395–9.

14. Hoffmann-Riem M, Diener W, Benninger C, Rating D, Unnebrink K, Stephani U, et al. Nonconvulsive status epilepticus—a possible cause of mental retardation in patients with Lennox-Gastaut syndrome. Neuropediatrics. 2000;31(4):169–74.

15. Bennett MR, Hacker PM. Emotion and cortical-subcortical function: conceptual developments. Prog Neurobiol. 2005;75(1):29–52.

16. Vignoli A, La Briola F, Peron A, Turner K, Vannicola C, Saccani M, et al. Autism spectrum disorder in tuberous sclerosis complex: searching for risk markers. Orphanet J Rare Dis. 2015;10:154.

17. Berkvens JJ, Veugen I, Veendrick-Meekes MJ, Snoeijen-Schouwenaars FM, Schelhaas HJ, Willemsen MH, et al. Autism and behavior in adult patients with Dravet syndrome (DS). Epilepsy Behav. 2015;47:11–6.

18. Saemundsen E, Ludvigsson P, Hilmarsdottir I, Rafnsson V. Autism spectrum disorders in children with seizures in the first year of life—a population-based study. Epilepsia. 2007;48(9):1724–30.

19. Hara H. Autism and epilepsy: a retrospective follow-up study. Brain and Development. 2007;29(8):486–90.

20. Matsuo M, Maeda T, Sasaki K, Ishii K, Hamasaki Y. Frequent association of autism spectrum disorder in patients with childhood onset epilepsy. Brain and Development. 2010;32(9):759–63.

21. Amiet C, Gourfinkel-An I, Bouzamondo A, Tordjman S, Baulac M, Lechat P, et al. Epilepsy in autism is associated with intellectual disability and gender: evidence from a meta-analysis. Biol Psychiatry. 2008;64(7):577–82.

22. Woolfenden S, Sarkozy V, Ridley G, Coory M, Williams K. A systematic review of two outcomes in autism spectrum disorder—epilepsy and mortality. Dev Med Child Neurol. 2012;54(4):306–12.

23. Berg AT, Plioplys S, Tuchman R. Risk and correlates of autism spectrum disorder in children with epilepsy: a community-based study. J Child Neurol. 2011;26(5):540–7.

24. Tuchman R, Cuccaro M, Alessandri M. Autism and epilepsy: historical perspective. Brain and Development. 2010;32(9):709–18.

25. Knickmeyer RC, Gouttard S, Kang C, Evans D, Wilber K, Smith JK, et al. A structural MRI study of human brain development from birth to 2 years. J Neurosci. 2008;28(47):12176–82.

26. Kurokawa T, Yokomizo Y, Lee S, Kusuda T. Clinical features of epilepsy with pervasive developmental disorder. Brain and Development. 2010;32(9):764–8.

27. Meng H, Xu HQ, Yu L, Lin GW, He N, Su T, et al. The SCN1A mutation database: updating information and analysis of the relationships among genotype, functional alteration, and phenotype. Hum Mutat. 2015;36(6):573–80.

28. Zhou P, He N, Zhang JW, Lin ZJ, Wang J, Yan LM, et al. Novel mutations and phenotypes of epilepsy-associated genes in epileptic encephalopathies. Genes Brain Behav. 2018. https://doi.org/10.1111/gbb.12456.

29. Allen AS, Berkovic SF, Cossette P, Delanty N, Dlugos D, Eichler EE, et al. De novo mutations in epileptic encephalopathies. Nature. 2013;501(7466):217–21.

30. Carvill GL, Heavin SB, Yendle SC, McMahon JM, O'Roak BJ, Cook J, et al. Targeted resequencing in epileptic encephalopathies identifies de novo mutations in CHD2 and SYNGAP1. Nat Genet. 2013;45(7):825–30.

31. Srivastava S, Sahin M. Autism spectrum disorder and epileptic encephalopathy: common causes, many questions. J Neurodev Disord. 2017;9:23.

32. Chonchaiya W, Au J, Schneider A, Hessl D, Harris SW, Laird M, et al. Increased prevalence of seizures in boys who were probands with the FMR1 premutation and co-morbid autism spectrum disorder. Hum Genet. 2012;131(4):581–9.

3

Exploring the heterogeneity of neural social indices for genetically distinct etiologies of autism

Caitlin M. Hudac[1*], Holly A. F. Stessman[2], Trent D. DesChamps[1], Anna Kresse[3], Susan Faja[4], Emily Neuhaus[3], Sara Jane Webb[1,3], Evan E. Eichler[2,5] and Raphael A. Bernier[1,3]

Abstract

Background: Autism spectrum disorder (ASD) is a genetically and phenotypically heterogeneous disorder. Promising initiatives utilizing interdisciplinary characterization of ASD suggest phenotypic subtypes related to specific likely gene-disrupting mutations (LGDMs). However, the role of functionally associated LGDMs in the neural social phenotype is unknown.

Methods: In this study of 26 children with ASD ($n = 13$ with an LGDM) and 13 control children, we characterized patterns of mu attenuation and habituation as children watched videos containing social and nonsocial motions during electroencephalography acquisition.

Results: Diagnostic comparisons were consistent with prior work suggesting aberrant mu attenuation in ASD within the upper mu band (10–12 Hz), but typical patterns within the lower mu band (8–10 Hz). Preliminary exploration indicated distinct social sensitization patterns (i.e., increasing mu attenuation for social motion) for children with an LGDM that is primarily expressed during embryonic development. In contrast, children with an LGDM primarily expressed post-embryonic development exhibited stable typical patterns of lower mu attenuation. Neural social indices were associated with social responsiveness, but not cognition.

Conclusions: These findings suggest unique neurophysiological profiles for certain genetic etiologies of ASD, further clarifying possible genetic functional subtypes of ASD and providing insight into mechanisms for targeted treatment approaches.

Keywords: Autism spectrum disorders (ASD), Likely gene-disrupting mutations, Electroencephalography (EEG), Social cognition, Mu rhythm attenuation, Social perception, Molecular subtyping

Background

The significant etiologic and phenotypic heterogeneity of autism spectrum disorder (ASD) [1] has made it challenging to target underlying mechanisms of ASD pathology. Considering that more than 1000 genes have been implicated in ASD [1, 2], recent initiatives have targeted genetic pathways [3, 4] and rare de novo likely gene-disrupting mutations (LGDMs) [5]. As such, a burgeoning "genetics-first" approach has been proposed to improve identification and characterization of genetic subtypes of individuals with

ASD [6]. For instance, genetics-first studies have identified phenotypically distinct subtypes of autism for *CHD8* [7] and *DYRK1A* [8, 9] based upon behavioral and physical features within both children and animal models. However, the relevant contribution of genetic risk to aspects of the ASD phenotype (i.e., social communicative impairments) is poorly understood, especially for low-functioning individuals with ASD.

Recent work supports social perception as a possible neural index related to the hallmark social deficits in ASD [10–15]. Although the neural indices have been targeted in relation to copy number variations, such as the 16p11.2 locus [16, 17], little is known about neural patterns associated with LGDMs, likely due to the wide

* Correspondence: chudac@uw.edu
[1]Department of Psychiatry and Behavioral Sciences, University of Washington, CHDD Box 357920, Seattle, WA 98195, USA
Full list of author information is available at the end of the article

range of variability of specific gene expression across LGDMs. Our objective was to examine patterns of neural heterogeneity associated with LGDMs by completing a series of diagnostic and genetics-guided analyses of social perception. We hypothesized a diagnostic approach would indicate atypical social perception in ASD, consistent with theories of social brain dysfunction in ASD [15]. Then, as a preliminary exploration, we predicted that the heterogeneity associated with LGDMs would indicate potentially divergent patterns of social perception based upon LGDM function. Following work suggesting distinct functional roles for genes strongly expressed during embryonic development [5, 18], we tested children with and without a LGDM associated with embryonic development as a possible functional neurodevelopment pathway that contributes to a shared phenotype. There is a growing body of evidence suggesting early embryonic disruptions may be related to impairments in social behavior (e.g., lack of interest in conspecific proximity) [19, 20] and/or dysfunctional information encoding (i.e., intellectual or developmental delays) [21, 22]. The current study sought to add to this literature by addressing whether individuals with an embryonically expressed LGDM exhibit dysfunctional information habituation within the social domain.

We opted to target mu attenuation, which is specifically sensitive to detecting the movements associated with biological motion and is known as a reliable index of social perception in typical populations [23, 24]. Mu rhythm is typically defined as neural activity oscillations within the 8–12-Hz frequency range of electroencephalography (EEG) across electrodes above the sensorimotor cortex. During the observation and execution of biological motion, the underlying neural assemblies of the mu rhythm desynchronize [25, 26]. This desynchronization results in the reduction of oscillatory power (i.e., *attenuation* of the signal), with a greater reduction for conditions with social significance (i.e., biological motion relative to nonbiological motion) in children and adults; for a review, see [27].

In ASD, several studies suggest atypical mu attenuation in ASD (e.g., no discrimination for social relative to nonsocial observed motion) [12, 28–30] while other studies indicate no difference in ASD compared to typical controls [31–33]. Recent work by Dumas and colleagues [34] suggests that this discrepancy may be driven by the functional significance of the lower and upper mu rhythm bands. Notably, there is evidence that the lower mu rhythm (8–10 Hz) is more responsive to observed motion than the upper mu rhythm (10–12 Hz) [35], which may be indicative of bottom-up sensory processing [36, 37]. Previous studies also implicate that upper mu (or alpha) is more sensitive to top-down cognitive processing, such as self-monitoring within social contexts [38] or increasing cognitive demands [39, 40].

It is also possible that conflicting mu attenuation results reflect the underlying heterogeneity in ASD, potentially driven by genetic etiology. For instance, both disrupted social cognition and information habituation are associated with embryonically expressed LGDMs (e.g., *ADNP* [21], *POGZ* [22]). Yet, it is unclear whether social information habituation is also disrupted and the extent to which this profile is unique to children with an embryonically expressed LGDM. To date, only one study has tested the rate at which mu attenuation is modulated (i.e., habituates, sensitizes) in ASD [17]. In that study, children with ASD and an ASD-associated deletion or duplication at the *16p11.2* locus demonstrated divergent dynamic patterns of mu attenuation providing additional insight into the relationship between ASD-associated copy number variations (CNVs) and social neural phenotypes.

This study sought to characterize social motion discrimination in ASD within the upper and lower mu bands continuously over time to capture dynamic neural social indices that may be associated with LGDMs expressed in embryonic development. We tested mu attenuation and habituation first via diagnostic comparisons between typically developing (TYP) and ASD children and, second, via genetics-guided comparisons between children with and without LGDMs expressed preferentially in embryonic development (LGDM E+ vs. LGDM E–). Based upon prior work [12, 28–30], we predicted a lack of social motion discrimination in ASD relative to TYP and anticipated no habituation to either condition in ASD, consistent with [17]. We predicted that children with an embryonically expressed ASD-associated LGDM might have a more severely impacted social profile relative to LGDM E–, in part due to embryonic development as a (more) critical period for regulation of gene expression in support of brain development [41]. Lastly, we evaluated relationships between the neural social indices and individual predictors of social and cognitive behavioral features to better assess the specificity of mu attenuation to capture social processing.

Methods
Participants and clinical procedures
Thirty-nine children age 6–19 years participated in this study (see Table 1 for full characterization details). ASD-LGDM children ($n = 13$) were recruited to enroll in this study following participation in the Simons Simplex Collection or following independent genetic screening that identified a de novo ASD-associated LGDM with family-based exome sequencing studies [5] or companion molecular inversion probe-based (MIP) targeted resequencing of potential ASD loci [42, 43]. Post hoc clustering, based upon the functional role of the LGDM, tested genetically guided patterns of neural heterogeneity. Per Iossifov and colleagues [5, 18], LGDMs consisted of five genes primarily expressed

in embryonic development (*ADNP* [44], *DYRK1A*, n = 3 [8], *MED13L* [5], *SETBP1* [45], and *SETD2*, n = 2 [46]) and four genes primarily expressed post-embryonic development (*CHD8*, n = 2 [7], *DSCAM* [42], *GRIN2B* [47], and *SCN2A* [48]). Comparison cases included equal number of age- and gender-matched children with idiopathic ASD (ASD-NON) and typical development (TYP). ASD-NON and TYP children were recruited from individuals who had previously completed other research projects within the research laboratory. None of the ASD-NON cases had an identified ASD-associated LGDM or otherwise specified ASD genetic events (e.g., ASD-associated copy number variation). TYP participants were defined as children without any parent-reported psychiatric or neurodevelopmental diagnoses and a lack of features of autism or subclinical communication concerns on the Social Responsiveness Scale-2 (SRS-2; i.e., all TYP participants scored under a *T*-score of 60) [49]. There were no differences in SRS-2 scores for ASD-LGDM or ASD-NON, $F(1,24) = 0.008$, $p = .93$. All research procedures conformed to regulations in accordance with the local ethical review board. Written informed consent was obtained from each parental representative(s). All children verbally assented to participate in the procedures, and written assent was obtained from children with a mental age of 7 or greater.

See Additional file 1: Table S1 for full clinical characterization of ASD participants. Diagnoses of autism were confirmed using the Autism Diagnostic Interview-Revised (ADI-R) [50, 51] and the Autism Diagnostic Observation Schedule-2 (ADOS-2) [49, 52]. Verbal and nonverbal IQ (VIQ, NVIQ) was assessed using the Wechsler Abbreviated Scale of Intelligence [10] or the Differential Ability Scales-Second Edition [50], depending on age. Due to the severe intellectual disabilities within the ASD-LGDM cases, IQ ratio scores (n = 3) were substituted when standard IQ deviation scores were not available. The ASD-LGDM cases were more cognitively impaired than both comparison groups in VIQ and NVIQ, $F(1,24)$'s > 23.21, p's < .001. Thus, VIQ and NVIQ were included in the statistical models

to account for known variation in IQ and explicitly tested as part of our third objective. We recognize that cognitive differences between LGDM and comparison groups (TYP, ASD-NON) is a limitation of our study; however, evidence suggests that mu attenuation during passive social perception is not linked to cognitive abilities [33]. In addition, the genetics-guided comparisons between LGDM E+ and LGDM E− were matched on age, IQ, autism severity (i.e., via the ADOS-2 score), and adaptive behavior (i.e., via the Vineland Adaptive Behavior Scales-2 [53]), $F(1,11)$'s < 2.15, $p > .17$.

Identification of genetic variants

Small-molecule molecular inversion probes (smMIPs) [54] were designed to the coding portions of *CHD8*, *DSCAM*, *DYRK1A*, *GRIN2B*, *SCN2A*, *SETBP1*, *SETD2*, *ADNP*, and *MED13L* with a 5-bp single-molecule tag using a scoring algorithm described previously [55] in order to identify single-nucleotide variants (SNVs) and insertions/deletions (INDELs). Oligonucleotides (IDT, Coralville, IA) were ordered, and probes were pooled at an equal molar ratio and phosphorylated (1X pool). After initial testing, poor-performing smMIPs were repooled and phosphorylated in either a 10X or a 50X pool. A final working probe pool was created by combining the three pools so that the final concentration of each smMIP in the 10X and 50X initial pools was a 10- or 50-fold excess relative to the 1X pool. Genomic DNA capture, exonuclease treatment, and PCR amplification of each library were performed as previously described [42] with 120 ng of genomic DNA input. smMIP concentration was based on a ratio of 800 copies of each MIP to each haploid genome copy, based on the 1X pool concentration. We pooled barcoded libraries together and purified the pools with 0.8X AMPure XP beads (Beckman Coulter, Brea, CA) according to the manufacturer's protocol. Pools were quantified in duplicate using the Qubit dsDNA HS Assay (Life Technologies, Grand Island, NY). All samples were sequenced on an Illumina MiSeq (Reagent Kit 300V2) or HiSeq 2000 according to the manufacturer's instructions. Sequencing reads were

Table 1 Participant characterization

Group	N (n female)	Age M (SD)	VIQ M (SD)	Range	NVIQ M (SD)	Range	SRS M (SD)	Range
TYP	13 (3)	11.30 (3.79)	118.54 (12.07)	99–146	110.46 (7.91)	98–128	43.54 (3.73)	37–51
ASD-NON	13 (3)	10.26 (3.59)	104.62 (18.74)	66–134	109.54 (18.71)	85–138	74.62 (10.15)	62–90
ASD-LGDM	13 (3)	13.38 (2.92)	54.54 (32.45)	16–136	53.08 (30.42)	22–137	74.15 (16.31)	45–103
LGDM E+	7 (2)	8.23 (3.39)	51.83 (22.32)	24–84	48.67 (22.31)	22–86	81 (17.62)	55–103
LGDM E−	6 (1)	9.08 (3.10)	56.86 (40.96)	16–136	56.86 (37.41)	31–137	68.29 (13.65)	45–84

Participant characterization is provided for comparison groups (typical development, TYP; autism spectrum disorder nonrelated to a known genetic etiology, ASD-NON) and likely gene-disruptive mutations (LGDM), as well as the genetically guided clustering of LGDM with (E+) and without (E−) a primary role in embryonic development

Abbreviations: *VIQ* verbal intelligence quotient, *NVIQ* nonverbal intelligence quotient, *SRS-2* Social Responsiveness Scale-2

analyzed using the mipgen analysis pipeline as described previously [55]. SNVs and INDELs were called using freebayes/0.9.14 and required a minimum of 8X coverage with a variant quality (QUAL) score greater than 20. Severe events (nonsense, frameshift, splice, and INDELs) were validated by Sanger sequencing.

In order to detect large CNVs, all samples (ASD-LGDM and ASD-NON) were run on custom genome-wide arrays (Agilent Technologies, Santa Clara, CA). Events for all ASD-LGDM samples have been previously published [56]. See Additional file 2: Table S2 for full genetic characterization of ASD participants.

Social motion task

The objective of the social motion task was to examine the neural response to moving stimuli as it pertains specifically to social, biological agents more so than non-social, nonbiological objects. In the same paradigm and procedures as Hudac et al. [17], each child watched 12 total minutes of silent motion, alternating between conditions of social motion (i.e., hands clapping, animated person dancing), nonsocial motion (i.e., tubes swinging, animated ball bouncing), and no motion (i.e., the two empty backgrounds of motion videos). In this way, we can distinguish between the neural response for social and nonsocial motions, both relative to a baseline without motion. Each of the six 60-s videos was observed twice in one of two possible stimuli presentation orders. Between videos, participants were directed to take a break and the experimenter initiated the next video after confirmation that the participant was ready. Children were seated approximately 75 cm from a video monitor and were instructed to sit still and attend to the videos. Video stimuli were displayed using E-Prime 2.0 software (Psychology Software Tools, Inc., Pittsburgh, PA) at a size of 27 cm by 36.8 cm and subtended a visual angle of 20.4° by 27.6°.

Electrophysiological recording

Continuous electroencephalogram (EEG) was recorded from a high-density 128-channel geodesic net using Net Station 4.3.1 software integrated with a 200-series high-impedance amplifier (Electrical Geodesics, Inc,, Eugene, OR). Electrode impedances were below 50 kΩ to maximize the signal-to-noise ratio, within the standard range for high-impedance amplifiers. During collection, EEG signals were referenced to the vertex electrode, analog filtered (0.1 Hz high-pass, 100 Hz elliptical low-pass), amplified, and digitized with a sampling rate of 500 Hz. A photocell recorded and marked the precise onset time of each video. During acquisition, researchers observed and marked periods containing movement and/or improper attention (e.g., participant looking away).

Electrophysiological preprocessing

Methodological decisions were consistent with our previous study [17] and standard practices for processing EEG data [57]. Following data collection, continuous EEG was segmented into 2-s epochs starting with the onset of each 1-min video in order to generate 30 epochs per video. Epochs marked during acquisition as contaminated by movement or improper attention were removed. Automatic artifact detection rejected channels containing voltage shifts greater than 100 μV for each trial. In addition, trained research assistants reviewed and verified the automated artifact detection to ensure the data were sufficiently clean. If the channel was rejected for more than 50% of epochs (i.e., signifying poor data recording for that channel specifically), the channel was marked as a bad channel. After artifact detection, bad channels were corrected via interpolation from neighboring channels. Epochs were re-referenced to the average reference, excluding the rim channels due to the increased amount of noise from channels consistent with prior work (e.g., [58, 59]) in order to reduce the contribution of noise to the average reference.

Of the 120 possible epochs for each condition, all groups had more than 71.7% of artifact-free data for each condition (Table 2). Pairwise group comparisons indicated that both ASD groups had fewer artifact-free epochs for the nonsocial condition compared to TYP, but there were no differences between ASD-LGD and ASD-NON groups. There were no significant two-tailed Pearson correlations between the number of artifact-free epochs and cognitive predictors (VIQ, $r = .31$, $p = .13$; NVIQ, $r = .25$, $p = .23$) or ASD symptom severity ($r = -.25$, $p = .22$) for the ASD groups. In other words, the amount of data loss is fairly comparable across groups, and missing data due to artifact rejection is largely unrelated to the behavioral phenotype (i.e., missing at random). However, to ensure equal numbers of epochs were included from each group and individual, statistical analyses were restricted to the first 30 epochs for each condition with artifact-free data for each child.

Spectral analysis

To create neural indices of social perception, we computed power attenuation relative to the average baseline (no motion) for the first 30 artifact-free epochs in each condition (social, nonsocial) across central electrodes. Spectral power was calculated using fast Fourier transforms (FFTs) in MATLAB (version 7.12.0, R2011a; Natick, MA) on each 2-s epoch. Each power spectra was averaged across standard [12, 24] central electrodes clustered around the C3 (31, 32, 37, 38, 42, 43, 53, and 54) and C4 (80, 81, 87, 88, 94, 104, 105, and 106) positions. These electrodes are across to the sensorimotor region of the brain, thought to correspond to the mirror neuron

Table 2 Artifact-free EEG data by group and condition

Mean (SD)	Social	Nonsocial
TYP	107.1 (21.4)	106.3 (14.5)
ASD-NON	98.8 (19.5)	92.1 (17.3)
ASD-LGDM	91.4 (28.5)	86 (24.8)
Group differences	Social	Nonsocial
TYP vs. ASD-LGDM	$t(24) = -1.59, p = .13$	$t(24) = -2.55, p = .018$
TYP vs. ASD-NON	$t(24) = 1.03, p = .32$	$t(24) = 2.27, p = .032$
ASD-NON vs. ASD-LGDM	$t(24) = -.78, p = .44$	$t(24) = -.72, p = .48$

Mean and standard deviations for the amount of acceptable, artifact-free epochs are presented for each group by condition. Results of independent-samples t tests are reported for pairwise comparisons between groups. Bold font highlights significant group differences.
Abbreviations: TYP typical development, *ASD* autism spectrum disorder, *NON* no known likely gene-disrupting mutation, *LGDM* likely gene-disrupting mutation

system. Power attenuation was computed as the natural log of the ratio between the power of social motion or nonsocial motion epoch and the power of the individual's average response during the no-motion condition. Subsequently, a value of zero represents no power attenuation relative to baseline [e.g., ln(condition/rest) = 0], and larger negative values represent greater power attenuation (i.e., social motion < rest). Only the first 30 artifact-free epochs in each condition (social, nonsocial) were included to ensure that each individual contributed an equal number of epochs. Power spectra included lower mu (8–10 Hz) and upper mu (10–12 Hz).

Data analysis strategies

All analyses were conducted via SAS 9.3 (SAS Institute) using restricted maximum likelihood (REML) and Satterthwaite denominator degrees of freedom. A series of multilevel models were generated using PROC MIXED to describe the variances and covariances of attenuation, separately for each analysis and the two mu bands. All models included a random intercept for each individual.

As we were interested in dynamic changes in power attenuation varying by condition across exposure to the video (i.e., trial order), the final models included fixed effects for condition (0 = nonsocial), ASD diagnosis (diagnostic comparison model) or genetic group (genetics-guided comparison model), time (0 = trial 30, the last epoch), and subsequent interactions. Subject predictors were included as fixed effects to test additional contribution by each child's age (0 = 12 years), FSIQ (0 = 100), VIQ (0 = 100), NVIQ (0 = 100), and gender (0 = male). None of the subject predictors significantly contributed to the models, $Fs < 3.14$, $ps > .086$. However, all subject predictor fixed effects remained in the model to account for potential contributions to group variances.

Results

By modeling dynamic changes over time (i.e., trial order), we were able to measure the rate by which mu attenuation habituates (becomes more positive over time) or sensitizes (becomes more negative over time). Specifically, neural indices were measured as the power attenuation difference between social and nonsocial conditions with the Tukey correction.

Diagnostic comparisons (TYP and ASD)

We first examined mu attenuation related to social discrimination (social vs. nonsocial motion differences) using a diagnostic comparison of typical development and ASD. Full model results for each comparison are reported in Table 3.

Average mu attenuation for each group is illustrated in Fig. 1. Omnibus tests (see Table 3) for both mu bands indicated main effects of condition, such that there was more mu attenuation for social relative to nonsocial motion. As expected, the TYP group exhibited social discrimination with greater social than nonsocial attenuation within both lower mu, $F(1,4635) = 11.70$, $p = .0006$, and upper mu, $F(1,4635) = 20.87$, $p < .0001$. In contrast, the ASD group only exhibited this pattern of social discrimination within lower mu, $F(1,4635) = 7.22$, $p = .0073$, and no discrimination within upper mu, $F(1,4635) = 0.23, p = .63$.

The omnibus tests also indicated a main effect of slope, such that mu attenuation habituated over the course of the experiment (i.e., collapsing across condition). Both groups exhibited different social and nonsocial slopes within lower mu [TYP: $F(1,4635) = 19.21$, $p < .0001$; ASD: $F(1,4635) = 7.16, p = .0075$], such that both groups habituated to nonsocial motion (TYP slope = .007; ASD slope = .004) more quickly than social motion (TYP slope = .005; ASD slope = 0). Within upper mu, only the TYP group had different dynamic patterns, [TYP: $F(1,4635) = 11.11$, $p = .0009$; ASD: $F(1,4635) = 0.29, p = .59$]. Neither group habituated or sensitized to social motion (slopes = 0), but only the TYP group habituated to nonsocial motion (TYP slope = .006, ASD slope = .003). Figure 2 illustrates the relative condition discrimination across trial order, highlighting in the ASD group both the increasing difference between social and nonsocial lower mu attenuation and the lack of discrimination in upper mu attenuation.

Table 3 Diagnostic comparison MLM results

Effect	Lower mu	Upper mu
Condition	$F(1,4635) = 27.88, p < .0001$	$F(1,4635) = 9.43, p = .002$
Group	$F(1,35) = 1.35, p = .254$	$F(1,34.9) = 0.66, p = .423$
Condition by group	$F(1,4635) = 4.75, p = .029$	$F(1,4635) = 6.32, p = .012$
Slope	$F(1,4635) = 19.64, p < .0001$	$F(1,4635) = 11, p < .001$
Slope by condition	$F(1,4635) = 3.21, p = .073$	$F(1,4635) = 3.86, p = .049$
Slope by group	$F(1,4635) = 4.85, p = .028$	$F(1,4635) = 2.43, p = .119$
Slope by condition by group	$F(1,4635) = 0.47, p = .495$	$F(1,4635) = 0.13, p = .717$
VIQ	$F(1,33) = 0.24, p = .631$	$F(1,33) = 1.83, p = .186$
NVIQ	$F(1,33) = 1.66, p = .207$	$F(1,33) = 1.92, p = .175$
Age	$F(1,33) = 1.16, p = .290$	$F(1,33) = 1.71, p = .200$
Gender	$F(1,33) = 2.07, p = .160$	$F(1,33) = 2.9, p = .098$

Multilevel model results for diagnostic comparison by group (TYP vs. ASD) for lower mu (8–10 Hz) and upper mu (10–12 Hz) attenuation. Bold denotes significant effect

Genetics-guided comparisons of the LGDM group (E− vs. E+)

Next, we sought to explore whether these patterns were consistent within a subsample of the ASD group with a known genetic etiology of ASD. In particular, we were interested in post hoc clustering comparisons based upon gene function given prior work targeting functional classes of LGDMs [5, 18]. To this extent, we evaluated mu attenuation related to social discrimination within the LGDM group to compare LGDMs associated with and without strong gene expression during embryonic development (LGDM E+ vs. LGDM E−).

Full model results are reported in Table 4, and patterns of average mu attenuation and dynamic changes over trial order are illustrated in Figs. 3 and 4, respectively. Omnibus tests (see Table 4) indicated that there were no condition, group, or slope effects within upper mu; thus, we focus here on the lower mu band. A main effect of condition indicated that both LGDM E+ and LGDM E− groups exhibited social discrimination with greater social than nonsocial attenuation within lower mu.

Omnibus tests (see Table 4) indicated slopes differed by condition and by group. Both groups exhibited different social and nonsocial slopes within lower mu [LGDM E−: $F(1,1541) = 4.89$, $p = .027$; LGDM E+: $F(1,1541) = 7.52$, $p = .0062$]. Neither group habituated or sensitized to nonsocial motion (slopes = 0), and the LGDM E− group also did not habituate or sensitize to social motion (slope = 0). However, the LGDM E+ group sensitized to social motion (slope = −.007), such that condition discrimination initially indicated more mu attenuation for nonsocial motion and ended with more mu attenuation for social motion at the end of the experiment. In other words, similar to typical development, both LGDM groups exhibited more social mu attenuation by the end of the experiment, but this effect was only shown after a delayed amount of time in the LGDM E+ group.

Relationships between neural indices and individual differences

Lastly, we wanted to determine the specificity of this measure of neural indices in relation to social and cognitive behavioral features for each child. Due to the known variability of nonclinical populations [60], we included all subjects in this analysis. We examined relationships to condition discrimination (i.e., the amount of difference

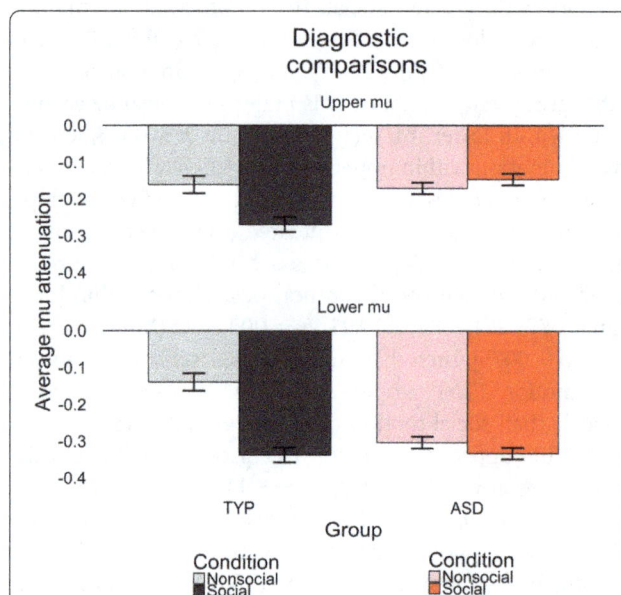

Fig. 1 Diagnostic comparisons of overall mu attenuation between TYP and ASD. Power attenuation for social (*dark black/dark red*) and nonsocial (*light pink/light gray*) motions is averaged and plotted for typically developing children (*TYP, black/gray*) and children with ASD (*ASD, red/pink*). Error bars reflect 1 standard deviation

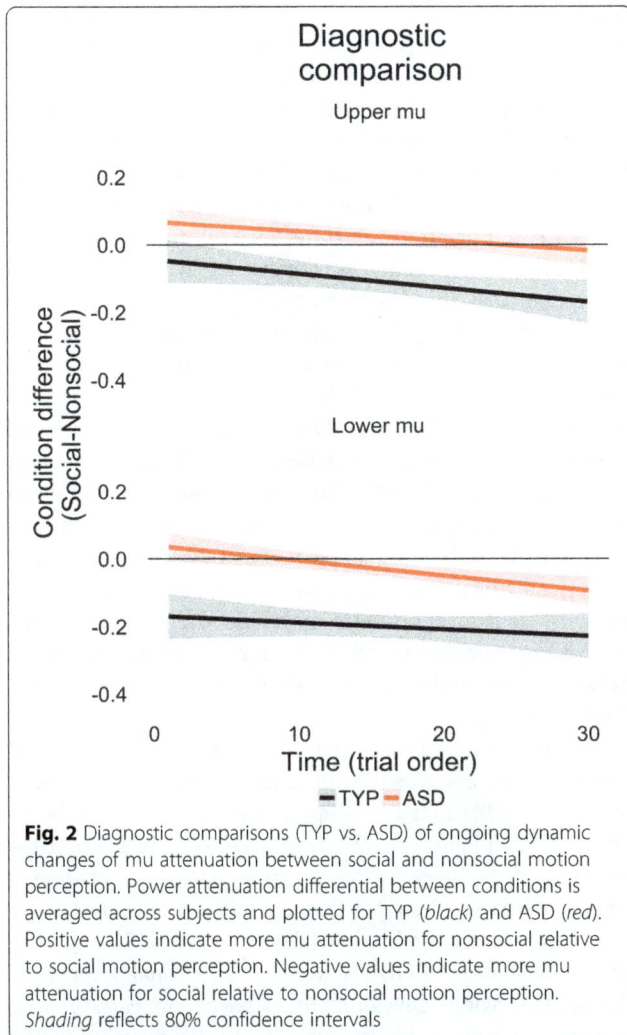

Fig. 2 Diagnostic comparisons (TYP vs. ASD) of ongoing dynamic changes of mu attenuation between social and nonsocial motion perception. Power attenuation differential between conditions is averaged across subjects and plotted for TYP (*black*) and ASD (*red*). Positive values indicate more mu attenuation for nonsocial relative to social motion perception. Negative values indicate more mu attenuation for social relative to nonsocial motion perception. *Shading* reflects 80% confidence intervals

between social and nonsocial mu attenuation). Partial correlation analyses ($p < .05$, controlling for age and NVIQ) indicated that condition discrimination was related to better overall social responsiveness (SRS-2) [49] for both lower mu, $r(35) = .42$, $p = .011$, and upper mu, $r(35) = .39$, $p = .017$ (Fig. 5). There were no significant associations between cognitive measures (VIQ, NVIQ) and condition discrimination within lower or upper mu as tested by Pearson correlations, p's > .15.

Discussion

Social impairments are a hallmark of ASD, yet phenotypic and genetic heterogeneity is thought to contribute to discrepant evidence in the literature. We explore a neural mechanism associated with ASD by considering patterns of social discrimination as measured by mu attenuation over time for children with different genetic etiologies. From the diagnostic comparisons, we show aberrant patterns of mu attenuation in ASD are specific to the upper mu band, while the lower mu band reflects less atypical patterns, consistent with prior work [34]. The dynamic patterns indicate that children with ASD show an increasing lower mu difference between social and nonsocial motions, which may help resolve diagnostic inconsistencies within the literature. For instance, prior evidence of atypical mu attenuation in ASD between observed motion conditions (i.e., social relative to nonsocial motion, as in the current study) [12, 28–30] has relied on individual averages. Our findings suggest that the discrimination pattern may not be evident if there are too few trials (i.e., before children with ASD habituated to nonsocial motion observations). Although it is a concern that children with ASD did contribute fewer trials than the typical controls, the eventual condition differentiation in ASD (i.e., noted by approximately

Table 4 LGDM comparison MLM results

Effect	Lower mu	Upper mu
Condition	**$F(1,1541) = 12.18, p < .001$**	$F(1,1541) = 0.69, p = .406$
Group	$F(1,9.33) = 0.24, p = .634$	$F(1,7.79) = 0.03, p = .865$
Condition by group	$F(1,1541) = 0.01, p = .914$	$F(1,1541) = 0.06, p = .809$
Slope	$F(1,1541) = 0.01, p = .904$	$F(1,1541) = 0.52, p = .469$
Slope by condition	**$F(1,1541) = 4.14, p = .042$**	$F(1,1541) = 0.04, p = .849$
Slope by group	**$F(1,1541) = 4.11, p = .043$**	$F(1,1541) = 2.98, p = .084$
Slope by condition by group	$F(1,1541) = 1.55, p = .213$	$F(1,1541) = 0.16, p = .687$
VIQ	$F(1,7) = 0.71, p = .426$	$F(1,7) = 2.71, p = .144$
NVIQ	$F(1,7) = 1.6, p = .246$	$F(1,7) = 0.86, p = .385$
Age	$F(1,7) = 0.09, p = .776$	$F(1,7) = 0.08, p = .785$
Gender	$F(1,7) = 1.56, p = .252$	$F(1,7) = 4.41, p = .074$

Multilevel model results for genetically guided comparison by group (LGDM E+ vs. LGDM E−) for lower mu (8–10 Hz) and upper mu (10–12 Hz) attenuation. Bold denotes significant effect
Abbreviations: *LGDM E+* likely gene-disrupting mutations primarily expressed during embryonic development, *LGDM E−* likely gene-disrupting mutations not primarily expressed during embryonic development

Genetics-guided comparisons

Upper mu

Lower mu

Fig. 3 Genetics-guided comparisons of overall mu attenuation between LGDM E+ and LGDM E−. Power attenuation for social (*dark green/orange*) and nonsocial (*light green/yellow*) motions is averaged and plotted for children with an LGDM that is primarily expressed during embryonic development (*LGDM E+, orange/yellow*) and children with an LGDM that is not primarily expressed during embryonic development (*LGDM E−, light green/dark green*). *Error bars* reflect 1 standard deviation

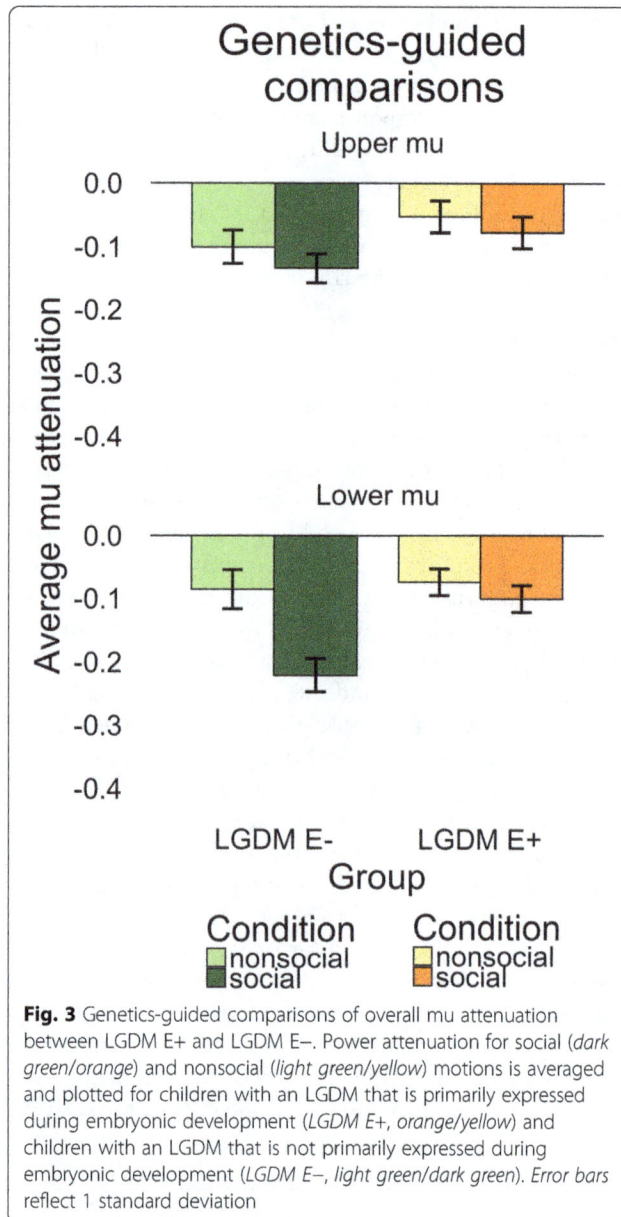

trial 15 in Fig. 2) indicates that our study had a sufficient number of trials.

Mu attenuation has been proposed to reflect a human corollary to the mirror neuron system [24, 61], which describes activation recorded over the sensorimotor cortex during both action execution and observation of human actions. Although it is possible that mu attenuation reflects the conductance of occipital or posterior alpha rhythm more broadly (i.e., responsivity to general motion information) [62], our results indicate differentiation of social and nonsocial motions. One working hypothesis of ASD suggests mirror neuron system deficits that disrupt neural correlates supporting the action/observation system, subsequently eliciting atypical mu attenuation [63].

Aligned with this theory, other evidence suggest that atypical functioning of the mirror neuron system may lead to a downstream effect of poor imitative abilities [33] or disrupted higher order social cognitive abilities (i.e., theory of mind) [64]. However, it is important to note that similar to prior work by Dumas and colleagues, we found mu attenuation diagnostic differences within the upper mu band (10–12 Hz), but no group difference within the lower mu band (8–10 Hz). This is consistent with prior work suggesting that this lower frequency may reflect primary sensory processing [36, 37] that habituates over the course of the exposure. Yet, sensory processing of biological motion occurred more rapidly in the TYP group compared to longer processing in the ASD group, perhaps indicative of functional connectivity reductions related to social cognition [65]. Our results offer further evidence of atypical mu attenuation patterns in ASD, although unique neural mechanisms underlying atypical social discrimination may be derived from specific genetic etiologies. In other words, a mirror neuron hypothesis may indeed describe a subset of children with ASD, while a more general, distributed network of neural correlates may be impacted in other ASD subgroups.

As part of a preliminary analysis, we examined the neural social indices associated with different functional genetic roles of LGDMs as a first step to explore a possible shared neural social phenotype. We implemented a post hoc clustering strategy in order to examine potential convergent pathways between LGDMs that are and are not functionally expressed during embryonic development [18, 66]. The choice to cluster LGDMs around functional expression during embryonic development is based on early genetic regulatory control supporting regional differentiation within the embryonic brain [67, 68], including key social neural structures (e.g., amygdala). We had predicted that the LGDM within the embryonic development group would have a more severely disrupted neural social index due to evidence from animal and human models indicating significant impairments related to social behavior [19, 20] and/or information encoding [21, 22]. The results indicated that children with an LGDM primarily expressed during embryonic development exhibit sensitization of lower mu attenuation to social motion. In other words, these children initially exhibited more mu attenuation for nonsocial motion, but eventually demonstrate more for social motion. This pattern was distinct from children with an LGDM not primarily expressed during embryonic development that exhibited greater lower mu attenuation discrimination throughout the entire experiment (i.e., greater mu attenuation to social than nonsocial motion beginning at the first few trials).

Our results suggest that social motion perception may be conserved despite early genetic disruption, though the delayed processing supports the notion of potentially

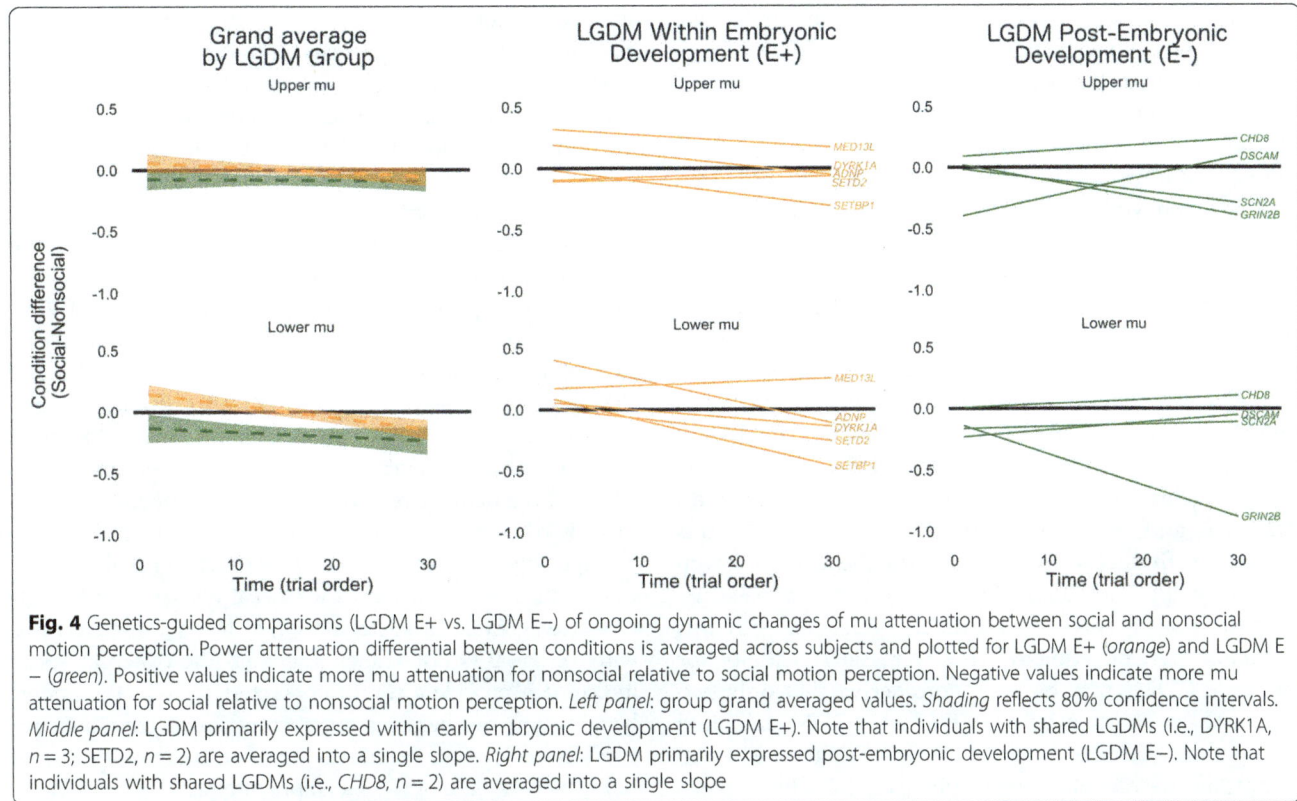

Fig. 4 Genetics-guided comparisons (LGDM E+ vs. LGDM E−) of ongoing dynamic changes of mu attenuation between social and nonsocial motion perception. Power attenuation differential between conditions is averaged across subjects and plotted for LGDM E+ (*orange*) and LGDM E − (*green*). Positive values indicate more mu attenuation for nonsocial relative to social motion perception. Negative values indicate more mu attenuation for social relative to nonsocial motion perception. *Left panel*: group grand averaged values. *Shading* reflects 80% confidence intervals. *Middle panel*: LGDM primarily expressed within early embryonic development (LGDM E+). Note that individuals with shared LGDMs (i.e., DYRK1A, n = 3; SETD2, n = 2) are averaged into a single slope. *Right panel*: LGDM primarily expressed post-embryonic development (LGDM E−). Note that individuals with shared LGDMs (i.e., *CHD8*, n = 2) are averaged into a single slope

delayed information processing. It is important to note that this delay was specific to the social motion condition (increasing neural response over time) but not the nonsocial motion condition (i.e., no change over time), which may help clarify the mechanism by which prior models [19, 20] derive impaired social behavior. An interpretation of the results may be that children with an LGDM primarily expressed during embryonic development are increasing

their attention to, or interest in, social stimuli after an initial period, which may reflect a delayed social engagement (e.g., motivation or salience). One explanation may be that the impact of embryonic genes on social perception is greater [69], suggesting that functional timing of genetic expression may differentially affect the neural social phenotype. Importantly, these findings align with genetics research indicating that ASD genes converge on several select pathways

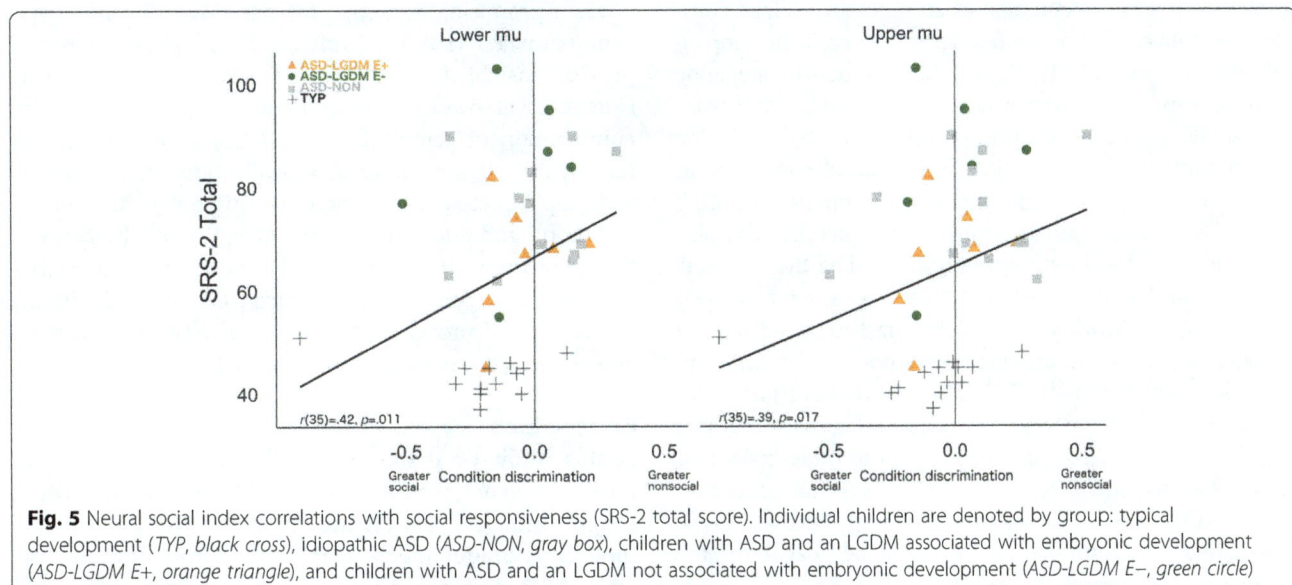

Fig. 5 Neural social index correlations with social responsiveness (SRS-2 total score). Individual children are denoted by group: typical development (*TYP, black cross*), idiopathic ASD (*ASD-NON, gray box*), children with ASD and an LGDM associated with embryonic development (*ASD-LGDM E+, orange triangle*), and children with ASD and an LGDM not associated with embryonic development (*ASD-LGDM E−, green circle*)

[70, 71], which may help to further explain the underlying neural social heterogeneity.

An important limitation of the current study is the continued genetic heterogeneity despite functionally classifying the expression of LGDM within early development. Within our LGDM groups, there are only several children with a shared LGDM (i.e., *SETD2*, $n = 2$; *DYRK1A*, $n = 2$; *CHD8*, $n = 2$). Thus, the discoveries of this work are not to be taken as firm conclusions, but rather considered in order to motivate and guide continued use of a genetics-first approach to elucidate potential etiological mechanisms of ASD. For instance, most of the children within the early embryonic LGDM group exhibit the social sensitization pattern described here (six out of eight cases; see Additional file 3: Figure S1 for individual patterns), except for one child with *MED13L* and one child with *DYRK1A*. In part, this qualitative finding is consistent with the overall group clustering approach indicating delayed social processing, suggesting a potential neural index associated with this particular genetic etiology. However, the specificity for specific LGDMs may be poor, considering that only two out of three children with a *DYRK1A* LGDM exhibited this pattern. Similar to prior work linking core social symptoms to biomarkers of ASD [11, 72–76], we encourage the use of this data as a way to bridge the gap between genetic and phenotypic characterization as a means to facilitate the discovery of ASD etiological mechanisms and accelerate progress for ASD therapeutic interventions.

It may be surprising that our task elicited mu attenuation during nonsocial motion observation (i.e., ball bouncing, tubes swinging) that is not biological and subsequently should not be simulated within the action/observation system. However, to a large extent, the majority of studies implementing mu attenuation as an outcome utilized comparisons between self-executed, social observed, and nonsocial observed motion. It may be the case that by engaging the motor execution system during these tasks, the threshold for the action/observation system is elevated, reducing the amount of mu attenuation for nonsocial comparisons. In fact, neural regions implicated in mu suppression during execution vs. observation [77] involve regions that also play a role in general motion perception, including the occipital, premotor, and somatosensory cortices. Moreover, this study replicated prior work with this same task that indicated a modest degree of mu attenuation to nonsocial motion, in addition to social motion [17]. We posit that our task measured more globally distributed neural differences between social and nonsocial motions compared to other tasks that have used self-initiated actions to target the premotor cortex. Of note, this passive viewing task is more conducive for children with reduced capacity for following behavioral instructions (i.e., to make self-

initiated motions), while still providing a robust neural index, which specifies individual patterns.

The neural social indices were correlated with features of social cognition (i.e., social responsiveness), particularly with the lower mu band. This finding is compelling evidence that these indices accurately capture subtle levels of social impairments in vivo, as opposed to relying on parental reports (e.g., SRS-2). Additionally, average patterns of mu attenuation were unaffected by general cognition, despite drastic cognitive differences for children with a LGDM. Although this may not negate a contributory role of cognitive ability for higher-order operations related to social motion (e.g., action prediction), this evidence from this study suggests that motion perception is intact for children with lower cognitive abilities (i.e., cognitive scores under 50). Much of the existing research investigating neural social indices is restricted to children and adults with moderate to average cognitive capabilities. The majority of ASD-LGDM cases with low verbal IQ show typical mu attenuation patterns (i.e., greater for social motion in five out of eight cases with verbal IQ < 50). Taken together, these neural social indices can provide a robust characterization of the underlying neural mechanisms supporting social cognition, regardless of level of cognitive function, thereby improving our understanding of the social phenotype.

This study is the first to use a genetics-first approach to explore the genetic etiologies of autism associated with severe LGDMs in the context of neural social indices. Our use of a unique statistical method to measure ongoing dynamic changes associated with social motion perception demonstrates the utility of this method to better understand underlying processes relevant to ASD and LGDMs. Although this study is limited by a small sample size and thus should be considered exploratory, the analysis of neural social phenotypes based on functional clustering offers a promising approach for narrowing in on convergent pathways that may reflect shared phenotypes and provide insight for targeted treatment [5, 18]. Future research will need to take into account the variety and combination of genetic functional roles. Ongoing efforts to recruit a larger, more genetically homogenous group will help target specific functional outcomes during early childhood and adolescence. However, due to the rarity of this population, these preliminary results are informative and can help guide future research by better describing the functional processes during social motion perception and similar processes that are impaired in ASD.

Conclusions

In this study, we demonstrated distinct neural social indices for genetic etiologies of ASD, providing critical insight into the underlying mechanisms of ASD pathology. A unique mechanism was identified for children with ASD and genetic etiology associated with early embryonic development, based upon level of mu attenuation related to social discrimination and patterns over time (i.e., habituation). Our findings implicate genetic heterogeneity as a possible reason for divergent findings in the literature and distinguish the manner by which neural social indices differ between groups and over time. We emphasize the need to continue to discover how phenotypic profiles align within children in specific genotypic subgroups of ASD. Taken together, we predict that future work pursuing phenotypic characterization via the integration of genetic, neural, and behavioral information will continue to inform our understanding of ASD subtypes and will have broad implications for our ability to adopt precision medicine strategies.

Additional files

Additional file 1: Clinical characterization for children with ASD is provided. Abbreviations: M, male; F, female; LGD, likely gene-disrupting; +, present; -, absent; NC, not completed. (XLS 47 kb)

Additional file 2: Genetic characterization for children with ASD is provided. Bold font highlights likely gene-disrupting mutations (LGD) associated with ASD. Abbreviations: +, present; -, absent; NC, not completed; (M), missense, (N), nonsense; (S), splice; (FS), frameshift; (IV) intronic variant. (XLSX 25 kb)

Additional file 3: Individual slopes from genetics-guided comparisons (LGDM E+ vs LGDM E-) of ongoing dynamic changes of mu attenuation between social and nonsocial motion perception. Power attenuation differential between conditions is averaged within subjects and plotted for LGDM E+ (orange) and LGDM E- (green). Individuals with shared LGDMs (i.e., *CHD8, DYRK1A, SETD2*) are distinguished by "_n". Positive values indicate more mu attenuation for nonsocial relative to social motion perception. Negative values indicate more mu attenuation for social relative to nonsocial motion perception. Left panel: LGDM primarily expressed within early embryonic development (LGDM E+). Right panel: LGDM primarily expressed post-embryonic development (LGDM E-). (TIFF 32871 kb)

Acknowledgements
We would like to thank the children and families for their participation in this study. We are grateful to all of the families at the participating Simons Simplex Collection (SSC) sites, as well as the principal investigators (A. Beaudet, R. Bernier, J. Constantino, E. Cook, E. Fombonne, D. Geschwind, R. Goin-Kochel, E. Hanson, D. Grice, A. Klin, D. Ledbetter, C. Lord, C. Martin, D. Martin, R. Maxim, J. Miles, O. Ousley, K. Pelphrey, B. Peterson, J. Piggot, C. Saulnier, M. State, W. Stone, J. Sutcliffe, C. Walsh, Z. Warren, E. Wijsman). We appreciate obtaining access to phenotypic data on SFARI Base. E.E.E. is an investigator of the Howard Hughes Medical Institute. The computerized dancer stimuli were provided courtesy of Nick Neave and Kristofor McCarty at Northumbria University.

Funding
Research reported in this publication was supported by the National Institute of Mental Health (MH100047, Bernier; MH10028, Webb/Bernier; and MH101221, Eichler), by the National Institute of Child Health and Human Development to the University of Washington's Center on Human Development and Disability (U54 HD083091), and in part by a grant from the Simons Foundation (SFARI 303241, Eichler). H.A.F.S. was supported in part by the NHGRI Interdisciplinary Training in Genome Science Grant (T32HG00035).

Authors' contributions
RAB contributed to the conceptualization and methodology. CMH and HAFS contributed to the formal analysis. TDD, AK, SF, and EN contributed to the investigation. RAB and EEE contributed to the resources. CMH and RAB wrote the original draft. All authors performed the review and editing. CMH contributed to the visualization. SJW, EEE, and RAB supervised the study. EEE and RAB contributed to the project administration and funding acquisition. All authors read and approved the final manuscript.

Competing interests
E.E.E. is on the scientific advisory board (SAB) of DNAnexus, Inc. and is a consultant for Kunming University of Science and Technology (KUST) as part of the 1000 China Talent Program. All other authors do not have competing interests.

Author details
[1]Department of Psychiatry and Behavioral Sciences, University of Washington, CHDD Box 357920, Seattle, WA 98195, USA. [2]Department of Genome Sciences, University of Washington School of Medicine, Seattle, WA 98195, USA. [3]Center for Child Health, Behavior, and Disabilities, Seattle Children's Research Institute, Seattle, WA 98145, USA. [4]Boston Children's Hospital and Division of Developmental Medicine, Harvard School of Medicine, Boston, MA 02215, USA. [5]Howard Hughes Medical Institute, Seattle, WA 98195, USA.

References
1. Geschwind DH. Advances in autism. Annu Rev Med. 2009;60:367–80.
2. Betancur C. Etiological heterogeneity in autism spectrum disorders: more than 100 genetic and genomic disorders and still counting. Brain Res. 2011;1380:42–77.
3. Bill BR, Geschwind DH. Genetic advances in autism: heterogeneity and convergence on shared pathways. Curr Opin Genet Dev. 2009;19:271–8.
4. Geschwind DH, State MW. Gene hunting in autism spectrum disorder: on the path to precision medicine. Lancet Glob Health. 2015;14(11):1109–20.
5. Iossifov I, O'Roak BJ, Sanders SJ, Ronemus M, Krumm N, Levy D, et al. The contribution of de novo coding mutations to autism spectrum disorder. Nature. 2014;515:216–21.
6. Higdon R, Earl RK, Stanberry L, Hudac CM, Montague E, Stewart E, et al. The promise of multi-omics and clinical data integration to identify and target personalized healthcare approaches in autism spectrum disorders. OMICS. 2015;19:197–208. Available from: http://online.liebertpub.com/doi/10.1089/omi.2015.0020.
7. Bernier R, Golzio C, Xiong B, Stessman HA, Coe BP, Penn O, et al. Disruptive CHD8 mutations define a subtype of autism early in development. Cell. 2014;158:1–14. Elsevier Inc.
8. van Bon B, Hoischen A, Hehir-Kwa J, de Brouwer A, Ruivenkamp C, Gijsbers A, et al. Intragenic deletion in DYRK1A leads to mental retardation and primary microcephaly. Clin Genet. 2011;79:296–9.
9. van Bon BWM, Coe BP, Bernier R, Green C, Gerdts J, Witherspoon K, et al. Disruptive de novo mutations of DYRK1A lead to a syndromic form of autism and ID. Molecular Psychiatry. 2016;21:126–32. Nature Publishing Group.
10. Wechsler D. Wechsler Abbreviated Scale of Intelligence (WASI). San Antonio: The Psychological Corporation; 1999.

11. Kaiser MD, Hudac CM, Shultz S, Lee SM, Cheung C, Berken AM, et al. Neural signatures of autism. Proc Natl Acad Sci. 2010;107:21223–8.

12. Bernier R, Dawson G, Webb S, Murias M. EEG mu rhythm and imitation impairments in individuals with autism spectrum disorder. Brain Cogn. 2007;64:228–37.

13. Webb SJ, Merkle K, Murias M, Richards T, Aylward E, Dawson G. ERP responses differentiate inverted but not upright face processing in adults with ASD. Soc Cogn Affect Neurosci. 2012;7:578–87. Oxford University Press.

14. Gordon I, Vander Wyk BC, Bennett RH, Cordeaux C, Lucas MV, Eilbott JA, et al. Oxytocin enhances brain function in children with autism. Proc Natl Acad Sci. 2013;110:20953–8.

15. Pelphrey KA, Shultz S, Hudac CM, Vander Wyk BC. Research review: Constraining heterogeneity: the social brain and its development in autism spectrum disorder. J Child Psychol Psychiatry. 2011;52:631–44. Available from: http://doi.wiley.com/10.1111/j.1469-7610.2010.02349.x.

16. Berman JI, Chudnovskaya D, Blaskey L, Kuschner E, Mukherjee P, Buckner R, et al. Abnormal auditory and language pathways in children with 16p11.2 deletion. Neuroimage Clin. 2015;9:50–7. Elsevier B.V.

17. Hudac CM, Kresse A, Aaronson B, DesChamps TD, Webb SJ, Bernier RA. Modulation of mu attenuation to social stimuli in children and adults with 16p11. 2 deletions and duplications. J Neurodevelopmental Dis. 2015;7(1):25.

18. Iossifov I, Levy D, Allen J, Ye K, Ronemus M, Lee Y-H, et al. Low load for disruptive mutations in autism genes and their biased transmission. Proc Natl Acad Sci. 2015;112(41):E5600-7.

19. Rampersad M, Gerlai R. Impairment of social behaviour persists two years after embryonic alcohol exposure in zebrafish: a model of fetal alcohol spectrum disorders. Behav Brain Res. 2015;292:102–8. Elsevier B.V.

20. Selemon LD, Zecevic N. Schizophrenia: a tale of two critical periods for prefrontal cortical development. Translational Psychiatry. 2015;5:e623–11. Nature Publishing Group.

21. Malishkevich A, Amram N, Hacohen-Kleiman G, Magen I, Giladi E, Gozes I. Activity-dependent neuroprotective protein (ADNP) exhibits striking sexual dichotomy impacting on autistic and Alzheimer's pathologies. Nat Publ Group. 2015;5:e501–9.

22. Stessman HAF, Willemsen MH, Fenckova M, Penn O, Hoischen A, Xiong B, et al. Disruption of POGZ is associated with intellectual disability and autism spectrum disorders. Am J Hum Genet. 2016;98:541–52.

23. Muthukumaraswamy SD, Johnson BW. Changes in rolandic mu rhythm during observation of a precision grip. Psychophysiol. 2004;41:152–6. Available from: http://doi.wiley.com/10.1046/j.1469-8986.2003.00129.x.

24. Muthukumaraswamy SD, Johnson BW, McNair NA. Mu rhythm modulation during observation of an object-directed grasp. Cogn Brain Res. 2004;19:195–201.

25. Arroyo S, Lesser RP, Gordon B, Uematsu S, Jackson D, Webber R. Functional significance of the mu rhythm of human cortex: an electrophysiologic study with subdural electrodes. Electroencephalogr Clin Neurophysiol. 1993;87:76–87. Available from: http://linkinghub.elsevier.com/retrieve/pii/001346949390114B.

26. Pfurtscheller G, Neuper C. Motor imagery activates primary sensorimotor area in humans. Neurosci Lett. 1997;239:65–8.

27. Fox NA, Bakermans-Kranenburg MJ, Yoo KH, Bowman LC, Cannon EN, Vanderwert RE, et al. Assessing human mirror activity with EEG mu rhythm: a meta-analysis. Psychol Bull. 2016;142:291–313. American Psychological Association.

28. Pineda JA, Brang D, Hecht E, Edwards L, Carey S, Bacon M, Futagaki C, Suk D, Tom J, Birnbaum C, Rork A. Positive behavioral and electrophysiological changes following neurofeedback training in children with autism. Res Autism Spectr Disord. 2008;2(3):557–81.

29. Oberman LM, McCleery JP, Hubbard EM, Bernier R, Wiersema JR, Raymaekers R, et al. Developmental changes in mu suppression to observed and executed actions in autism spectrum disorders. Soc Cogn Affect Neurosci. 2013;8:300–4. Oxford University Press.

30. Oberman LM, Hubbard EM, McCleery JP, Altschuler EL, Ramachandran VS, Pineda JA. EEG evidence for mirror neuron dysfunction in autism spectrum disorders. Brain Res Cogn Brain Res. 2005;24:190–8.

31. Raymaekers R, Wiersema JR, Roeyers H. EEG study of the mirror neuron system in children with high functioning autism. Brain Res. 2009;1304:113–21.

32. Fan Y-T, Decety J, Yang C-Y, Liu J-L, Cheng Y. Unbroken mirror neurons in autism spectrum disorders. J Child Psychol Psychiatry. 2010;51:981–8.

33. Bernier R, Aaronson B, McPartland J. The role of imitation in the observed heterogeneity in EEG mu rhythm in autism and typical development. Brain Cogn. 2013;82:69–75.

34. Dumas G, Soussignan R, Hugueville L, Martinerie J, Nadel J. Revisiting mu suppression in autism spectrum disorder. Brain Res. 2014;1585:108–19.

35. Frenkel-Toledo S, Bentin S, Perry A, Liebermann DG, Soroker N. Dynamics of the EEG power in the frequency and spatial domains during observation and execution of manual movements. Brain Res. 2013;1509:43–57.

36. Sacchet MD, LaPlante RA, Wan Q, Pritchett DL, Lee AKC, Hamalainen M, et al. Attention drives synchronization of alpha and beta rhythms between right inferior frontal and primary sensory neocortex. J Neurosci. 2015;35:2074–82.

37. Başar E. A review of alpha activity in integrative brain function: fundamental physiology, sensory coding, cognition and pathology. Int J Psychophysiol. 2012;86:1–24. Elsevier B.V.

38. Naeem M, Prasad G, Watson DR, Kelso JAS. Electrophysiological signatures of intentional social coordination in the 10-12 Hz range. Neuroimage. 2012; 59:1795–803.

39. Fink A, Schwab D, Papousek I. Sensitivity of EEG upper alpha activity to cognitive and affective creativity interventions. Int J Psychophysiol. 2011;82:233–9.

40. Fink A, Grabner RH, Neuper C, Neubauer AC. EEG alpha band dissociation with increasing task demands. Cogn Brain Res. 2005;24:252–9.

41. Patapoutian A, Reichardt LF. Roles of Wnt proteins in neural development and maintenance. Curr Opin Neurol. 2000;10:392–9. NIH Public Access.

42. O'Roak BJ, Stessman HA, Boyle EA, Witherspoon KT, Martin B, Lee C, et al. Recurrent de novo mutations implicate novel genes underlying simplex autism risk. Nat Commun. 2014;5:5595.

43. O'Roak BJ, Deriziotis P, Lee C, Vives L, Schwartz JJ, Girirajan S, et al. Exome sequencing in sporadic autism spectrum disorders identifies severe de novo mutations. Nat Genet. 2011;43:585–9.

44. Vandeweyer G, Helsmoortel C, Van Dijck A, Vulto-van Silfhout AT, Coe BP, Bernier R, et al. The transcriptional regulator ADNP links the BAF (SWI/SNF) complexes with autism. Kosho T, Miyake N, editors. Am J Med Genet C Semin Med Genet. 2014;166:315–26

45. Coe BP, Witherspoon K, Rosenfeld JA, van Bon BWM, Vulto-van Silfhout AT, Bosco P, et al. Refining analyses of copy number variation identifies specific genes associated with developmental delay. Nat Genet. 2014;46:1063–71. Available from: http://dx.doi.org/10.1038/ng.3092.

46. Lumish HS, Wynn J, Devinsky O, Chung WK. Brief report: SETD2 mutation in a child with autism, intellectual disabilities and epilepsy. J Autism Dev Disord. 2015;45(11):3764–70.

47   O'Roak BJ, Vives L, Girirajan S, Karakoc E, Krumm N, Coe BP, et al. Sporadic autism exomes reveal a highly interconnected protein network of de novo mutations. Nature. 2013;485:246–50. Nature Publishing Group.

48   Weiss LA, Escayg A, Kearney JA, Trudeau M, MacDonald BT, Mori M, et al. Sodium channels SCN1A, SCN2A and SCN3A in familial autism. Mol Psychiatry. 2003;8:186–94.

49   Constantino JN, Przybeck T, Friesen D, Todd RD. Reciprocal social behavior in children with and without pervasive developmental disorders. LWW; 2000;21:2–11

50   Elliott CD. Differential Ability Scales-II. Pearson: San Antonio; 2007.

51   Lord C, Rutter M, Le Couteur A. Autism Diagnostic Interview-Revised: a revised version of a diagnostic interview for caregivers of individuals with possible pervasive developmental disorders. J Autism Dev Disord. 1994;24:659–85.

52   Lord C, Rutter M, Goode S, Heemsbergen J, Jordan H, Mawhood L, et al. Autism diagnostic observation schedule: a standardized observation of communicative and social behavior. J Autism Dev Disord. 1989;19:185–212.

53   Sparrow SS, Cicchetti DV, Balla DA, Doll EA. Vineland-II, Vineland Adaptive Behavior Scales: Teacher Rating Form. 2006.

54   Hiatt JB, Pritchard CC, Salipante SJ, O'Roak BJ, Shendure J. Single molecule molecular inversion probes for targeted, high-accuracy detection of low-frequency variation. Genome Res. 2013;23:843–54. Cold Spring Harbor Lab.

55   Boyle EA, O'Roak BJ, Martin BK, Kumar A, Shendure J. MIPgen: optimized modeling and design of molecular inversion probes for targeted resequencing. Bioinformatics. 2014;30:2670–2.

56   Girirajan S, Dennis MY, Baker C, Malig M, Coe BP, Campbell CD, et al. Refinement and discovery of new hotspots of copy-number variation associated with autism spectrum disorder. Am J Hum Genet. 2013;92:221–37.

57   Webb SJ, Bernier R, Henderson HA, Johnson MH, Jones EJH, Lerner MD, et al. Guidelines and best practices for electrophysiological data collection, analysis and reporting in autism. J Autism Dev Disord. 2015;45:425–43.

58   Neuhaus E, Jones EJH, Barnes K, Sterling L, Estes A, Munson J, et al. The relationship between early neural responses to emotional faces at age 3

and later autism and anxiety symptoms in adolescents with autism. J Autism Dev Disord. 2016;46:1–14. Springer US.

59 Ding J, Sperling G, Srinivasan R. Attentional modulation of SSVEP power depends on the network tagged by the flicker frequency. Cerebral Cortex. 2006;16:1016–29.

60 Hobson HM, Bishop DVM. Mu suppression—a good measure of the human mirror neuron system? Cortex. 2016;82:290–310.

61 Pineda JA. The functional significance of mu rhythms: translating "seeing" and "hearing" into "doing". Brain Res Brain Res Rev. 2005;50:57–68.

62 Varela FJ, Toro A, John ER, Schwartz EL. Perceptual framing and cortical alpha-rhythm. Neuropsychologia. 1981;19:675–86.

63 Pineda JA, Hecht E. Mirroring and mu rhythm involvement in social cognition: are there dissociable subcomponents of theory of mind? Biol Psychol. 2009;80:306–14. Available from: http://linkinghub.elsevier.com/retrieve/pii/S0301051108002287.

64 Hamilton AF De C, Brindley RM, Frith U. Imitation and action understanding in autistic spectrum disorders: how valid is the hypothesis of a deficit in the mirror neuron system? Neuropsychologia. 2007;45:1859–68.

65 von dem Hagen EA, Stoyanova RS, Baron-Cohen S, Calder AJ. Reduced functional connectivity within and between "social" resting state networks in autism spectrum conditions. Soc Cogn Affect Neurosci. 2012;8:694–701.

66 Iossifov I, O'Roak BJ, Sanders SJ, Ronemus M, Krumm N, Levy D, et al. The contribution of de novo coding mutations to autism spectrum disorder. Nature. Nature Publishing Group; 2014;515:216–21.

67 Puelles L, Kuwana E, Puelles E, Bulfone A, Shimamura K, Keleher J, et al. Pallial and subpallial derivatives in the embryonic chick and mouse telencephalon, traced by the expression of the genes Dlx-2, Emx-1, Nkx-2.1, Pax-6, and Tbr-1. J Comp Neurol. 2000;424:409–38.

68 Puelles L, Rubenstein JLR. Forebrain gene expression domains and the evolving prosomeric model. Trends Neurosci. 2003;26:469–76.

69 Chang J, Gilman SR, Chiang AH, Sanders SJ, Vitkup D. Genotype to phenotype relationships in autism spectrum disorders. Nat Neurosci. 2014;18:191–8.

70 Robinson EB, St Pourcain B, Anttila V, Kosmicki JA, Bulik-Sullivan B, Grove J, et al. Genetic risk for autism spectrum disorders and neuropsychiatric variation in the general population. Nat Genet. 2016;48:552–5.

71 Krishnan A, Zhang R, Yao V, Theesfeld CL, Wong AK, Tadych A, et al. Genome-wide prediction and functional characterization of the genetic basis of autism spectrum disorder. Nat Neurosci. 2016;19:1454–62.

72 Veenstra-VanderWeele J, Blakely RD. Networking in autism: leveraging genetic, biomarker and model system findings in the search for new treatments. Neuropsychopharmacology. 2012;37:196–212. Nature Publishing Group.

73 Key AP, Ibanez LV, Henderson HA, Warren Z, Messinger DS, Stone WL. Positive affect processing and joint attention in infants at high risk for autism: an exploratory study. J Autism Dev Disord. 2015;45:4051–62. Springer US.

74 Wang F, Zhu AJ, Lajiness-O'Neill R, Bowyer S. Functional network connectivity: possible biomarker for autism spectrum disorders (ASD). 2015.

75 Neuhaus E, Bernier R, Beauchaine TP. Brief report: social skills, internalizing and externalizing symptoms, and respiratory sinus arrhythmia in autism. J Autism Dev Disord. 2014;44:730–7.

76 Spencer MD, Holt RJ, Chura LR, Suckling J, Calder AJ, Bullmore ET, et al. A novel functional brain imaging endophenotype of autism: the neural response to facial expression of emotion. Transl Psychiatry. 2011;1:e19–7. Nature Publishing Group.

77 Braadbaart L, Williams JHG, Waiter GD. Do mirror neuron areas mediate mu rhythm suppression during imitation and action observation? Int J Psychophysiol. 2013;89:99–105. Elsevier B.V.

4

An experimental study of executive function and social impairment in Cornelia de Lange syndrome

Lisa Nelson[1,4], Hayley Crawford[1,2]* , Donna Reid[1], Joanna Moss[1,3] and Chris Oliver[1]

Abstract

Background: Extreme shyness and social anxiety is reported to be characteristic of adolescents and adults with Cornelia de Lange syndrome (CdLS); however, the nature of these characteristics is not well documented. In this study, we develop and apply an experimental assessment of social anxiety in a group of adolescents and adults with CdLS to determine the nature of the social difficulties and whether they are related to impairments in executive functioning.

Methods: A familiar and unfamiliar examiner separately engaged in socially demanding tasks comprising three experimental conditions with a group of individuals with CdLS ($n = 25$; % male = 44; mean age = 22.16; $SD = 8.81$) and a comparable group of individuals with Down syndrome (DS; $n = 20$; % male = 35; mean age = 24.35; $SD = 5.97$). Behaviours indicative of social anxiety were coded. The Behavior Rating Inventory of Executive Function-Preschool version, an informant measure of executive function, was completed by participants' caregivers.

Results: Significantly less verbalisation was observed in the CdLS group than the DS group in conditions requiring the initiation of speech. In the CdLS group, impairments in verbalisation were not associated with a greater degree of intellectual disability but were significantly correlated with impairments in both planning and working memory. This association was not evident in the DS group.

Conclusions: Adolescents and adults with CdLS have a specific difficulty with the initiation of speech when social demands are placed upon them. This impairment in verbalisation may be underpinned by specific cognitive deficits, although further research is needed to investigate this fully.

Keywords: Executive function, Social anxiety, Cornelia de Lange syndrome, Down syndrome

Background

Research has revealed a spectrum of profiles of sociability across genetic syndromes that appears unrelated to degree of intellectual disability. This spectrum includes a heightened level of sociability evident in Angelman, Williams and Down syndromes (DS), and social anxiety in Fragile X (FXS) and Turner syndromes [1–4]. In this study, we aim to identify the nature of aspects of the social impairment of Cornelia de Lange syndrome (CdLS) and the association between social anxiety and executive function impairments.

CdLS affects approximately 1 in 40,000 live births [5] and is associated with intellectual disability as well as specific physical characteristics, including distinctive facial features and limb abnormalities. CdLS is primarily caused by a deletion in the NIPBL gene located on chromosome 5 [6–8] with fewer cases being caused by mutations on the SMC3 gene on chromosome 10 [9], the SMC1A gene [10], the RAD21 gene [11], and the HDAC8 gene [12]. CdLS is associated with mild to profound intellectual disability [13] and a discrepancy between expressive and receptive language skills [13–15].

To date, the social impairment in CdLS has been characterised by social communication difficulties, selective

* Correspondence: Hayley.crawford@coventry.ac.uk
[1]Cerebra Centre for Neurodevelopmental Disorders, School of Psychology, University of Birmingham, B15 2TT, Edgbaston, UK
[2]Faculty of Health and Life Sciences, Coventry University, Coventry CV1 5FB, UK
Full list of author information is available at the end of the article

mutism, social anxiety and extreme shyness [16–21]. Our recent research has indicated that individuals with CdLS display less sociability than those with Angelman syndrome, DS and Rubinstein-Taybi syndrome and similar sociability to those with FXS and autism spectrum disorder (ASD), two neurodevelopmental disorders similarly associated with social withdrawal and social anxiety [20]. Children with CdLS have also demonstrated lower levels of social motivation and enjoyment than those with Angelman and Cri du Chat syndromes [22].

Interestingly, both social anxiety and sociability reported in CdLS may be dependent on the demands of the social situation presented. Richards and colleagues [19] investigated the behavioural presentation of social anxiety in children with CdLS compared to children with Cri du Chat syndrome. Although no overall differences emerged on the frequency or duration of behaviours indicative of social anxiety, individuals with CdLS were significantly more likely to display social anxiety-related behaviors immediately before and after eye contact and speech. This suggests that the nature and\or level of social demand may play a role in the presentation of social anxiety in individuals with CdLS. In addition, fine-grained analysis conducted by Moss and colleagues [20] revealed that individuals with CdLS were reported to be more sociable than individuals with FXS and ASD during three out of four social situations with an unfamiliar adult. This research also indicated that individuals with CdLS and other genetic syndromes are significantly more sociable when interacting with a familiar versus unfamiliar adult [20]. The current study aims to further understanding of the social impairment in CdLS by investigating the effect of the familiarity of an interacting adult, and the nature of social demand, on social anxiety-related behaviour.

There is still no 'gold-standard' experimental measure of sociability. However, there has been a move towards the experimental assessment of social impairments in the intellectual disability research literature. This has been most notable in the FXS literature (e.g. [23, 24–26]). Several studies on FXS have employed experimental conditions to provide a more detailed picture of social anxiety and the behavioural responses to specific social situations. It has also allowed researchers to determine if there are specific social situations (antecedents) that evoke social anxiety-related behaviours. Some of this research has also investigated differences in social behaviour as a function of both the familiarity of the interacting adult [27] and the examiner's behaviour [28]. On the basis of this published research, it is clear that experimental methodology involving manipulations of social demand is an effective way to gain a detailed picture of social impairments in individuals who have an intellectual disability. However, careful consideration of the nature of the social tasks is important. One important consideration is the examination of the behaviour of the other person in the interaction which has not been evaluated in the FXS literature on social anxiety. Research in other genetic syndromes, such as DS and Angelman syndromes, has considered the importance of the inter-play between participant and adult behaviour [29–32]. For example, in a study of 13 children with Angelman syndrome, Horsler and colleagues [29] demonstrated that smiling, touch, eye contact and speech from adults were important factors in eliciting smiling and laughing in participants. The present study aims to explore this through behavioural observation of the interacting adult, as well as the participant.

In addition to documenting the phenomenology of social impairment in CdLS, it is also important to consider the cognitive processes that may be associated with the social impairments in this group. Existing literature on a number of neurodevelopmental disorders suggests that specific social impairments are associated with specific executive function processes. The literature on ASD, for example, has generated a wealth of information implicating 'theory of mind' deficits in underpinning socio-behavioural impairments characteristic of the disorder [33]. Interestingly, research has demonstrated that theory of mind deficits in FXS are likely to be accounted for by impairments in working memory [34]. More recent research has also identified that specific executive processes may be related to the social impairments reported in ASD. For example, a study examining the association between executive functioning and joint attention impairments in children with ASD found that ventromedial test performance was strongly associated with joint attention skills [35]. These studies demonstrate that social impairments may be subserved by impairments in executive functioning.

In the current study, the relationship between executive functioning and social impairments were examined in order to identify whether impairments in social interactions in CdLS may be associated with specific cognitive impairments. As no gold-standard assessment of social anxiety exists for this population, the study employed novel experimental conditions which manipulate systematically both the *nature of social demand* and the *familiarity of the other person in the interaction*, so these effects on participants' behaviour, including expressive language, can be examined. The behaviour of the other person in the interaction was also examined. A similar approach has been employed in younger children with CdLS before, highlighting the success of this methodological approach in this population [22]. As DS is associated with a well-delineated phenotype [4, 36, 37], the current study employed a contrast group of individuals with DS to control for the effect of degree of disability and expressive language difficulties. Importantly, chronological age is likely to be an important factor in social impairment. Existing literature indicates an increase in social anxiety and a reduction in sociability with chronological age, with these social impairments being particularly prominent in late adolescence and early adulthood. Therefore, the current study assessed social impairment in adolescents and adults [17, 20].

To summarise, the aims of the current study were to:

1. Investigate whether the familiarity of the interacting adult (hereinafter referred to as examiner) and the nature of social demand impacts differentially on behaviour indicative of social anxiety in adolescents and adults with CdLS and a matched group of participants with DS. It was hypothesised that the CdLS participant group would show more behaviours indicative of social anxiety than the DS group, and that these behaviours would be more prominent in conditions involving an unfamiliar examiner and in conditions with communication demands.

2. Investigate the association between social anxiety and executive function in participants with CdLS, compared to participants with DS. It was hypothesised that compromised executive function would be correlated with social anxiety. Whether or not this would be syndrome-specific was not possible to predict due to limited literature.

Methods
Participants
Twenty-five participants with CdLS (11 males and 14 females) aged between 13 and 42 years (mean age = 22.16; SD = 8.81) and 20 participants with DS (7 males and 13 females) aged between 15 and 33 years (mean age = 24.35; SD = 5.97) took part in this study. Individuals with CdLS were recruited both directly through a research database held at the Cerebra Centre for Neurodevelopmental Disorders, University of Birmingham and indirectly through the CdLS Foundation (UK and Ireland), the parent support group. Participants with DS were recruited through the Cerebra Centre participant database.

The inclusion criteria were as follows: a diagnosis of the relevant syndrome from an appropriate professional, aged 12 years or over, able to speak more than 30 words, mobile, and a self-help score on the Wessex Scale [38] of seven or more (maximum score is 9), indicating that they were able or at the upper end of partly able in terms of self-help skills, or had a receptive vocabulary age equivalent score on the Vineland Adaptive Behavior Scale [VABS; 39] of 40 months or more. Individuals with CdLS who had speech but only used it in certain situations (selective mutism) were still eligible for the study.

A comparison of the group demographics and key characteristics demonstrated that the two groups did not differ significantly in terms of age, gender, receptive language and adaptive behaviour (see Table 1).

Measures
Parents/primary caregivers of participants completed the following measures:

Demographic questionnaire
A demographic questionnaire was used to obtain information regarding participants' age, gender and diagnostic status (whether a diagnosis had been made and by whom).

The Vineland Adaptive Behavior Scale [39]
This semi-structured interview was administered to participant's parents in order to obtain information regarding participants' adaptive behaviour skills. There are four domains: Communication, Daily Living Skills, Socialisation, and Motor Skills. Each domain is divided into three further subdomains. An overall Adaptive Behavior Composite may also be derived. Internal consistency ranges from .83–.94 across the domains and .69–.89 across the subdomains.

Behavior Rating Inventory of Executive Function-Preschool Version (BRIEF-P; [40])
The BRIEF-P is an informant-based questionnaire used to examine potential deficits in several areas of executive function. The questionnaire consists of 63 items. For each item, the informant rates whether a specific behaviour has been a problem for their child over the previous 6 months using a 3-point Likert scale (never, sometimes, always). The BRIEF-P is made up of five domains: Inhibit, Shift, Emotional Control, Working Memory, Plan/Organise. Higher scores on the BRIEF-P are suggestive of greater perceived deficits. The psychometric properties of the BRIEF-P appear robust. Studies have demonstrated that the measure captures profiles of executive functioning that differ across various disorders, including attention-deficit hyperactivity disorder and ASD [41]. Although the BRIEF-P was designed for individuals who are younger than the participants in the current study, it was deemed a more appropriate measure than the BRIEF (5–18 years) based on the suitability of the items for the participant's level of intellectual disability. An informant measure of executive function was used in the current study, rather than a performance-based measure. Informant-based measures have been described to tap into how participants interpret and react to a situation without being directed to perform a specific task or being taught a rule [42]. This suggests that informant measures, such as the BRIEF-P, capture participant's everyday executive

Table 1 A comparison of demographic information and key characteristics between the Cornelia de Lange and Down syndrome groups. Comparison between participants on: Chronological age, gender, receptive language ability as measured by the British Picture Vocabulary Scale, and adaptive behaviour as measured by the Vineland Adaptive Behavior Scale. Data from the BRIEF-P are also presented here

	CdLS (n = 25)	DS (n = 20)	p
Age (years)			
Mean (SD)	22.16 (8.81)	24.35 (5.97)	.35
Range	13–42	15–33	
Gender			
% Male	44	35	.54
Receptive Language (British Picture Vocabulary Scale)			
Raw score mean (SD)	67.12 (19.96)	69.25 (22.30)	.74
Age equivalence in years mean (SD)	6.16 (2.12)	6.45 (2.68)	.69
Adaptive behaviour (VABS)			
Communication standard score mean (SD)	50.44 (17.58)	50.80 (24.01)	.96
Daily living skills standard score mean (SD)	56.56 (14.18)	57.20 (10.36)	.88
Socialisation domain standard score mean (SD)	57.52 (18.00)	53.40 (25.61)	.59
Adaptive Behavior Composite standard score mean (SD)	54.64 (16.58)	51.33 (18.68)	.56
Executive Function (BRIEF-P)			
Inhibit subscale mean (SD)	26.57 (5.70)	24.37 (4.87)	.192
Shift subscale mean (SD)	19.70 (4.00)	17.11 (4.25)	.049
Emotional control subscale mean (SD)	18.07 (4.47)	15.42 (4.00)	.053
Working memory subscale mean (SD)	29.91 (6.75)	27.44 (6.12)	.234
Plan/organise subscale mean (SD)	17.30 (3.38)	16.16 (3.42)	.283

function skills, as opposed to best possible performance on a task, which was deemed important for the current study.

The British Picture Vocabulary Scale—second edition (BPVS-II; [43])

The BPVS-II was used to assess receptive vocabulary. The assessment comprises 168 items. The administration of the test allows basal and ceiling levels to be established without needing to administer the entire test. For each item, the participant is required to select one of four pictures from a stimulus booklet that most accurately represents the meaning of the word spoken by the examiner. The test has been standardised on typically developing individuals and it has been reported to be psychometrically robust with good validity and reliability.

Social Tasks

The Social Tasks were designed to assess whether behaviours indicative of social anxiety are evoked by various social situations. The Social Tasks comprised one control condition and three experimental conditions. The experimental conditions are designed to place increasing

social demands upon the participant. The experimental conditions are *Voluntary Social Interaction, Required Social Interaction* and *Performance*. They were administered as follows:

1. The control condition is a modified version of the 'Break' condition from modules three and four of the Autism Diagnostic Observation Schedule (ADOS; [44]). During this condition, the participant and examiner are sat at a table. The participant is given some items (paper and pens, newspaper, magazine and some puzzles) to engage with, whilst the examiner either does some work or reads a magazine. The examiner is still in close proximity to the participant during this condition to control for the presence of the examiner in the experimental conditions. The control condition lasts for approximately 4 min.

2. The Voluntary Social Interaction condition involves the examiner showing the participant a series of 20 holiday photographs and making pre-determined comments about every other photograph. Here, the participant is provided with the opportunity to make a comment about the photographs or respond

to a comment made by the examiner, but there is no explicit expectation for them to do so. This condition is not timed and finishes after the last photograph has been shown to the participant.

3. The Required Social Interaction condition involves a conversation between the examiner and participant, whereby the examiner asks the participant a series of questions and the participant *is* explicitly expected to respond to them. The conversation also provides the participant with the opportunity to initiate conversation with the examiner by asking the examiner questions. The examiner predominantly leads this condition because they ask the participant questions in order to maintain the conversation. The Required Social Interaction condition lasts for approximately 4 min.

4. The Performance condition is a modified version of the 'Cartoons' condition from the ADOS [44] and utilises both sets of cartoons from the ADOS. The examiner tells the participant the story in one of the cartoons and then asks the participant to stand up and tell them the story back. This procedure is then repeated for a second cartoon. The participants are expected to stand up and re-tell or 'perform' a story on their own without guidance. Only if the participant shows difficulty with retelling the story does the examiner prompt. This condition is not timed and finishes after the participant has presented both cartoons.

A familiar examiner and an unfamiliar examiner carried out the four conditions separately, in order to identify whether there was an effect of familiarity on the Social Tasks. The familiar examiner was someone the participant sees at least three times a week, e.g. their main caregiver, their teacher, their support worker, etc. The unfamiliar examiner was a trained confederate involved in the project who had never met the participant. The order of conditions and whether the familiar examiner or unfamiliar examiner administered the conditions first were counterbalanced.

Real-time coding of social tasks

The literature on observational indicators of social anxiety in both typically developing children and individuals with intellectual disabilities was examined to identify indicators of social anxiety [23–25, 27, 45–51]. Behaviours previously identified in existing literature as indicators of social anxiety were coded during each condition of the Social Tasks. Several examiner behaviours are also coded during the conditions and used in the analysis to provide a more detailed picture of the nature of the interaction between the examiner and the participant. All behaviours are operationally defined. Table 2

shows all the behaviours that were included in the analysis. Behaviours were coded using Obswin 3.2 [52]. The Voluntary Social Interaction and Performance conditions were coded for the full length of time that they had been recorded for because these conditions were dependent on other factors, i.e. the Voluntary Social Interaction condition finished once all 20 photographs had been shown to the participant and the Performance condition finished once the participant had explained the story in both cartoons. The first 4 min of the control condition and the Required Social Interaction condition were coded so that the duration of these conditions were matched across the groups. Some behaviours were coded as durations (i.e. behaviours with an onset and an offset) and some were coded as events (i.e. behaviours of such short duration that only their occurrence is recorded). Table 2 shows whether behaviours were coded as events or durations.

The following three variables were coded in addition to the participant and examiner outcome behaviours: examiner off camera, participant off camera and participant's hands off camera. These variables affected whether several outcome variables could be coded during a condition, e.g. if the participant was off camera, then 'participant looks at examiner' could not be coded. For the purpose of calculating more accurate durations and frequencies of outcome behaviours, if any of these three variables occurred for 10% or more of the time in a condition then the outcome behaviours affected by these variables were recalculated to only take into account the time when these behaviours could be coded, e.g. if a participant's hands were off the camera for 15% of time during a condition, then 'participant fidgets' was only coded during the 85% of time during which the participant's hands could be seen.

Inter-rater reliability was conducted on all behaviours coded in the Social Tasks for 26.67% of participants (25% of Down syndrome participants and 28% of CdLS participants). Agreement between two independent raters was calculated using Cohen's Kappa co-efficient based on 5-s interval-by-interval basis. The mean level of agreement across the participant behaviours was .64 (range .48 to .82). The mean level of agreement across the examiner behaviours was .59 (range .44 to .85). This reliability was considered to be moderate—very good [53].

Procedure

All participants were visited at their home. The first assessment to be conducted on all research visits was the Social Tasks so that the researcher acting as the unfamiliar examiner would have had minimal contact with the participant. The Social Tasks were always conducted in a room with a table and only the participant and familiar or

Table 2 Operationalised definitions of behaviours coded as control variables; and participant and examiner behaviours used in the analysis

Behaviour	Operationalised definitions
Participant verbalisation	
Participant verbalisation (duration)	The participant's speech; These may be utterances (e.g. 'erm'), words, phrases or sentences. The person may use speech for the purpose of communication with someone else, e.g. asking a question, making a comment, answering a question or the speech may be used when the person is talking to himself or herself. The participant's speech may be intelligible or unintelligible.
Participant question (event)	The participant asks the examiner a question. For example, 'Did you drive here?'
Participant offers information (event)	The participant spontaneously (not in response to a question) offers information. The information may or may not be about them. For example, 'I went to the beach on holiday' or 'the cartoon is funny'.
Participant verbal response (event)	The participant responds verbally to a question, statement, comment, prompt or request made by the examiner by providing information. N.b. this code also includes the participant's description of the cartoons in the Cartoon condition.
Participant non-verbal behaviour	
Participant positive facial expression (duration)	The participant demonstrates a positive facial expression, for example, laughing or smiling. Facial expression must clearly indicate expression of pleasure in activity or conversation. Facial expression may or may not be directed towards the examiner.
Participant looks at examiner (duration)	The participant looks in the direction of the examiner's eyes or face.
Participant nod/shake (event)	The participant responds to a question, statement, comment or prompt made by the examiner, by nodding their head to indicate 'yes' or shaking their head to indicate 'no'. This *does not* include use of Makaton or British Sign Language.
Participant descriptive gestures (duration)	The participant uses movements of their arms or hands to help them describe something.
Participant fidget (duration)	The participant displays restless, repetitive, non-rhythmic, non-functional motor movements, such as, moving their hands, touching their face or hair or moving an object, or wriggling in their seat. This code *does not* include stereotyped behaviours, which are *rhythmic*, unusual seemingly purposeless movements of their body or objects (based on Lesniak-Karpiak, Mazzocco & Ross, 2003 [23]).
Examiner verbalisation	
Examiner verbalisation (duration)	The examiner's speech; These may be utterances (e.g. 'erm'), words, phrases or sentences. The person may use speech for the purpose of communication with someone else, e.g. asking a question, making a comment, answering a question or the speech may be used when the person is talking to himself or herself. The examiner's speech may be intelligible or unintelligible.
Examiner question (event)	The examiner asks the participant a question, which requires a response from the participant. For example' What books do you like?'
Examiner prompt (event)	The examiner prompts the participant to respond by repeating or slightly paraphrasing the original question, request, comment or piece of information.
Examiner verbal response (event)	The examiner responds to the participant's verbal question, comment, statement or offering of information using verbal communication to give the appropriate information.
Examiner Offers information (event)	The examiner spontaneously (not in response to a question) offers information. The information may or may not be about themselves. For example 'I came from Birmingham'. N.b. this code also includes the examiner's description of the cartoons in the Cartoon condition.
Behaviours coded as control variables	
Participant engage with task (duration)	The participant looks at and/or touches an object allocated for a condition. This may be reading a magazine / newspaper, colouring with felt tips, listening to the radio in the 'Break' condition; looking at or touching the photographs in the 'Photograph' condition; looking at or touching the cartoon in the 'Cartoon' condition. Objects that have not been incorporated as part of the social presses *should not* be coded, e.g. if the person is drinking from a cup or mug, which is on the table. This code *does not* apply to the 'Conversation' condition because no objects are required for this condition.
Examiner looks at participant (duration)	The examiner is looking in the direction of the participant's eyes or face.

unfamiliar examiner were present. The Social Task conditions were counterbalanced so that there were no order effects across the groups.

After the Social Tasks were completed, the BPVS-II [43] was administered. The VABS-II [39] was administered to either the participant's main caregiver or key worker at a convenient time for them, during the research visit day. After the research visits had taken place, footage from the Social Tasks was coded.

Data analysis

A preliminary analysis was conducted to ensure that the Social Tasks were administered uniformly across groups. The duration of the condition, the duration of the participant engaging in the task and the duration of the examiner looking at the participant were examined. See Table 3 for differences on these variables. The majority of differences were not significant ($p < .05$). The differences that were significant were marginal differences which could not be controlled for given the need to keep the conditions as representative of naturalistic social situations as possible. These analyses show that any significant differences identified between the groups in any of the behavioural outcome variables are not due to differences in the administration of the Social Tasks.

The data for almost all the outcome variables were not normally distributed across all conditions (Kolmogrov-Smirnov test; $p < .05$) and consequently non-parametric tests were employed throughout the analysis. The analyses examined the effect of group (CdLS, DS), nature of demand (Voluntary Social Interaction, Required Social Interaction, Performance) and familiarity (unfamiliar examiner, familiar examiner) on the outcome variables. Participant outcome variables included verbal behaviours (verbalisation, question-asking, offering of information, and responses) and non-verbal behaviours (positive facial expression, looking to the examiner, nodding/shaking head, gestures, and fidgeting). Examiner outcome variables included verbal behaviour (verbalisation, question-asking, prompting, responses, and offering of information). See Table 2 for operationalised definitions of each outcome variable.

Results

Preliminary analysis: comparison between the control condition and experimental conditions

An analysis was conducted initially for each group to ensure that participant outcome variables examined in the experimental conditions were evoked by social demands. Consequently, pairwise Wilcoxon rank sum tests were conducted separately for each group to compare each participant outcome variable between the control condition and each of the experimental conditions.[1] All but one[2] of the analyses were significant with all the outcome variables being observed for significantly longer in the experimental conditions than the control condition, demonstrating that the outcome variables being examined in the current study were evoked by the social demands of the experimental conditions.

Comparison of outcome variables on social tasks
Participant behaviour

Figure 1 shows median duration/frequency of the participant outcome variables for both the CdLS and DS groups. A more conservative alpha level ($p < .005$) was employed for this set of analyses.

The analysis revealed a two-way interaction between group and nature of demand for participant verbalisation. The CdLS group showed significantly less verbalisation than the DS group in both the familiar and unfamiliar Voluntary Social Interaction conditions ($U = 108$, $p < .005$; $U = 65$, $p < .001$) and both the

Table 3 Differences between the Cornelia de Lange syndrome and Down syndrome groups on control variables

Behaviour	Condition	CdLS median (IQR)	DS median (IQR)	U	Z	p
Duration of condition	Familiar voluntary social interaction	341 (361.50)	355 (200.00)	236.5	−.02	.98
	Unfamiliar voluntary social interaction	225 (105.50)	228.5 (84.25)	217	−.75	.45
	Familiar required social interaction	240 (.50)	240 (6.00)	218	−.59	.56
	Unfamiliar required social interaction	240 (.00)	240 (0.00)	236	−.74	.46
	Familiar performance	151 (161.00)	109 (121.00)	173	−1.53	.13
	Unfamiliar performance	142 (112.00)	125 (62.00)	150.5	−2.06	<.05
Participant engage in task	Familiar voluntary social interaction	89.67 (25.44)	97.97 (5.23)	89	−3.52	<.001
	Unfamiliar voluntary social interaction	96.15 (19.95)	96.63 (5.68)	180.5	−1.59	.11
	Familiar required social interaction	N/A				
	Unfamiliar required social interaction	N/A				
	Familiar performance	87.5 (17.39)	97.16 (11.33)	145.5	−2.18	<.05
	Unfamiliar performance	92.91 (27.41)	95.49 (4.72)	192.5	−1.07	.29
Examiner looks at participant	Familiar voluntary social interaction	27.05 (19.77)	22.04 (13.44)	186	−1.22	.22
	Unfamiliar voluntary social interaction	21.36 (28.20)	37.27 (18.17)	134	−2.65	<.01
	Familiar required social interaction	94.58 (18.34)	97.5 (14.59)	181	−1.34	.18
	Unfamiliar required social interaction	95.83 (10.63)	94.79 (7.40)	248.5	−.03	.97
	Familiar performance	0 (5.80)	0 (28.30)	233	−.14	.89
	Unfamiliar performance	0 (43.44)	0 (0.00)	149	−2.48	<.05

N/A not applicable

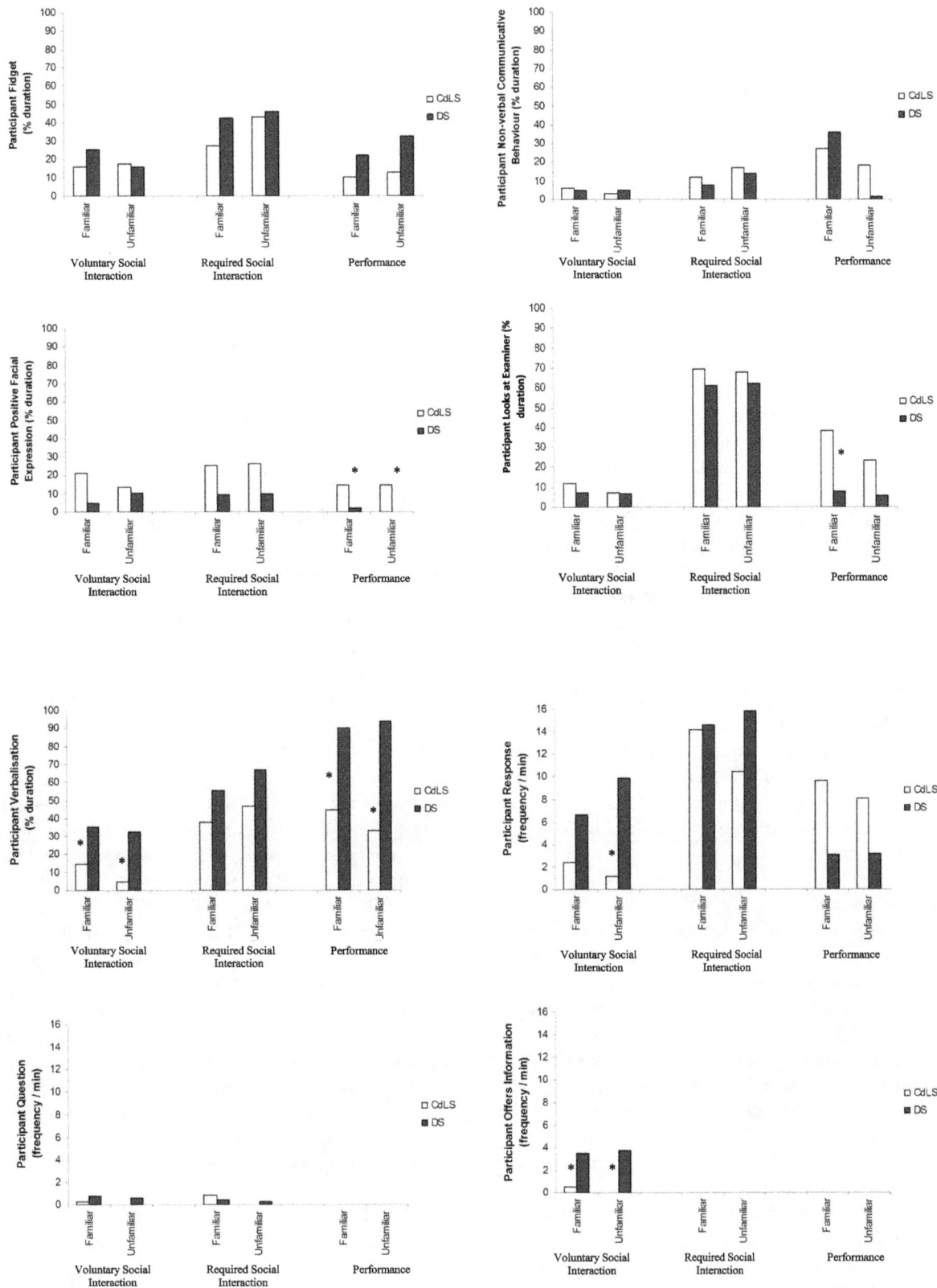

Fig. 1 Participant outcome variables for the Down syndrome and Cornelia de Lange syndrome groups; *asterisk* indicates significant between-groups difference (*p* < .005)

familiar and unfamiliar Performance conditions ($U = 77.5$, $p < .001$; $U = 109$, $p < .005$). The difference in verbalisation between the groups in the unfamiliar Required Social Interaction condition approached significance ($p = .006$).

An analysis of the type of participant verbalisation shown in the Voluntary Social Interaction and Performance conditions revealed that there was a significant difference between the groups in the type of verbalisation shown in the Voluntary Social Interaction condition only. The DS group demonstrated significantly more offering of information than the CdLS group in both the familiar and unfamiliar Voluntary Social Interaction conditions ($U = 62$, $p < .001$; $U = 46$, $p < .001$) and also responded significantly more often than the CdLS group in the unfamiliar Voluntary Social Interaction condition ($U = 73$, $p < .001$). The analyses also revealed a main effect of familiarity for participant verbalisation in the Required Social Interaction condition for the DS group. Interestingly, the DS group actually showed significantly more verbalisation in the unfamiliar Required Social Interaction condition than in the familiar Required Social Interaction condition ($z = -3.14$, $p < .005$).

Surprisingly, the analysis also showed significantly more positive facial expression by the CdLS group in comparison to the DS group in the familiar and unfamiliar Performance conditions ($U = 113$, $p < .005$; $U = 75$, $p < .001$). The analysis also revealed that the CdLS group looked at the examiner for a significantly longer duration than the DS group in the familiar Performance condition ($U = 99$, $p = .001$). Finally, the analysis demonstrated that there was no significant difference in fidgeting or non-verbal communicative behaviour between the two groups, in any condition.

Examiner behaviour

Figure 2 shows the median duration/ frequency of the examiner outcome variables for both the CdLS and DS groups. An analysis of examiner verbalisation revealed a two-way interaction between group and nature of demand as significant differences were found between the two groups in the Voluntary Social Interaction condition and the Performance condition, but not in the Required Social Interaction condition. Significantly more verbalisation was shown by the familiar and unfamiliar examiners when interacting with the CdLS group in the Performance condition when compared to the DS group ($U = 23$, $p < .001$; $U = 43$, $p < .001$). In the Voluntary Social Interaction conditions, significantly more verbalisation was also shown by the familiar examiners with the CdLS group in comparison to the DS group ($U = 112$, $p < .005$). The unfamiliar examiners, however, showed significantly more verbalisation with the DS participants than the CdLS participants in this condition ($U = 119$, $p < .005$).

An analysis of the type of examiner verbalisation shown in the Voluntary Social Interaction and Performance conditions revealed that familiar and unfamiliar examiners used significantly more prompts ($U = 70$, $p < .001$; $U = 85.5$, $p < .001$) and responses ($U = 32$, $p < .001$; $U = 67$, $p < .001$) with the CdLS group than the DS group in the Performance condition. In the Voluntary Social Interaction conditions, the familiar examiners gave significantly more prompts ($U = 107.5$, $p < .005$) and offering of information ($U = 100$, $p < .005$) to the CdLS group than the DS group, whilst the unfamiliar examiners gave significantly more questions ($U = 106$, $p < .005$) and responses ($U = 97$, $p < .001$) to the DS group than the CdLS group.

Association between social impairments and cognitive functioning in Cornelia de Lange syndrome

As the current study has identified a specific impairment in verbalisation for the CdLS group, this was correlated with a measure of executive functioning. For the purpose of this analysis, the mean duration of participant verbalisation across the familiar and unfamiliar Performance conditions was used for examining the relationship between verbalisation and executive functioning because this condition placed the highest social (and thus cognitive) demands on participants. In addition, mean participant verbalisation across the Performance conditions was correlated with age, receptive and expressive language and adaptive behaviour in order to examine whether these broader developmental variables were also related to verbalisation in either group. A series of Spearman's correlations were conducted for this analysis. Table 4 shows the results for these correlations.

The analysis revealed that only receptive language (measured by the BPVS) was significantly, positively correlated with verbalisation in the CdLS group. In the DS group, both language and adaptive behaviour were significantly correlated with verbalisation. The pattern of correlations observed for the DS group was expected given that as verbalisation increases, adaptive behaviour would also be expected to increase. The dissociation of the relationship between verbalisation and adaptive behaviour in the CdLS group suggested that these individuals may have a specific cognitive impairment that is related to language and was independent of global development of adaptive behaviour.

Table 5 shows the correlations between mean verbalisation and the BRIEF-P subscales for the CdLS and DS groups. A series of Spearman's correlations[3] between mean verbalisation across the Performance conditions and subscale scores on the BRIEF-P revealed that there were significant associations between the duration of verbalisation and working memory, and the duration of verbalisation and planning in the CdLS group but these

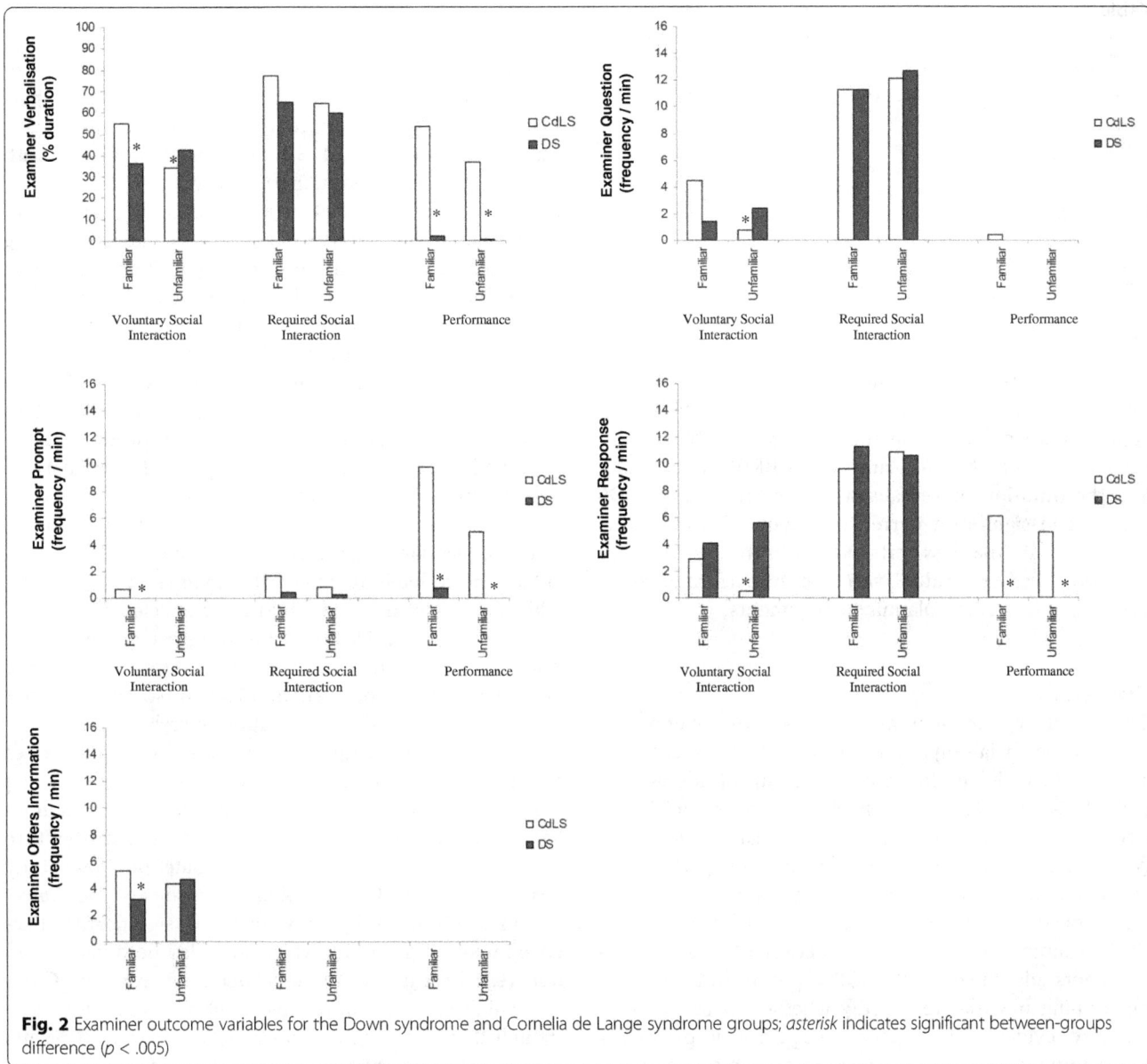

Fig. 2 Examiner outcome variables for the Down syndrome and Cornelia de Lange syndrome groups; *asterisk* indicates significant between-groups difference ($p < .005$)

Table 4 Correlations between mean participant verbalisation across the Performance conditions and age, receptive and expressive language and adaptive behaviour for the Cornelia de Lange syndrome and Down syndrome groups

	CdLS mean participant verbalisation	DS mean participant verbalisation
Chronological age (years)	.30	.16
BPVS raw score	.53**	.81**
VABS communication domain standard score	−.16	.76**
VABS daily living skills domain standard score	.30	.75**
VABS socialisation domain standard score	.27	.59*

*$p < .05$
**$p < .01$

Table 5 Correlations between mean participant verbalisation across the Performance conditions and BRIEF-P subscales for both the Cornelia de Lange syndrome and Down syndrome groups

BRIEF-P subscale	CdLS mean participant verbalisation	DS mean participant verbalisation
Inhibit	.41	−.24
Shift	−.26	.07
Emotional control	−.31	−.12
Working memory	−.57**	.10
Plan/organise	−.62**	−.07

*$p < .05$
**$p < .01$

associations were not evident in the DS group. The correlation between the Inhibit subscale and verbalisation approached significance in the CdLS group. No significant correlations between any of the BRIEF-P subscales and the duration of verbalisation was found in the DS group. The significant correlations found for the CdLS group indicate that less verbalisation in the Performance condition was associated with poorer performance on working memory and planning assessments.

Discussion

This novel experimental study assessed the phenomenology of the social impairment in verbal adolescents and adults with CdLS in contrast to a group of adolescents and adults with DS. This is the first study on social anxiety in CdLS to employ a robust factorial, experimental design, placing different social demands on participants whilst varying familiarity, in order to examine which factors evoked behaviours indicative of social anxiety. The study examined the relationship between any social impairments identified in the CdLS group and cognitive functioning in order to identify whether there was preliminary evidence for specific cognitive impairments underpinning specific social impairments in this group.

The most striking difference identified between the two groups was in the duration of participant verbalisation. The CdLS group showed significantly less verbalisation than the DS group in the familiar and unfamiliar Voluntary Social Interaction and Performance conditions, whilst no significant group difference was observed in the Required Social Interaction condition where there was an explicit expectation to verbalise. It appears that there are specific social demands in the Voluntary Social Interaction and Performance conditions which reduce verbalisation in the CdLS group. The two conditions which showed group differences in verbalisation rely more heavily on participants being able to initiate speech, so it may be that this is a particular difficulty for the CdLS group. For example, verbalisation in the Voluntary Social Interaction condition relies on

participants being able to initiate speech to comment (offering information) on photographs or respond to a comment made by the examiner on a photograph (response), and there is no explicit expectation for the participant to do this. Taken together, these findings suggest that individuals with CdLS have a specific difficulty with the initiation of speech, particularly when the expectation to do so is implicit, which results in a marked reduction in verbalisation when social demands involving the initiation of speech are placed upon individuals with CdLS. Interestingly, participants with CdLS also looked at the examiner for longer than the DS group, indicating that participants with CdLS are not demonstrating complete social withdrawal, but rather the lack of social motivation is specific to verbalisation. It is unlikely that these differences in verbalisation were a product of expressive language deficits in the CdLS as the two participant groups did not differ on the Expressive Language Subdomain of the VABS. Although not a direct measure of expressive language, this measure, completed by parents, is more likely to reflect the abilities of participants with CdLS due to the elevated rates of selective mutism in this population. However, future research should examine this further to disentangle the effects of expressive language abilities on verbalisation in social situations which differ in terms of expectation of verbalisation.

This is the first empirical evidence showing a reduction in speech, in adolescents and adults with CdLS that may be due to a specific difficulty in the initiation of speech. These findings contribute to the sparse literature on social impairments in CdLS. To date, only one study has been published on the phenomenology of social anxiety in CdLS and this study found no significant difference in communication, which included both verbal and non-verbal communication, between children with CdLS and children in a comparable contrast group [19]. Although these findings do appear to contrast with results reported in the current study, where we report significantly less verbalisation in individuals with CdLS compared to those with DS, these differences were particularly prominent in the Voluntary Social Interaction and Performance conditions. Interestingly, Richards and colleagues [19] reported that individuals with CdLS were significantly more likely to display social-anxiety related behaviours immediately before and after eye contact and speech, suggesting that social anxiety is heightened in CdLS, particularly at the point of speech initiation. The consistency of findings indicating that social anxiety in CdLS is mediated by the type of social situation is particularly interesting given the different ages of participants across samples. Specifically, the mean age of participants in the current study was 22 years, whereas the mean age of participants in Richards et al. [19] was 11 years. Socio-behavioural characteristics have been reported to change with age in CdLS, such that social anxiety increases and sociability decreases during early adulthood [17, 20].

The findings in the current study therefore indicate that specific social demands reduce verbalisation in individuals with CdLS, with the familiarity of the other person being relatively unimportant. However, more in-depth analysis regarding the type of verbalisation revealed some empirical evidence for the effect of familiarity in the Voluntary Social Interaction condition. Specifically, the CdLS group responded significantly less to comments made by the unfamiliar examiner than the DS group, yet no significant difference was found between the groups in responding to the familiar examiner in this condition. This suggests that the presence of an unfamiliar examiner caused a significant reduction in responses by the CdLS group, providing support for the effect of familiarity on social interactions in CdLS. These results support previous literature indicating that the familiarity of the other person in the interaction does affect sociability in adolescents and adults with CdLS [17, 20, 54].

Interestingly, no significant differences were found between the groups on some additional indicators of social anxiety such as fidgeting and non-verbal behaviour. In addition, the CdLS group actually showed significantly more positive facial expression with the familiar and unfamiliar examiners in the Performance condition and looked significantly longer at the familiar examiner in the Performance condition than the DS group. These are unexpected findings given that a longer duration of positive facial expression and a longer duration of looking in the direction of the examiner would not be expected if social anxiety was evident in the CdLS group. This supports the notion that the lack of social motivation or engagement in individuals with CdLS is specific to verbalisation and is not reflective of more global social withdrawal. It is likely that a specific communication problem affecting the initiation of speech makes it appear that individuals with CdLS show anxiety in social situations. Although this is possible, the reported effect of the presence of unfamiliar people on levels of sociability in the literature for individuals with CdLS would suggest that there is some anxiety-related difficulty in this group. Therefore, it may be that there is a communication problem which is enhanced by anxiety caused by the presence of unfamiliar people. A positive facial expression and looking in the direction of the examiner may then serve to compensate for the lack of verbalisation in demanding conditions or act as a coping strategy, prompting the examiner to speak on their behalf. This is supported by the fact that these behaviours were shown in the Performance condition where the most difficulties in verbalisation were evident.

Group differences were found in the duration of examiner verbalisation in the Voluntary Social Interaction and Performance conditions. Familiar and unfamiliar examiners showed significantly more verbalisation in the Performance condition with significantly more prompts and responses being used for the CdLS participants compared to the DS participants. It appears that the examiners tried to help the CdLS participants, although, this increase in verbalisation by examiners may have further increased the demands on the CdLS participants. The familiar examiners in the Voluntary Social Interaction condition also demonstrated this pattern of behaviour as familiar examiners used significantly more comments and prompts with the CdLS group. Interestingly, the Voluntary Social Interaction condition does not involve examiners prompting participants because there is no explicit expectation for participants to verbalise. Perhaps this indicates that the familiar examiners will try to prompt individuals with CdLS to verbalise whenever they can to encourage individuals to verbalise. This research indicates that further exploration of the extent to which participant social behaviour is governed by examiner behaviour is warranted.

There is currently no study of CdLS that examines how participant and examiner behaviour affect one another in social interactions. Therefore, this is the first study to contribute to the literature in this way. Further research examining the inter-play between participant and examiner behaviours would be useful to determine how these may affect one another. Research in other genetic syndromes has already demonstrated the inter-play between participant and adult behaviour. For example, increased laughing and smiling by individuals with Angelman syndrome is evoked by increased social interactions with adults and increased social contact from adults [1]. This type of research is important in CdLS because it may also help when devising intervention strategies, e.g. asking adults not to prompt the person if it increases further demands on them.

In addition to describing the social impairment in CdLS, the current study also examined whether social impairments observed in the CdLS group were related to specific cognitive impairments. The results indicated that reduction of verbalisations in the CdLS group was associated with impairments in both planning and working memory. This was further supported by the fact that this relationship was not evident in the DS group and the fact that verbalisation was not related to adaptive behaviour in the CdLS group. It cannot be assumed that the relationship between verbalisation and cognitive impairments is causal from the correlational analysis and the use of an informant-based measure of executive functioning. However, the fact that a significant association between these domains was present in the CdLS group, but not in the DS group, suggests that further investigations examining the relationship between planning, working memory and verbalisation in CdLS are needed to understand whether deficits in working memory and planning underpin the difficulties observed in verbalisation in this group. Interestingly, whilst the relationship between inhibition and verbalisation approached significance, verbalisation was not related to the inhibition and attention switching in the same way. One interpretation of these findings concerns the reliance on working memory and planning resources in a social exchange with regard to holding conversational information in mind, and planning a response. Inhibition may similarly be required to restrict prepotent verbal responses; however, attention shifting and emotional control may not be relied upon to the same extent for the verbalisation aspect of a social exchange.

There were several limitations to the current study that may affect the interpretation of the findings. Only behavioural indicators of social anxiety were employed in the current study which meant that it was difficult to fully determine whether a reduction in verbalisation in the CdLS group was due to or affected by anxiety caused by the presence of unfamiliar people. Physiological measures have been used in combination with behavioural indicators of social anxiety in the FXS literature [24, 25] to provide a more accurate picture about whether the behaviours shown in this group are anxiety-related. Any future research on social anxiety in CdLS should try to incorporate physiological measures as well as behavioural indicators. Furthermore, although preliminary analyses indicate differences in social behaviour between the control condition and experimental conditions, which points to the integrity of the Social Tasks, validation of the measure in a typically developing population would further demonstrate that the conditions differed in social pressure. An additional limitation to the present study is the lack of information available about any anti-anxiety medication that participants may have been taking at the time of data collection. Another drawback is that the levels of social anxiety in adolescents and adults with CdLS may be under-reported. Two individuals with CdLS were recruited for the current study but withdrew before the research visits because parents reported that both individuals were experiencing significant anxiety about being visited by an unfamiliar person. The fact that these and other individuals with CdLS may not have taken part in the current study due to anxiety about being visited by an unfamiliar person indicates that the effect of unfamiliar people on levels of anxiety may be under-reported in this study.

Conclusions

Despite the limitations, this study has still provided several important findings that contribute to the literature on social impairments in CdLS. The results suggest that adolescents and adults with CdLS have a specific difficulty with the initiation of speech that leads to a reduction in verbalisation when social demands involving the initiation of speech are placed upon individuals. Although, the evidence was not conclusive in the current study, adolescents and adults with CdLS seem to show increased anxiety in the presence of unfamiliar people which causes a further reduction in speech. The results from the current study also indicate that there is a syndrome-environment interaction between verbalisation in adolescents and adults with CdLS and verbalisation in examiners interacting with them. It seems that a reduction in verbalisation in adolescents and adults with CdLS is related to increased verbalisation in examiners interacting with them. It may be that this increased examiner verbalisation causes further demands on verbalisation in people with CdLS and increases the cognitive and social demand. The study also provided some preliminary evidence for a relationship between verbalisation, working memory and planning in CdLS. Research is needed to examine the pathway from cognition to behaviour in CdLS in order to identify the cause of the verbal impairment identified in this study and use this to develop helpful prevention and intervention strategies. Furthermore, a clearer understanding of the association between anxiety and verbalisation in this group is needed to understand how these factors impact upon each other.

Endnotes

[1]A mean score was taken across the three experimental conditions.
[2]A significant difference was not found in positive facial expression ($p = .02$) for the DS group between the familiar control condition and the mean of the experimental conditions. This was due to the low level of positive facial expression shown by the group in the experimental conditions.
[3]Pearson's Partial correlations between mean participant verbalisation and the BRIEF-P subscales, whilst controlling for BPVS scores in the CdLS group and BPVS and VABS in the DS group, showed the same findings as the Pearson's correlations.

Abbreviations
ADOS: Autism Diagnostic Observation Schedule; ASD: Autism spectrum disorder; BPVS: British Picture Vocabulary Scale; BRI: Behavioural Regulation Index; BRIEF-P: Behaviour Rating Inventory of Executive Function-Preschool Version; CdLS: Cornelia de Lange syndrome; DS: Down syndrome; FXS: Fragile X syndrome; GEC: Global Executive Function Composite; MI: Metacognition Index; VABS: Vineland Adaptive Behavior Scale

Acknowledgements
The authors would like to thank all the participants and families who took part in this research, and the Cornelia de Lange Foundation for helping with the recruitment of participants.

Funding
This research was funded by Cornelia de Lange Syndrome Foundation, UK and Ireland and Cerebra.

Authors' contributions

LN was involved in the study design, data collection of the CdLS group, data analysis and initial drafting of the manuscript. HC revised the manuscript and drafted it for submission. DR was involved in data collection of the DS group. JM was involved in study design and editing the revised manuscript. CO was involved in study design, data analysis, data interpretation and editing of the revised manuscript. All authors read and approved the final manuscript.

Competing interests

The authors declare that they have no competing interests.

Author details

[1]Cerebra Centre for Neurodevelopmental Disorders, School of Psychology, University of Birmingham, B15 2TT, Edgbaston, UK. [2]Faculty of Health and Life Sciences, Coventry University, Coventry CV1 5FB, UK. [3]Institute of Cognitive Neuroscience, University College London, 17 Queen Square, London WC1N 3AR, UK. [4]Derby Royal Hospital, Uttoxeter Road, Derby DE22 3NE, UK.

References

1. Oliver C, Horsler K, Berg K, Bellamy G, Dick K, Griffiths E. Genomic imprinting and the expression of affect in Angelman syndrome. What's in the smile? J Child Psychol Psychiatry. 2007;48:571–9.

2. Jones W, Bellugi U, Lai Z, Chiles M, Reilly J, Lincoln A, Adolphs R II. Hypersociability in Williams syndrome. Cognitive Neuroscience. 2000;12:30–46.

3. Cordeiro L, Ballinger E, Hagerman R, Hessl D. Clinical assessment of DSM-IV anxiety disorders in fragile X syndrome: prevalence and characterization. J Neurodev Disord. 2011;3:57–67.

4. Kasari C, Freeman SF. Task-related social behavior in children with Down syndrome. Am J Ment Retard. 2001;106:253–64.

5. Beck B. Epidemiology of Cornelia de Lange's syndrome. Acta Paediatr. 1976;65:631–8.

6. Gillis LA, McCallum J, Kaur M, DeScipio C, Yaeger D, Mariani A, Kline AD, Li H-H, Devoto M, Jackson LG. NIPBL mutational analysis in 120 individuals with Cornelia de Lange syndrome and evaluation of genotype-phenotype correlations. Am J Hum Genet. 2004;75:610–23.

7. Krantz ID, McCallum J, DeScipio C, Kaur M, Gillis LA, Yaeger D, Jukofsky L, Wasserman N, Bottani A, Morris CA. Cornelia de Lange syndrome is caused by mutations in NIPBL, the human homolog of Drosophila melanogaster Nipped-B. Nat Genet. 2004;36:631–5.

8. Miyake N, Visser R, Kinoshita A, Yoshiura K-I, Niikawa N, Kondoh T, Matsumoto N, Harada N, Okamoto N, Sonoda T. Four novel NIPBL mutations in Japanese patients with Cornelia de Lange syndrome. Am J Med Genet A. 2005;135:103–5.

9. Deardorff MA, Kaur M, Yaeger D, Rampuria A, Korolev S, Pie J, Gil-Rodríguez C, Arnedo M, Loeys B, Kline AD. Mutations in cohesin complex members SMC3 and SMC1A cause a mild variant of Cornelia de Lange syndrome with predominant mental retardation. Am J Hum Genet. 2007;80:485–94.

10. Musio A, Selicorni A, Focarelli ML, Gervasini C, Milani D, Russo S, Vezzoni P, Larizza L. X-linked Cornelia de Lange syndrome owing to SMC1L1 mutations. Nat Genet. 2006;38:528–30.

11. Minor A, Shinawi M, Hogue JS, Vineyard M, Hamlin DR, Tan C, Donato K, Wysinger L, Botes S, Das S, del Gaudio D. Two novel RAD21 mutations in patients with mild Cornelia de Lange syndrome-like presentation and report of the first familial case. Genet Med. 2014;537:279–84.

12. Deardorff MA, Bando M, Nakato R, Watrin E, Itoh T, Minamino M, Saitoh K, Komata M, Katou Y, Clark D, et al. HDAC8 mutations in Cornelia de Lange syndrome affect the cohesin acetylation cycle. Nature. 2012;489:313–7.

13. Berney TP, Ireland M, Burn J. Behavioural phenotype of Cornelia de Lange syndrome. Arch Dis Child. 1999;81:333–6.

14. Hyman P, Oliver C, Hall S. Self-injurious behaviour, self-restraint, and compulsive behaviours in Cornelia de Lange syndrome. Am J Ment Retard. 2002;107

15. Oliver C, Arron K, Sloneem J, Hall S. Behavioural phenotype of Cornelia de Lange syndrome: case-control study. Br J Psychiatry. 2008;193:466–70.

16. Goodban MT. Survey of speech and language skills with prognostic indicators in 116 patients with Cornelia de Lange syndrome. Am J Med Genet. 1993;47:1059–63.

17. Collis L, Oliver C, Moss J. Low mood and social anxiety in Cornelia de Lange syndrome. J Intellect Disabil Res. 2006;50:792.

18. Moss J, Oliver C, Berg K, Kaur G, Jephcott L, Cornish K. Prevalence of autism spectrum phenomenology in Cornelia de Lange and Cri du Chat syndromes. Am J Ment Retard. 2008;113:278–91.

19. Richards C, Moss J, O'Farrell L, Kaur G, Oliver C. Social anxiety in Cornelia de Lange syndrome. J Autism Dev Disord. 2009;39:1155–62.

20. Moss J, Nelson L, Powis L, Waite J, Richards C, Oliver C. A comparative study of sociability in Angelman, Cornelia de Lange, Fragile X, Down and Rubinstein-Taybi Syndromes and Autism Spectrum Disorder. American Journal on Intellectual and Developmental Disabilities. 2016;121:465–486.

21. Richards C, Jones C, Groves L, Moss J, Oliver C. Prevalence of autism spectrum disorder phenomenology in genetic disorders: a systematic review and meta-analysis. The Lancet Psychiatry. 2015;2:909–16.

22. Moss J, Howlin P, Hastings RP, Beaumont S, Griffith GM, Petty J, Tunnicliffe P, Yates R, Villa D, Oliver C. Social behavior and characteristics of autism spectrum disorder in Angelman, Cornelia de Lange, and Cri du Chat syndromes. Am J Intellect Dev Disabil. 2013;118:262–83.

23. Lesniak-Karpiak K, Mazzocco MMM, Ross JL. Behavioral assessment of social anxiety in females with Turner or fragile X syndrome. J Autism Dev Disord. 2003;33:55–67.

24. Hessl D, Glaser B, Dyer-Friedman J, Reiss AL. Social behavior and cortisol reactivity in children with fragile X syndrome. J Child Psychol Psychiatry. 2006;47:602–10.

25. Hall S, DeBernardis M, Reiss AL. Social escape behaviors in children with fragile X syndrome. J Autism Dev Disord. 2006;36:935–47.

26. Hall S, Lightbody AA, Huffman LC, Lazzeroni LC, Reiss AL. Physiological correlates of social avoidance behavior in children and adolescents with fragile X syndrome. J Am Acad Child Adolesc Psychiatry. 2009;48:320–9.

27. Cohen IL, Fisch GS, Sudhalter V, Wolf-Schein EG, Hanson D, Hagerman R, Jenkins EC, Brown WT. Social gaze, social avoidance, and repetitive behavior in fragile X males: a controlled study. Am J Ment Retard. 1988;92:436–46.

28. Kover ST, McDuffie A, Abbeduto L, Brown WT. Effects of sampling contect on spontaneous expressive language in males with fragile X syndrome or Down syndrome. J Speech Lang Hear Res. 2012;55:1022–38.

29. Horsler K, Oliver C. Environmental influences on the behavioural phenotype of Angelman syndrome. Am J Ment Retard. 2006;111:311–21.

30. de Falco S, Venuti P, Esposito G, Bornstein MH. Mother-child and father-child emotional availability in families of children with Down syndrome. Parenting: Science and Practice. 2009;9:198–215.

31. Oliver C, Demetriades L, Hall S. The effect of environmental events on smiling and laughing behavior in Angelman syndrome. Am J Ment Retard. 2002;107:194–200.

32. Venuti P, de Falco S, Esposito G, Bornstein MH. Mother-child play: children with Down syndrome and typical development. Am J Intellect Dev Disabil. 2009;114:274–8.

33. Baron-Cohen S, Leslie AM, Frith U. Does the autistic child have a 'theory of mind'? Cognition. 1985;21:37–46.

34. Grant CM, Apperly I, Oliver C. Is theory of mind understanding impaired in males with fragile X syndrome? J Abnorm Child Psychol. 2007;35:17–28.

35. Dawson G, Meltzoff AN, Osterling J, Rinaldi J, Brown E. Children with autism fail to orient to naturally occurring social stimuli. J Autism Dev Disord. 1998;28:479–85.

36. Gibbs MV, Thorpe JG. Personality stereotype of noninstitutionalized Down syndrome children. Am J Ment Defic. 1983;102:228–37.

37. Kasari C, Sigman M. Expression and understanding of emotion in atypical development. In: Lewis M, Sullivan MW, editors. *Emotional development in atypical children*. Hillsdale: Erlbaum; 1996.

38. Kushlick A, Blunden R, Cox C. A method of rating behaviour characteristics for use in large scale surveys of mental handicap. Psychol Med. 1973;3:466–78.

39. Sparrow SS, Cicchetti DV, Balla DA. Vineland-II adaptive behavior scales: survey forms manual. Circle Pines: AGS Publishing; 2005.

40. Gioia GA, Espy KA, Isquith PK: BRIEF-P: Behavior rating inventory of executive function-preschool version: professional manual. Psychological assessment resources; 2003.

41. Gioia GA, Isquith PK, Kenworthy L, Barton R. Profiles of everyday executive function in acquired and developmental disorders. Child Neuropsychol. 2002;8:121–37.

42. Toplak ME, West RF, Stanovich KE. Practitioner review: do performance-based measures and ratings of executive function assess the same construct? J Child Psychol Psychiatry. 2013;54:131–43.

43. Dunn LM, Whetton C, Burley J. The British picture vocabulary scale, second edition testbook. NFER: Windsor; 1997.

44. Lord C, Rutter M, DiLavore P, Risi S. Autism diagnostic observation schedule: manual. Los Angeles: Western Psychological Services; 2002.

45. Fydrich T, Chambless DL, Perry KJ, Buergener F, Beazley MB. Behavioral assessment of social performance: a rating system for social phobia. Behav Res Ther. 1998;36:995–1010.

46. Conger JC, Farrell AD. Behavioral components of heterosocial skills. Behav Ther. 1981;12:41–55.

47. Glass CR, Arnkoff DB. Behavioral assessment of social anxiety and social phobia. Clin Psychol Rev. 1989;9:75–90.

48. Glennon B, Weisz JR. An observational approach to the assessment of anxiety in young children. J Consult Clin Psychol. 1978;46:1246–57.

49. Millbrook JM, Farrell AD, Wallander JL, Curran JP. Behavioral components of social skills: a look at subject and confederate behaviors. Behavioural Assessment. 1986;8:203–20.

50. Monti PM, Boice R, Fingeret AL, Zwick WR, Kolko D, Munro S, Grunberger A. Midi-level measurement of social anxiety in psychiatric and non-psychiatric samples. Behavior Research and Therapy. 1984;22:651–60.

51. Trower P, Yardley K, Bryant BM, Shaw P. The treatment of social failure: a comparison of anxiety-reduction and skills acquisition procedures on two social problems. Behav Modif. 1978;2:41–60.

52. Martin N, Oliver C, Hall S. Obswin: software for the collection and analysis of observational data. Birmingham: University of Birmingham; 1988.

53. Altman DG. Practical statistics for medical research. London: Chapman & Hall; 1991.

54. Kline AD, Grados M, Sponseller P, Levy HP, Balagowidow N, Schoedel C, Rampolla J, Clemens DK, Krantz ID, Kimball A, et al. Natural history of aging in Cornelia de Lange syndrome. Am J Med Genet C Semin Med Genet. 2007;145C:248–60.

5

Auditory repetition suppression alterations in relation to cognitive functioning in fragile X syndrome: a combined EEG and machine learning approach

Inga Sophia Knoth[1,2*], Tarek Lajnef[3,4], Simon Rigoulot[1,2,3,4,5], Karine Lacourse[2], Phetsamone Vannasing[2], Jacques L. Michaud[2,6], Sébastien Jacquemont[2], Philippe Major[2], Karim Jerbi[3,4,5,7,8] and Sarah Lippé[1,2,3,4,5]

Abstract

Background: Fragile X syndrome (FXS) is a neurodevelopmental genetic disorder causing cognitive and behavioural deficits. Repetition suppression (RS), a learning phenomenon in which stimulus repetitions result in diminished brain activity, has been found to be impaired in FXS. Alterations in RS have been associated with behavioural problems in FXS; however, relations between RS and intellectual functioning have not yet been elucidated.

Methods: EEG was recorded in 14 FXS participants and 25 neurotypical controls during an auditory habituation paradigm using repeatedly presented pseudowords. Non-phased locked signal energy was compared across presentations and between groups using linear mixed models (LMMs) in order to investigate RS effects across repetitions and brain areas and a possible relation to non-verbal IQ (NVIQ) in FXS. In addition, we explored group differences according to NVIQ and we probed the feasibility of training a support vector machine to predict cognitive functioning levels across FXS participants based on single-trial RS features.

Results: LMM analyses showed that repetition effects differ between groups (FXS vs. controls) as well as with respect to NVIQ in FXS. When exploring group differences in RS patterns, we found that neurotypical controls revealed the expected pattern of RS between the first and second presentations of a pseudoword. More importantly, while FXS participants in the ≤ 42 NVIQ group showed no RS, the > 42 NVIQ group showed a delayed RS response after several presentations. Concordantly, single-trial estimates of repetition effects over the first four repetitions provided the highest decoding accuracies in the classification between the FXS participant groups.

Conclusion: Electrophysiological measures of repetition effects provide a non-invasive and unbiased measure of brain responses sensitive to cognitive functioning levels, which may be useful for clinical trials in FXS.

Keywords: Fragile X syndrome, Intellectual disability, EEG, Repetition suppression, Machine learning, Habituation, IQ, Cognition

Background

Fragile X Syndrome (FXS) is a neurodevelopmental genetic disorder, which causes cognitive and behavioural deficits. FXS is caused by a mutation of the *FMR1* ('fragile X mental retardation 1') gene located on the X chromosome [1] that prevents expression of the fragile X mental retardation protein (FMRP) [2]. The majority of individuals affected by FXS have an intellectual disability (ID), ranging from mild to severe in males and from mild to moderate in females [3]. Cognitive impairments are often found in language, executive functions and visuo-spatial and social-cognitive domains [4]. Particular impairments are found in auditory working memory span and working memory for words [5]. Many of the symptoms found in FXS are typical of autistic spectrum disorders (ASD), [6] including aberrant behaviours,

* Correspondence: IngaSophia.Knoth@gmail.com
[1]Neuroscience of Early Development (NED), 90 Avenue Vincent-D'indy, Montreal, QC H2V 2S9, Canada
[2]Research Center of the CHU Sainte-Justine Mother and Child University Hospital Center, 3175 Chemin Côte Ste-Catherine, Montreal, QC H3T 1C5, Canada
Full list of author information is available at the end of the article

emotional instability and hyperarousal to sensory stimulation [4], especially in the auditory modality [7].

Deficits in auditory processing likely contribute to behavioural hypersensitivity and hyperexcitability to auditory stimulation reported in FXS individuals [8–10] and may be involved in abnormal language development as suggested by studies investigating autism [7, 11, 12]. Electroencephalography (EEG) studies revealed alterations in auditory evoked potentials (AEPs) reflecting basic auditory processing deficits in FXS [13–18]. These deficits are perhaps impairing the generation of memory traces, a concept reflecting the memorization of a learnt stimulus, which is required for stimulus discrimination [18] and may thus be related to a lack of habituation. EEG alterations in FXS have been found not only in basic auditory processing, but also in later event-related potential (ERP) components reflecting cognitive processes. A classic protocol to elicit cognitive ERPs is the oddball paradigm: trains of frequent standard stimuli are randomly interspersed with rare deviant stimuli eliciting a particular response, such as the Mismatch Negativity (MMN) in passive tasks and the P3 in active tasks in which a response to the infrequent stimuli is required [19]. Amplitudes of MMN and P3 components are attenuated in FXS [16–18], suggesting poor memory trace formation of the standard stimulus [20] as well as attention deficits [21].

Repetition suppression (RS) describes a phenomenon in which stimulus repetitions result in diminished brain activity in response to the standard stimulus. Using EEG, auditory RS in FXS has been assessed by comparing responses to early and late standard tones in oddball paradigms [15, 18] and by analysing a maximum of four sequential presentations of a standard tone [9, 13]. Both paradigms consistently show a lack of N1/P2 amplitude suppression in FXS. Recently, Ethridge et al. [9] analysed single-trial time–frequency in addition to AEP habituation and reported a decrease of RS in N1 amplitude together with alterations in both power and phase locking index in several frequency bands in FXS [9].

Whereas impairments in RS have been repeatedly found in FXS [9, 13, 15, 18, 22, 23], it has not yet been investigated with regard to cognitive functioning. In an exploratory analysis, Ethridge et al. suggested that reductions in RS were associated with parental reports of auditory hypersensitivity and social problems in FXS participants [9]. In support of these findings, Bruno et al. found impairments in RS to be correlated to higher autism symptoms in FXS [22]. However, no reference to ID severity has been made. Given that RS appears to be associated with auditory perceptual learning [24] and learning being a prerequisite for cognitive functioning, we expect RS patterns to vary in FXS with regard to IQ. Further, habituation, the behavioural pendant to repetition suppression,

has been found to predict later IQ in infant populations [25], suggesting a possible link between RS and IQ.

In order to reveal the distinct patterns of repetition effects in FXS participants in relation to cognition, we used a passive listening paradigm presenting ten standards without deviants, allowing measurement of a delayed repetition effect with more repetitions. In addition, we extended the investigation of RS from basic sensory components, as performed previously, to stimuli mimicking words. Processing of such stimuli is typically reflected in early as well as late components such as the N400 [26]. In fact, loss of N400 RS in response to spoken target words was found in fragile X-associated tremor/ataxia syndrome (FXTAS) [27]. We aimed at controlling for familiarity by using novel complex auditory stimuli in order to avoid semantic information that might bias cerebral processing and elicit late cognitive components such as the N400 [2, 28].

Auditory RS can also be studied in FXS animal models [29] supporting the relevance of RS as a translational biomarker for therapeutic approaches [30, 31]. Lovelace et al. demonstrated that a class of enzymes targeted by FMRP is directly involved in RS in *FMR1* KO mice [29]. In line with this, Bruno and colleagues [22] used fMRI and found impaired RS to visual face/gaze stimuli in the left fusiform gyrus directly correlated to lower, less typical levels of FMRP in FXS participants. Importantly, Schneider et al. used RS as an outcome measure in a clinical trial and found an improvement of RS in the N1/P2 complex in response to late vs. early sinusoidal tones in FXS participants after 3 months of minocycline treatment [15], pointing to the possibility of rescuing RS in humans as it was found in *FMR1* KO mice [29]. To further explore the clinical potential of this measure, we also used a machine learning approach to quantify the accuracy of single-trial RS features in the prediction of cognitive functioning levels in FXS participants.

Methods

Participants

A total of 19 FXS participants and 29 neurotypical controls participated in the experiment. Five FXS participants and three controls were excluded from analysis due to extensive movement artifacts. The 14 remaining FXS participants were compared to 26 neurotypical controls with a similar age distribution. Table 1 displays the demographics of the study population. Medication was reported by the parents, and all FXS participants were on a stable dose since at least 6 months before testing. Diagnoses of comorbidities were obtained from the medical file at the hospital and were based on psychiatric and/or neuropsychological evaluations. Medication and comorbidities are detailed in Table 2.

Patient recruitment was based on DNA analyses previously conducted in the genetics department of the CHU

Table 1 Demographics of the study population

Variable	FXS participants	Neurotypical controls
N	14 (4♀)	26 (11♀)
Age range	9–32 years	9–32 years
Mean age (SD)	15.5 (± 6.06)	17.1 (± 6.1)
NVIQ range	32–93	87–129
Mean NVIQ (SD)	48 (± 14.12)	113 (± 10.41)

Sainte-Justine Mother and Child University Hospital Center in Montreal. Neurotypical controls were recruited using posters at the Sainte-Justine Hospital and the University of Montreal and by classified ads on selected websites. Normal hearing and normal or corrected-to-normal vision was reported in all participants. All participants were francophone, right-handed and born at term. Non-verbal intelligence was examined using the non-verbal Leiter-R International Performance Scale [32] for all FXS participants as well as neurotypical children and adolescents and the Wechsler Abbreviated Scale of Intelligence (WASI) [33] for neurotypical adults only. Autistic behaviour in FXS participants was quantified using the repetitive behavior questionnaire [34] and the aberrant behavior checklist [35], which were completed by the parents. Results from these questionnaires are reported in [14]. The study protocol was reviewed and approved by the ethics, administrative and scientific committees at the Sainte-Justine's Hospital Research Center. Procedures undertaken were explained to participants and parents or legal caregivers, and written informed consent was obtained.

Apparatus

Testing took place in a dark soundproof experimental chamber in the Sainte-Justine hospital. A Dell GX150 PC was used to present the stimuli via E-Prime 1.0 (Psychology

Table 2 Characteristics of the FXS NVIQ median-split subgroups

Variable	≤ 42 NVIQ group	> 42 NVIQ group
N	8 (0 female)	6 (4 female)
Age range	9–32 years	10–22 years
Mean age (SD)	16.38 (± 7.37)	14.34 (± 4.08)
NVIQ range	32–42	52–93
Mean NVIQ (SD)	38 (± 3.64)	62 (± 10.02)
Medication	N = 6 Methylphenidate (36–45 mg qd) (4) Amphetamine mixed salts (50 mg qd) (1) Venlafaxine (75 mg qd) (1)	N = 3 Methylphenidate (36–50 mg qd) (2) Atomoxetine (25–40 mg qd) (2) Citalopram (20 mg qd) (1)
Comorbidities	Autistic spectrum disorder (4) Attention-deficit hyperactivity disorder (6)	Autistic spectrum disorders (1) Attention deficit hyperactivity disorder (3)

Software Tools Inc. Pittsburgh, PA, USA). Two speakers (Optimus XTS 24, Boston, MA, USA) were placed laterally at a 30-cm distance from the subject's ears.

Stimuli

Eighteen different two-syllable pseudowords were chosen from the BELEC [36] and ODÉDYS-II [37] paediatric batteries and recorded in a soundproof chamber while spoken by a native French-speaking woman. Adobe Audition 3.0 (Adobe Systems Inc., San Jose, CA, USA) was used for recording and normalization to − 3 dB SPL. Pseudowords had an average length of 930 ms and ranged between 800 and 1300 ms.

Procedure

Participants chose among five movies for children that they watched without sound and without subtitles during EEG installation and stimuli presentation in order to enhance acceptance of the procedure and reduce movement artefacts through fixation on the screen. The same pseudoword was presented successively ten times each with an inter-stimulus interval of 250 ms at 70 dB SPL intensity and 16-bit resolution. In total, 18 trials with different pseudowords were presented in sequential order with an inter-trial interval of 250 ms in a passive listening paradigm. The order of pseudowords was fixed across participants in order to avoid pseudowords starting with a similar sound to be presented in succession.

A 128 electrode dense array EEG was used for recording (Electrical Geodesics System Inc., Eugene, OR, USA). Impedances were maintained under 40 kΩ [38], and during recording, Cz was used as reference. Signals were acquired and processed by a G4 Macintosh computer using NetStation Software (Version 2.0). EEG data was digitalized at a sampling rate of 250 Hz, and an analog bandpass filter of 0.01−100 Hz was applied. Off-line analyses were carried out with BrainVision Analyser software, version 2.0 (Brain Products, Munich, Germany). Data were digitally filtered with a 1–50 Hz filter and re-referenced to an average reference. Thirty electrodes containing muscular artefacts, around the neck and face, were removed for all participants. Blink artefacts were removed using a semi-automatic independent component analysis (ICA) [39] (see Additional file 1 for details). EEG signal was segmented into 800-ms epochs after stimulus onset. Algorithmic artefact marking of voltage exceeding ± 100 μV was followed by visual data inspection of segmented data in which epochs with artefacts were rejected manually. An average of 178/180 segments were kept for control participants and 174/180 for FXS participants.

EEG signal processing

Data was exported to a commercial software package (MATLAB 6.1, The MathWorks Inc., Natick, MA, 2000)

using BrainVision solutions. Signal energy (E) was used as a measure of total signal amplitude in order to detect repetition effects as in [40]. Signal energy measures allowed the inclusion of a larger age range compared to ERP component analyses, since it is less affected by maturational changes found in AEP components [41].

Signal energy is defined as $E = \Sigma\,|amp|2$ where amp is the amplitude value (μV) of all EEG data points contained in a segmented trial. The time series of each presentation p (1 to 10) were normalized relative to the standard deviation of its series of ten presentations (the repetition series) of the pseudoword stimulus s (1 to 18) for each participant and channel. The objective was to normalize the time series of each pseudoword s (the series of ten presentations of s) to make the standard deviation of each pseudoword the same. Subsequently, the energy was computed for all ten presentations ($1 \le n \le 10$) of pseudowords. A detailed explanation of the signal energy computation can be found in the Additional file 1.

Spatial principal component analysis

In order to identify spatial regions of interest (ROIs) relevant for the task performed in our samples, we used the properties of principal component analysis (PCA) [42–45]. For each group of participants (FXS participants and controls), we performed a separate spatial PCA (Varimax rotation, SPSS statistics, version 20, IBM Corp., Armonk, NY, USA) with 99 electrode sites as dependent variables, participants (14 in the FXS and 26 in the control group) and presentations (10) as observations [46]. Specific details of the spatial PCA factor loadings can be found in Additional file 1.

The spatial PCA yielded 12 factors for the FXS and 15 for the control group. The first five factors explained 60% of the data variance for the control group, and the first two factors explained 62% of the variance for the FXS group. Seven regions of interest were identified from these factors (see Fig. 1): central and left frontal areas based on the two factors for the FXS group and left temporal, fronto-central, right frontal, right temporal and occipital areas based on the five factors for the control group.

Statistical analysis
Linear mixed models
Statistical analyses were performed using SPSS statistics, version 23 (IBM Corp., Armonk, NY, USA). Linear mixed models (LMM) were used to understand how group membership (FXS vs. control) and NVIQ predicted signal energy changes across repetitions. Further, age was assessed as predictor in order to account for the large age range in our sample. A LMM approach was chosen over traditional repeated measures analysis in order to account for unbalanced design, enable random intercepts and slopes, allow for nonlinear modeling of energy changes across repetitions and select an appropriate covariance structure for the repetition effects [47–50].

The model used for this study was determined by a series of steps to determine model fit [47] that can be found in Additional file 1. Finally, LMM analysis was performed using maximum likelihood for estimation method [47] and predictors group, NVIQ and age were added sequentially, verifying if model fit was improved by the addition of each predictor using chi-square likelihood ratio test [47]. Finally, covariance structure was selected by comparing model fit between available structures using Akaike's Information Criterion (AIC) [47].

Based on significant interactions, further LMMs were performed, exploring signal energy changes across presentations in FXS and controls separately following the same series of steps described above for each model. Bonferroni-corrected post hoc paired comparisons were performed for significant main effects. Significance level was set to 5% ($p = 0.05$). In order to explore significant interactions and reveal patterns of RS, a NVIQ median-split was performed dividing the FXS group into two subgroups (≤ 42 and > 42 NVIQ).

Classification of NVIQ subgroups in FXS using single-trial RS features
A machine learning approach was used in order to specifically investigate whether differences in RS effects can predict differences in cognitive capacities (i.e. NVIQ levels) within the FXS group. Importantly, we chose to explore this question using a binary classification approach (to decode between NVIQ median-split subgroups) based on single-

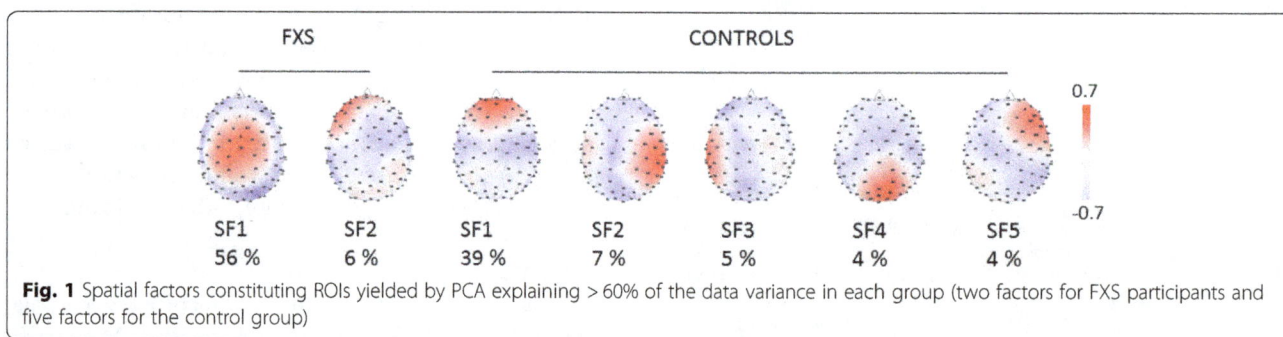

Fig. 1 Spatial factors constituting ROIs yielded by PCA explaining > 60% of the data variance in each group (two factors for FXS participants and five factors for the control group)

trial differences in EEG energy between consecutive presentations (18 trials across 14 FXS participants, i.e. $n = 252$). In addition to addressing the limitation of small sample size, which precludes a standard statistical analysis, a successful single-trial classification of FXS participants (i.e. based on 252 samples) would provide an important demonstration of the sensitivity of RS. The features used in the classification consisted of differences in energy between P1 and subsequent presentations as well as differences between P2 and subsequent presentations. Because they capture single-trial changes in energy between first (or second) stimulus presentations and subsequent presentations, these features were designed to account for repetition effects. A total of 17 such features were calculated for each of the seven ROIs, yielding 119 features in total.

We ran the single-trial classifications using a leave-two-subject-out cross-validation across the group of FXS participants, which is equivalent to a K-fold cross-validation where all 36 trials from two participants (one from each subgroup) are used as test set in each fold. Given that the NVIQ based division of the FXS group yielded a subgroup with NVIQ ≤ 42 ($n = 8$) and another with NVIQ > 42 ($n = 6$), we used a bootstrap approach to repeatedly run the classification on balanced classes. This led to running 28 classifications (all options of picking subgroups of 6 among 8 participants) with 216 samples (6×18 trials). In other words, in each fold, a model is trained on single-trial RS features from ten participants (5 per NVIQ subgroup) and tested on the single trials from the two remaining participants (1 from each class). The mean decoding accuracy (DA) of each single feature was used as a measure of classification performance.

Several classification algorithms were tested including k-th nearest neighbor (KNN), linear discriminant analysis (LDA) and support vector machine (SVM). Although the performances were reasonably similar, SVM (with radial basis function kernel) provided the best decoding results and was thus used in this study.

Given that the decoding problem investigated here is a binary classification, the theoretical chance level for the DA is 50%. However, a reliable assessment of the accuracy of machine learning decoding accuracy requires an evaluation in terms of statistical significance. We therefore evaluated the statistical significance of all reported DAs using the binomial cumulative distribution [51], followed by Bonferroni correction across the number of explored features to correct for multiple comparisons. This conservative approach indicated that a decoding accuracy is considered statistically significant at $p < 0.05$ or $p < 0.01$ if it exceeds 62.96 or 64.35% respectively.

Results

Characteristics of the population
FXS participants had a lower NVIQ ($M = 51$, ± 15.46) than the control group ($M = 113$, ± 10.79) ($t_{(23)} = -15.5$,

$p = 0.0001$). Based on our NVIQ measures, one participant (14 years, NVIQ = 93, female) did not present an ID. The rest presented an ID ranging from mild to severe. For some analyses, the FXS group was split into subgroups using a median-split at 42 NVIQ. Characteristics of the NVIQ-FXS subgroups can be found in Table 2. NVIQ differed significantly between the two FXS subgroups ($t_{(12)} = -5.6$, $p = 0.001$) with a mean of 38 (± 3.64) vs. 62 (± 10.02). EEG segments kept for analysis did not differ significantly between control and FXS participants ($t_{(15)} = -2.1$, $p = 0.058$) or between the two NVIQ FXS subgroups ($t_{(8)} = -1.9$, $p = 0.099$).

Linear mixed models
Baseline model: intercept, slope and polynomial structure
The construction of the model was started with a simple repeated measures (repetition (10) × ROI (7)) model with energy as outcome variable and repetition and ROI as fixed effects and without any predictors that served as baseline model. Using the chi-square likelihood ratio test, best fit for the baseline model was found using a random slope but not intercept and a linear model (see Additional file 1 for details).

Predictors
The first predictor added to the model was group (FXS vs. control) in order to verify if information about group membership improves model fit. Repetition, ROI and group were entered as fixed effects as well as interactions between repetition and ROI; repetition and group; and repetition, group and ROI. A random slope term accounted for inter-individual differences in trajectory changes across repetitions. Adding the predictor 'group' improved the model significantly [χ^2 (70, $N = 40$) = 103, $p < 0.01$]. Whereas no significant main effect was found for group and ROI, repetition yielded a significant effect (F (9, 395.4) = 5.77, $p = 0.0001$), meaning that signal energy significantly changed across stimulus repetitions. A significant interaction was found between repetition and group (F (9, 395.4) = 3.75, $p = 0.0001$), suggesting that signal energy repetition effects differed between groups. No interactions were found between ROI and repetition or ROI, group and repetition.

Then, NVIQ was added as a second predictor and fixed effect to the model. Interactions between NVIQ and repetition as well as between NVIQ, repetition and group were added to the existing interactions. The model improved significantly [χ^2 (20, $N = 40$) = 43, $p < 0.01$] with the inclusion of the predictor 'NVIQ'. In this model, the main effect for repetition was not significant any more (F (9, 596) = 1.43, $p = 0.174$) and neither were the other main effects (ROI, IQ, group). A significant interaction was found between repetition and group (F (9, 596) = 2.09, $p = 0.029$), as well as between repetition and NVIQ (F (9,

602) = 2.05, $p = 0.032$) and repetition, NVIQ and group (F (10, 417) = 2.57, $p = 0.005$), suggesting that repetition effect differences between groups varied with NVIQ.

Finally, age was added as predictor and fixed effect to the model. Adding age as predictor diminished model fit according to AIC and differed not significantly from the previous model [χ^2 (40, $N = 40$) = 41, $p < 0.9$].

Thus, we concluded that a random slope model with group and NVIQ as predictors presents the best fit for the data. All available covariance structures were tested, and first-order autoregressive covariance structure provided the best model fit according to AIC. Based on the significant interactions between group and repetitions, we decided to build separate models for FXS and controls in order to examine their distinct repetition effect patterns.

Controls

The test statistics for the baseline model can be found in Additional file 1. A significant main effect was found for repetition (F (9, 273.3) = 9.31, $p = 0.0001$), meaning that signal energy significantly changed between repetitions, but not for ROI. A significant interaction was found between ROI and repetition (F (54, 1253) = 1.52, $p = 0.01$). A Bonferroni-corrected post hoc test showed a significant reduction in energy between the first and all following presentations of a pseudoword (see Table 3 for mean values and t statistics). Figure 2 shows energy across presentations for the control group. The addition of NVIQ as predictor did not improve the model significantly [χ^2 (10, $N = 26$) = 15, $p > 0.05$].

FXS

The baseline model is described in Additional file 1. In the baseline model, with fixed effects for repetition, ROI and the interaction between repetition and ROI, a significant effect could be found for repetition (F (9, 133.5) = 2.02, $p = 0.042$), meaning that signal energy changed significantly between repetitions. No main effect could be found for ROI, and the interaction between repetition and ROI was also not found to be significant.

Then, we added NVIQ as predictor and fixed effect to the model, as well as interactions between repetition and NVIQ. The model improved significantly with the addition of NVIQ as a predictor [χ^2 (10, $N = 14$) = 20, $p < 0.05$]. A main effect for repetition was found (F (9, 207) = 1.99, $p = 0.042$), but not for ROI or NVIQ. The interaction between repetition and NVIQ was found to be significant (F (9, 216.6) = 2.36, $p = 0.015$), suggesting that repetition effects in signal energy differed with respect to NVIQ. Bonferroni-corrected post hoc tests showed no significant changes in energy between the ten presentations. In order to explore the significant interaction between repetition and NVIQ, we decided to split

the FXS group into subgroups using a median-split at 42 NVIQ.

> 42 NVIQ FXS subgroup

The baseline model is detailed in Additional file 1. A significant main effect was found for repetition (F (9, 58.9) = 3.76, $p = 0.001$), meaning signal energy changed between repetitions. No main effect was found for ROI or the interaction between ROI and repetition. Bonferroni-corrected post hoc tests showed a significant reduction in energy between presentation 2/3 and later presentations. Test statistics can be found in Table 3. Figure 2 shows energy across presentations for the > 42 NVIQ subgroup.

≤ 42 NVIQ FXS subgroup

No significant main effect was found for repetition or ROI, and the interaction between ROI and repetition was not significant. Energy across presentations for the ≤ NVIQ FXS subgroup is illustrated in Fig. 2. Signal energy did not change significantly between repetitions in the ≤ 42 NVIQ FXS group.

Single-trial RS classification results: NVIQ FXS subgroups

Training an SVM to classify ≤ 42 NVIQ FXS vs. > 42 NVIQ FXS participants based on single-trial EEG repetition effects yielded significant decoding accuracies across four ROIs, mainly over frontal and central regions (Fig. 3). The best predictions of FXS subgroup based on the EEG single-trial data, in other words the highest decoding accuracy, was observed over the frontal-right ROI. More precisely, this was achieved using single-trial RS changes observed between the first and fourth presentations (FR 1–4), yielding 65.2% correct classification, and also between the second and fourth presentations (FR 2–4), with 64.4% correct classifications. The other features that provided statistically significant decoding were obtained with RS measured in the following three ROIs: C 1–2, FC 1–4 and TL 1–3.

Discussion

In this study, we confirm alterations in the repetition effect brain responses of FXS patients. Differences in repetition effects according to NVIQ in FXS participants were demonstrated for the first time. Neurotypical controls showed the expected pattern of RS between the first and second presentations of a pseudoword and a stable response to subsequent presentations. In FXS participants, NVIQ was a significant predictor of RS patterns. When further exploring this result by separating FXS patients into two groups, we observed RS after four repetitions of a pseudoword in the > 42 NVIQ group, whereas no RS could be found in the FXS participants presenting more cognitive impairment according to their NVIQ scores (≤ 42 NVIQ). Our single-trial

Table 3 Mean energy (±SD) for each presentation and participant group and t statistics for significant energy differences between presentations (Bonferroni corrected p-values for multiple comparisons)

Presentations	Controls	FXS ≤ 42 NVIQ	FXS > 42 NVIQ
1	213.2 (± 16)	207.6 (± 16.2)	216.5 (± 25.9)
2	192.2 (± 9.8)	202 (± 16.1)	223.5 (± 17.7)
1 vs. 2	$t_{(471)} = 7.5, p = 0.0001$		
3	199.8 (± 11.8)	195.3 (± 14.5)	220 (± 29.5)
1 vs. 3	$t_{(304)} = 4.2, p = 0.001$		
4	195.3 (± 10.8)	201.2 (± 22.1)	186.9 (± 8.2)
1 vs. 4	$t_{(258)} = 5.6, p = 0.0001$		
2 vs. 4			$t_{(74)} = 5.2, p = 0.004$
3 vs. 4			$t_{(101)} = 2.7, p = 0.0001$
5	201.6 (± 10.8)	190.8 (± 16.7)	192.7 (± 22.2)
1 vs. 5	$t_{(249)} = 3.6, p = 0.013$		
6	195.4 (± 12.3)	193.1 (± 18.1)	195.1 (± 19.4)
1 vs. 6	$t_{(247)} = 5.5, p = 0.0001$		
7	198.7 (± 14.7)	191.3 (± 15.5)	192.6 (± 19.2)
1 vs. 7	$t_{(247)} = 4.5, p = 0.0001$		
8	195.3 (± 16.9)	192.9 (± 13.7)	186.7 (± 18.6)
1 vs. 8	$t_{(247)} = 5.6, p = 0.0001$		
2 vs. 8			$t_{(44)} = 2.8, p = 0.009$
9	202.1 (± 14.6)	202.2 (± 23.7)	185.7 (± 11.5)
1 vs. 9	$t_{(247)} = 3.4, p = 0.023$		
2 vs. 9			$t_{(42)} = 3.7, p = 0.015$
3 vs. 9			$t_{(43)} = 2.4, p = 0.043$
10	196.7 (± 13.7)	213.4 (± 30.9)	188.7 (± 21.7)
1 vs. 10	$t_{(247)} = 5.1, p = 0.0001$		
2 vs. 10			$t_{(42)} = 2.3, p = 0.038$

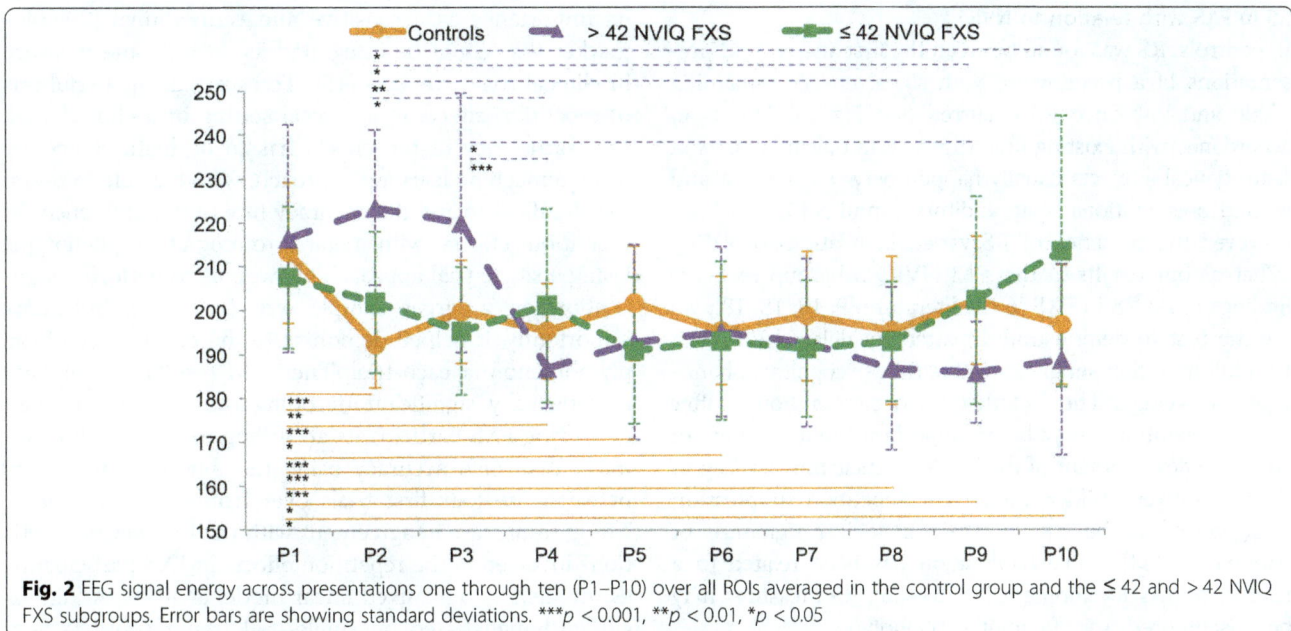

Fig. 2 EEG signal energy across presentations one through ten (P1–P10) over all ROIs averaged in the control group and the ≤ 42 and > 42 NVIQ FXS subgroups. Error bars are showing standard deviations. ***$p < 0.001$, **$p < 0.01$, *$p < 0.05$

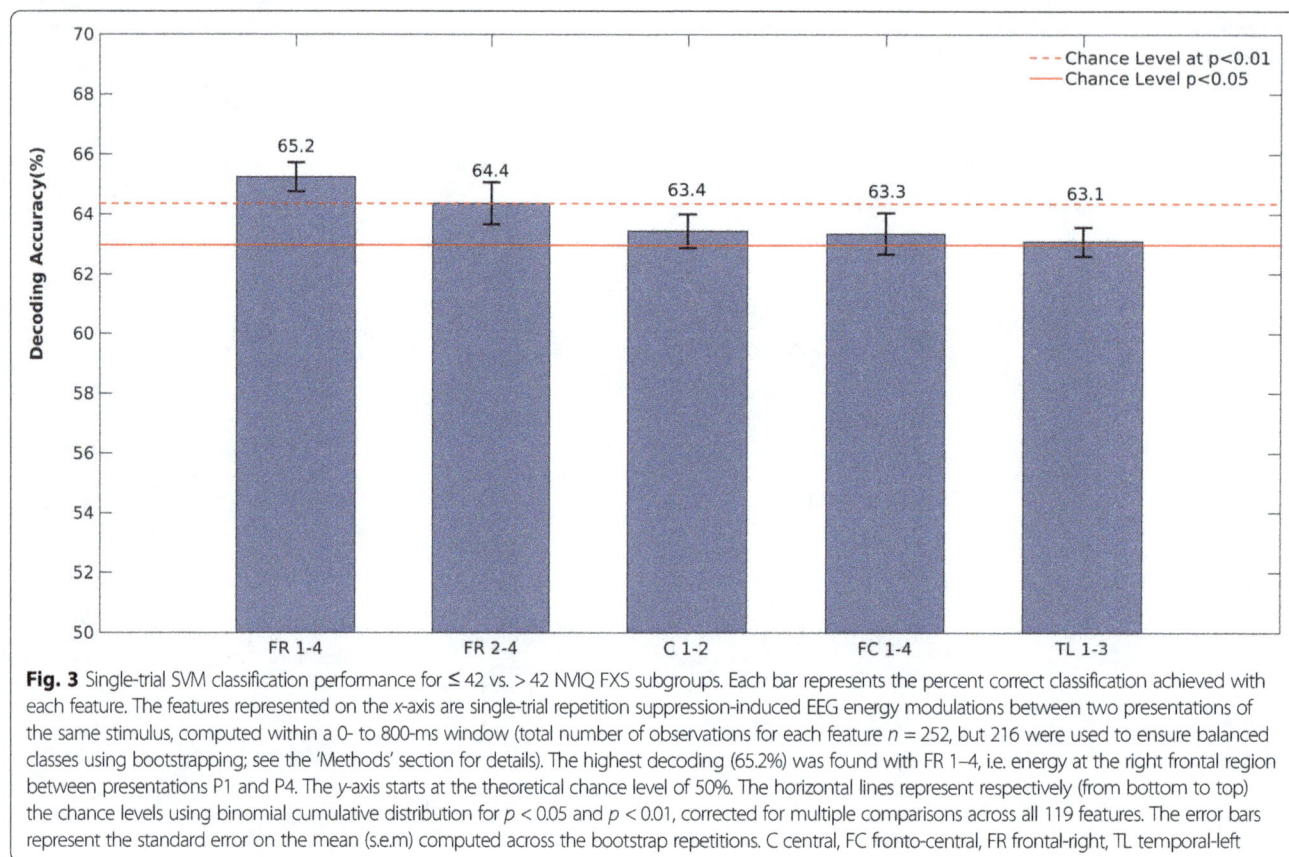

Fig. 3 Single-trial SVM classification performance for ≤ 42 vs. > 42 NVIQ FXS subgroups. Each bar represents the percent correct classification achieved with each feature. The features represented on the x-axis are single-trial repetition suppression-induced EEG energy modulations between two presentations of the same stimulus, computed within a 0- to 800-ms window (total number of observations for each feature $n = 252$, but 216 were used to ensure balanced classes using bootstrapping; see the 'Methods' section for details). The highest decoding (65.2%) was found with FR 1–4, i.e. energy at the right frontal region between presentations P1 and P4. The y-axis starts at the theoretical chance level of 50%. The horizontal lines represent respectively (from bottom to top) the chance levels using binomial cumulative distribution for $p < 0.05$ and $p < 0.01$, corrected for multiple comparisons across all 119 features. The error bars represent the standard error on the mean (s.e.m) computed across the bootstrap repetitions. C central, FC fronto-central, FR frontal-right, TL temporal-left

machine learning approach further revealed that repetition effects can accurately categorize FXS participants according to their level of cognitive functioning.

RS in FXS with relation to NVIQ

In controls, RS was found between the first and second presentations of a pseudoword with signal energy remaining stable and low once RS occurred (see Fig. 2). This is in accordance with existing literature stating that RS effects in neurotypical subjects usually happen between the first and second presentations of an auditory stimulus [52]. In FXS, however, the presence of RS varied in relation to NVIQ. Whereas our results in the ≤ 42 NVIQ subgroup replicate findings of no RS in FXS in the literature [9, 13, 15, 18], we are the first to demonstrate a pattern of delayed RS in an FXS full mutation subgroup with a milder cognitive phenotype on average. The fact that RS occurs, although after several repetitions, may be an important building block of cognitive development of these FXS participants, leading to a comparatively milder phenotype. Repetition suppression is suggested to be the electrophysiological signature of habituation [53]. Since habituation has been related to a later cognitive development [25, 54–56], RS measures may be a useful predictor of cognitive phenotype.

The relation of RS with auditory hypersensitivity, social problems [9], autism symptoms and FMRP levels [22] in FXS individuals and animal models [29] has been previously reported. Our findings add the factor of cognitive functioning to the existing literature, further underlining its importance as a sensitive and translational [29] biomarker that could be integrated as an outcome measure in clinical trial protocols [15]. To ascertain the usefulness of repetition effects in a clinical setting or a clinical trial, the consistency of the effects has to be high. Hence, by using a machine learning approach, we were able to reveal the significance and the accuracy rate of the differences in repetition effects with regard to cognitive phenotype. Using a single trial approach allowed us to perform classification on a larger sample size ($n = 252$), but most importantly, it helped demonstrate the consistency of the phenomenon at each trial. The SVM results demonstrate a statistically significant decoding rate ($p < 10^{-5}$) when classifying FXS participants according to their NVIQ with more than 65% accuracy using the difference in energy between the four first trials over fronto-central regions. These results are in agreement with the number of repetitions involved in the repetition effects in FXS participants, as revealed by our mixed linear model analyses. Additionally, although based on single-trial training and testing, the cross-validation scheme applied here (cf. the 'Methods' section) ensured a strict separation of participants across testing and training conditions. In other words, our machine learning findings reveal the feasibility of classifier generalization across participants with single-trial RS training and testing. These findings may suggest that the proposed method may be used to train a model for fast predictions (e.g. a few trials) in totally naïve FXS participants in particular with larger training sets. In general, our classification results confirm the distinct patterns of repetition effects in the FXS cognitive level subgroups and reveal the potential of our measure in a clinical setting.

Mechanisms underlying impaired RS in FXS

Different mechanisms have been proposed to explain RS and its disruption in FXS. Simple, passive listening paradigms with short ISIs are designed to assess RS mediated through refractory properties of the neuronal network [9, 57]. The refractory system in FXS may be impaired through less synchronized and more widely excitable local synaptic networks due to exaggerated long-term depression found in *FMR1* KO mice [2] leading to weakened connections in neuronal circuits [9].

Another more cognitive theory accounting for RS is the sharpening model, proposing that repeated information leads to a 'sharpening' of information presentation in the cortex [13, 58–60]. While novel stimuli activate large non-specific populations of neurons, repeated stimuli exposure results in fewer firing neurons, with the response of these few neurons being more specific and thus sharper. The 'predictive coding' model is a neural network model [61] that explains sharpening through an interplay between bottom-up sensory input and top-down expectations in hierarchically organized sensory systems, ranging from the primary areas receiving sensory information from thalamic nerve projections to the frontal cortex generating a predictive percept [62]. RS is thereby the physiological correlate of a reduction in prediction error in response to a repeatedly presented stimulus that is achieved by modifying connections between hierarchical levels through synaptic plasticity [63]. Four phenomena identified in *FMR1* KO mice, closely entwined with deficient synaptic plasticity, might be involved in disrupted RS with regard to the sharpening theory: (1) hyperexcitable neurons [30], in interplay with (2) delayed and weaker inhibition [64], (3) less sharply selective neurons [30] with broader frequency-tuning curves [31] and, finally, (4) abnormal dendrite morphology that is closely related to defects in circuit plasticity [65]. Long dendritic spines with immature morphologies and higher spine density suggest a failure in the synapse maturation process [66, 67]. Recently, an interest was developed regarding synaptic BK channels that are crucial for short-term habituation and directly interact with FMRP [31, 68–71]. The BK channel seems

to be involved in the abnormal dendritic spine phenotype [69], learning deficits [70] and hyperexcitabilty in FXS [71]. These mechanisms might be less affected in less severe ID FXS subgroups, since they are expected to have higher levels of FMRP.

Another factor that might mediate NVIQ-related differences in RS is attention, since the > 42 NVIQ group can be expected to pay more attention to the auditory stimulation. Attention-based prediction of up-coming stimuli modulated by the ventral striatum and the prefrontal cortex are central in the predictive coding model of RS [72, 73]. Concordantly, our group showed through transcranial direct current stimulation (tDCS) over the dorsolateral prefrontal cortex (DLPC) an enhancement of RS when the DLPC was excited and a reduction of RS when the DLPC was inhibited [40, 74]. Dorsolateral caudate circuitry has been found abnormal and related to cognitive and behavioural deficits in FXS [75]. Recent reports highlight the contribution of hippocampal memory activity in predictive coding [76–78], whereas a larger hippocampal size has been associated with worse memory in FXS [79].

Lastly, recent studies by Van der Molen et al. and Wang et al. have suggested that the lack of RS in FXS might be the result of uncoordinated neuronal synchronization patterns, since an imbalance between slow and fast oscillatory activity has been found in FXS [80, 81]. Elevated baseline levels of gamma power in FXS were interpreted as increased 'background neural noise' that contributed to impairments in synchronizing gamma frequency activity when necessary, leading to hyperexcitable and disorganized cortical networks [9]. These results underline the importance of comparing evoked responses against baseline levels in order to differentiate them from high neural background noise. Consequently, we normalized the time series of each presentation of a stimulus in our energy measures and examined the non-phase locked energy response relative to all ten presentations (see the 'Methods' section).

Main factors of spatial PCA

Given that previous EEG studies found different scalp distributions of ERPs in FXS and controls [13, 15, 17, 18], we conducted a separate spatial PCA analysis for FXS and controls in order to identify all ROIs relevant for the performed task in our study population. Interestingly, the spatial PCA differed not only in location, but also in number of factors. The concentration of activity in the central and frontal areas in FXS is in line with what has been found in previous studies which found a more frontal distribution of AEPs [13] and higher AEP/ERP amplitudes over central electrodes in FXS [15], whereas no differences were found over the posterior and occipital sites when compared to controls [18]. This focus of auditory hyperexcitability over fronto-central sites in FXS might contribute to the fact that these two factors (central, left frontal) explain a major part of the data variance whereas spatial components of activity in the control group appears more distributed and complex, having a total of five factors explaining the majority of the data variance. Further, altered functional connectivity and brain network activation has been found in FXS, with increased spatial spreading of phase synchronised activity, which may account for a more unitary activation pattern [80, 81].

Pseudoword learning and NVIQ

Language is typically a major deficit in FXS individuals, although receptive vocabulary is described as a relative strength in their cognitive domain [82]. In this study, cognitive functioning of FXS participants was evaluated using the non-verbal Leiter-R since it eliminates language deficit confounds. Furthermore, it can estimate NVIQ as low as 30, whereas a floor effect would have been expected when using most other batteries. The fact that repetition effects in response to pseudowords are predictors of NVIQ may suggest that repetition effects are of core importance for cognitive development, independent of the modality being investigated. As such, alterations of the repetition effects have been found in not only the auditory but also the visual modality [22, 23].

Conflation between sex and NVIQ effects in FXS

Sex is an important confounding variable when investigating cognitive functioning in FXS. Given that females have a milder phenotype than males with FXS [3], all of our female FXS participants fell into the > 42 NVIQ subgroup and we did not have not enough statistical power to compare RS between male and female participants in this subgroup. Given the fundamental biological differences between males and females presenting FXS, such as but not limited to FMRP levels, our study may have shown differences in RS as much in relation to sex as to NVIQ. Our results show that the more cognitively affected a FXS participant is, the less likely they are to show RS. Female FXS participants, who are generally less affected, are more likely to show some RS, although delayed.

Limitations and perspectives

Due to difficulties inherent to rare disease studies, our sample size is small, especially in the exploratory analysis in the median-split subgroups. Thus, single-trial machine learning was added in order to verify if our results would be confirmed with a completely different analysis approach. Studies investigating EEG in FXS often have small sample sizes, since difficulties in EEG recordings are a common problem [83]. These problems result in selection bias, since participants with severe ID and intense behavioural problems can rarely be tested, and as such, we are not able to investigate the full spectrum of FXS. Less invasive EEG setups, such as wireless nets and home

recordings, may enable an adaptation of study procedures for this population. In this study, we demonstrated that reliable results could be obtained with a very short test (5 min), supporting the feasibility of EEG for FXS participants in a clinical setting.

We included a rather large age range (9–32 years) to avoid further reducing the sample size. Electrophysiological activity is known to change with age, and maturation effects might present a confounding variable in our analysis. Also, RS effects in specific AEP components are difficult to compare across age groups since morphology, amplitudes and latencies change with maturation [84]. Signal energy is less affected by maturational changes found in AEP components, since it summarizes all amplitude values within a given time window and thus allows for a global examination of repetition effects across presentations, independent of specific AEP components [40]. Further, the LMM approach can take variations in intercept and slope between participants into account. When entered as a possible predictor in our LMM, age did not significantly improve model fit, suggesting that age did not contribute to the explanation of repetition effects. Lastly, we controlled for age by using a control group with a similar age distribution.

Similarly, FXS participants in the ≤ 42 NVIQ subgroup showed more autism symptoms, such as repetitive and aberrant behaviour, even though no statistical differences were found due to a lack of power for multiple testing. Segments containing movement artifacts were removed for all participants, and no significant difference for segments kept was found between FXS subgroups. As mentioned above, attention deficits in FXS participants could have perhaps disrupted RS. Although both subgroups present ADHD comorbidities, the severity of attention deficits may differ between groups.

A study evaluating the effect of these confounding variables would require a large N of different ID and autism populations as well as enough variability on all the variables to match and compare participants. This could most realistically be done in a multi-centric setting. Further, FMRP levels of FXS participants would have been of interest, since they likely represent a mediating factor between underlying neuronal alterations and severity of cognitive, behavioural and RS deficits.

Medication

The majority of our FXS population was medicated with different psychoactive drugs. Since psychoactive drugs are known to influence parameters of electrophysiological activity, it is possible that drug effects are masking or creating effects found in our sample. Type of medication and dosage differed between all FXS participants, rendering a detailed examination of drug effects difficult due to small sample sizes in each subgroup.

However, both FXS NVIQ subgroups contain a comparable amount of medicated and non-medicated individuals (see Table 2), suggesting that neither of the effects found in either group can solely be attributed to medication.

Meaning of the median-split

It is important to underline that the median-split at a NVIQ of 42 was used as a statistical tool in order to explore the interaction between group, NVIQ and repetition effects revealed by the LMM. Repetition effects appeared to differ relative to NVIQ, but further analyses were necessary to get an idea of how patterns of RS change with NVIQ. Given the small sample size, a median-split was chosen, in order to have a similar N in each subgroup. Since two individuals had an NVIQ of 42, they were both included in the ≤ 42 subgroup, whereas the lowest NVIQ in the > 42 group has an NVIQ of 52, rendering the separation between both groups to ten NVIQ points. However, this artificial NVIQ cut point is not clinically meaningful. Considering that NVIQ covaries significantly with RS in FXS, it is to be expected that participants further away from the split-point present a better model fit than participants close to a NVIQ of 42/ 52 who are more likely to be located somewhere between the two patterns explored in the median-split analyses.

Conclusion

Due to their sensitivity, EEG measures may be a promising treatment biomarker. One important asset of such a biomarker is its independence from task comprehension, which is inherent to classic cognitive testing. Further clinical trials are needed to demonstrate direct treatment effects on cognition. We propose presentation-by-presentation EEG repetition effects as a sensitive tool in order to display modifications in brain processes relevant to cognitive and behavioural development in FXS.

Abbreviations

AEP: Auditory evoked potential; ASD: Autism spectrum disorder; C: Central ROI; CHU: University Hospital Center; DA: Decoding accuracy; DLPC: Dorsolateral prefrontal cortex; EEG: Electroencephalography; ERP: Event-related potential; FC: Fronto-central ROI; FMR1: Fragile X mental retardation 1; fMRI: Functional magnetic resonance imaging; FMRP: Fragile X mental retardation protein; FR: Frontal-right ROI; FXS: Fragile X syndrome; ICA: Independent component analysis; ID: Intellectual disability; IQ: Intelligence quotient; KNN: k-th nearest neighbor; KO: Knockout; LDA: Linear discriminant analysis; LMM: Linear mixed model; mGluRs: Metabotropic glutamate receptors; MMN: Mismatch negativity; NVIQ: Non-verbal IQ; PCA: Principal component analysis; RE: Repetition enhancement; RF: Random forest; ROIs: Regions of interest; RS: Repetition suppression; SVM: Support vector machine; tDCS: Transcranial direct current stimulation; TL: Temporal left ROI; WASI: Wechsler Abbreviated Scale of Intelligence

Acknowledgements

We would like to thank all of our participants and their families as well as the Fragile X Québec Association for their continuous collaboration and support. We thank Emilie Sheppard for providing her voice for the auditory stimuli and Patricia Laniel and Maude Joannette for their help in the acquisition of EEG data.

Funding

This research was supported by a Scottish Rite Charitable Foundation grant to Sarah Lippé (grant number TSRCFC-12112) and a Fragile X Foundation of Canada grant awarded to Sarah Lippé and Sébastien Jacquemont. Karim Jerbi acknowledges the funding from the Canada Research Chairs program and NSERC Discovery Grant [RGPIN-2015-04854]. The funding body had no role in the design, collection, analysis and interpretation of the data and in writing the manuscript.

Authors' contributions

IK participated in the study design; coordinated the study; carried out the recruitment, EEG recording, EEG and statistical analysis; and drafted the manuscript. TL designed and applied the classification methods and helped in drafting the manuscript. SR participated in the study design, carried out the spatial principal component analysis, helped with the statistical analysis and helped in drafting the manuscript. KL designed the analysis tools, calculated the signal energy and helped in drafting the manuscript. PV participated in the EEG recordings and analysis. JLM participated in the DNA analysis and study design. SJ participated in the study design and helped with the recruitment. PM examined the EEGs for epileptic activity. KJ participated in the study design, designed and applied the classification tools and helped in drafting the manuscript. SL conceived the study, participated in its design and helped in drafting the manuscript. All authors read and approved the final manuscript.

Competing interests
The authors declare that they have no competing interests.

Author details

[1]Neuroscience of Early Development (NED), 90 Avenue Vincent-D'indy, Montreal, QC H2V 2S9, Canada. [2]Research Center of the CHU Sainte-Justine Mother and Child University Hospital Center, 3175 Chemin Côte Ste-Catherine, Montreal, QC H3T 1C5, Canada. [3]Department of Psychology, Université de Montréal, 90 Avenue Vincent-D'indy, Montreal, QC H2V 2S9, Canada. [4]Centre de Recherche en Neuropsychologie et Cognition (CERNEC), 90 Avenue Vincent-D'indy, Montreal, QC H2V 2S9, Canada. [5]International Laboratory for Brain, Music and Sound Research (BRAMS), 1430 Boul Mont-Royal, Montreal, QC H2V 2J2, Canada. [6]Faculty of Medicine, Université de Montréal, 2900 boulevard Édouard-Montpetit, Montréal, QC H3T 1J4, Canada. [7]Centre de Recherche de l'Institut Universitaire en Santé Mentale de Montréal (CRIUSMM), 7401 Rue Hochelaga, Montréal, QC H1N 3M5, Canada. [8]Centre de Recherche de l'Institut Universitaire de Gériatrie de Montréal (CRIUGM), 4565, chemin Queen-Mary, Montreal, QC H3W 1W5, Canada.

References

1. Penagarikano O, Mulle JG, Warren ST. The pathophysiology of fragile X syndrome. Annu Rev Genomics Hum Genet. 2007;8:109–29.
2. Bear MF, Huber KM, Warren ST. The mGluR theory of fragile X mental retardation. Trends Neurosci. 2004;27(7):370–7.
3. Hessl D, Nguyen DV, Green C, Chavez A, Tassone F, Hagerman RJ, Senturk D, Schneider A, Lightbody A, Reiss AL, et al. A solution to limitations of cognitive testing in children with intellectual disabilities: the case of fragile X syndrome. J Neurodev Disord. 2009;1(1):33–45.
4. Schneider A, Hagerman RJ, Hessl D. Fragile X syndrome—from genes to cognition. Dev Disabil Res Rev. 2009;15(4):333–42.
5. Ornstein PA, Schaaf JM, Hooper SR, Hatton DD, Mirrett P, Bailey DB Jr. Memory skills of boys with fragile X syndrome. Am J Ment Retard. 2008; 113(6):453–65.

6. Bailey DB Jr, Raspa M, Bishop E, Holiday D. No change in the age of diagnosis for fragile X syndrome: findings from a national parent survey. Pediatrics. 2009;124(2):527–33.

7. Rotschafer SE, Razak KA. Auditory processing in fragile X syndrome. Front Cell Neurosci. 2014;8:19.

8. Baranek GT, Roberts JE, David FJ, Sideris J, Mirrett PL, Hatton DD, Bailey DB Jr. Developmental trajectories and correlates of sensory processing in young boys with fragile X syndrome. Phys Occup Ther Pediatr. 2008;28(1):79–98.

9. Ethridge LE, White SP, Mosconi MW, Wang J, Byerly MJ, Sweeney JA. Reduced habituation of auditory evoked potentials indicate cortical hyper-excitability in fragile X syndrome. Transl Psychiatry. 2016;6:e787.

10. Rogers SJ, Hepburn S, Wehner E. Parent reports of sensory symptoms in toddlers with autism and those with other developmental disorders. J Autism Dev Disord. 2003;33(6):631–42.

11. Nieto Del Rincon PL. Autism: alterations in auditory perception. Rev Neurosci. 2008;19(1):61–78.

12. Roberts TP, Cannon KM, Tavabi K, Blaskey L, Khan SY, Monroe JF, Qasmieh S, Levy SE, Edgar JC. Auditory magnetic mismatch field latency: a biomarker for language impairment in autism. Biol Psychiatry. 2011;70(3):263–9.

13. Castren M, Paakkonen A, Tarkka IM, Ryynanen M, Partanen J. Augmentation of auditory N1 in children with fragile X syndrome. Brain Topogr. 2003;15(3):165–71.

14. Knoth IS, Vannasing P, Major P, Michaud JL, Lippe S. Alterations of visual and auditory evoked potentials in fragile X syndrome. Int J Dev Neurosci. 2014;36:90–7.

15. Schneider A, Leigh MJ, Adams P, Nanakul R, Chechi T, Olichney J, Hagerman R, Hessl D. Electrocortical changes associated with minocycline treatment in fragile X syndrome. J Psychopharmacol. 2013;27(10):956–63.

16. St Clair DM, Blackwood DH, Oliver CJ, Dickens P. P3 abnormality in fragile X syndrome. Biol Psychiatry. 1987;22(3):303–12.

17. Van der Molen MJ, Van der Molen MW, Ridderinkhof KR, Hamel BC, Curfs LM, Ramakers GJ. Auditory and visual cortical activity during selective attention in fragile X syndrome: a cascade of processing deficiencies. Clin Neurophysiol. 2012;123(4):720–9.

18. Van der Molen MJ, Van der Molen MW, Ridderinkhof KR, Hamel BC, Curfs LM, Ramakers GJ. Auditory change detection in fragile X syndrome males: a brain potential study. Clin Neurophysiol. 2012;123(7):1309–18.

19. Luck SJ. An introduction to the event-related potential technique. Cambridge: MIT Press; 2005.

20. Näätanen R, Paavilainen P, Rinne T, Alho K. The mismatch negativity (MMN) in basic research of central auditory processing: a review. Clin Neurophysiol. 2007;118(12):2544–90.

21. Polich J. Updating P300: an integrative theory of P3a and P3b. Clin Neurophysiol. 2007;118(10):2128–48.

22. Bruno JL, Garrett AS, Quintin EM, Mazaika PK, Reiss AL. Aberrant face and gaze habituation in fragile X syndrome. Am J Psychiatry. 2014; 171(10):1099–106.

23. Rigoulot S, Knoth IS, Lafontaine MP, Vannasing P, Major P, Jacquemont S, Michaud JL, Jerbi K, Lippé S. Altered visual repetition suppression in fragile X syndrome: new evidence from ERPs and oscillatory activity. Int J Dev Neurosci. 2017;59:52–59.

24. Garrido MI, Kilner JM, Kiebel SJ, Stephan KE, Baldeweg T, Friston KJ. Repetition suppression and plasticity in the human brain. NeuroImage. 2009;48(1):269–79.

25. Kavšek M. Predicting later IQ from infant visual habituation and dishabituation: a meta-analysis. J Appl Dev Psychol. 2004;25(3):369–93.

26. Kutas M, Federmeier KD. Thirty years and counting: finding meaning in the N400 component of the event-related brain potential (ERP). Annu Rev Psychol. 2011;62:621–47.

27. Yang JC, Chi L, Teichholtz S, Schneider A, Nanakul R, Nowacki R, Seritan A, Reed B, DeCarli C, Iragui VJ, et al. ERP abnormalities elicited by word repetition in fragile X-associated tremor/ataxia syndrome (FXTAS) and amnestic MCI. Neuropsychologia. 2014;63:34–42.

28. Deacon D, Dynowska A, Ritter W, Grose-Fifer J. Repetition and semantic priming of nonwords: implications for theories of N400 and word recognition. Psychophysiology. 2004;41(1):60–74.

29. Lovelace JW, Wen TH, Reinhard S, Hsu MS, Sidhu H, Ethell IM, Binder DK, Razak KA. Matrix metalloproteinase-9 deletion rescues auditory evoked potential habituation deficit in a mouse model of fragile X syndrome. Neurobiol Dis. 2016;89:126–35.

30. Rotschafer S, Razak K. Altered auditory processing in a mouse model of fragile X syndrome. Brain Res. 2013;1506:12–24.

31. Sinclair D, Oranje B, Razak KA, Siegel SJ, Schmid S. Sensory processing in autism spectrum disorders and fragile X syndrome—from the clinic to animal models. Neurosci Biobehav Rev. 2016;76(pt B):235–53.

32. Roid GH, Miller LJ. Leiter International Performance Scale—Revised: examiner's manual. In: Roid GH, Miller LJ, editors. Leiter International Performance Scale—revised edn. Wood Dale: Stoelting Co.; 1997.

33. Wechsler D. Wechsler Abbreviated Scale of Intelligence. San Antonio: The Psychological Corporation; 1999.

34. Lam KSL, Aman MG. The Repetitive Behavior Scale-Revised: independent validation in individuals with autism spectrum disorders. J Autism Dev Disord. 2007;37(5):855–66.

35. Aman MG, Singh NN, Stewart AW, Field CJ. The aberrant behavior checklist: a behavior rating scale for the assessment of treatment effects. Am J Ment Defic. 1985;89(5):485–91.

36. Mousty P, Leybaert J, Alegria J, Content A, Morais J. BELEC. Batterie d'évaluation du langage écrit et de ces troubles. Bruxelles: De Boeck; 1994.

37. Jacquier-Roux M, Valdois S, Zorman M, Lequette C, Pouget G. ODÉDYS Outil de DÉpistage des DYSlexies Version 2. Université Pierre Mendes France: Laboratoire de Psychologie et Neurocognition; 2009.

38. Tucker DM. Spatial sampling of head electrical fields: the geodesic sensor net. Electroencephalogr Clin Neurophysiol. 1993;87(3):154–63.

39. Plank M. Ocular correction ICA. In: Brain product press release 49: brain product press release 49; 2013. p. 1–4.

40. Lafontaine MP, Lacourse K, Lina JM, McIntosh AR, Gosselin F, Theoret H, Lippe S. Brain signal complexity rises with repetition suppression in visual learning. Neuroscience. 2016;326:1–9.

41. Ceponiene R, Rinne T, Näätänen R. Maturation of cortical sound processing as indexed by event-related potentials. Clin Neurophysiol. 2002;113(6):870–82.

42. Rigoulot S, Delplanque S, Despretz P, Defoort-Dhellemmes S, Honore J, Sequeira H. Peripherally presented emotional scenes: a spatiotemporal analysis of early ERP responses. Brain Topogr. 2008;20(4):216–23.

43. Rigoulot S, Fish K, Pell MD. Neural correlates of inferring speaker sincerity from white lies: an event-related potential source localization study. Brain Res. 2014;1565:48–62.

44. Spencer KM, Dien J, Donchin E. A componential analysis of the ERP elicited by novel events using a dense electrode array. Psychophysiology. 1999; 36(3):409–14.

45. Spencer KM, Dien J, Donchin E. Spatiotemporal analysis of the late ERP responses to deviant stimuli. Psychophysiology. 2001;38(2):343–58.

46. Pourtois G, Delplanque S, Michel C, Vuilleumier P. Beyond conventional event-related brain potential (ERP): exploring the time-course of visual emotion processing using topographic and principal component analyses. Brain Topogr. 2008;20(4):265–77.

47. Field A. Discovering statistics using IBM SPSS statistics. Thousand Oaks: Sage; 2013.

48. Kaushal N, Rhodes RE. Exercise habit formation in new gym members: a longitudinal study. J Behav Med. 2015;38(4):652–63.

49. Shek DT, Ma CM. Longitudinal data analyses using linear mixed models in SPSS: concepts, procedures and illustrations. ScientificWorldJournal. 2011;11:42–76.

50. West BT. Analyzing longitudinal data with the linear mixed models procedure in SPSS. Eval Health Prof. 2009;32(3):207–28.

51. Combrisson E, Jerbi K. Exceeding chance level by chance: the caveat of theoretical chance levels in brain signal classification and statistical assessment of decoding accuracy. J Neurosci Methods. 2015;250:126–36.

52. Rosburg T, Zimmerer K, Huonker R. Short-term habituation of auditory evoked potential and neuromagnetic field components in dependence of the interstimulus interval. Exp Brain Res. 2010;205(4):559–70.

53. Snyder KA, Keil A. Repetition suppression of induced gamma activity predicts enhanced orienting toward a novel stimulus in 6-month-old infants. J Cogn Neurosci. 2008;20(12):2137–52.

54. Colombo J, Mitchell DW. Infant visual habituation. Neurobiol Learn Mem. 2009;92(2):225–34.

55. Rankin CH, Abrams T, Barry RJ, Bhatnagar S, Clayton DF, Colombo J, Coppola G, Geyer MA, Glanzman DL, Marsland S, et al. Habituation revisited: an updated and revised description of the behavioral characteristics of habituation. Neurobiol Learn Mem. 2009;92(2):135–8.

56. Rose DH, Slater A, Perry H. Prediction of childhood intelligence from habituation in early infancy. Intelligence. 1986;10(3):251–63.

57. Budd TW, Barry RJ, Gordon E, Rennie C, Michie PT. Decrement of the N1 auditory event-related potential with stimulus repetition: habituation vs. refractoriness. Int J Psychophysiol. 1998;31(1):51–68.

58. Desimone R. Neural mechanisms for visual memory and their role in attention. Proc Natl Acad Sci U S A. 1996;93(24):13494–9.

59. Grill-Spector K, Henson R, Martin A. Repetition and the brain: neural models of stimulus-specific effects. Trends Cogn Sci. 2006;10(1):14–23.

60. Wiggs CL, Martin A. Properties and mechanisms of perceptual priming. Curr Opin Neurobiol. 1998;8(2):227–33.

61. Friston K. A theory of cortical responses. Philos Trans R Soc Lond Ser B Biol Sci. 2005;360(1456):815–36.

62. Summerfield C, Egner T, Greene M, Koechlin E, Mangels J, Hirsch J. Predictive codes for forthcoming perception in the frontal cortex. Science. 2006;314(5803):1311–4.

63. Baldeweg T. Repetition effects to sounds: evidence for predictive coding in the auditory system. Trends Cogn Sci. 2006;10(3):93–4.

64. Gibson JR, Bartley AF, Hays SA, Huber KM. Imbalance of neocortical excitation and inhibition and altered UP states reflect network hyperexcitability in the mouse model of fragile X syndrome. J Neurophysiol. 2008;100(5):2615–26.

65. Portera-Cailliau C. Which comes first in fragile X syndrome, dendritic spine dysgenesis or defects in circuit plasticity? Neuroscientist. 2012;18(1):28–44.

66. Irwin SA, Galvez R, Greenough WT. Dendritic spine structural anomalies in fragile-X mental retardation syndrome. Cereb Cortex. 2000;10(10):1038–44.

67. Irwin SA, Patel B, Idupulapati M, Harris JB, Crisostomo RA, Larsen BP, Kooy F, Willems PJ, Cras P, Kozlowski PB, et al. Abnormal dendritic spine characteristics in the temporal and visual cortices of patients with fragile-X syndrome: a quantitative examination. Am J Med Genet. 2001;98(2):161–7.

68. Deng PY, Rotman Z, Blundon JA, Cho Y, Cui J, Cavalli V, Zakharenko SS, Klyachko VA. FMRP regulates neurotransmitter release and synaptic information transmission by modulating action potential duration via BK channels. Neuron. 2013;77(4):696–711.

69. Hebert B, Pietropaolo S, Meme S, Laudier B, Laugeray A, Doisne N, Quartier A, Lefeuvre S, Got L, Cahard D, et al. Rescue of fragile X syndrome phenotypes in Fmr1 KO mice by a BKCa channel opener molecule. Orphanet J Rare Dis. 2014;9:124.

70. Typlt M, Mirkowski M, Azzopardi E, Ruettiger L, Ruth P, Schmid S. Mice with deficient BK channel function show impaired prepulse inhibition and spatial learning, but normal working and spatial reference memory. PLoS One. 2013;8(11):e81270.

71. Zhang Y, Bonnan A, Bony G, Ferezou I, Pietropaolo S, Ginger M, Sans N, Rossier J, Oostra B, LeMasson G, et al. Dendritic channelopathies contribute to neocortical and sensory hyperexcitability in Fmr1(-/y) mice. Nat Neurosci. 2014;17(12):1701–9.

72. Bar M, Kassam KS, Ghuman AS, Boshyan J, Schmid AM, Dale AM, Hamalainen MS, Marinkovic K, Schacter DL, Rosen BR, et al. Top-down facilitation of visual recognition. Proc Natl Acad Sci U S A. 2006;103(2):449–54.

73. O'Doherty J, Dayan P, Schultz J, Deichmann R, Friston K, Dolan RJ. Dissociable roles of ventral and dorsal striatum in instrumental conditioning. Science. 2004;304(5669):452–4.

74. Lafontaine MP, Theoret H, Gosselin F, Lippe S. Transcranial direct current stimulation of the dorsolateral prefrontal cortex modulates repetition suppression to unfamiliar faces: an ERP study. PLoS One. 2013;8(12):e81721.

75. Peng DX, Kelley RG, Quintin EM, Raman M, Thompson PM, Reiss AL. Cognitive and behavioral correlates of caudate subregion shape variation in fragile X syndrome. Hum Brain Mapp. 2014;35(6):2861–8.

76. Bosch SE, Jehee JF, Fernandez G, Doeller CF. Reinstatement of associative memories in early visual cortex is signaled by the hippocampus. J Neurosci. 2014;34(22):7493–500.

77. Hindy NC, Ng FY, Turk-Browne NB. Linking pattern completion in the hippocampus to predictive coding in visual cortex. Nat Neurosci. 2016;19(5):665–7.

78. Kok P, Jehee JF, de Lange FP. Less is more: expectation sharpens representations in the primary visual cortex. Neuron. 2012;75(2):265–70.

79. Molnar K, Keri S. Bigger is better and worse: on the intricate relationship between hippocampal size and memory. Neuropsychologia. 2014;56:73–8.

80. van der Molen MJ, Stam CJ, van der Molen MW. Resting-state EEG oscillatory dynamics in fragile X syndrome: abnormal functional connectivity and brain network organization. PLoS One. 2014;9(2):e88451.

81. Wang J, Ethridge LE, Mosconi MW, White SP, Binder DK, Pedapati EV, Erickson CA, Byerly MJ, Sweeney JA. A resting EEG study of neocortical hyperexcitability and altered functional connectivity in fragile X syndrome. J Neurodev Disord. 2017;9:11.

82. Abbeduto L, Brady N, Kover ST. Language development and fragile X syndrome: profiles, syndrome-specificity, and within-syndrome differences. Ment Retard Dev Disabil Res Rev. 2007;13(1):36–46.

83. Devitt NM, Gallagher L, Reilly RB. Autism spectrum disorder (ASD) and fragile X syndrome (FXS): two overlapping disorders reviewed through electroencephalography—what can be interpreted from the available information? Brain Sci. 2015;5(2):92–117.

84. Fox AM, Anderson M, Reid C, Smith T, Bishop DV. Maturation of auditory temporal integration and inhibition assessed with event-related potentials (ERPs). BMC Neurosci. 2010;11:49.

6

Delta rhythmicity is a reliable EEG biomarker in Angelman syndrome: a parallel mouse and human analysis

Michael S. Sidorov[1,2,3], Gina M. Deck[4,5,8], Marjan Dolatshahi[4,5], Ronald L. Thibert[4], Lynne M. Bird[6,7], Catherine J. Chu[4,5*] and Benjamin D. Philpot[1,2,3*]

Abstract

Background: Clinicians have qualitatively described rhythmic delta activity as a prominent EEG abnormality in individuals with Angelman syndrome, but this phenotype has yet to be rigorously quantified in the clinical population or validated in a preclinical model. Here, we sought to quantitatively measure delta rhythmicity and evaluate its fidelity as a biomarker.

Methods: We quantified delta oscillations in mouse and human using parallel spectral analysis methods and measured regional, state-specific, and developmental changes in delta rhythms in a patient population.

Results: Delta power was broadly increased and more dynamic in both the Angelman syndrome mouse model, relative to wild-type littermates, and in children with Angelman syndrome, relative to age-matched neurotypical controls. Enhanced delta oscillations in children with Angelman syndrome were present during wakefulness and sleep, were generalized across the neocortex, and were more pronounced at earlier ages.

Conclusions: Delta rhythmicity phenotypes can serve as reliable biomarkers for Angelman syndrome in both preclinical and clinical settings.

Keywords: Angelman syndrome, Biomarker, Delta, EEG, Mouse model, Outcome measure, UBE3A

Background

Angelman syndrome (AS) is a neurodevelopmental disorder characterized by developmental delay, impaired speech and motor skills, and high comorbidity with epilepsy [1]. Loss-of-function mutations in the maternal copy of the imprinted *UBE3A* gene cause AS [2, 3], while maternal duplications in the same region (15q11-13) are linked to autism [4–6]. Recent work has identified multiple approaches with preclinical therapeutic potential for AS: antisense oligonucleotides and topoisomerase inhibitors have the potential to unsilence paternal *UBE3A* and re-express UBE3A protein; gene therapy provides a direct method of expressing *UBE3A*; mechanism-based approaches downstream of *UBE3A* include GABA$_A$ agonists (THIP/gaboxadol) and modulation of αCaMKII; other approaches include altering diet [7–12]. Many of these approaches are in the pipeline for upcoming clinical trials. It is therefore critically important to develop biomarkers for AS that are clinically relevant, objectively quantifiable, highly penetrant, and have strong face validity between animal models and patient populations. Such biomarkers need not have predictive or diagnostic value, as AS diagnoses are confirmed genetically [13], but rather their value would lie primarily in their use as outcome measures.

Electroencephalography (EEG) has revealed consistent signatures of AS, which have been described by clinical reports and case studies spanning nearly 30 years [14–22]. EEG abnormalities in AS include rhythmic delta, rhythmic theta, and epileptiform spike-wave discharges. Increased delta rhythmicity is the most common EEG phenotype in AS (~84% of patients) [21], and of these phenotypes, it is the most specific for AS relative to other syndromes [20]. Multiple variants of delta activity have been described based on brain region and waveform characteristics [20], yet every

* Correspondence: cjchu@mgh.harvard.edu; bphilpot@med.unc.edu
[4]Department of Neurology, Massachusetts General Hospital, Boston, MA 02114, USA
[1]Department of Cell Biology and Physiology, University of North Carolina, Chapel Hill, NC 27599, USA
Full list of author information is available at the end of the article

variant of delta, by definition, has a common oscillation frequency of ~2–4 cycles per second. Clinical studies typically report delta abnormalities in a binary fashion, being present or absent, but in some cases have further subdivided delta abnormalities into being continuous or intermittent [17]. To date, no study has quantified delta rhythmicity in AS, quantitatively compared AS individuals to a neurotypical control group, or quantitatively tracked developmental and state-dependent (sleep/wake) changes in delta oscillations in AS. Principled characterization of these features, and validation in a mouse model, are critical for development of delta rhythms as a biomarker.

AS model mice ($Ube3a^{m-/p+}$) have genetic construct validity with the human condition and thus provide a powerful preclinical model. Silencing of the paternal $Ube3a$ allele is conserved from humans to mice; thus $Ube3a^{m-/p+}$ mice, like individuals with AS, have minimal functional UBE3A protein [23]. Using parallel quantitative methods, we analyzed delta rhythmicity in AS model mice and human EEG data. We found that increased delta power provides a robust and reliable biomarker with strong face validity between the AS mouse model and a patient population, 4–11 years old. Additionally, quantitative methods allowed for a novel study of delta "dynamics," a measure of how delta rhythms vary over time across a single recording session. Delta activity is more dynamic, both in AS mice and AS individuals. Children with AS exhibited enhanced delta activity across all EEG electrode placements. The enhanced delta power and dynamics were present during both wakefulness and sleep and were observed at all ages tested but most pronounced in younger children. Overall, this study corroborates qualitative clinical descriptions of delta oscillations in AS individuals [14–22], provides the first quantitative assessment of delta rhythmicity in AS individuals and comparison with a neurotypical reference group, and validates this biomarker in a mouse model. Delta rhythmicity thus has promise as a preclinical and clinical biomarker for AS and as an outcome measure for AS clinical trials.

Methods
Study design
Our prespecified goal was to quantify delta power in AS: first in a mouse model, then in a patient population. We refined analysis methods during mouse studies and used these parameters for subsequent human EEG data analysis. We allowed for the possibility that mouse studies would shift our area of interest to other frequencies (e.g., theta) that have also been reported as abnormal in AS [14, 17, 20, 21, 24]; however, because mouse studies confirmed delta abnormalities with largely normal power in other frequency bands, we entered human studies with the original prespecified hypothesis that delta power is increased. We became interested in a secondary experimental question—the dynamics of delta abnormalities in AS—during mouse studies. Therefore,

based on our mouse work (Figs. 1 and 2, Additional files 1: Figure S1 and 2: Figure S2) and clinical reports [14–22], we began human EEG studies with a clear hypothesis: delta power and dynamics are quantitatively increased in children with AS. We thus avoided problems with circularity and data selection that may arise when a study "fishes" for a phenotype with no predefined hypothesis [25].

Mouse studies were conducted on AS model mice ($Ube3a^{m-/p+}$) and wild-type littermate controls, with experimenters blind to genotype. Human studies were retrospective analyses of AS and neurotypical EEG data. Human subjects were children with a genetic diagnosis of AS who had EEGs between 2006 and 2014 at the San Diego site (Rady Children's Hospital San Diego: RCHSD) of the AS Natural History Study (ClinicalTrials.gov identifier: NCT00296764), and an age- and sex-matched sample of neurotypical controls who had EEGs at Massachusetts

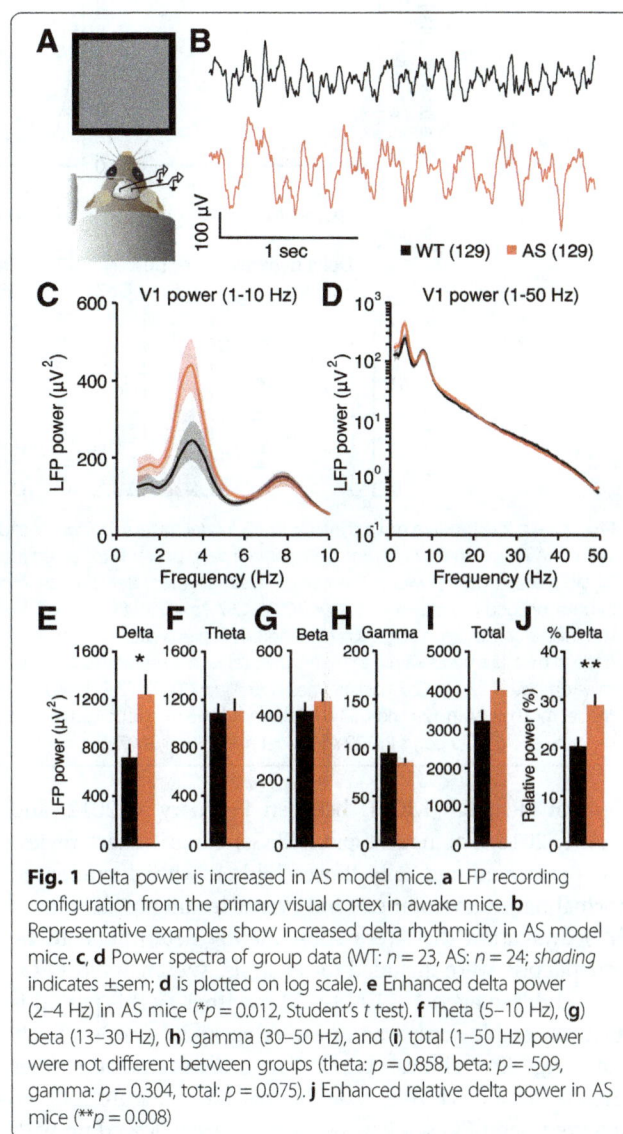

Fig. 1 Delta power is increased in AS model mice. **a** LFP recording configuration from the primary visual cortex in awake mice. **b** Representative examples show increased delta rhythmicity in AS model mice. **c, d** Power spectra of group data (WT: $n = 23$, AS: $n = 24$; shading indicates ±sem; **d** is plotted on log scale). **e** Enhanced delta power (2–4 Hz) in AS mice (*$p = 0.012$, Student's t test). **f** Theta (5–10 Hz), (**g**) beta (13–30 Hz), (**h**) gamma (30–50 Hz), and (**i**) total (1–50 Hz) power were not different between groups (theta: $p = 0.858$, beta: $p = .509$, gamma: $p = 0.304$, total: $p = 0.075$). **j** Enhanced relative delta power in AS mice (**$p = 0.008$)

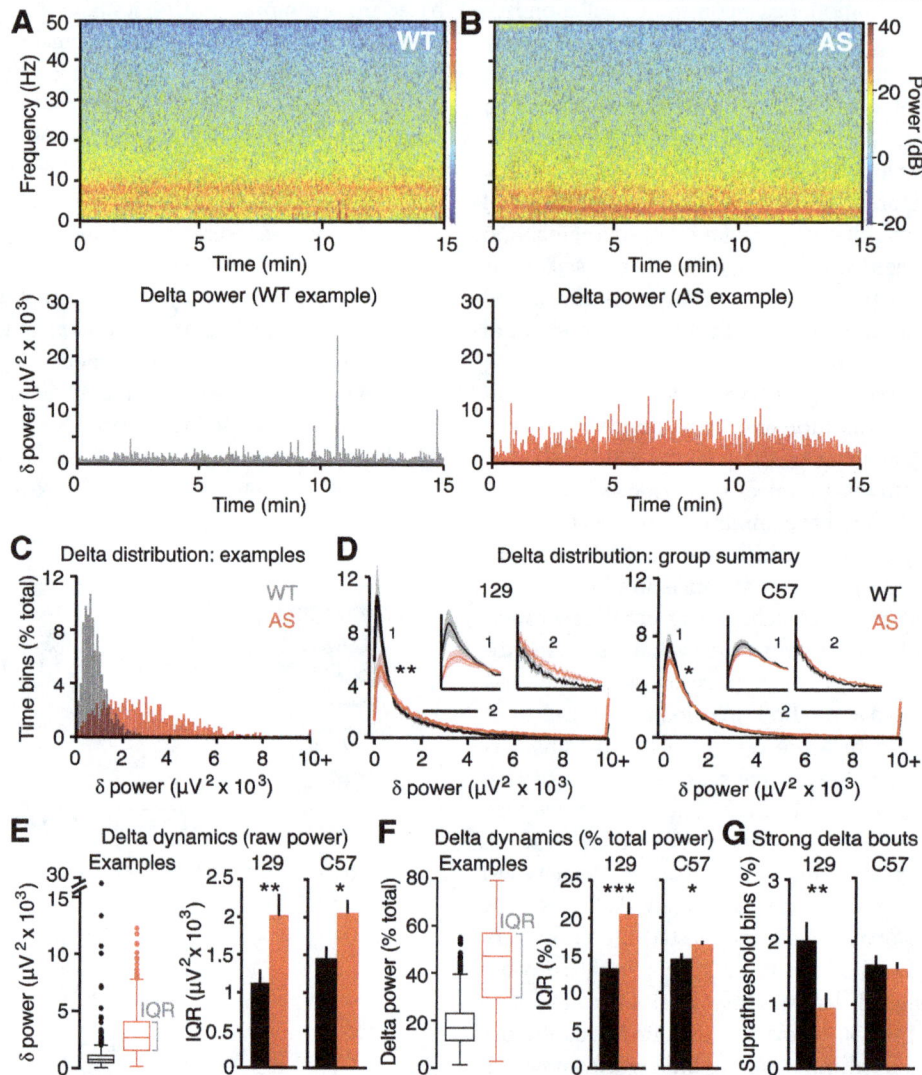

Fig. 2 Delta rhythms are more dynamic in AS model mice. **a, b** *Top*: spectrograms show rhythmicity across time in single LFP sessions in representative WT and AS mice on a 129 background. *Bottom*: delta power is extracted from the spectrogram during each 2-s time bin for representative examples. **c** Distributions of delta power across a single session for representative examples used in **a** and **b**. **d** Group analyses reveal differences in delta distributions in both 129 and C57 strains (129: *p = 0.0005, C57: *p = 0.0198, K-S tests). *Inset 1* spans (in $\mu V^2 \times 10^3$) 0–1 on the *x-axis*; *inset 2* spans 2–8. **e** Quantification of within-session delta dynamics. *Box plots* indicate representative examples used in **a** and **b**. Interquartile range (*IQR*) measures the spread of the middle 50% of delta measurements within a session. *Dots* represent suprathreshold bins where delta > Q3 + 1.5*IQR. Group analyses reveal increased IQR in AS model mice on both 129 and C57 backgrounds (129: **p = 0.0093, C57: *p = 0.010). **f** Calculating IQR based on relative delta power within each 2-s bin reveals AS model mice on both 129 and C57 backgrounds have increased within-session delta dynamics (129: ***p = 0.0008, C57: *p = 0.021). **g** There are fewer suprathreshold delta bouts in 129 AS model mice (**p = 0.007) but not C57 AS model mice (p = 0.74) compared to WT littermates

General Hospital (MGH) between February 1, 2012, and May 1, 2012. For neurotypical EEGs, clinical chart review was performed and only those children with documented normal neurodevelopment and events leading to diagnostic EEG evaluation that were subsequently determined to be nonepileptic were included for analysis. We analyzed EEGs from children aged 4–11 (48–132 months), as this period is relatively stable compared to earlier ages [26] and is a likely age range for clinical trials. For cross-sectional studies (Figs. 3, 4, and 5a, b, e, f, Additional file 3: Figure S3), we analyzed one EEG session per subject. We followed up with

longitudinal studies in a subset of children where multiple EEG sessions were available (Fig. 5c, d). In the longitudinal group, we analyzed two EEGs outside of our initial age parameters, both from children aged 11–12.

Because delta rhythms are a feature of slow-wave sleep and AS individuals have abnormal sleep patterns [1, 27], sleep during EEG sessions was a potential confounding variable. Therefore, an experienced clinical neurophysiologist manually categorized wake and non-REM sleep epochs using standard criteria [28]. We made AS versus neurotypical comparisons separately for periods of sleep and periods of wakefulness.

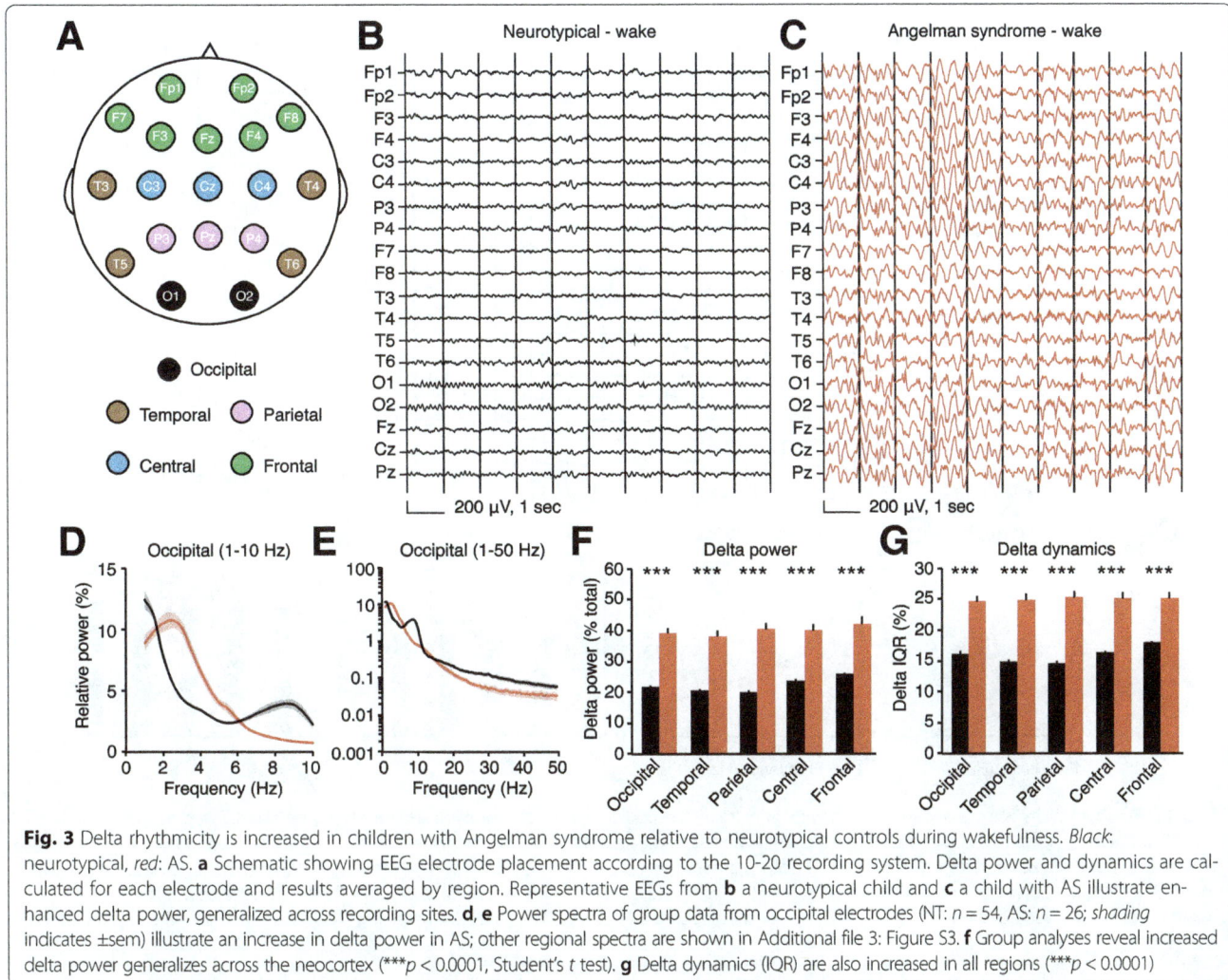

Fig. 3 Delta rhythmicity is increased in children with Angelman syndrome relative to neurotypical controls during wakefulness. *Black*: neurotypical, *red*: AS. **a** Schematic showing EEG electrode placement according to the 10-20 recording system. Delta power and dynamics are calculated for each electrode and results averaged by region. Representative EEGs from **b** a neurotypical child and **c** a child with AS illustrate enhanced delta power, generalized across recording sites. **d**, **e** Power spectra of group data from occipital electrodes (NT: $n = 54$, AS: $n = 26$; *shading* indicates ±sem) illustrate an increase in delta power in AS; other regional spectra are shown in Additional file 3: Figure S3. **f** Group analyses reveal increased delta power generalizes across the neocortex (***$p < 0.0001$, Student's t test). **g** Delta dynamics (IQR) are also increased in all regions (***$p < 0.0001$)

Our mouse sample size was determined a priori. Our retrospective human EEG sample sizes (wake and sleep) were determined by availability of de-identified data. All data exclusion criteria were defined prospectively for both mouse and human studies. For mouse studies, individual sessions were excluded (blind to genotype) only in rare cases where a headcap detached during a recording session or where movement artifacts were continuous and pervasive. Outliers in which total raw power (1–50 Hz) exceeded 2 SD from the group mean were excluded (number of outliers per group—129/WT, 2/25; 129/AS, 0/24; C57/WT, 1/31; C57/AS, 1/40). For human studies, individual electrodes were excluded in cases of excessive noise or poor connections. EEG recordings with less than 100 s of sleep or wake were excluded [29].

Mouse LFP methods
Animals
All mouse protocols were approved by the Institutional Animal Care and Use Committee of the University of North Carolina at Chapel Hill. Mice were group-housed on a 12:12 light/dark cycle with ad libitum access to food and water. Male and female mice were used for experiments in equal genotypic ratios. Female $Ube3a^{m+/p-}$ × male $Ube3a^{m+/p+}$ breeders generated littermate experimental $Ube3a^{m-/p+}$ (AS) and $Ube3a^{m+/p+}$ wild-type (WT) mice. We maintained separate 129 and C57BL/6 colonies, each congenic for 10+ generations. Ype Elgersma (Erasmus Medical Center) provided the 129 mice, and Jackson Labs (Bar Harbor, ME) provided the C57BL/6 mice (JAX #: 016590).

Surgeries and LFP recordings
Surgery and local field potential (LFP) recordings were conducted as previously described [30], with only minor modifications. We anesthetized adult mice and implanted tungsten microelectrodes (FHC) bilaterally in layer 4 of the primary visual cortex (coordinates relative to lambda, in mm, 0 A/P, +3.2–3.3 M/L, –0.47 D/V). We implanted a silver ground wire in the cerebellum and head-fixed mice using a steel headpost attached to

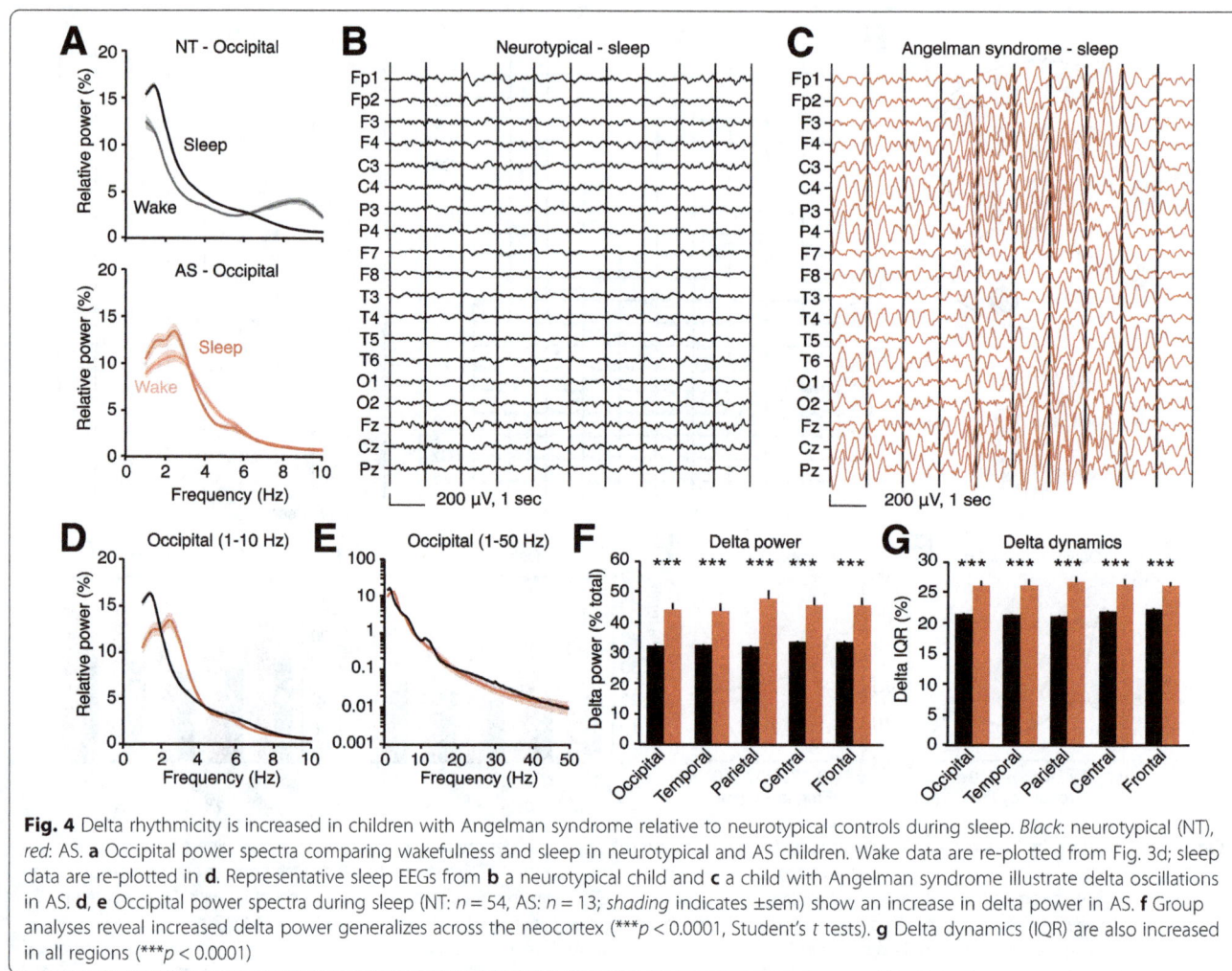

Fig. 4 Delta rhythmicity is increased in children with Angelman syndrome relative to neurotypical controls during sleep. *Black*: neurotypical (NT), *red*: AS. **a** Occipital power spectra comparing wakefulness and sleep in neurotypical and AS children. Wake data are re-plotted from Fig. 3d; sleep data are re-plotted in **d**. Representative sleep EEGs from **b** a neurotypical child and **c** a child with Angelman syndrome illustrate delta oscillations in AS. **d, e** Occipital power spectra during sleep (NT: $n = 54$, AS: $n = 13$; *shading* indicates ±sem) show an increase in delta power in AS. **f** Group analyses reveal increased delta power generalizes across the neocortex (***$p < 0.0001$, Student's t tests). **g** Delta dynamics (IQR) are also increased in all regions (***$p < 0.0001$)

the skull anterior to the bregma. Electrodes and head-posts were held in place by headcaps made from dental cement (Metabond). Following surgeries, mice recovered for at least 2 days prior to 2 days of habituation (15 min) to the recording apparatus. We then recorded LFP continuously for 15 min on three consecutive days following habituation. Mice were head-fixed during all recordings and viewed a static gray screen in an otherwise dark, quiet environment. We amplified data 1000× using single-channel amplifiers (Grass Technologies), digitized data using a Micro 1401 digitizer (CED), and acquired data at 4 kHz using Spike2 software (CED). We applied analog 0.1-Hz high-pass and 100-Hz low-pass filtration during data acquisition and digital 1-Hz high-pass filtration (second-order Butterworth) after data acquisition. The roll-off of the high-pass Butterworth filter did not impinge onto the delta range of interest (2–4 Hz). Ages of mice on the first day of LFP recording ranged from P85 to P114 and averaged 94.0 ± 1.2 days (129) and 100.0 ± 0.8 days (C57).

LFP analysis

Sample size ("n") represents the number of mice. For each mouse, we averaged processed data from the left and right hemispheres within a session, then averaged results across three sessions. For sessions with movement artifacts, we selected the longest continuous period with no artifacts present for analysis. We analyzed spectral power using a fast Fourier transform (FFT) of the continuous signal, resulting in frequency bins of 0.5 Hz. We determined relative power by expressing power in a given frequency band as a percentage of the total power between 1 and 50 Hz. A disadvantage of using relative power is that by definition, total power must summate to 100%, so a genotype difference in one frequency band (e.g., delta) may also manifest as relative genotype differences in other frequency bands (see "Results"). Thus, it is difficult to appropriately assess differences in relative power in frequency bands other than delta (Additional file 2: Figure S2). We defined delta as 2–4 Hz, theta as 5–10 Hz, beta as 13–30 Hz, and gamma as 30–50 Hz.

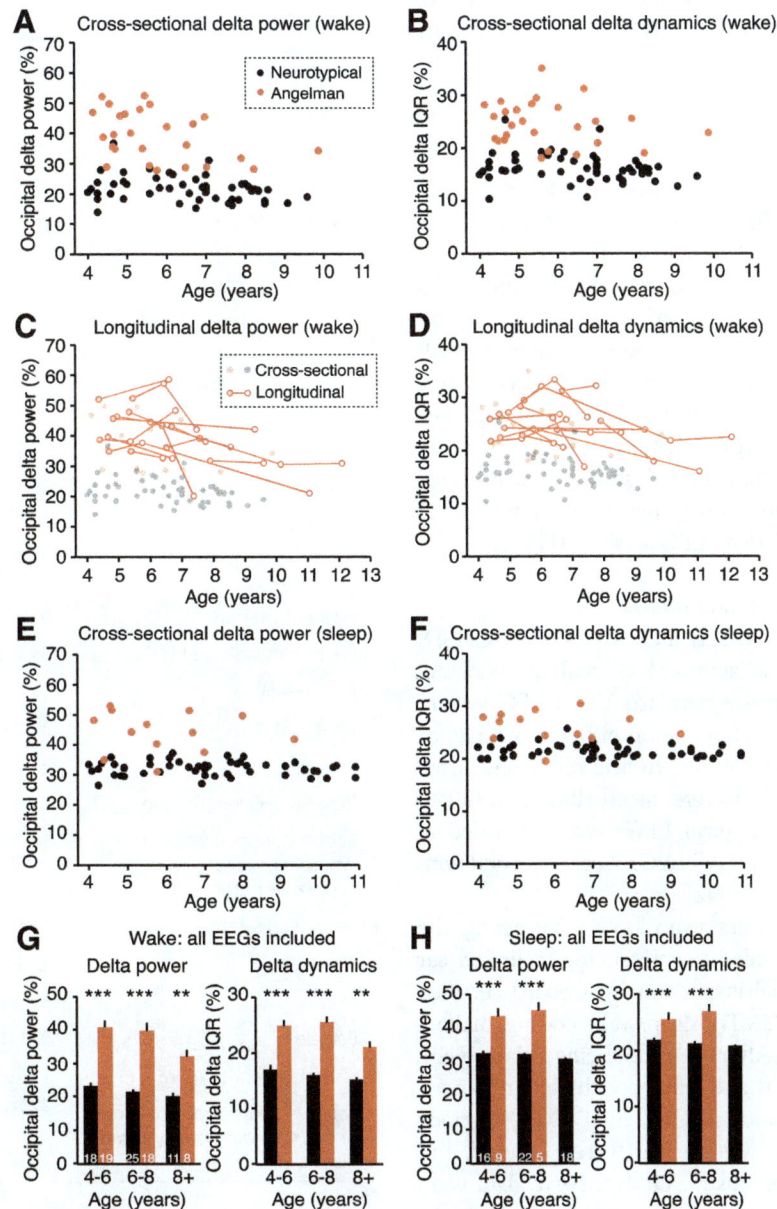

Fig. 5 Delta phenotypes are stronger at earlier ages in children with Angelman syndrome. **a** Increased occipital delta power in children with AS is age-dependent during wakefulness (NT: $n = 54$, AS: $n = 26$). **b** Occipital delta dynamics as a function of age in neurotypical and AS children. Longitudinal studies in a subset of AS patients show that **c** delta power and **d** delta dynamics decrease as a function of age ($n = 12$ children, $n = 31$ sessions). **e** Delta power during sleep (NT: $n = 54$, AS: $n = 13$) and **f** delta dynamics during sleep do not show statistical age dependence. **g**, **h** Analysis of grouped cross-sectional and longitudinal occipital delta power and dynamics during wakefulness and sleep. **g** Delta power during wakefulness was increased in AS at ages 4–6, 6–8, and 8+ (two-way ANOVA and post hoc Bonferroni: ***$p < 0.0001$, **$p = 0.0002$). Delta dynamics (IQR) during wakefulness were increased in AS at ages 4–6, 6–8, and 8+ (***$p < 0.0001$, **$p = 0.0007$). Sample sizes are represented in *bars*. **h** Delta power and dynamics during sleep were increased in AS at ages 4–6 and 6–8 (***$p < 0.0001$)

For each LFP electrode, we assessed delta dynamics (Fig. 2) by quantifying the spread of delta power in all 2-s bins with a 1-s overlap. We generated box plots of raw and relative delta power using 2-s bins for the duration of each recording and quantified three parameters: mean, interquartile range (IQR), and outliers, defined as Q1 – 1.5*IQR or Q3 + 1.5*IQR. Mean delta power calculated by averaging

bins was statistically indistinguishable from delta power calculated by FFT on the entire signal (mean of bins—WT, $20.0 \pm 2.2\%$; AS, $29.0 \pm 2.4\%$; FFT of the entire signal—WT, $20.3 \pm 2.0\%$; AS, $28.9 \pm 2.3\%$, represented in Fig. 1j). IQR represents the spread between the middle 50% of delta measurements, and we used this as a readout of within-session delta dynamics. Suprathreshold outliers represent bouts of "strong delta." We wrote custom MATLAB scripts to analyze delta dynamics and used Spike2 software for basic spectral analyses.

Human EEG methods
Data sources
All EEG studies and analyses were performed with institutional review board (IRB) approval. We analyzed EEGs from 28 children with AS (14 males, 14 females) and 72 neurotypical controls (42 males, 30 females). During EEGs, 26/28 AS individuals had periods of wake and 13/28 had periods of sleep. During EEGs, 54/72 neurotypical individuals had periods of wake and 54/72 had periods of sleep. These samples (Table 1) represent the cross-sectional data analyzed in Fig. 3 (wake), Fig. 4 (sleep), Additional file 3: Figure S3, and Fig. 5a, b, e, f. For longitudinal studies, we analyzed repeat EEGs from 12 AS individuals, resulting in a total of 45 wake EEG sessions and 15 sleep EEG sessions (Fig. 5c, d).

Data acquisition, processing, and analysis
Both neurotypical EEGs (MGH) and AS EEGs (RCHSD) were performed using the standard clinical method. All data were recorded using the standard 10-20 EEG system using a common physical reference on either Bio-Logic or Xltek systems. The location of the physical reference varied between sites; therefore, we re-referenced all data to linked ears ((A1 + A2) / 2). Neurotypical EEGs were recorded at 200, 250, 500, or 512 Hz, and AS EEGs were recorded with a sampling rate of 256 or 512 Hz.

We processed all raw data from both sites using the same pipeline, which included re-referencing to linked ear reference, filtering, manual inspection by a board-certified neurophysiologist (CJC, GMD), sleep/wake coding, artifact removal, and analysis. After re-referencing, data were broken into sleep (NREM) and wake epochs by an experienced clinical neurophysiologist (CJC, GMD, MD). Periods in which wake/sleep state was unclear were excluded, and periods of REM sleep were also excluded. Next, data were digitally filtered (second-order Butterworth): 1-Hz high-pass, 100-Hz low-pass, and 60-Hz notch. Movement artifacts were manually marked and excluded. We used EEGLAB [31] as a viewer to assess sleep state and identify artifacts. Observers were not blind to genotype during EEG inspection, sleep/wake coding, and artifact removal.

After processing, we used custom MATLAB scripts to analyze all data. Neurotypical and AS EEGs were batch-processed using the same programs at the same time. We slightly modified scripts from mouse LFP analysis for human EEG analysis. For each of 19 recording electrodes, we generated power spectra and calculated delta power and delta dynamics. We group-averaged results from neighboring electrodes to assess delta phenotypes by region (Fig. 3a): occipital (O1, O2), temporal (T3, T4, T5, T6), parietal (P3, Pz, P4), central (C3, Cz, C4), and frontal (Fp1, Fp2, F3, Fz,

Table 1 Characteristics of study subjects

	Neurotypical	Angelman
Total patients	72	28
Age (years)	7.0 ± 0.2	5.8 ± 0.3
Male	42 (58%)	14 (50%)
Female	30 (42%)	14 (50%)
Molecular diagnosis	N/A	Class 1 deletion: 7 Class 2 deletion: 10 UBE3A mutation: 6 Atypical deletion: 2 Uniparental disomy: 1 Imprinting defect: 1 Abnormal DNA methylation, negative for deletion: 1
History of seizures	0 (0%)	26 (93%)
Patients with wake in EEG	54 (75%)	26 (93%)
Age (years)	6.6 ± 0.3	5.8 ± 0.3
Male	30 (56%)	14 (54%)
Female	24 (44%)	12 (46%)
Wakeful EEG length (min)	7.9 ± 1.0	18.2 ± 2.3
Seizures under control at time of first recording or no seizure history	54 (100%)	24 (92%)
Patients with sleep in EEG	54 (75%)	13 (46%)
Age (years)	7.1 ± 0.3	6.0 ± 0.4
Male	32 (59%)	8 (62%)
Female	22 (41%)	5 (38%)
Sleep EEG length (min)	13.6 ± 0.8	22.0 ± 2.4
Seizures under control at time of first recording or no seizure history	54 (100%)	12 (92%)

F4, F8). We quantified relative power in all human data analyses to account for variability in the amplitude of raw signals (higher variability than seen in mouse). Sleep/wake coding and artifact removal resulted in noncontinuous signals. We did not concatenate processed signals together; instead, we analyzed all 2-s bins (with 1-s overlap) of active signal. We averaged spectra and delta power from all active bins. This approach diverged slightly from mouse LFP analysis, where we performed spectral analysis on the continuous signal. However, as noted above, adapting these methods to mice resulted in no change in the values of delta.

Statistical analysis
In mouse, we compared power (raw or relative, as noted) in a given band of interest (delta, gamma, etc.) using Student's

t tests (Fig. 1e–i, Additional files 1: Figure S1C, D and 2: Figure S2D–J). We compared group delta distributions using a Kolmogorov-Smirnov (K-S) test (Fig. 2f). We assessed delta dynamics (IQR) and the number of strong delta bouts using Student's *t* tests (Fig. 2g–i). In human, we compared delta power and delta dynamics (IQR) within each region using Student's *t* tests (Figs. 3f, g and 4f, g). We assessed the effects of age and genotype on delta power and dynamics in a cross-sectional sample using a two-way ANOVA with age (as a continuous measure) and genotype as factors (Fig. 5a, b, e, f). As there was a significant main effect of age on delta power in the total sample, we used a post hoc one-way ANOVA with age (as a continuous measure) as a factor to the age dependence of delta power within the AS group (Fig. 5a). We assessed the effect of age on delta in a longitudinal sample using a linear mixed model examining the fixed main effect of age on either power or dynamics, including the random effect of age nested in each subject in order to account for individual differences in the ages and age intervals of each repeated measure (Fig 5c, d). We assessed the effects of age and genotype in a combined sample containing all EEG sessions using a two-way ANOVA with age and genotype as factors; we used Bonferroni tests to make post hoc comparisons between groups within each age range (Fig. 5g, h). We used GraphPad Prism and JMP software (SAS) to perform statistical analyses.

Results

Angelman syndrome model mice have increased delta power

We previously showed that deletion of *Ube3a* from GABAergic neurons, but not glutamatergic neurons, increased delta rhythmicity and caused an exaggerated increase in seizure susceptibility compared to AS model mice with pan-cellular loss of the maternal *Ube3a* allele ($Ube3a^{m-/p+}$) [30]. While these studies provided insights into the importance of *Ube3a* loss in GABAergic neurons to hyperexcitability phenotypes in AS, it is critically important to fully assess whether $Ube3a^{m-/p+}$ mice accurately reflect clinical EEG phenotypes and to establish objective measures in both the preclinical mouse model and the clinical AS population. Towards this goal, we first quantified delta in $Ube3a^{m-/p+}$ mice and wild-type littermate controls ($Ube3a^{m+/p+}$). Because delta rhythmicity was reported to be strong in the occipital cortex in humans with AS [20, 21], we implanted electrodes into layer 4 of the primary visual cortex and recorded local field potentials (LFPs) (Fig. 1a). Direct brain implantation distinguishes LFP recordings from traditional scalp EEG and provides a more accurate reflection of local neural activity [32]. To approximate a resting state, we recorded LFP in awake, head-fixed mice viewing a static gray screen in a dark, quiet environment to which they were previously habituated. We compared AS model mice to wild-type littermates separately in two commonly used mouse strains in AS research: 129 and C57BL/6.

AS model mice on a 129 background showed enhanced delta (2–4 Hz) power (Fig. 1b–e). Genotypic differences in LFP power were restricted to the delta band (Fig. 1f–i). LFP power within a band of interest is often represented as a fraction of total power (relative power), and we found that relative delta power was also significantly increased in AS model mice (Fig. 1j). However, for other frequency bands, genotypic differences in relative power must be interpreted with caution: because total power must summate to 100%, increases in delta (which normally accounts for a dispro-portionate ~20% of total power) may also manifest in artifactual or misleading relative power differences in other bands. For example, AS model mice displayed statistically decreased relative theta and relative gamma power (Additional file 1: Figure S1), despite normal raw power in these bands. Therefore, raw and relative analyses of delta power may be interchangeable in AS model mice, but group differences in relative power outside of delta can be misleading if delta itself shows group differences.

Delta power in the primary visual cortex was not significantly different between WT and AS mice on a C57BL/6 background (Additional file 2: Figure S2A–F). AS mice showed a trend towards increased raw power in the 3–5 Hz range (Additional file 2: Figure S2G) and a statistically significant increase in relative 3–5 Hz power (Additional file 2: Figure S2H). Total power (1–50 Hz) was not different as a function of genotype (Additional file 2: Figure S2I). Surprisingly, gamma power (both raw and relative) was decreased in AS mice on a C57 background (Additional file 2: Figure S2J, K). Beta power (both raw and relative) were not different as a function of genotype (Additional file 2: Figure S2L, M).

Angelman syndrome model mice exhibit more dynamic delta oscillations

We sought to understand the nature of increased delta power in AS model mice. Broadly, the overall increase in delta power in AS could be driven by (a) short bouts of very strong delta, (b) a consistent moderate increase in delta, or (c) a more complex pattern. We thus quantified the distribution of delta power across time within individual recordings. First, we quantified delta power during every 2-s window of continuous LFP recordings (Fig. 2a, b) and analyzed the distribution of these measurements (Fig. 2c, d). On both 129 and C57 backgrounds, WT and AS mice had statistically different distributions of delta power over time, with AS distributions shifted towards having more periods of stronger delta. However, this approach—group averaging of individual delta distributions—is unable to determine whether group differences between WT and AS are driven by within-animal differences or across-animal differences. Therefore, we assessed delta variability, or dynamics, within single recording sessions. Within each session, we represented delta power in every 2-s window as a box plot. We quantified delta dynamics in two ways: (1) interquartile range (IQR), as a proxy for the range of "typical" delta, and (2) fraction of suprathreshold bins (where threshold = Q3 + 1.5*IQR), as a way to assess the amount of "strong" delta bouts (Fig. 2e, f). AS mice showed increased IQR, indicating that delta power is more dynamic within a session. Delta was more dynamic in AS mice on both 129 and C57 backgrounds, using both raw and relative power as measures (Fig. 2e, f). There was no increase in the number of strong delta bouts in AS mice on either background (Fig. 2g), indicating that delta power phenotypes in AS model mice were not driven by discrete bouts of abnormally strong delta oscillations. There were actually fewer strong delta bouts in AS mice relative to WT, but this was likely driven by increased IQR in these mice, resulting in a higher threshold for defining a strong bout. Overall, we found that delta power was more variable across time (i.e., "dynamic") within single recording sessions in AS model mice.

Children with Angelman syndrome exhibit enhanced delta power and dynamics

Employing similar methods used to quantify mouse LFPs, we compared delta power and dynamics from retrospective clinical EEGs in children with AS and age-matched neurotypical controls. EEG recordings contained periods of both wakefulness and sleep, presenting a potential confound. Children with AS have severe sleep disturbances [1], potentially biasing their EEG recordings towards wakefulness. Indeed, 15/47 total EEGs from AS individuals included periods of sleep (32%), while 54/72 total EEGs from neurotypical individuals included periods of sleep (75%). Because enhanced delta is a signature of slow-wave sleep [33], we separately analyzed EEG in wake and sleep states between groups. Another potential confound was the high incidence of epilepsy (80-95%) in AS patient populations [1]. In our sample, 26/28 AS individuals (93%) had a history of seizures (1 no seizures, 1 unknown), and no neurotypical individuals had a history of seizures (Table 1; for raw data, see Additional file 4). However, most (24/26) children with a history of seizures were on at least one medication at the time of their first EEG, and most (24/26) children's seizures were under control at the time of their first EEG (1 with persistent seizures, 1 unknown).

We quantified delta power and dynamics for each EEG electrode and group-averaged neighboring electrodes by region (Fig. 3a). During wakefulness, children with AS ($n = 26$) showed strongly increased delta power and delta dynamics relative to neurotypical controls ($n = 54$) (Fig. 3b–g; Additional files 3: Figure S3 and 5: Figure S4A–C). Delta power and dynamics were increased in every spatially defined region, suggesting

that delta phenotypes generalize across the neocortex. While delta phenotypes were present across all recording areas in group-averaged data, individual recordings did show some spatially restricted delta bouts (Additional file 5: Figure S4D–F). As expected, periods of manually identified sleep showed increased delta power relative to periods of wakefulness in both AS and neurotypical children (Fig. 4a; compare Figs. 3f and 4f). During sleep, delta power and dynamics were increased in children with AS ($n = 13$) relative to neurotypical controls ($n = 54$) in all regions (Fig. 4b–g; Additional file 3: Figure S3). Manual inspection of traces revealed that our sample included other EEG signatures, such as "notched" delta (Additional file 5: Figure S4G–I), that have been previously reported in children with AS [20]. As some antiepileptic medications are known to cause EEG slowing [34], we confirmed that the two children with AS not taking medication displayed elevated delta power (awake occipital relative delta power in NT, $21.7 \pm 0.6\%$; in AS, $39.3 \pm 1.6\%$; in child 1, age 4, 49.6%; in child 2, age 5, 52.1%). Thus, it is not likely that delta phenotypes in children with AS were caused by antiepileptic medications.

Delta power in Angelman syndrome is age-dependent

Our initial sample (analyzed in Figs. 3 and 4) included one EEG session per child, age 4–11. This cross-sectional sample showed an age-dependent decrease in occipital delta power during wakefulness, independent of genotype (Fig. 5a; two-way ANOVA, main effect of genotype: $p < 0.0001$, main effect of age: $p = 0.0011$). Occipital delta power decreased with age in children with AS ($p = 0.041$, post hoc test); this result supports qualitative clinical observations from a sample of children with AS ranging in age from 0.4 to 25 years [21]. However, there was no statistical difference in delta power trajectories between AS and neurotypical groups (genotype × age interaction: $p = 0.0801$). Occipital delta dynamics during wakefulness (Fig. 5b) also varied with genotype ($p < 0.001$), though there was not a statistically significant effect of age on dynamics ($p = 0.069$) or an interaction between genotype and age ($p = 0.769$).

If delta phenotypes are to be a useful biomarker in AS, they must remain stable or follow a predictable developmental trajectory within subjects. We thus quantified delta power and dynamics longitudinally in a subset of AS individuals from the original sample, where follow-up EEG recordings were available. We analyzed longitudinal EEGs (two to four per child) from 13/28 children, spanning up to 7 years. Twelve of 13 children had multiple recordings with periods of wakefulness; only two of 13 had multiple recordings with periods of sleep. Within subjects, there was a significant main effect of age on delta power during wakefulness ($p < 0.0001$), confirming that individuals showed developmental trajectories of reduced delta in line with cross-sectional data (Fig. 5c). Longitudinal assessment also revealed a significant main effect of age on delta dynamics (IQR) in children with AS ($p = 0.0003$; Fig. 5d). During sleep, cross-sectional analyses revealed that delta power in AS individuals was not significantly age-dependent (Fig. 5e; two-way ANOVA, main effect of genotype: $p < 0.0001$, main effect of age: $p = 0.458$, genotype × age interaction: $p = 0.658$). Additionally, delta dynamics during sleep were not significantly age-dependent (Fig. 5f; main effect of genotype: $p < 0.0001$, main effect of age: $p = 0.259$, genotype × age interaction: $p = 0.645$).

Overall, cross-sectional and longitudinal analyses indicated that during wakefulness, delta phenotypes in AS were more pronounced at earlier ages. We next sought to determine whether enhanced delta rhythms persisted in older children despite the developmental trajectory in AS individuals towards reduced delta. Overall, we compared 44 awake EEGs from 26 children with AS (combined cross-sectional and longitudinal data) to 54 wake EEGs, one per neurotypical child, and assessed delta phenotypes in three age ranges (in years): 4–6, 6–8, and 8+. During wakefulness, delta power and delta dynamics were significantly increased at all ages in children with AS (Fig. 5g). During sleep (AS: $n = 15$ sessions from 13 children; NT: $n = 54$ sessions, one per child), delta power and dynamics were significantly increased at age 4–6 and age 6–8; we analyzed only one sleep EEG from a child with AS older than 8 (Fig. 5h).

Discussion

Rhythmic delta is the most pervasive EEG abnormality in AS, but delta phenotypes have not been previously quantified. If delta oscillations are to be an effective biomarker, quantitative methods are required to track acute or longitudinal changes in rhythmicity. Here, we used spectral analyses to confirm that delta abnormalities in AS model mice mirror clinical reports from the AS patient population (Fig. 1). Using similar methods, we quantified robust delta phenotypes in children with AS across the neocortex during wake and sleep (Figs. 3 and 4), showing that the enhanced delta phenotype scales in a state-dependent manner. The enhanced delta activity in AS individuals followed a predictable developmental trajectory across subjects and within subjects (Fig. 5). While delta phenotypes were stronger at earlier ages, they persisted in all age groups tested (4–11 years), demonstrating that delta activity may be useful as a longitudinal biomarker, in addition to its utility as an acute biomarker in young children. Spectral analyses revealed increased dynamics, or variability, of delta oscillations within single sessions in both AS model mice and children with AS (Figs. 2 and 4). This phenotype had not been described in a patient population

and would be difficult to visualize and assess clinically without quantitative methods.

With multiple approaches currently being developed for clinical trials in AS, reliable and robust biomarkers are needed. Characteristics of a strong disease biomarker also include face validity and evidence for reversibility in a mouse model. Here, we showed that abnormal delta rhythmicity is conserved between mouse models and patient populations in AS, and prior work showed that increased delta power may be reversed in AS model mice by embryonic reinstatement of the UBE3A protein in a subset of neurons [30]. To date, phenotypic behaviors have been characterized in AS model mice with varying reliability [35] and include sensory, motor, and learning impairments [11, 23]. Taken together, mouse behavioral phenotypes generally resemble human symptoms, but their direct face validity is limited and, thus, are not ideal biomarkers. One exception to this rule is seizures, which may be robustly and reliably induced in AS mouse models [23, 30]. However, the use of seizures as a biomarker in AS children is limited; seizures are typically treated with antiepileptic medications and are controlled to a great extent in the majority of children [36]. Delta rhythmicity represents a robust, reliable biomarker with strong face validity between mouse models and patient populations.

We observed strain differences in delta phenotypes in AS model mice: delta power (2–4 Hz) was increased in AS on a 129 background (Fig. 1), but not on a C57BL/6 background (Additional file 2: Figure S2), despite a trend towards increased power in the 3–5-Hz band. Despite statistically normal delta power, AS model mice on a C57BL/6 background did show increased delta dynamics (Fig. 2). Thus, while delta power phenotypes may be strain-specific, abnormal delta dynamics are preserved across two commonly used strains for AS research. Strain differences in delta power are not surprising, as behavioral differences have also been noted between AS mice on 129 and C57BL/6 backgrounds [35].

Quantitative assessment of retrospective human EEG data revealed a robust increase in delta power in children with AS. These results support clinical reports [14–22], and our data validate the utility of quantifying delta activity pre- and post-intervention to track acute and sustained consequences of therapeutic interventions. Spectral analyses also address the nature of delta abnormalities in AS in a manner not possible by clinician review. Our study of within-session delta dynamics revealed that delta oscillations are more variable in AS, but are not confined to intermittent bouts.

Clinically, delta abnormalities have been observed in both posterior (73% of patients) and anterior (59%) regions [21], with potential differences in the type of delta seen by region [37]. We found that delta phenotypes (increased power and dynamics) generalized across the neocortex in a large sample (Figs. 3 and 4). However, spatially restricted runs of delta were observed within individual recordings (Additional file 5: Figure S4). Additionally, while spectral analyses provide an unbiased method to quantify power within a band of interest, a disadvantage of their use is an inability to dissociate subtle variants of delta, such as notched delta (Additional file 5: Figure S4), which have been noted in clinical studies of AS [17, 20, 22]. Thus, spectral analyses are best suited for quantifying broad delta biomarkers. We chose to focus on delta rhythmicity because it is the most common EEG abnormality in AS and the most specific abnormality to AS relative to related disorders [20, 24]. However, interictal epileptiform discharges and theta abnormalities have also been widely reported [14, 17, 20, 21, 38]. Epileptiform discharges are typically coincident with rhythmic delta [37] and are therefore likely captured by using delta power as a biomarker; our analyses did not distinguish epileptiform discharges in the 2–4-Hz frequency band from background delta rhythms. Increased theta (~4–6 Hz in human) has been noted in ~30–60% of children with AS (Additional file 5: Figure S4), but is age-dependent and rarely observed beyond age 8 [17, 20, 21]. Thus, we were not surprised to see normal theta in adult AS model mice (Fig. 1, Additional file 2: Figure S2). Quantitative assessment of theta and other bands in human EEG data were complicated by our a priori hypothesis that delta is increased and by the limits imposed by quantifying relative power (see "Results" or "Methods").

Enhanced delta rhythmicity is a signature of slow-wave sleep, and our quantification confirmed that delta rhythms are indeed increased in neurotypical individuals during sleep epochs (Fig. 4). In AS individuals, delta rhythms are also increased during sleep relative to wakefulness, and thus, the enhanced delta phenotypes are preserved and scaled with state changes. These data show that it is critical to identify and separate wakeful and sleep epochs during EEG recordings but that delta remains an effective biomarker when making state-specific comparisons. Enhanced delta does not appear to broadly disrupt sleep architecture. Children with AS show typical sleep architecture such as sleep spindles and vertex waves. While there may be some disruption in sleep architecture, these appear to be minor compared to the significant effects of sleep-activated discharges on sleep architecture.

In addition to generalizing across sleep and wake, delta phenotypes in AS are also present across childhood development. We found a developmental reduction in delta power in AS; however, delta phenotypes persisted in all age ranges tested, to 12 years (Fig. 5). Thus, delta remains a valid biomarker throughout childhood and may be used as interventions and clinical trials are likely

to occur in children of all ages. It is not clear whether the developmental attenuation of delta phenotypes is directly linked to loss of UBE3A. The attenuation of delta activity may be related to a secondary feature of AS, such as improvements in epilepsy and sleep at older ages [39]. It is also not yet known how delta phenotypes correlate with clinical features of AS such as epilepsy severity, sleep, and behavioral, cognitive, and motor impairments. However, in mice, cell type-specific manipulations of UBE3A that increase delta power also increase seizure susceptibility, and those that do not affect delta also do not affect seizures [30].

Our work represents the first direct comparison of EEGs from children with AS and neurotypical controls. However, an inherent limit of our retrospective EEG analyses was that AS data and neurotypical data were gathered at two different sites. We processed and analyzed all data in parallel and were encouraged by the robustness of phenotypes, but future prospective studies should be designed to recruit AS and control patients to a single site. In addition, intellectual disability in children with AS presents a potential confound, as EEG slowing has been associated with cognitive impairment in several populations [40, 41]. Future work comparing AS to other reference groups (i.e., nonsyndromic seizure, intellectual disability, autism) will be critical to understanding the extent to which other disorders may exhibit delta phenotypes. AS may be considered an autism-like disorder, as a subset of children with AS also meet the diagnostic criteria for autism [42–44]. Quantitative EEG methods have characterized some spectral and coherence phenotypes in nonsyndromic autism [29, 45–51], yet the genetic heterogeneity of nonsyndromic autism introduces challenges in finding common EEG biomarkers. However, recent work has identified EEG signatures of Dup15q syndrome, a syndromic form of autism caused by duplication of the 15q11-13 genetic region which includes *UBE3A* [4–6]. The most profound EEG abnormality in Dup15q is increased beta rhythmicity, which is normal in AS model mice (Fig. 1, Additional files 1: Figure S1 and 2: Figure S2), but decreased delta power has also been noted in Dup15q individuals [52–54]. Thus, bidirectional changes in *UBE3A* gene dosage are linked to mirror symmetric changes in delta power, suggesting a critical role for UBE3A protein in regulating delta-generating brain circuits.

Fragile X syndrome, another single-gene disorder associated with autism, provides a case study in the importance of defining reliable biomarkers for use as clinical outcome measures. A series of mechanism-based pharmacological studies in mice sought to normalize synaptic protein synthesis, a key pathological feature of Fragile X [55–57]. Pharmacological interventions directed towards normalizing protein synthesis were highly successful in correcting Fragile X phenotypes in mice [58–60], ultimately leading to multiple phase 2 clinical trials [61, 62].

These well-designed and well-powered trials ultimately failed because no improvements were seen in predefined behavioral endpoints [63]. While other aspects of these studies were also relevant to their outcomes, such as the age of children enrolled and the duration of treatments, this work provides a rationale to develop biologically based, quantitative, robust, and repeatable outcome measures for clinical trials. We propose that delta rhythmicity meets these criteria for Angelman syndrome.

Conclusions

Delta rhythmicity phenotypes are quantifiable and robust in children with Angelman syndrome and in mouse models of the disorder. Delta phenotypes have strong face validity between mouse models and patient populations; thus, future mechanistic studies of delta rhythms in mice will have high translational potential. In patient populations, delta phenotypes have value as biomarkers to chart progression of AS and as clinical outcome measures.

Additional files

Additional file 1: Figure S1. Quantifying relative power preserves delta phenotypes in AS model mice, but complicates interpretations in other bands. (A, B) Relative power in 129 mice (WT: $n = 23$, AS: $n = 24$), plotted as a fraction of total power (1–50 Hz). Quantification of relative (C) theta, (D) beta, and (E) gamma power. Relative theta and gamma are significantly decreased in AS model mice on a 129 background (theta: *$p = 0.013$, beta: $p = .209$, gamma: **$p = 0.0007$, Student's t test). (PDF 131 kb)

Additional file 2: Figure S2. Strain differences in the primary visual cortex LFP power in Angelman syndrome model mice. (A, B) Power spectra of group data (WT: $n = 30$, AS: $n = 39$; shading indicates ±sem) from the primary visual cortex in C57BL/6 mice. (C, D) Power spectra, measured relative to total power. (E) Raw and (F) relative delta power are not different between WT and AS (raw: $p = 0.277$, relative: #$p = 0.073$, Student's t tests). (G) Raw power in the 3–5-Hz band is not different between WT and AS (#$p = 0.077$). (H) Relative power in the 3–5-Hz band is significantly increased in AS model mice (**$p = 0.0052$). (I) Total power (1–50 Hz) is not different between groups ($p = 0.460$). (J) Raw and (K) relative gamma power are decreased in AS model mice on a C57BL/6 background (raw: *$p = 0.022$, relative: ***$p = 0.00074$). (L) Raw and (M) relative beta power are not different between groups (raw: $p = .476$, relative: $p = .166$) (PDF 179 kb)

Additional file 3: Figure S3. Power spectra from all regions during epochs of wake and sleep. Black: neurotypical (NT), red: AS. During wakefulness (NT: $n = 54$, AS: $n = 26$), (A) occipital, (B) temporal, (C) parietal, (D) central, and (E) frontal spectra. During sleep (NT: $n = 54$, AS: $n = 13$), (F) occipital, (G) temporal, (H) parietal, (I) central, and (J) frontal spectra. (PDF 896 kb)

Additional file 4: Seizure and medication history for children with AS. This file is a table that provides the following information for each child with AS where it was available: (1) age at EEG, (2) gender, (3) molecular diagnosis, (4) history of seizures (yes/no), (5) age of onset of seizures, (6) seizures controlled at the time of EEG (yes/no), (7) types of seizures in the past, and (8) medications at the time of EEG. (XLS 36 kb)

Additional file 5: Figure S4. Examples of EEG variants in children with Angelman syndrome. (A–C) Three examples of enhanced delta oscillations generalized across the neocortex. (D) An example of delta oscillations restricted to posterior electrodes. (E) An example of delta oscillations restricted to frontal electrodes. (F) An example of delta

oscillations restricted to frontal electrodes over the left hemisphere. (G, H) Examples of notched delta. (I) An example of theta oscillations. (PDF 9020 kb)

Abbreviations
AS: Angelman syndrome; EEG: Electroencephalography; IQR: Interquartile range; LFP: Local field potential

Acknowledgements
We thank April Levin (Boston Children's), Rob Komorowski (MIT), Mark Shen (UNC), and Alana Campbell (UNC) for thoughtful discussion and advice. We thank Thorfinn Riday (Paris Descartes) for contribution of preliminary data and technical advice.

Funding
Work was supported by NINDS (R01 NS085093), the Simons Foundation (SFARI grant #274426), the Angelman Syndrome Foundation, and the Angelman Syndrome Alliance to BDP and by NINDS (K23-NS092923) to CJC. MSS was supported by a training fellowship (NICHD T32 HD040127).

Authors' contributions
MSS and BDP designed mouse studies and wrote the manuscript. MSS, CJC, and RLT designed human EEG analyses. MSS conducted mouse studies and analyzed both mouse and human data. LMB provided AS patient data. CJC provided neurotypical patient data. GMD, MD, and CJC defined sleep and wake epochs in human data. All authors read and approved the final manuscript.

Competing interests
The authors declare that they have no competing interests.

Author details
Department of Cell Biology and Physiology, University of North Carolina, Chapel Hill, NC 27599, USA. ²Carolina Institute for Developmental Disabilities, University of North Carolina, Chapel Hill, NC 27599, USA. ³Neuroscience Center, University of North Carolina, Chapel Hill, NC 27599, USA. ⁴Department of Neurology, Massachusetts General Hospital, Boston, MA 02114, USA. ⁵Harvard Medical School, Boston, MA 02215, USA. ⁶Department of Pediatrics, University of California, San Diego, CA, USA. ⁷Division of Dysmorphology/Genetics, Rady Children's Hospital, San Diego, CA, USA. ⁸Present Address: The Neurology Foundation, Rhode Island Hospital and Warren Alpert School of Medicine at Brown University, Providence, RI 02903, USA.

References
1. Thibert RL, Larson AM, Hsieh DT, Raby AR, Thiele EA. Neurologic manifestations of Angelman syndrome. Pediatr Neurol. 2013;48:271–9.
2. Kishino T, Lalande M, Wagstaff J. UBE3A/E6-AP mutations cause Angelman syndrome. Nat Genet. 1997;15:70–3.
3. Matsuura T, Sutcliffe JS, Fang P, Galjaard RJ, Jiang YH, Benton CS, Rommens JM, Beaudet AL. De novo truncating mutations in E6-AP ubiquitin-protein ligase gene (UBE3A) in Angelman syndrome. Nat Genet. 1997;15:74–7.
4. Miles JH. Autism spectrum disorders—a genetics review. Genet Med. 2011;13:278–94.
5. Moreno-De-Luca D, Sanders SJ, Willsey AJ, Mulle JG, Lowe JK, Geschwind DH, State MW, Martin CL, Ledbetter DH. Using large clinical data sets to infer pathogenicity for rare copy number variants in autism cohorts. Mol Psychiatry. 2013;18:1090–5.
6. DiStefano C, Gulsrud A, Huberty S, Kasari C, Cook E, Reiter LT, Thibert R, Jeste SS. Identification of a distinct developmental and behavioral profile in children with Dup15q syndrome. J Neurodev Disord. 2016;8:19.
7. Meng L, Ward AJ, Chun S, Bennett CF, Beaudet AL, Rigo F. Towards a therapy for Angelman syndrome by targeting a long non-coding RNA. Nature. 2015;518:409–12.

8. Huang HS, Allen JA, Mabb AM, King IF, Miriyala J, Taylor-Blake B, Sciaky N, Dutton Jr JW, Lee HM, Chen X, et al. Topoisomerase inhibitors unsilence the dormant allele of Ube3a in neurons. Nature. 2012;481:185–9.

9. Daily JL, Nash K, Jinwal U, Golde T, Rogers J, Peters MM, Burdine RD, Dickey C, Banko JL, Weeber EJ. Adeno-associated virus-mediated rescue of the cognitive defects in a mouse model for Angelman syndrome. PLoS One. 2011;6, e27221.

10. Egawa K, Kitagawa K, Inoue K, Takayama M, Takayama C, Saitoh S, Kishino T, Kitagawa M, Fukuda A. Decreased tonic inhibition in cerebellar granule cells causes motor dysfunction in a mouse model of Angelman syndrome. Sci Transl Med. 2012;4:163ra157.

11. van Woerden GM, Harris KD, Hojjati MR, Gustin RM, Qiu S, de Avila FR, Jiang YH, Elgersma Y, Weeber EJ. Rescue of neurological deficits in a mouse model for Angelman syndrome by reduction of alphaCaMKII inhibitory phosphorylation. Nat Neurosci. 2007;10:280–2.

12. Ciarlone SL, Grieco JC, D'Agostino DP, Weeber EJ. Ketone ester supplementation attenuates seizure activity, and improves behavior and hippocampal synaptic plasticity in an Angelman syndrome mouse model. Neurobiol Dis. 2016;96:38–46.

13. Margolis SS, Sell GL, Zbinden MA, Bird LM. Angelman syndrome. Neurotherapeutics. 2015;12:641–50.

14. Boyd SG, Harden A, Patton MA. The EEG in early diagnosis of the Angelman (happy puppet) syndrome. Eur J Pediatr. 1988;147:508–13.

15. Viani F, Romeo A, Viri M, Mastrangelo M, Lalatta F, Selicorni A, Gobbi G, Lanzi G, Bettio D, Briscioli V, et al. Seizure and EEG patterns in Angelman's syndrome. J Child Neurol. 1995;10:467–71.

16. Casara GL, Vecchi M, Boniver C, Drigo P, Baccichetti C, Artifoni L, Franzoni E, Marchiani V. Electroclinical diagnosis of Angelman syndrome: a study of 7 cases. Brain Dev. 1995;17:64–8.

17. Laan LA, Renier WO, Arts WF, Buntinx IM, vd Burgt IJ, Stroink H, Beuten J, Zwinderman KH, van Dijk JG, Brouwer OF. Evolution of epilepsy and EEG findings in Angelman syndrome. Epilepsia. 1997;38:195–9.

18. Minassian BA, DeLorey TM, Olsen RW, Philippart M, Bronstein Y, Zhang Q, Guerrini R, Van Ness P, Livet MO, Delgado-Escueta AV. Angelman syndrome: correlations between epilepsy phenotypes and genotypes. Ann Neurol. 1998;43:485–93.

19. Buoni S, Grosso S, Pucci L, Fois A. Diagnosis of Angelman syndrome: clinical and EEG criteria. Brain Dev. 1999;21:296–302.

20. Valente KD, Andrade JQ, Grossmann RM, Kok F, Fridman C, Koiffmann CP, Marques-Dias MJ. Angelman syndrome: difficulties in EEG pattern recognition and possible misinterpretations. Epilepsia. 2003;44:1051–63.

21. Vendrame M, Loddenkemper T, Zarowski M, Gregas M, Shuhaiber H, Sarco DP, Morales A, Nespeca M, Sharpe C, Haas K, et al. Analysis of EEG patterns and genotypes in patients with Angelman syndrome. Epilepsy Behav. 2012;23:261–5.

22. Korff CM, Kelley KR, Nordli Jr DR. Notched delta, phenotype, and Angelman syndrome. J Clin Neurophysiol. 2005;22:238–43.

23. Jiang YH, Armstrong D, Albrecht U, Atkins CM, Noebels JL, Eichele G, Sweatt JD, Beaudet AL. Mutation of the Angelman ubiquitin ligase in mice causes increased cytoplasmic p53 and deficits of contextual learning and long-term potentiation. Neuron. 1998;21:799–811.

24. Wang PJ, Hou JW, Sue WC, Lee WT. Electroclinical characteristics of seizures-comparing Prader-Willi syndrome with Angelman syndrome. Brain Dev. 2005;27:101–7.

25. Kriegeskorte N, Simmons WK, Bellgowan PS, Baker CI. Circular analysis in systems neuroscience: the dangers of double dipping. Nat Neurosci. 2009;12:535–40.

26. Chu CJ, Leahy J, Pathmanathan J, Kramer MA, Cash SS. The maturation of cortical sleep rhythms and networks over early development. Clin Neurophysiol. 2014;125:1360–70.

27. Bruni O, Ferri R, D'Agostino G, Miano S, Roccella M, Elia M. Sleep disturbances in Angelman syndrome: a questionnaire study. Brain Dev. 2004;26:233–40.

28. Silber MH, Ancoli-Israel S, Bonnet MH, Chokroverty S, Grigg-Damberger MM, Hirshkowitz M, Kapen S, Keenan SA, Kryger MH, Penzel T, et al. The visual scoring of sleep in adults. J Clin Sleep Med. 2007;3:121–31.

29. Matlis S, Boric K, Chu CJ, Kramer MA. Robust disruptions in electroencephalogram cortical oscillations and large-scale functional networks in autism. BMC Neurol. 2015;15:97.

30. Judson MC, Wallace ML, Sidorov MS, Burette AC, Gu B, van Woerden GM, King IF, Han JE, Zylka MJ, Elgersma Y, et al. GABAergic neuron-specific loss of Ube3a causes Angelman syndrome-like EEG abnormalities and enhances seizure susceptibility. Neuron. 2016;90:56–69.

31. Delorme A, Makeig S. EEGLAB: an open source toolbox for analysis of single-trial EEG dynamics including independent component analysis. J Neurosci Methods. 2004;134:9–21.

32. Buzsaki G, Anastassiou CA, Koch C. The origin of extracellular fields and currents—EEG, ECoG, LFP and spikes. Nat Rev Neurosci. 2012;13:407–20.

33. McCormick DA, Bal T. Sleep and arousal: thalamocortical mechanisms. Annu Rev Neurosci. 1997;20:185–215.

34. Duncan JS. Antiepileptic drugs and the electroencephalogram. Epilepsia. 1987;28:259–66.

35. Huang HS, Burns AJ, Nonneman RJ, Baker LK, Riddick NV, Nikolova VD, Riday TT, Yashiro K, Philpot BD, Moy SS. Behavioral deficits in an Angelman syndrome model: effects of genetic background and age. Behav Brain Res. 2013;243:79–90.

36. Shaaya EA, Grocott OR, Laing O, Thibert RL. Seizure treatment in Angelman syndrome: a case series from the Angelman Syndrome Clinic at Massachusetts General Hospital. Epilepsy Behav. 2016;60:138–41.

37. Laan LA, Vein AA. Angelman syndrome: is there a characteristic EEG? Brain Dev. 2005;27:80–7.

38. Mandel-Brehm C, Salogiannis J, Dhamne SC, Rotenberg A, Greenberg ME. Seizure-like activity in a juvenile Angelman syndrome mouse model is attenuated by reducing Arc expression. Proc Natl Acad Sci U S A. 2015;112:5129–34.

39. Larson AM, Shinnick JE, Shaaya EA, Thiele EA, Thibert RL. Angelman syndrome in adulthood. Am J Med Genet A. 2015;167A:331–44.

40. Morita A, Kamei S, Mizutani T. Relationship between slowing of the EEG and cognitive impairment in Parkinson disease. J Clin Neurophysiol. 2011;28:384–7.

41. Benz N, Hatz F, Bousleiman H, Ehrensperger MM, Gschwandtner U, Hardmeier M, Ruegg S, Schindler C, Zimmermann R, Monsch AU, Fuhr P. Slowing of EEG background activity in Parkinson's and Alzheimer's disease with early cognitive dysfunction. Front Aging Neurosci. 2014;6:314.

42. Trillingsgaard A, Ostergaard JR. Autism in Angelman syndrome—an exploration of comorbidity. Autism. 2004;8:163–74.

43. Bonati MT, Russo S, Finelli P, Valsecchi MR, Cogliati F, Cavalleri F, Roberts W, Elia M, Larizza L. Evaluation of autism traits in Angelman syndrome: a resource to unfold autism genes. Neurogenetics. 2007;8:169–78.

44. Peters SU, Horowitz L, Barbieri-Welge R, Taylor JL, Hundley RJ. Longitudinal follow-up of autism spectrum features and sensory behaviors in Angelman syndrome by deletion class. J Child Psychol Psychiatry. 2012;53:152–9.

45. Righi G, Tierney AL, Tager-Flusberg H, Nelson CA. Functional connectivity in the first year of life in infants at risk for autism spectrum disorder: an EEG study. Plos One. 2014;9.

46. Duffy FH, Als H. A stable pattern of EEG spectral coherence distinguishes children with autism from neuro-typical controls—a large case control study. BMC Med. 2012;10:64.

47. Peters JM, Taquet M, Vega C, Jeste SS, Fernandez IS, Tan J, Nelson CA, Sahin M, Warfield SK. Brain functional networks in syndromic and non-syndromic autism: a graph theoretical study of EEG connectivity. BMC Med. 2013;11.

48. Gabard-Durnam L, Tierney AL, Vogel-Farley V, Tager-Flusberg H, Nelson CA. Alpha asymmetry in infants at risk for autism spectrum disorders. J Autism Dev Disord. 2015;45:473–80.

49. Coben R, Clarke AR, Hudspeth W, Barry RJ. EEG power and coherence in autistic spectrum disorder. Clin Neurophysiol. 2008;119:1002–9.

50. Heunis TM, Deng CA, de Vries PJ. Recent advances in resting-state electroencephalography biomarkers for autism spectrum disorder—a review of methodological and clinical challenges. Pediatr Neurol. 2016;61:28–37.

51. Jeste SS, Frohlich J, Loo SK. Electrophysiological biomarkers of diagnosis and outcome in neurodevelopmental disorders. Curr Opin Neurol. 2015;28:110–6.

52. Al Ageeli E, Drunat S, Delanoe C, Perrin L, Baumann C, Capri Y, Fabre-Teste J, Aboura A, Dupont C, Auvin S, et al. Duplication of the 15q11-q13 region: clinical and genetic study of 30 new cases. Eur J Med Genet. 2014;57:5–14.

53. Urraca N, Cleary J, Brewer V, Pivnick EK, McVicar K, Thibert RL, Schanen NC, Esmer C, Lamport D, Reiter LT. The interstitial duplication 15q11.2-q13 syndrome includes autism, mild facial anomalies and a characteristic EEG signature. Autism Res. 2013;6:268–79.

54. Frohlich J, Senturk D, Saravanapandian V, Golshani P, Reiter LT, Sankar R, Thibert RL, DiStefano C, Huberty S, Cook EH, Jeste SS. A quantitative electrophysiological biomarker of duplication 15q11.2-q13.1 syndrome. PLoS One. 2016;11, e0167179.

55. Bear MF, Huber KM, Warren ST. The mGluR theory of fragile X mental retardation. Trends Neurosci. 2004;27:370–7.

56. Qin M, Kang J, Burlin TV, Jiang CH, Smith CB. Postadolescent changes in regional cerebral protein synthesis: an in vivo study in the Fmr1 null mouse. J Neurosci. 2005;25:5087–95.

57. Qin M, Schmidt KC, Zametkin AJ, Bishu S, Horowitz LM, Burlin TV, Xia ZY, Huang TJ, Quezado ZM, Smith CB. Altered cerebral protein synthesis in fragile X syndrome: studies in human subjects and knockout mice. J Cereb Blood Flow Metab. 2013;33:499–507.

58. Michalon A, Sidorov M, Ballard TM, Ozmen L, Spooren W, Wettstein JG, Jaeschke G, Bear MF, Lindemann L. Chronic pharmacological mGlu5 inhibition corrects fragile X in adult mice. Neuron. 2012;74:49–56.

59. Henderson C, Wijetunge L, Kinoshita MN, Shumway M, Hammond RS, Postma FR, Brynczka C, Rush R, Thomas A, Paylor R, et al. Reversal of disease-related pathologies in the fragile X mouse model by selective activation of GABAB receptors with arbaclofen. Sci Transl Med. 2012;4:152ra128.

60. Osterweil EK, Chuang SC, Chubykin AA, Sidorov M, Bianchi R, Wong RK, Bear MF. Lovastatin corrects excess protein synthesis and prevents epileptogenesis in a mouse model of fragile X syndrome. Neuron. 2013;77:243–50.

61. Berry-Kravis EM, Hessl D, Rathmell B, Zarevics P, Cherubini M, Walton-Bowen K, Mu Y, Nguyen DV, Gonzalez-Heydrich J, Wang PP, et al. Effects of STX209 (arbaclofen) on neurobehavioral function in children and adults with fragile X syndrome: a randomized, controlled, phase 2 trial. Sci Transl Med. 2012;4:152ra127.

62. Berry-Kravis E, Des Portes V, Hagerman R, Jacquemont S, Charles P, Visootsak J, Brinkman M, Rerat K, Koumaras B, Zhu L, et al. Mavoglurant in fragile X syndrome: results of two randomized, double-blind, placebo-controlled trials. Sci Transl Med. 2016;8:321ra325.

63. Jeste SS, Geschwind DH. Clinical trials for neurodevelopmental disorders: at a therapeutic frontier. Sci Transl Med. 2016;8.

7

Oscillatory motor patterning is impaired in neurofibromatosis type 1: a behavioural, EEG and fMRI study

Gilberto Silva[1,2†], Isabel Catarina Duarte[1,2†], Inês Bernardino[1], Tânia Marques[1], Inês R. Violante[3] and Miguel Castelo-Branco[1,2*] (iD)

Abstract

Background: Neurofibromatosis type1 (NF1) is associated with a broad range of behavioural deficits, and an imbalance between excitatory and inhibitory neurotransmission has been postulated in this disorder. Inhibition is involved in the control of frequency and stability of motor rhythms. Therefore, we aimed to explore the link between behavioural motor control, brain rhythms and brain activity, as assessed by EEG and fMRI in NF1.

Methods: We studied a cohort of 21 participants with NF1 and 20 age- and gender-matched healthy controls, with a finger-tapping task requiring pacing at distinct frequencies during EEG and fMRI scans.

Results: We found that task performance was significantly different between NF1 and controls, the latter showing higher tapping time precision. The time-frequency patterns at the beta sub-band (20–26 Hz) mirrored the behavioural modulations, with similar cyclic synchronization/desynchronization patterns for both groups. fMRI results showed a higher recruitment of the extrapyramidal motor system (putamen, cerebellum and red nucleus) in the control group during the fastest pacing condition.

Conclusions: The present study demonstrated impaired precision in rhythmic pacing behaviour in NF1 as compared with controls. We found a decreased recruitment of the cerebellum, a structure where inhibitory interneurons are essential regulators of rhythmic synchronization, and in deep brain regions pivotally involved in motor pacing. Our findings shed light into the neural underpinnings of motor timing deficits in NF1.

Keywords: Neurofibromatosis type 1, Inhibition, EEG, fMRI, Motor coordination

Background

Neurofibromatosis type 1 (NF1) is the most common autosomal dominant neurogenetic condition with an estimated prevalence of 1 in 3000 individuals [1–3]. The disorder is caused by mutations in the NF1 gene that encodes neurofibromin. This protein is involved in cell proliferation and differentiation [4], and its loss may explain abnormalities in the brain structure, which include increased volume of the cortical and subcortical structures, and white and gray matter abnormalities [5–9].

Behavioural difficulties are also frequent and encompass a wide range of cognitive deficits, which include perceptual impairments, attention and learning disabilities [10–12]. Moreover, there is a tendency for those symptoms to persist or even increase in severity with age [2].

Motor skill and time perception impairments have been reported in NF1 children [13]. Debrabant and colleagues [14] studied temporal perception (motor timing indexed by the reaction time decrease upon presentation of predictable stimuli). They found that the clinical group responded with an increased reaction time to such temporally predictable stimuli (as defined by regular interstimulus intervals) when compared to typically developing children [14]. Accordingly, a comprehensive study by Hyman on motor and cognitive function in NF1 showed that fine motor coordination

---

* Correspondence: mcbranco@fmed.uc.pt
†Equal contributors
[1]CNC.IBILI, Institute for Biomedical Imaging and Life Sciences, University of Coimbra, 3000-548 Coimbra, Portugal
[2]ICNAS, CIBIT, Institute for Nuclear Sciences Applied to Health, University of Coimbra, 3000-548 Coimbra, Portugal
Full list of author information is available at the end of the article

deficits and slowing of motor speed were present in approximately 20 and 30% of the NF1 cohort, respectively [10]. Using a more broad motor performance test battery, Rietman and colleagues found that 61% of the studied cohort had motor problems [15].

Although knowledge on the cognitive and behavioural deficits in NF1 is increasing, the neural mechanisms underlying such impairments are still poorly understood. Previous studies addressing other cognitive domains have proposed that abnormalities in the balance of the excitatory and the inhibitory activity underlie a basic disease mechanism.

Initial studies in mouse models of NF1 indicated that lack of neurofibromin causes increased GABA (γ-aminobutyric acid)-mediated neurotransmission and showed a relationship between enhanced inhibitory activity and behavioural profile [16–18]. However, studies in human patients have shown a pattern of GABA alterations that include reduced GABA levels and $GABA_A$ receptor density [19–21]. In order to reconcile these differences across species, a recent study investigated pre- and post-synaptic GABA levels in an NF1 mouse model employing magnetic resonance spectroscopy (the only technique available to measure GABA levels in vivo in humans) combined with molecular approaches [22]. This study showed that the pattern of GABA alterations in mice is region specific and that this pattern is not always consistent across species. Thus, although mutations in the NF1 gene do seem to impact the GABA system and those can have behavioural and cognitive consequences [21], their pattern across species and brain regions do not seem to be trivial. Importantly, lower GABA levels may still be consistent with enhanced inhibitory activity. This is the case for example in the hippocampus, where low GABA levels coexist with very high post-synaptic receptor density [22] and increased inhibitory post-synaptic potentials [18].

Here, we hypothesized that rhythmic taping performance is impaired in NF1 and that it is related to abnormal physiology and brain activity patterns. Inhibition is involved in the function of motor central pattern generators—neuronal circuits that when activated can produce rhythmic motor patterns [23]—and in the control of frequency and stability of motor rhythms [24, 25]. We therefore aimed to explore the link between behavioural control of motor rhythms, brain oscillations and brain activity in regions involved in motor pacing. To reach that goal, we choose a finger-tapping task so we can precisely measure the participant's performance either during functional magnetic resonance imaging (fMRI) or electroencephalography (EEG). We used synchronous and asynchronous finger-tapping tasks. The latter requires alternated finger tapping, which implies interhemispheric inhibitory control, in contrast with the synchronous

variant. In both synchronous and asynchronous conditions, finger tapping was performed in incremental rates, 1, 3 and 5 Hz, to vary the performance load. The latter frequency has been shown to be the most discriminative of disease states in cerebellar disorders (in particular genetic ataxias) where rhythmic motor control is impaired [26]. We hypothesized that the NF1 cohort would perform worse at rhythmic pacing than the healthy group, and we aimed to identify the neural correlates of such impaired temporal patterning. Since oscillatory pacing can be related to the modulation of populations of inhibitory interneurons [27, 28], we expected that behavioural differences would be reflected in the power of the beta band. We used the same pacing paradigm during functional scans to induce effects in the BOLD (blood-oxygen-level dependent) signal in motor-related areas during task performance. We aimed to unravel the neural underpinnings of abnormal motor coordination.

Methods

Subjects

Twenty-one adults with NF1 were recruited from a database used in previous studies [19] and in collaboration with the Portuguese Association of Neurofibromatosis. They all had a definite diagnosis of NF1 in accordance with the criteria of the National Institutes of Health (National Institutes of Health Consensus Development Conference, 1988). The control group (20 age- and gender-matched participants) was recruited via advertisement in the local community. Exclusion criteria for all participants included psychiatric disorders, neurologic illness affecting brain function other than NF1, brain tumor burden, intelligence quotient (IQ) lower than 75, epilepsy and traumatic brain injury. One control was excluded due to neurological illness. None of the NF1 patients were diagnosed with ADHD or had a formal diagnosis of learning disabilities. None of the participants were taking medication for treating anxiety or depression in the year before the study, and none of them were ever medicated with anticonvulsants.

All the participants but one were right-handed as assessed by the Edinburgh Handedness Inventory [29] and had normal or corrected to normal visual acuity. Intellectual function was assessed by using the Portuguese-adapted version of the Wechsler Adult Intelligence Scale-3rd edition (WAIS-III) [30]. Two control participants were unavailable to complete the IQ assessment. Full-scale IQ values were in the normal range for the NF1 patients (mean IQ ± SD 104. 4 ± 13.7). All the participants performed the standard Stroop Colour and Word Test [31] composed by two congruent conditions [word (W) and colour (C)] and one incongruent (interference) condition [colour-word (CW)]. Participants had 45 s to complete each task condition. An Interference Index was calculated according to the method proposed by Golden [31]: incongruent score (IG) = CW

– [(W × C)/(W + C)]. Groups did not differ regarding this index (independent-samples t tests, $p > .05$), indicating similar ability to control over the interference effect.

Three participants were excluded from the EEG analysis. One due to a malfunction in the trigger recording system and two due to differences in the cap system (ground positioning and channel locations). Two participants exceeded the limits of movement during the functional magnetic resonance (3 mm in, at least, one axis), and thus were excluded from that analysis. Our final sample for the EEG analysis was composed of 19 patients with NF1 and 19 controls. The clinical group ($n = 19$, 10 females, age range 23.8–51.8, mean age ± standard deviation [SD] 36.1 ± 6.7) and the control group ($n = 19$, 11 females, age range 22.5–55.0, mean age ± SD 37.1 ± 7.2) were matched for age ($U = 160.0$, $p = 0.549$) and gender (χ^2 (1) = .106, $p = 0.744$). The final sample for the fMRI analysis was composed of 19 patients with NF1 and 20 controls. The clinical group ($n = 19$, 11 females, age range 23.8–51.8, mean age ± standard deviation [SD] 36.5 ± 7.0) and the control group ($n = 20$, 12 females, age range 22.5–55.0, mean age ± SD 36.8 ± 7.1) were matched for age ($U = 182.5$, $p = 0.833$) and gender (χ^2 (1) = .018, $p = 0.894$).

Task

Participants performed a previously validated audio-paced tapping paradigm [26] at three incremental frequencies (1, 3 and 5 Hz). Participants were asked to tap using both

index fingers either simultaneously ("synchronous" condition) or alternating the tapping ("alternating" or "asynchronous" condition) as prompted by a cue shown in a computer screen ("A" for the alternating condition and an "S" for the synchronous condition). All participants were familiarized with the task and the interface before the beginning of the recording sessions. The paradigm was designed and presented using the Psychophysics Toolbox 3 [32, 33], running on Matlab R2013b (MathWorks, Natick, MA, USA).

For the fMRI task, a total of 24 blocks of the motor paradigm, 8 per frequency (4 synchronous and 4 alternating), were presented. Block duration was 9 s either for the finger tapping or for the baseline. The cues were presented in a 698.40 × 392.85 mm LCD monitor (NordicNeuroLab, Bergen, Norway), placed ~ 156 cm away from the participants' head. Audio was provided through MR-compatible headphones. Behavioural data (tapping timings) were recorded using the MRI-compatible response box Lumina LP-400 (Cedrus Corporation, San Pedro, CA, USA).

Regarding the EEG acquisition, we acquired four runs, each composed of five repetitions of the main sequence (1, 3 and 5 Hz, each frequency executed in two variations, synchronous and alternating). Blocks lasted 12 s and were composed by a baseline period of 3 s (where the participant fixated the central cross and did not execute any movements) and 9 s of task (see Fig. 1). The cueing

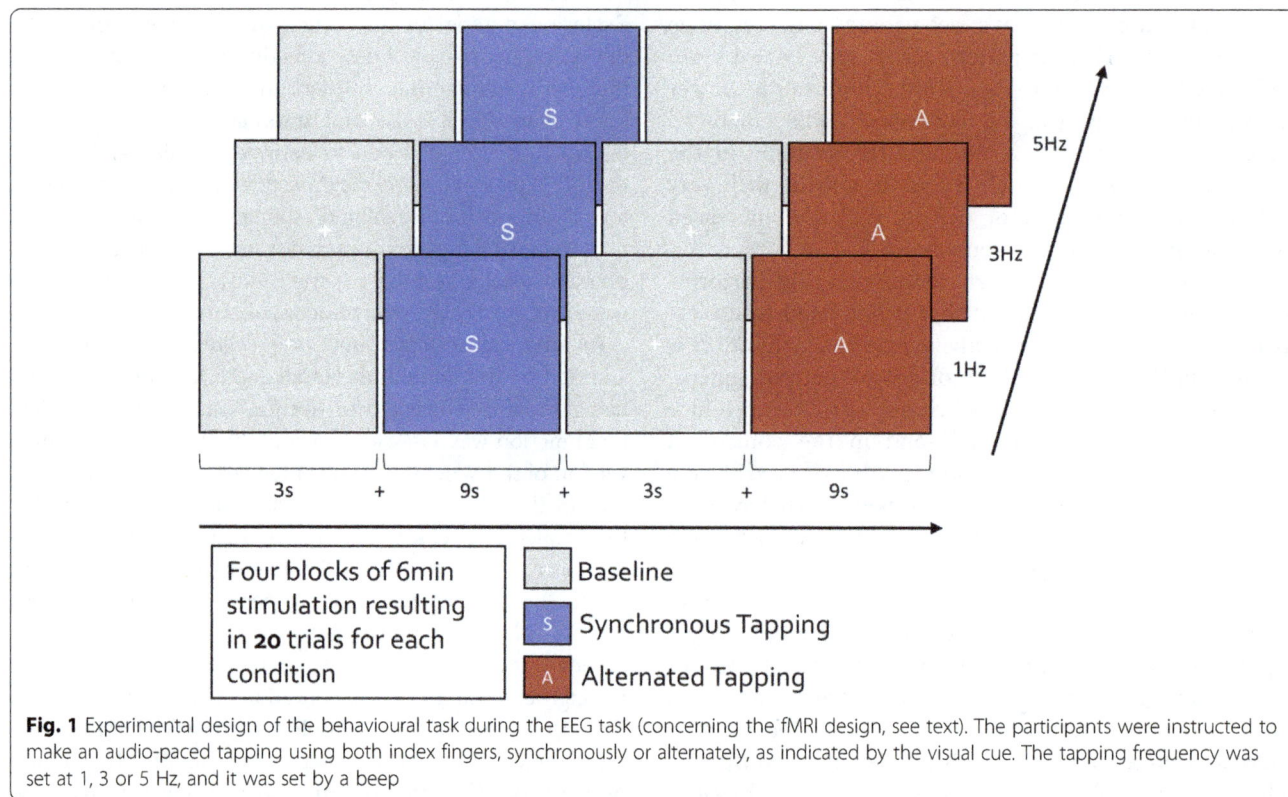

Fig. 1 Experimental design of the behavioural task during the EEG task (concerning the fMRI design, see text). The participants were instructed to make an audio-paced tapping using both index fingers, synchronously or alternately, as indicated by the visual cue. The tapping frequency was set at 1, 3 or 5 Hz, and it was set by a beep

paradigm was presented in a laptop placed ~ 50 cm in front of the participant. Participants were instructed to fixate the centre of the screen during the EEG task, and behavioural data were recorded using the "Z" and "M" buttons of a common keyboard.

MR recordings and analysis

MR scans were acquired in a 3T Magnetom Tim Trio scanner (Siemens, Erlangen, Germany), using a 12-channel birdcage head coil. A T1-weighted magnetization-prepared rapid gradient echo sequence was acquired with a repetition time of 2530 ms, echo time of 3.42 ms, resolution of 1 mm^3 isotropic voxel, flip angle of 7°, matrix size 256×256 and a field of view of 256×256 mm. Functional data were acquired using echo-planar imaging sequences, using voxel size 3 mm^2 and slice thickness of 3 mm, no gap between slices, 43 slices acquired parallel to the anterior commissure-posterior commissure line, repetition time 3000 ms, echo time 30 ms, flip angle of 90°, matrix size 256×256 and a field of view of 256×256 mm. In total, 147 volumes were acquired. A T2-weighted fluid attenuation inversion recovery sequence was used to identify unidentified bright objects, and it was acquired using a 1 mm^3 voxel, repetition time 5 s, echo time 388 ms, inversion time 1.8 s, field of view 250×250 mm, matrix size 256×256 and160 slices.

The complete processing pipeline and analysis of the functional data was done using BrainVoyager QX 2.8.2 (Brain Innovation, Maastricht, The Netherlands). Data were corrected for (1) slice scanning time differences using cubic spline interpolation, (2) motion artifacts by combining trilinear and sinc function based methods for interpolation in the three axes and (3) filtered in the time domain using an approach with Fourier basis set using 2 cycles per time course. Functional data were automatically co-registered to the anatomical T1 (and manually verified) and subsequently normalized to the Talairach atlas. Spatial smoothing was applied using a Gaussian kernel with a full width at half maximum of 6 mm. Statistical analyses were performed at the group level using a general linear model approach. The predictor's model was obtained by convolution of the box-car function with a standard 2-gamma hemodynamic response function. Motion parameters were also included in the model as regressors of no interest. Random effects analysis (RFX) was performed, and the results were corrected for multiple comparisons using false discovery rate (FDR) with a fixed p value of 0.05 and minimum cluster extension of 20 voxels.

EEG recordings and analysis

Electroencephalographic signals were recorded using a 64 electrodes cap (QuickCap, NeuroScan, USA) with electrodes placed according to the extended 10/20 system. In order to ensure the quality of the signal, all electrode impedances were kept below 20 kΩ. The continuous signal was amplified and recorded at a sampling rate of 1 kHz, low pass filter at 200 Hz, through a SynAmps2/RT amplifier. Data were acquired using Scan 4.5 (NeuroScan, Compumedics, Charlotte, NC), and the acquisition reference was set to an electrode located at a half distance between CZ and FCZ.

The processing was performed using the EEGlab toolbox [34] for Matlab (MathWorks, Natick, MA). The EEG signal was downsampled to 400 Hz and digitally filtered between 1 and 100 Hz. A notch filter (47.5–52.5 Hz) was applied, and epochs from – 3000 to 9000 ms were obtained locked to the stimuli onset. Epoch rejection was done automatically by scanning the entire dataset using a rejection threshold of 120 μV for all electrodes followed by visual inspection to ensure the data was free from artifacts. Channels with abnormal noise activity were interpolated using spherical spline interpolation. The HEO/VEO channels were excluded from further analysis, and the recordings were re-referenced to the average of all remaining channels. We proceeded to epoch division by trigger data, i.e. we separated the time-frequency epochs by sub-task type (1, 3 and 5 Hz tapping, synchronous and alternated). All the participants met the minimum criterion (more than 40%) of the trials per condition available for analysis.

Time-frequency decomposition was done using the function *pop_newtimef()*, with Morlet wavelet, beginning with a 7-cycle at 6 Hz and increasing linearly with frequency (maximum of 30 cycles at 50 Hz). We calculated 400 timepoints (with an effective time window from – 2600 to 6080 ms) and set the baseline from the beginning of the epoch until 100 ms before the onset of the stimulus. Electrodes corresponding to motor areas were clustered (FC1, FC2, CZ, C1, C3, C2 and C4). We truncated the time analysis intervals (from – 2000 to 6000 ms) in order to avoid boundary effects on time-frequency spectra.

Further analysis was performed in the time-course variation for three sub-bands of mu, beta and gamma frequencies (respectively, 8–12, 20–26 and 40–44 Hz intervals). Beta range (20–26 Hz range) was defined around the desynchronization peak that matches the motor pattern. The choice of the interval of low gamma was based on our previous work [35–37] and was set up to 44 Hz to avoid power line interferences in the time-frequency analysis. The bands were not juxtaposed, in order to avoid information contamination between bands. Frequency-domain evaluations were performed specifically for beta sub-band variations, since they exhibit a marked sinusoidal profile, matching motor responses. For that, we computed the power per subject at the exact frequency of tapping.

Statistics for group comparisons

Measurements of motor performance were done in data recorded during EEG recordings because larger amounts of data could be recorded. The statistical comparison between groups was performed using one-way multivariate ANOVAs (MANOVAs) to determine whether there are any differences between the independent variable (group) based on the dependent continuous variables (tapping at three different frequencies: 1, 3 and 5 Hz), for synchronous and asynchronous conditions. Similarly,

we used MANOVA to test group differences on EEG data.

Results

Behavioural results

Tapping time histograms reflecting the distribution of motor responses in the synchronous condition are presented in Fig. 2. The histograms indicate a reduction in tapping time precision in patients with NF1 compared to the healthy control group as indexed by the sharper curve around the cued tapping time in the control group. To quantify this effect, we computed the power at the ideal tapping frequency as a measure of motor performance precision. Higher power values correspond

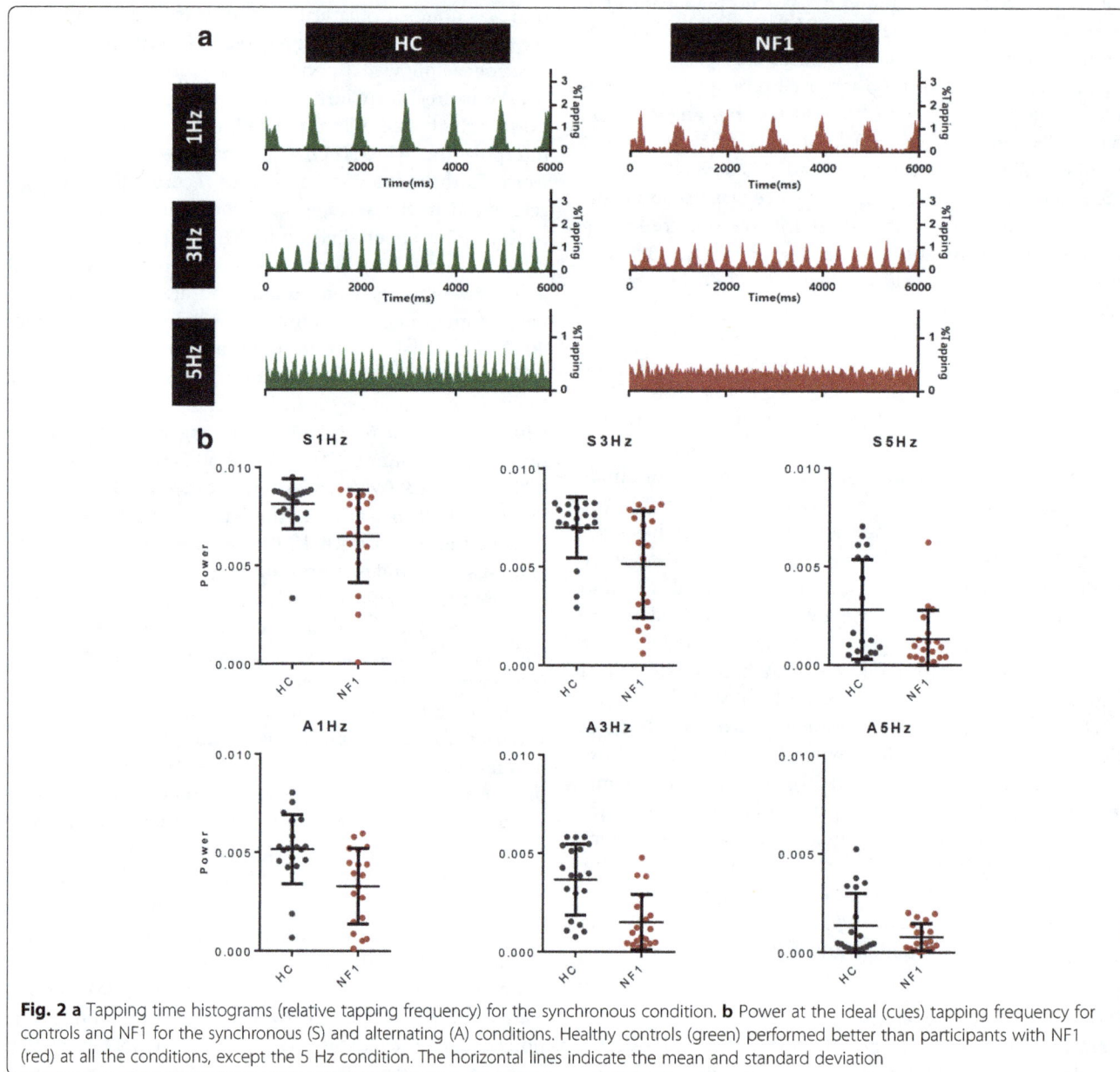

Fig. 2 a Tapping time histograms (relative tapping frequency) for the synchronous condition. **b** Power at the ideal (cues) tapping frequency for controls and NF1 for the synchronous (S) and alternating (A) conditions. Healthy controls (green) performed better than participants with NF1 (red) at all the conditions, except the 5 Hz condition. The horizontal lines indicate the mean and standard deviation

to higher participant's ability to keep tapping at the required frequency.

For the synchronous condition, we found, as assessed by MANOVA, a statistically significant difference between controls and NF1 patients, $F (3, 34) = 6.10$, $p = 0.041$; Wilk's $\Lambda = 0.787$. These differences in behavioural performance were significant at all tested frequencies of 1, 3 and 5 Hz (respectively, $F (1, 36) = 7.14$, $p = 0.011$; $F (1, 36) = 6.61$, $p = 0.014$; and $F (1, 36) = 4.887$, $p < 0.034$).

For the asynchronous condition, MANOVA also yielded statistically significant differences between groups, $F (3,34) = 6.104$, $p = 0.02$; Wilk's $\Lambda = 0.650$. Subsequent analyses revealed that these effects were mainly derived from differences at 1 and 3 Hz (respectively, $F (1, 36) = 9.84$, $p = 0.003$ and $F (1, 36) = 17.01$, $p < 0.001$).

We followed up this analysis by performing ROC (receiver operating characteristic) curve analysis to further investigate which frequencies better discriminated between patients ($n = 18$) and controls ($n = 19$), Fig. 3. Synchronous 1 Hz tapping and alternated 3 Hz tapping were the most suitable to separate patients with NF1 from controls (respectively, area ± standard deviation 0. 7729 ± 0.0781, $p = 0.012$ and 0.8421 ± 0.0622, $p < 0.01$, corrected for multiple comparisons), such that the alternated test at 3 Hz achieved a sensitivity of 84% with 74% specificity.

EEG results

Time-frequency analysis in the motor cluster (electrodes FC1, FC2, CZ, C1, C3, C2 and C4) was performed for both groups. Plots for the synchronous condition at 1 Hz are presented in Fig. 4. Both groups exhibit a marked cyclic synchronization/desynchronization pattern in the *mu* and *beta* range, which are known to be tightly related with the behavioural execution of movements.

To statistically compare the groups concerning this synchronization/desynchronization pattern in the 8–12 Hz (corresponding to mu band) and 20–26 Hz range (the peak of beta range, corresponding to the desynchronization peak matching the motor pattern, see above), we computed the power for the specific frequency of the task per subject. We did not find statistical differences in the power between groups across any of these motor pacing frequencies.

fMRI results

Our analysis only identified differences between healthy controls and patients with NF1 at 5 Hz, as presented in Fig. 5 ($t(76) > 3.26$, $p < 0.05$, multiple comparison FDR corrected, minimum cluster size of 20 voxels). The control group presented a higher recruitment of the putamen, cerebellum (anterior lobe), red nucleus, medial prefrontal cortex and auditory cortex, bilaterally. The left superior parietal lobule showed higher activation in the group of patients with NF1 than controls. All findings are detailed in Table 1.

Discussion

In the present study, we aimed to understand the neural basis of rhythmic motor pacing deficits in NF1, using a comprehensive set of approaches, including behavioural assessment, EEG and fMRI. We studied a cohort of participants with NF1 and healthy controls during a simple motor task requiring pacing at distinct frequencies during EEG recording and fMRI scans.

We found that NF1 patients were significantly impaired in the behavioural precision of rhythmic pacing. Their tapping times showed larger dispersion and therefore decreased power at the cued pacing frequency. Time-frequency analysis revealed similar oscillatory patterns across groups that mirrored motor behaviour. Accordingly, the power at the beta sub-band matched the motor

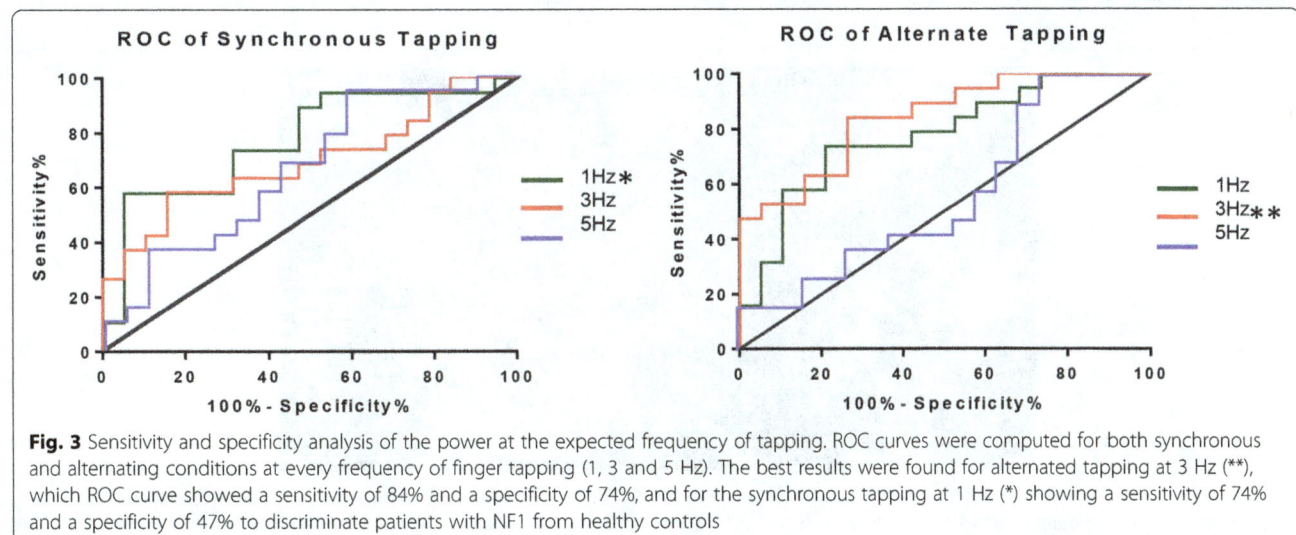

Fig. 3 Sensitivity and specificity analysis of the power at the expected frequency of tapping. ROC curves were computed for both synchronous and alternating conditions at every frequency of finger tapping (1, 3 and 5 Hz). The best results were found for alternated tapping at 3 Hz (**), which ROC curve showed a sensitivity of 84% and a specificity of 74%, and for the synchronous tapping at 1 Hz (*) showing a sensitivity of 74% and a specificity of 47% to discriminate patients with NF1 from healthy controls

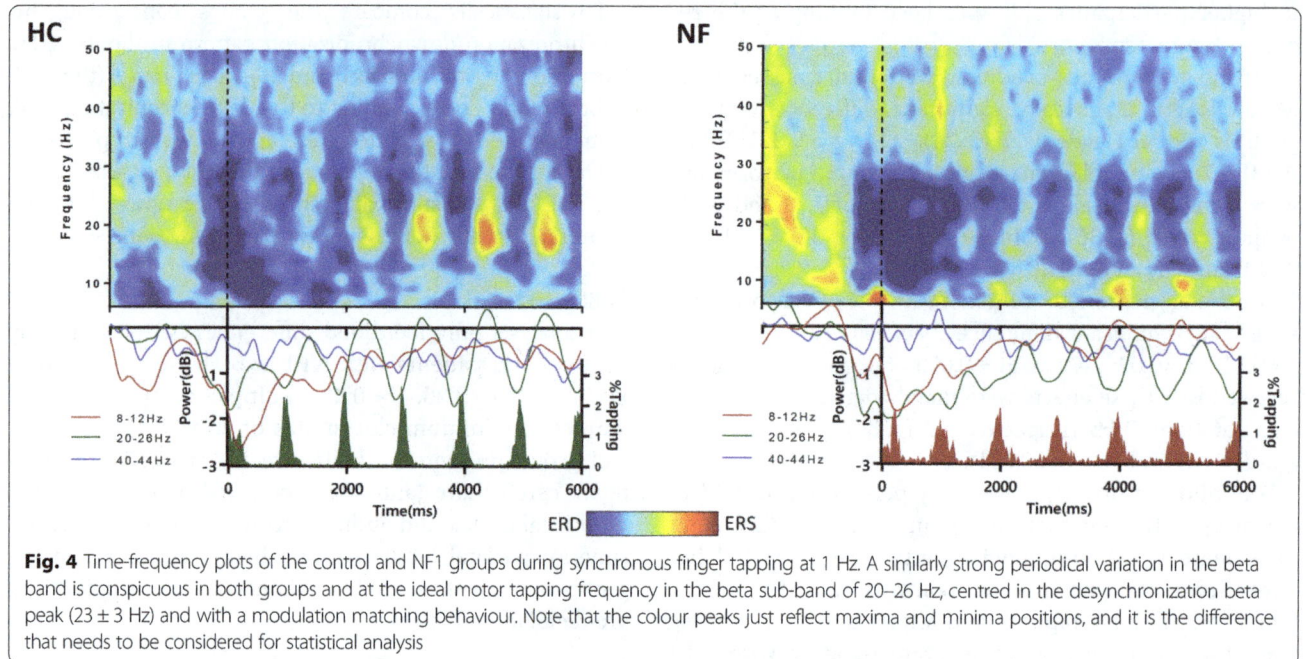

Fig. 4 Time-frequency plots of the control and NF1 groups during synchronous finger tapping at 1 Hz. A similarly strong periodical variation in the beta band is conspicuous in both groups and at the ideal motor tapping frequency in the beta sub-band of 20–26 Hz, centred in the desynchronization beta peak (23 ± 3 Hz) and with a modulation matching behaviour. Note that the colour peaks just reflect maxima and minima positions, and it is the difference that needs to be considered for statistical analysis

behavioural patterning. BOLD signals evoked by the task suggested group differences in the deep brain regions pivotally involved in motor pacing, not reachable by EEG, such as the basal ganglia and the cerebellum.

Power at the cued frequency as potentially relevant clinical measure

The histograms of tapping times of both groups showed clear group differences. The tapping distribution of the healthy control group resulted in sharper curves with higher amplitude near the ideal (cued) tapping frequency. As the responses were sparser in time, the curve of NF1 participants was broader and, consequently, the amplitude was lower than the control group curve. The statistical analysis of the power at the cued tapping

frequency demonstrated that performance was statistically different between groups across all frequencies in the synchronous task and at 1 and 3 Hz in the asynchronous task. ROC curve analysis showed the best discrimination for alternate tapping at 3 Hz. This analysis showed a sensitivity of 84% and a specificity of 74% to discriminate patients with NF1 from healthy controls. The alternate tapping variant poses larger cognitive control demands and inhibition from the contralateral hemisphere as opposed to the synchronous tapping. Our results suggest that the combination of 3 Hz and the alternate variant task rendered this task more sensitive to detect impairments in the NF1 cohort.

Impaired performance during motor tests has been often reported in NF1 [10, 13–15, 38–41] but not in the

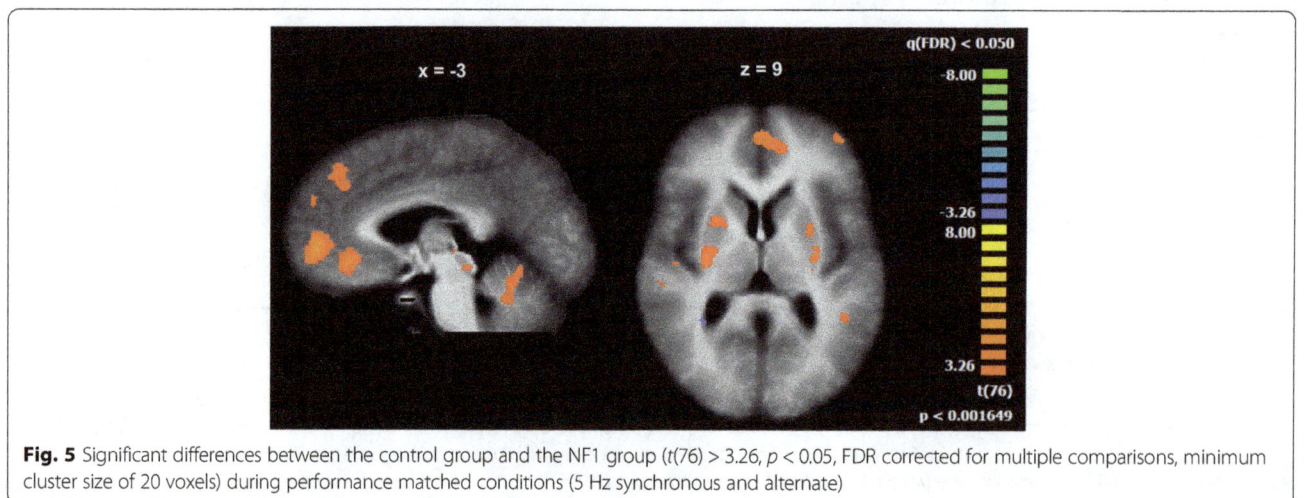

Fig. 5 Significant differences between the control group and the NF1 group ($t(76) > 3.26$, $p < 0.05$, FDR corrected for multiple comparisons, minimum cluster size of 20 voxels) during performance matched conditions (5 Hz synchronous and alternate)

Table 1 Regions differentially recruited by the control group and the NF1 group ($t(76) > 3.26$, $p < 0.05$, FDR corrected for multiple comparisons, minimum cluster size of 20 voxels) during the fastest tapping conditions (5 Hz synchronous and 5 Hz alternate tapping). The clusters are described by their hemisphere (H), peak voxel coordinates in Talairach space, the t and p values in the peak voxel and the number of voxels (n)

Region	H	Peak x	y	z	t	p	n
Putamen	R	30	− 13	7	4.30	0.000027	33
Putamen	L	− 30	− 10	14	3.93	0.000119	25
Cerebellum	R	15	− 40	− 26	4.02	0.000084	39
Cerebellum	R,L	0	− 52	− 26	3.90	0.000135	40
Red nucleus	R,L	9	− 19	− 2	4.75	0.000004	55
Medial prefrontal cortex	R, L	− 3	50	4	5.16	0.000001	223
Medial frontal gyrus	L	− 9	29	31	4.24	0.000035	92
Middle frontal gyrus	L	− 24	17	43	4.58	0.000008	28
Middle frontal gyrus	L	− 43	50	7	4.35	0.000022	47
Posterior cingulate gyrus	L	− 9	− 49	32	3.71	0.000275	26
Auditory cortex	R	51	− 28	16	5.16	0.000001	75
Auditory cortex	L	− 42	− 28	19	5.80	< 0.000001	57
Superior temporal gyrus	R	57	− 10	1	5.34	< 0.000001	36
Superior temporal gyrus	L	− 57	− 43	− 8	4.44	0.000015	92
Middle temporal gyrus	L	− 60	− 22	− 20	5.43	< 0.000001	217
Parahippocampal gyrus	L	− 27	5	− 26	4.46	0.000014	54
Precentral gyrus	R	15	− 28	67	5.88	< 0.000001	26
Superior parietal lobule	L	− 30	− 58	43	− 4.57	0.000009	50
White matter	R	24	− 46	15	− 4.62	0.000007	39
White matter	L	− 27	20	25	4.17	0.000047	33

context of rhythmic pacing. Along with the motor deficits, a wide array of impairments in other cognitive domains is known, as executive dysfunction [3, 10, 39], and it is believed that there is a common biological mechanism underlying all these deficits. There is however the concern whether executive dysfunction could underlie observed motor deficits [40, 41]. However, this is an unlikely explanation for our results because our groups were matched in executive function, as measured by a Stroop task. Moreover, we used a task without working memory load and no need to memorize motor sequences.

Studies on mouse models suggest that abnormal neurodevelopmental mechanisms in NF1 can result from an imbalance on the excitatory and the inhibitory drive [16, 18, 22], and this may also be the case for the observed changes in rhythmic motor pacing.

Cyclic pattern of behavioural and EEG power curves
The time-frequency analysis of the signal over the sensorimotor cortex showed a strong periodical variation in the beta band, which closely matches the behavioural data. This is a well-established spectral pattern (including also the so-called post-movement beta rebound); beta oscillations over the motor cortex showed increased desynchronization at the beginning of a movement and increased synchronization after the movement (~ 300 to 1000 ms) [42]. Therefore, a rhythmic finger-tapping task was expected to produce a synchronization/desynchronization cyclic pattern in the beta band with the same frequency as the tapping movement.

A relation between beta oscillations and inhibitory activity was demonstrated before by Gaetz and colleagues. They found that the level of GABA, an inhibitory neurotransmitter, in the motor cortex correlated with the power of the post-movement beta transient increase [27]. Jensen and co-workers further found that benzodiazepines, which are GABAergic agonists, modulate beta sources by increasing the power of the beta oscillations at rest over the primary sensorimotor cortex [28]. Modulations in beta oscillations are linked to the behaviour of inhibitory interneurons and thus have been related to the underlying excitation/inhibition balance [42, 43]. Future work should further test whether this putative link between GABA and abnormal beta activity is suggestive of impaired cortical inhibition and can be related to the behavioural impairments we found here.

A critical role for regions involved in motor pacing: the basal ganglia and cerebellum

Functional neuroimaging data analysis showed group differences at the fastest frequency (5 Hz). This pacing rhythm was previously demonstrated to best discriminate between healthy participants and patients with genetic disorders leading to cerebellar atrophy and impaired rhythmic motor control [26]. Here, the group contrast revealed higher recruitment of subcortical structures of the extrapyramidal motor system in the control group, namely the putamen, cerebellum and red nucleus. The synchronization between the audio pacing stimuli and the motor action requires complex information processing involving diverse functions such as timing, temporal prediction, sequence processing and sensory-motor integration [44]. This implies the recruitment of a wide network involving the primary auditory cortex, motor cortex, basal ganglia and cerebellar circuits. The putamen, as part of basal ganglia, plays an important role in motor control [45], and it is known to be parametrically modulated by movement frequency [46]. The red nucleus is a pivotal region in motor function and shows significant functional connectivity with the cerebellum [47]. It is also generally accepted that the cerebellum plays a role in rhythmic synchronization, by processing timing information, as required by the present task [44, 48]. In the cerebellum, inhibitory interneurons are essential regulators of motor coordination [49]. The pattern of differences found in the cerebellum, a structure which is dominated by inhibitory physiology, is consistent with the inhibitory/excitatory imbalance theory in NF1. The task required the participant to keep continuous monitoring of his/her own motor pacing performance, which may explain the activation of the dorsolateral prefrontal regions. As the level of motor demand increases, the effort required to perform the task also increases. It is known that there is an increase in prefrontal cortex activity with the increasing of the cognitive control demands [50] that is intrinsically related to the role of PFC in monitoring and top-down control [51]. This may explain the observed differential activation in fronto-striatal networks in our study.

The group differences identified for the auditory cortex and superior parietal lobe are quite intriguing. Sensorimotor synchronization implies pacing and time prediction. As our motor paradigm is audio paced, this process starts with the sensory input and with attentional deployment in parietal cortex. This suggests that sensorimotor integration and synchronization are also impaired in NF1.

Conclusions

In the present study, we aimed to investigate the neural basis of putative rhythmic motor pacing deficits in NF1 by comprehensively exploring behavioural motor control, brain rhythms and brain activity in neurofibromatosis type 1.

Our study demonstrates impaired precision in rhythmic pacing behaviour and sheds light into the neural underpinnings of motor timing deficits in NF1, in particular concerning the basal ganglia and the cerebellum.

Abbreviations

BOLD: Blood-oxygen-level dependent; EEG: Electroencephalography; FDR: False discovery rate; fMRI: Functional magnetic resonance imaging; GABA: γ-Aminobutyric acid; IQ: Intelligence quotient; NF1: Neurofibromatosis type 1; RFX: Random effects analysis; ROC: Receiver operating characteristic; SD: Standard deviation

Acknowledgements

The authors would like to thank all the participants who took part in the project.

Funding

This work was supported by grant BIGDATIMAGE, CENTRO-01-0145-FEDER-000016, and financed by Centro 2020 FEDER, COMPETE, FLAD Life Sciences Ed 2 2016, COMPETE, POCI-01-0145-FEDER-007440, FCT. UID/NEU/04539/2013-2020, PAC – MEDPERSYST, POCI-01-0145-FEDER-016428, H2020-STIPED Project number: 731827 to MCB.

Authors' contributions

IRV, IB, ICD and MCB conceived and designed the experiment. IB carried out the participants' recruitment. GS, IB and TM performed the experiments. GS and ICD analyzed the data. ICD, GS and MCB wrote the paper. All authors read and approved the paper content.

Competing interests

The authors declare that they have no competing interests.

Author details

[1]CNC.IBILI, Institute for Biomedical Imaging and Life Sciences, University of Coimbra, 3000-548 Coimbra, Portugal. [2]ICNAS, CIBIT, Institute for Nuclear Sciences Applied to Health, University of Coimbra, 3000-548 Coimbra, Portugal. [3]School of Psychology, Faculty of Health and Medical Sciences, University of Surrey, Guildford GU2 7XH, UK.

References

1.   Williams VC, Lucas J, Babcock MA, Gutmann DH, Korf B, Maria BL. Neurofibromatosis type 1 revisited. Pediatrics. 2009;123:124–33.

2. Kayl AE, Moore BD. Behavioral phenotype of neurofibromatosis, type 1. Ment Retard Dev Disabil Res Rev. 2000;6:117–24.

3. Gutmann DH, Ferner RE, Listernick RH, Korf BR, Wolters PL, Johnson KJ. Neurofibromatosis type 1. Nat Rev. 2017;3:1–18. https://doi.org/10.1038/nrdp.2017.4.

4. Lee DY, Yeh T, Emnett RJ, White CR, Gutmann DH. Neurofibromatosis-1 regulates neuroglial progenitor proliferation and glial differentiation in a brain region-specific manner. Genes Dev. 2010;24:2317–29.

5. Violante IR, Ribeiro MJ, Silva ED, Castelo-branco M. Gyrification, cortical and subcortical morphometry in neurofibromatosis type 1: an uneven profile of developmental abnormalities. J Neurodev Disord. 2013;5:1–13. https://doi.org/10.1186/1866-1955-5-3.

6. Moore BD, Slopis JM, Jackson EF, De Winter AE, Leeds NE. Brain volume in children with neurofibromatosis type 1 relation to neuropsychological status. Neurology. 2000;54:914–20.

7. Duarte JV, Ribeiro MJ, Violante IR, Cunha G, Silva E, Castelo-branco M. Multivariate pattern analysis reveals subtle brain anomalies relevant to the cognitive phenotype in neurofibromatosis type 1. Hum Brain Mapp. 2014;35:89–106.

8. Filippi CG, Watts R, Duy LAN, Cauley KA. Diffusion-tensor imaging derived metrics of the corpus callosum in children with neurofibromatosis type I. AJR Am J Roentgenol. 2013;200:44–9.

9. Koini M, Rombouts SARB, Veer IM, Van Buchem MA, Huijbregts SCJ. White matter microstructure of patients with neurofibromatosis type 1 and its relation to inhibitory control. Brain Imaging Behav. 2016; https://doi.org/10.1007/s11682-016-9641-3.

10. Hyman SL, Shores A, North KN. The nature and frequency of cognitive deficits in children with neurofibromatosis type 1. Neurology. 2005;65:1037–44.

11. Silva G, Ribeiro MJ, Costa GN, Violante IR, Ramos F, Saraiva J, et al. Peripheral attentional targets under covert attention lead to paradoxically enhanced alpha desynchronization in neurofibromatosis type 1. PLoS One. 2016;11: e0148600.

12. Bluschke A, Hagen M Von Der, Papenhagen K, Roessner V, Beste C. NeuroImage: Clinical conflict processing in juvenile patients with neuro fi bromatosis type 1 (NF1) and healthy controls—two pathways to success. NeuroImage Clin 2017;14:499–505. doi:https://doi.org/10.1016/j.nicl.2017.02.014.

13. Lorenzo J, Barton B, Acosta MT, North K. Mental, motor, and language development of toddlers with neurofibromatosis type 1. J Pediatr. 2011;158: 660–5. https://doi.org/10.1016/j.jpeds.2010.10.001.

14. Debrabant J, Plasschaert E, Caeyenberghs K, Vingerhoets G, Legius E, Janssens S, et al. Research in developmental disabilities deficient motor timing in children with neurofibromatosis type 1. Res Dev Disabil. 2014;35: 3131–8. https://doi.org/10.1016/j.ridd.2014.07.059.

15. Rietman AB, Oostenbrink R, Bongers S, Gaukema E, Van Abeelen S, Hendriksen JG, et al. Motor problems in children with neurofibromatosis type 1. J Neurodev Disord. 2017;9:1–10.

16. Costa RM, Federov NB, Kogan JH, Murphy GG, Stern J, Ohno M, et al. Mechanism for the learning deficits in a mouse model of neurobromatosis type 1. Nature. 2002;415:526–30.

17. Shilyansky C, Karlsgodt KH, Cummings DM, Sidiropoulou K, Hardt M, James AS, et al. Neurofibromin regulates corticostriatal inhibitory networks during working memory performance. Proc Natl Acad Sci USA. 2010;107:13141–6.

18. Cui Y, Costa RM, Murphy GG, Elgersma Y, Zhu Y, David H, et al. Neurofibromin regulation of ERK signaling modulates GABA release and learning. Cell. 2008;135:549–60.

19. Violante IR, Patricio M, Bernardino I, Rebola J, Abrunhosa AJ, Ferreira N, et al. GABA deficiency in NF1. Neurology. 2016;87:897–904.

20. Violante IR, Ribeiro MJ, Edden RAE, Guimarães P, Bernardino I, Rebola J, et al. GABA deficit in the visual cortex of patients with neurofibromatosis type 1: genotype–phenotype correlations and functional impact. Brain. 2013;136:918–25.

21. Ribeiro MJ, Violante IR, Bernardino I, Edden RAE, Castelo-Branco M. Abnormal relationship between GABA, neurophysiology and impulsive behavior in neurofibromatosis type 1. Cortex. 2015;64:194–208.

22. Gonçalves J, Violante IR, Sereno J, Leitão RA, Cai Y, Abrunhosa A, et al. Testing the excitation/inhibition imbalance hypothesis in a mouse model of the autism spectrum disorder: in vivo neurospectroscopy and molecular evidence for regional phenotypes. Mol Autism. 2017;8:1–8.

23. Marder E, Bucher D. Central pattern generators and the control of rythmic movements. Curr Biol. 2001;11:R986–96.

24. Nishimaru H, Kakizaki M. The role of inhibitory neurotransmission in locomotor circuits of the developing mammalian spinal cord. Acta Psychol. 2009;197:83–97.

25. Cinelli E, Mutolo D, Robertson B, Grillner S, Contini M, Pantaleo T, et al. GABAergic and glycinergic inputs modulate rhythmogenic mechanisms in the lamprey respiratory network. J Physiol. 2014;592:1823–38.

26. Duarte JV, Faustino R, Cunha G, Ferreira C, Janu C. Parametric fMRI of paced motor responses uncovers novel whole-brain imaging biomarkers in spinocerebellar ataxia type 3. Hum Brain Mapp. 2016;37:3656–68.

27. Gaetz W, Edgar JC, Wang DJ, Roberts TPL. Relating MEG measured motor cortical oscillations to resting γ-aminobutyric acid (GABA) concentration. NeuroImage. 2011;55:616–21. https://doi.org/10.1016/j.neuroimage.2010.12.077.

28. Jensen O, Goel P, Kopell N, Pohja M, Hari R, Ermentrout B. On the human sensorimotor-cortex beta rhythm: sources and modeling. NeuroImage. 2005; 26:347–55.

29. Oldfield RC. The assessment and analysis of handedness: the Edinburgh inventory. Neuropsychologia. 1971;9:97–113.

30. Rocha AM, Ferreira C, Barreto H, Moreira AR, Wechsler D. Manual for intelligence scale for adults - third edition (WAIS-III) - [Portuguese adaptation]. Lisbon: Cegoc-Tea; 2008.

31. Golden CJ. A manual for the clinical and experimental use of the Stroop color and word test. Chicago: Stoelting Co.; 1978.

32. Brainard DH. The Psychophysics Toolbox. Spat Vis. 1997;10:433–6.

33. Pelli DG. The VideoToolbox software for visual psychophysics: transforming numbers into movies. Spat Vis. 1997;10:437–42.

34. Delorme A, Makeig S. EEGLAB: an open source toolbox for analysis of single-trial EEG dynamics including independent component analysis. J Neurosci Methods. 2004;134:9–21.

35. Castelhano J, Rebola J, Leitão B, Rodriguez E, Castelo-Branco M. To perceive or not perceive: the role of gamma-band activity in signaling object percepts. PLoS One. 2013;8:e66363.

36. Castelhano J, Duarte IC, Wibral M, Rodriguez E, Castelo-Branco M. The dual facet of gamma oscillations: separate visual and decision making circuits as revealed by simultaneous EEG/fMRI. Hum Brain Mapp. 2014;35:5219–35.

37. Bernardino I, Castelhano J, Farivar R, Silva ED, Castelo-Branco M. Neural correlates of visual integration in Williams syndrome: gamma oscillation patterns in a model of impaired coherence. Neuropsychologia. 2013;51:1287–95.

38. Rowbotham I, Cate IMP, Sonuga-Barke EJS, Huijbregts SCJ. Cognitive control in adolescents with neurofibromatosis type 1. Neuropsychology. 2009;23:50–60.

39. Levine TM, Materek A, Abel J, Donnell MO, Cutting LE. Cognitive profile of neurofibromatosis type 1. Pediatr Neurol. 2006;13:8–20.

40. Remigereau C, Roy A, Costini O, Barbarot S, Bru M, Le GD. Praxis skills and executive function in children with neurofibromatosis type 1. Appl Neuropsychol Child. 2017:1–11. https://doi.org/10.1080/21622965.2017.1295856.

41. Huijbregts S, Swaab H, De Sonneville L. Cognitive and motor control in neurofibromatosis type I: influence of maturation and hyperactivity-inattention. Dev Neuropsychol. 2010;35:737–51.

42. Kilavik BE, Zaepffel M, Brovelli A, Mackay WA, Riehle A. The ups and downs of beta oscillations in sensorimotor cortex. Exp Neurol. 2013;245:15–26. https://doi.org/10.1016/j.expneurol.2012.09.014.

43. Whittington MA, Traub RD, Kopell N, Ermentrout B, Buhl EH. Inhibition-based rhythms: experimental and mathematical observations on network dynamics. Int J Psychophysiol. 2000;38:315–36.

44. Molinari M, Leggio MG, Thaut MH. The cerebellum and neural networks for rhythmic sensorimotor synchronization in the human brain. Cerbellum. 2007;6:18–23.

45. DeLong MR, Wichmann T. Circuits and circuit disorders of the basal ganglia. Neurol Rev. 2007;64:20–4.

46. Lehéricy S, Bardinet E, Tremblay L, Van de Moortele P-F, Pochon J-B, Dormont D, et al. Motor control in basal ganglia circuits using fMRI and brain atlas approaches. Cereb Cortex. 2006;16:149–61.

47. Nioche C, Cabanis EA, Habas C. Functional connectivity of the human red nucleus in the brain resting state at 3T. Am J Neuroradiol. 2009;30:396–403.

48. Ivry RB, Spencer RMC. The neural representation of time. Curr Opin Neurobiol. 2004;14:225–32.

49. Wulff P, Schonewille M, Renzi M, Viltono L, Sassoe M, Badura A, et al. Synaptic inhibition of Purkinje cells mediates consolidation of vestibulo-cerebellar motor learning. Nat Neurosci. 2009;12:1042–52.

50. Badre D. Cognitive control, hierarchy, and the rostro–caudal organization of the frontal lobes. Trends Cogn Sci. 2008;12:193–200.

51. Rae XCL, Hughes LE, Anderson MC, Rowe XB. The prefrontal cortex achieves inhibitory control by facilitating subcortical motor pathway connectivity. J Neurosci. 2015;35:786–94.

8

Classifying and characterizing the development of adaptive behavior in a naturalistic longitudinal study of young children with autism

Cristan Farmer[1], Lauren Swineford[1,2], Susan E. Swedo[1] and Audrey Thurm[1*]

Abstract

Background: Adaptive behavior, or the ability to function independently in ones' environment, is a key phenotypic construct in autism spectrum disorder (ASD). Few studies of the development of adaptive behavior during preschool to school-age are available, though existing data demonstrate that the degree of ability and impairment associated with ASD, and how it manifests over time, is heterogeneous. Growth mixture models are a statistical technique that can help parse this heterogeneity in trajectories.

Methods: Data from an accelerated longitudinal natural history study ($n = 105$ children with ASD) were subjected to growth mixture model analysis. Children were assessed up to four times between the ages of 3 to 7.99 years.

Results: The best fitting model comprised two classes of trajectory on the Adaptive Behavior Composite score of the Vineland Adaptive Behavior Scale, Second Edition—a low and decreasing trajectory (73% of the sample) and a moderate and stable class (27%).

Conclusions: These results partially replicate the classes observed in a previous study of a similarly characterized sample, suggesting that developmental trajectory may indeed serve as a phenotype. Further, the ability to predict which trajectory a child is likely to follow will be useful in planning for clinical trials.

Keywords: Autism spectrum disorders, Adaptive behavior, Longitudinal studies

Background

Autism spectrum disorder (ASD) is typically life-long, with impairments stemming from core symptoms that present early in development [1, 2]. ASD is frequently associated with intellectual disability [3], a diagnosis which requires deficits in adaptive behavior. However, regardless of cognitive function, individuals with ASD display deficits in adaptive functioning, both in the domains most directly affected by the core symptoms of ASD (e.g., socialization and communication) [4] and also more generally [5]. As such, adaptive functioning deficits have long been used to quantify the impairments in functioning required for the ASD diagnosis [6, 7] and to track

changes in functioning [8], including in the early years [9] (see [10] for a historical review in individuals with ASD and intellectual disability).

Adaptive function has been discussed as a promising outcome measure for a variety of neurodevelopmental and neuropsychiatric conditions [11–14] because it has clinical significance for both families and researchers [15]. Adaptive behavior has been used rarely as a primary outcome in treatment research (e.g., [16]), though it appears listed amongst secondary outcomes in a number of trials. These include double-blind, placebo-controlled drug studies [17, 18] as well as studies that include behavioral interventions [19]. Some of these studies used independent evaluators, blind to treatment group, to conduct the interviews with parents or caregivers [20, 21], while others use the parent rating form in an unblinded fashion (e.g., [22]). In fact, there has

* Correspondence: athurm@mail.nih.gov
[1]Pediatrics and Developmental Neuroscience Branch, National Institute of Mental Health, National Institutes of Health, Bethesda, MD 20892, USA
Full list of author information is available at the end of the article

been enough interest that researchers are investigating the best statistical methods for detecting change in adaptive functioning for future trials [23].

Most of our knowledge about adaptive behavior in individuals with ASD comes from cross-sectional studies, which suggest ASD-specific profiles that vary with factors such as age and IQ [15]. However, recently published data are making increasingly apparent that some phenotypic characteristics may be less stable over time than previously assumed [24]. This is based on the slower-than-expected, but not negligible, growth in skills as children age. Thus, it may not be the snapshot-in-time that best describes an individual, but rather his or her change over time; in other words, developmental trajectories themselves could serve as phenotypes [25].

We know less about the development of adaptive behavior in ASD than we do about its snapshot-in-time presentation, especially across longer periods during early to middle childhood. This dearth exists because there have been very few longitudinal studies of ASD beginning in the preschool period, and even fewer that report on longitudinal measurement of adaptive functioning. Available data indicate that on average, adaptive behavior deficits seem to persist into adulthood (for a review see [8]), and adaptive behavior in ASD is heterogeneous and variable, even within an individual. While adaptive behavior impairment has a generally predictable relationship with cognitive ability in samples of individuals with intellectual disability, the relationship appears to be more complicated

in individuals with ASD. Children with ASD who do not have intellectual disability may still have impaired adaptive function [5], while individuals with both ASD and intellectual disability may have relatively less impairment in adaptive function compared to their level of cognitive impairment [26].

Some longitudinal studies have attempted to parse samples based on this heterogeneity, though for the most part, their sample sizes were small, they used few assessment points or limited age ranges, and/or they were focused on very specific domains of adaptive behavior (see Table 1). One useful statistical method for the empirical description of heterogeneous data is growth mixture models (GMM), which provide a richer understanding of the data than do standard growth curve models [27]. The most basic form of these models, latent class growth curve analysis (LCGA, known by other names, such as a "semi-parametric and group-based approach" and by the name of the program often used to implement it, Proc Traj), has been used in a handful of investigations of *within-subject* adaptive behavior development in ASD. In one study, investigators analyzed three assessments (5, 8, and 15 years of age) from 152 individuals with ASD, finding evidence for two patterns of development in age equivalents of adaptive behavior domains: one with little growth across the time points, and the other with substantial but less-than-expected growth [28]. Another study of approximately 85 individuals, assessed between the ages of 2 and

Table 1 Vineland trajectory study summaries

Report	ASD, n	Age (years) at baseline	Length of follow-up (occasions)	Cognitive ability level at baseline	Summary of findings
Szatmari et al. [30] (overlaps with Flanagan et al. [42])	421	3.32 ± 0.75	Four assessments: baseline, 6 and 12 months post-baseline, and age 6 years	Merrill-Palmer-Revised Developmental Index (full-scale IQ): 57.23 ± 26.20	Three classes of ABC trajectory: lower/worsening, moderate/stable, and higher/improving
Anderson et al. [26]	144	2.46 ± 0.39	Six assessments at approximate ages of 2, 3, 5, 9, 18, and 21 years (plus parent report at 10 and 13 years) (not all time points used in all publications)	Non-verbal IQ: 62.4 ± 17.36	Outcome was Vineland socialization age equivalent. Two classes were observed for both groups. Autism—low and flat, and moderate with age-appropriate growth. PDD—moderate with faster than expected growth, and low with moderate growth
Bal et al. [32]	Autism: 93 PDD: 51	Autism: 2.43 ± 0.42 PDD: 2.43 ± 0.47		Mullen Scales of Early Learning Non-verbal mental age: 1.62 ± 0.56 years	Two classes of daily living skills age equivalents trajectory: high and low. While both gained skills over time, the low group gained at a slower rate.
Baghdadli et al. [28]	152	4.9 ± 1.3	Three assessments at approximately 5, 8, and 15 years	Did not use standard assessments. "cognition related to object (months)": 22.4 ± 11.9; "Cognition related to person (months)": 19.2 ± 10.8	Across the subdomains of adaptive behavior, two patterns of development in age equivalents were observed: one with little growth across the time points and the other with substantial but less-than-expected growth.
Current study	105	4.24 ± 1.30	Follow-up at 6-month intervals prior to the third birthday; annual follow-ups until 3 years of study participation	Full-scale developmental quotient: 49.88 ± 16.83	Two classes of ABC trajectory: low/decreasing, moderate/stable

PDD pervasive developmental disorder, not otherwise specified, *ABC* Adaptive Behavior Composite

19 years, revealed the same two patterns of development, this time in the daily living skills domain [29]. Using an overall standard score measure of adaptive behavior, findings from four assessments of an inception sample of 406 children with ASD suggested low/worsening, moderate/stable, and average/improving trajectories over the period of 3 to 6 years of age [30].

Current study

The goal of this longitudinal study (NCT00298246) was to identify subtypes of ASD based on medical and behavioral phenotypes. Adaptive behavior was a key construct which we expected to differentiate the participants, but this specific analysis was not proposed a priori. Rather, we set out to replicate and extend previous research on the heterogeneity of adaptive behavior in individuals with ASD, using more advanced statistical models and a study population unique in its age at assessment, density of assessments, and length of follow-up. In the current analysis, we use GMM to explain the heterogeneity in development of adaptive behavior in children with ASD. We hypothesized that this mixture model would better fit the data than a standard latent curve model, suggesting that variability in trajectories is better explained by two or more subpopulations, rather than one.

Methods

Participants and procedures

Informed consent for participation was obtained from the parents or legal guardians of participants, who were enrolled in a longitudinal natural history study of autism approved by an NIH Institutional Review Board (06-M-0102). Participants were recruited from the community based on diagnosed or suspected ASD. Recruitment sources included medical, educational, and other service providers, as well as general announcements. The study period was between 2006 and 2014. The primary inclusionary criterion was a DSM-IV-TR [1] diagnosis of autistic disorder, based on the gold standard diagnostic battery described below. Exclusionary criteria for this study were a primary language other than English, cerebral palsy, or unmanageable behavior problems that prevented participation in standardized testing procedures. A total of 106 participants with ASD were enrolled. Smaller groups with non-ASD developmental delay and typical development were enrolled but are not reported here.

The design of the study was accelerated longitudinal; at enrollment, participants were between the ages of 18 months and 7 years, exclusive (mean ± SD = 4.05 ± 1.28 years). Visits prior to the third birthday were spaced at 6-month intervals, and later visits were annual until the child completed at least 3 years of participation or

until the child's fifth birthday. For this analysis, data were restructured into a "wide" format (i.e., 1-year bands starting at 24 months). If an individual had more than one visit per age band, the earlier visit was retained.

Measures

Participants were evaluated by expert doctoral-level clinicians who met research reliability standards on the Autism Diagnostic Interview-Revised (ADI-R; [31]) and the Autism Diagnostic Observation Schedule (ADOS; [32]). The diagnosis of autistic disorder was made using the information from these instruments, as well as the DSM-IV-TR.

At each visit, participants were administered a test to assess cognitive ability, either the Mullen Scales of Early Learning [33] or the Differential Abilities Scales, Second Edition [34]. To facilitate comparison between the tests and to account for the inability of participants to achieve standard scores, we use developmental quotients (DQ; the ratio of mental age to chronological age) in place of conventional IQ.

Parents responded to several interviews and questionnaires, including the Child Behavior Checklist (CBCL; [35]) and the interview version of the Vineland Adaptive Behavior Scales, Second Edition (VABS; [36]). The VABS is a semi-structured interview that assesses adaptive behavior in several domains, summarized by the Adaptive Behavior Composite (ABC) standard score. ABC standard scores may range from 20 to 160, with a population mean of 100 and a standard deviation of 15. To facilitate comparison with existing studies, we used the ABC as our outcome measure.

This battery was repeated at all visits, excepting the ADI-R, which was conducted only at the first and last visits. Because the age band at study entry differed across participants, we could not evaluate baseline predictors of class membership. Instead, we plot observed contemporaneous data across several domains of interest (non-verbal and verbal DQ, ADOS Calibrated Severity Score (CSS), and CBCL Externalizing and Internalizing scores) by most likely class assignment.

Statistical analysis

We used GMM to evaluate the developmental trajectory of adaptive behavior in children with ASD and to characterize the heterogeneity in these trajectories. While this analytic approach has been commonly employed in other areas of the developmental literature, there have been limited applications in the developmental disability literature. Further, the method we used is more extensive and complete than previously published in the ASD literature (e.g., [28–30]). For this reason, we present a brief overview (for more in-depth and technical introductions, see [37, 38]) and we provide the necessary Mplus syntax in Additional file 1.

GMM is an extension of conventional latent growth modeling, a class of statistical procedures used in longitudinal investigations to characterize both intra- and interindividual variability in change. GMM may be particularly helpful in testing the assumption that the parameters from a standard growth model adequately describe data from two subpopulations (e.g., in physical growth curves, sex would be a known marker of subpopulation), especially when the explanation for heterogeneity is unknown. GMM treats this unknown as a latent variable problem, explained by an unobserved class variable. GMM provides information about whether the observed data are best explained by a single distribution of trajectory parameters (i.e., a latent class variable with only one class) or by a mixture of component distributions (i.e., a latent variable with two or more classes) [38].

Because the goal of GMM is to determine whether the data are best explained by one or more distributions, the first step is to establish the latent growth model (i.e., the best fitting model, assuming that there are no subpopulations reflected in the data). Subsequent GMM models will be compared to this "baseline" model to determine whether assuming a mixture of distributions, rather than a single distribution, improves fit.

GMMs of increasing complexity are then fit to the data. These models are distinguished by which parameters (i.e., mean, variance, and covariance of the intercept, slope, and/or quadratic terms) are allowed to vary, both within and between the classes. The simplest GMM is the latent class growth analysis (LCGA), which estimates only the mean values of the intercept, slope, and quadratic terms. These parameters are allowed to vary *between* classes, but not *within* (i.e., the variances, and therefore covariances, are constrained to zero). This means that all members of class 1 are constrained to have the same intercept, for example, but that intercept differs from those of the members of class 2. While it is possible that this preliminary model is appropriate, whether the variances and covariances should be constrained to zero is an empirical question. Thus, the remaining procedures entail the evaluation of at least four more models in the following sequence: (a) relax the within-class constraint on the variance of the intercept and slope factors (GMM1), (b) relax the within-class constraint on the covariance of the intercept and slope factors (GMM2), (c) relax the between-class constraint on the variance of the intercept and slope factors (GMM3), and (d) relax the between-class constraint on the covariance of the intercept and slope factors (GMM4). Each model specification is then evaluated for one, two, three, four or more classes, or until the model is no longer able to converge.

The best model is selected in an iterative process. First, the relative fit indices of all models are compared. In the current analyses, we used the following fit indices: the loglikelihood, the Bayesian information criterion, the adjusted Bayesian information criterion, Aikake's information criterion, and the consistent Aikake's information criterion. Bayes' factor and the approximate weight of evidence criterion were used to assist in the interpretation of information criteria. Finally, the Vuong-Lo-Mendell-Rubin likelihood ratio test (and an adjusted value) and the parametric bootstrap likelihood ratio test were used to assess the degree of improvement in model fit with additional classes. Each of these fit indices is described in Additional file 1.

Next, a handful of candidate models with the best profile of relative fit indices are further evaluated based on their classification quality and the degree of distinction between classes. In this study, we calculated entropy, the average posterior probability, the odds of correct classification, and the modal class assignment proportion for each class. The homogeneity and separation were calculated for each parameter that was allowed to vary and therefore characterize each class. The models were also evaluated for robustness to slight changes in the model specification; for example, does class assignment in the two-class solutions change significantly between the GMM1 and GMM2 specifications?

All GMM analyses were completed in Mplus version 7.4; other analyses and data management were performed in SAS/STAT version 9.3. We note that the maximum likelihood estimation with robust standard errors accommodates the missing data imposed by the age-cohort structure of the data. Because the results and fit indices for all 21 models are voluminous, they are reported in Additional file 1.

Results

Sparseness of data at age bands 2, 8, and 9 (see Additional file 1: Figure S1) was likely to cause convergence problems, so only age bands 3 through 7 (representing visits between the ages of 3 to 7.99 years) were used in this analysis. All 106 participants had at least one visit within these age bands, but we made the a priori choice to exclude from analysis one participant with data in age bands 3 and 4, who was an outlier with abnormally high ABC scores compared to other participants in the sample (see Additional file 1: Figure S2). Baseline demographic information, obtained at the first visit included in this analysis (not necessarily the participant's first study visit), for the remaining 105 participants is shown in Table 2. The number of study visits per participant ranged from one to five (median = 4) (see Additional file 1: Figure S1 for data coverage). Seven participants had only one visit.

Table 2 Participant demographics at baseline (*n* = 105)

	n (%)	Mean	Standard deviation
Male	91 (88)		
Age (years)	105 (100)	4.24	1.30
Maternal education			
High school	10 (10)		
Some college/college degree	63 (60)		
Graduate degree	28 (27)		
Not reported	4 (4)		
Full-scale developmental quotient	103 (98)	49.88	16.83
Non-verbal developmental quotient	103 (98)	58.39	16.87
Verbal developmental quotient	103 (98)	41.01	18.49
ADOS Calibrated Severity Score	103 (98)	7.66	1.40
Vineland Adaptive Behavior Composite	105 (100)	65.55	8.88
Full-scale DQ and Vineland ABC < 70	67 (64)		

The age cohorts 2, 8, and 9 were excluded from analysis and are therefore not reflected in this table. Thus, baseline in these analyses was not the first visit for all participants

Consistent with visual inspection, the best-fitting latent growth model was of quadratic form, where the variance in both the intercept and slope was estimated but was constrained to zero for the quadratic term. We used this baseline model for the remaining GMM analyses.

The full complement of fit indices for the GMM specifications is shown in Additional file 1: Table S1. Based on these results, the candidate models were the LCGA two-class, LCGA three-class, and the two-class solutions in the GMM1, GMM2, and GMM3 parameterizations. First, we reviewed the parameter estimates from each candidate model (Additional file 1: Table S2). The GMM parameterizations differ from LCGA in that they allow variation within the group on the intercept and slope factors. The within-class variance of the intercept, but not the slope, was large and significantly different from zero, suggesting that the GMM parameterizations might

be more reflective of the data than the LCGA. However, the covariance between the intercept and slope, which was allowed to be non-zero in the GMM2 parameterization, was not significant. Further, when the between-class variance was allowed in intercept and slope (GMM3), these parameters were non-significant. Considering that the mean estimates for the intercept and slope were similar for each class across the GMM parameterizations, the GMM1 appeared to be the best representation of the data.

Next, classification quality, as well as the homogeneity and separation of the resulting classes, was evaluated for the LCGA and GMM1 parameterizations (Additional file 1: Table S3). All models had acceptable classification quality, homogeneity, and separation. Thus, the selection of the GMM1 two-class solution, rather than the LCGA solution, was driven by the large and significant within-class variance of the intercept.

In the final model (Fig. 1), the low/decreasing class (class 1) was characterized by an ABC score of approximately 66 at age 3 years and a significant quadratic trajectory. The moderate/stable class (class 2) was characterized by a slightly higher age 3 score (about 72), with no change over the study period (i.e., slope and quadratic terms were non-significant) (see Additional file 1: Table S2). The model-estimated proportion of the sample in each class was 73 and 27%, respectively. To facilitate the comparison to published data, the observed means from the Szatmari et al. study were superimposed on the current study estimated class trajectories in Fig. 1.

The classes are descriptively characterized using other phenotypic data in Fig. 2. Modal class assignment was used to calculate the mean cognitive, ADOS CSS, and CBCL scores. Stronger non-verbal DQ relative to verbal DQ was characteristic of both classes, and in both classes, more change was observed over time in non-verbal DQ than in verbal DQ. However, for the moderate/stable class, average DQ scores increased over time, while average DQ

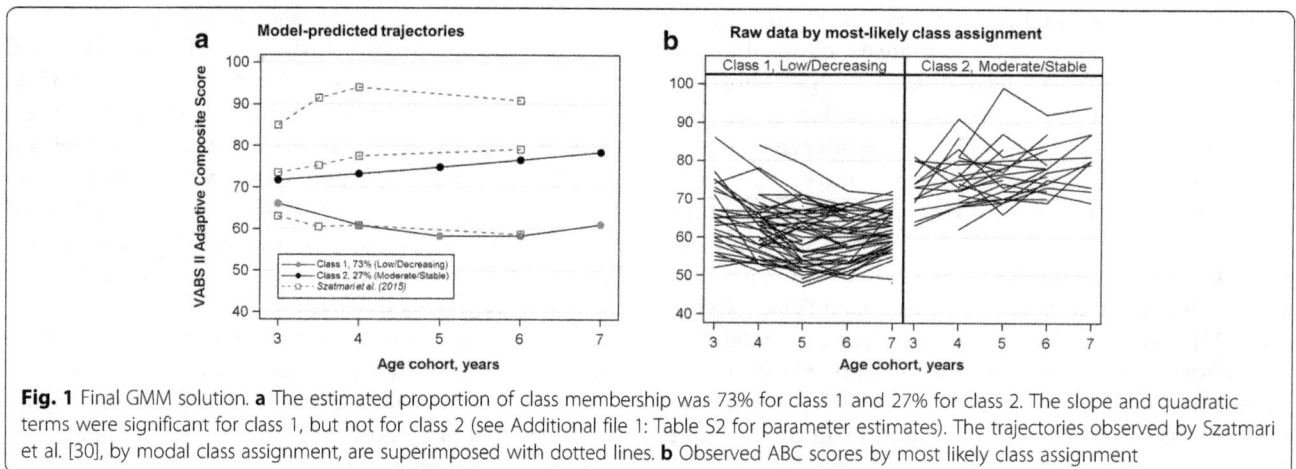

Fig. 1 Final GMM solution. **a** The estimated proportion of class membership was 73% for class 1 and 27% for class 2. The slope and quadratic terms were significant for class 1, but not for class 2 (see Additional file 1: Table S2 for parameter estimates). The trajectories observed by Szatmari et al. [30], by modal class assignment, are superimposed with dotted lines. **b** Observed ABC scores by most likely class assignment

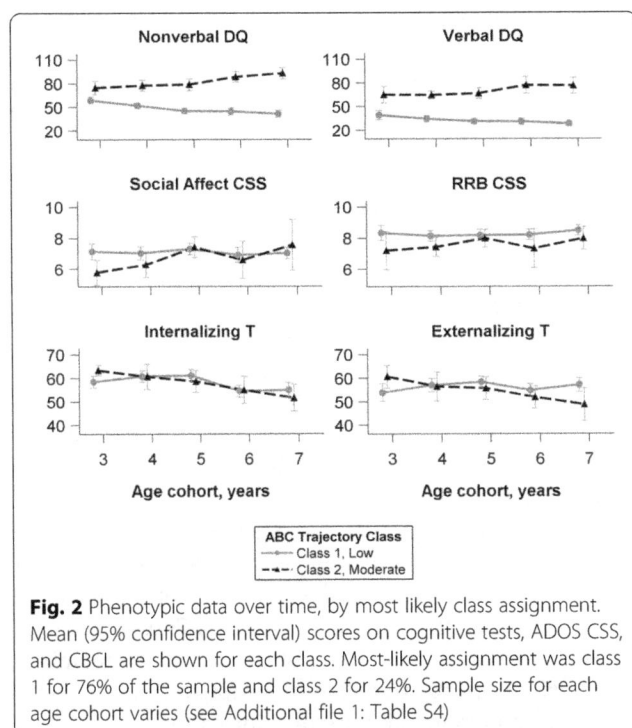

Fig. 2 Phenotypic data over time, by most likely class assignment. Mean (95% confidence interval) scores on cognitive tests, ADOS CSS, and CBCL are shown for each class. Most-likely assignment was class 1 for 76% of the sample and class 2 for 24%. Sample size for each age cohort varies (see Additional file 1: Table S4)

scores decreased over time for the low/decreasing class. No characteristic patterns were observed in ADOS CSS scores, which remained relatively stable over time, nor were the classes distinguished by CBCL Internalizing or Externalizing scores, though a general trend of decreasing over time was observed in both classes for the former.

Discussion

We used longitudinal data from children with ASD aged 3 to 7.99 years to explore heterogeneity in the development of adaptive behavior. About three quarters of the sample were assigned to a low/decreasing trajectory. The remainder of the sample were best classified in a trajectory exemplified by stable scores around 70 (moderate/stable). Thus, even within a sample likely to exhibit a high rate of intellectual disability later in childhood, we observed variability in the progression of adaptive function over time. Still, these data confirm previous findings that on average, young children with ASD are likely to exhibit significantly impaired adaptive function (based on age-referenced standard scores) during the preschool to school-age period, with only a minority exhibiting an improving trajectory [23, 30].

These two trajectories are reminiscent of patterns observed in studies of the development of cognitive ability; on average, children with more moderate scores tend to improve somewhat over time, while children with lower scores appear to fall further behind. The latter is to be expected with the use of standard scores; anything

less than on-pace gains in skills will result in decreasing standard scores over time. Decreasing standard scores over time are certainly not unique to ASD; similar trajectories have recently been described in various genetic disorders associated with intellectual disability, including fragile X syndrome, Williams syndrome, and tuberous sclerosis. This suggests that the presence of intellectual disability, rather than ASD specifically, may be the predominate explanatory factor for these declines. It is also possible that this pattern is reflective of psychometric properties of the VABS; with relatively fewer items at the lower extremes, stability in standard scores is difficult to achieve.

Adaptive behavior development does not exist in a vacuum, so it is essential to characterize subpopulations in terms of other phenotypic characteristics. Other studies have documented consistently that lower cognitive and language ability predicts less optimal trajectories of adaptive behavior [28–30]. This finding is echoed by data from cross-sectional or pre-post analytic designs (e.g., [9, 39, 40]). Given the strong correlations between measures of IQ and measures of adaptive behavior, it is unsurprising that changes in non-verbal and verbal DQ paralleled the adaptive behavior trajectory in our study. While IQ is not the only determinant of adaptive behavior, and studies have shown discrepancies between adaptive behavior scores and IQ scores may depend on IQ range [26, 41], it is well-established that cognitive impairment negatively affects the ability to carry out functions of daily life, above and beyond the effects of symptoms of ASD. However, while there was little difference in adaptive behavior and cognitive scores in the moderate/stable class, the average cognitive score in the low/decreasing class was much lower than the adaptive behavior score. This profile of relatively stronger adaptive behavior, compared to IQ, has been observed in other samples of individuals with low IQ [15, 42]. However, when IQ is not in the range of intellectual disability, adaptive behavior is often found to be lower than IQ in ASD [5], leading to the suggestion that the pattern is driven by deficits in social abilities [43]. The high proportion of children with low IQ and/or language impairment in our sample necessitated the use of ratio IQ scores, and this may have influenced our results by overemphasizing the effect of age (ratio IQs are divided by an ever-increasing denominator of chronological age). This may artificially delate IQ, resulting in lower ratio IQs than adaptive behavior scores in those with the lowest IQs.

The finding that the development of VABS composite scores over the preschool and early school-age years in our sample was best described by low/decreasing and moderate/stable classes was remarkably consistent with findings reported by Szatmari et al. and may be considered a partial replication, enhancing our confidence that these subpopulations exist. The wider age range in our study extends the Szatmari et al. findings, although a longer follow-up with denser sampling is necessary to confirm the short-term stabilizing trend observed after the age of 6 years in these data. In our sample, we did not find evidence for the "high functioning and improving" class described by Szatmari et al., which may reflect several factors, including ascertainment (they included participants referred to the longitudinal study directly from community referral centers, whereas our participants were mostly self-referral from the community) and diagnosis (they included DSM-IV-TR pervasive developmental disorder, not otherwise specified, while we required autistic disorder). Given that our sample had few participants with cognitive scores in the average range, we surmise that we simply did not sample the population represented by the "high functioning and improving" class in Szatmari et al. [30]. However, we do note that while the average IQ score in our sample was lower than that of Szatmari et al., mean IQs in both studies indicate similar levels of intellectual disability. Our slightly lower IQ likely reflects the more severely impaired cognitive profile of children already diagnosed with DSM-IV-TR autistic disorder (as opposed to an inception sample including pervasive developmental disorder, not otherwise specified). Thus, because our sample did not include many children with average IQs, these results are only generalizable to the subset of the ASD population with low IQ scores.

These data help to address the dearth of longitudinal natural history data on adaptive behavior in children with ASD and generally low cognitive ability. The most serious weaknesses of this study are its relatively small size, especially at the more extreme ages, and our inability to evaluate early predictors of class membership due to varying ages of study entry. Although we used the semi-structured survey interview form of the VABS, the necessary reliance on parent report may have biased results. However, a significant strength of this study is the analytic approach. While not novel in the broader child development literature, GMM has been implemented in few ASD studies, and when they have been used, researchers were likely to stop at the LCGA specification (e.g., [28–30]), limiting insights into data patterns that may not be obvious with traditional growth models.

Finally, we underscore the importance of these findings in relation to the ongoing search for appropriate outcome measures in intervention trials. Due to an emphasis on function as the most important outcome, adaptive behavior may become a more common primary and secondary target in clinical trials [44, 45]. We confirmed the presence of at least two subpopulations of adaptive behavior trajectories within ASD—children who are moderately impaired, but exhibit stable adaptive behavior standard scores over the early childhood and school-age years, and those who have more impaired scores that worsen over time. The reliable identification of the latter class would be advantageous for any clinical trial that uses adaptive behavior as an outcome. Specifically, researchers are investigating novel statistical methods to identify a "minimal clinically important difference" [23] in order to ease reliance on classical null hypothesis testing wherein significance is defined only by the difference from zero. Importantly, in some cases, this may actually be manifested as stability, or just minimal improvements in adaptive behavior standard scores (but growth in raw scores). The degree of meaningfulness may depend upon ability level [23] and may be further adjusted based on membership in an adaptive behavior trajectory subpopulation like those described herein. Szatmari et al. found that language and cognitive scores predicted class membership; it will be important to also explore whether the initial level of adaptive behavior had similarly predictive power. Future research, focused on the identification of predictors of membership, will help to translate descriptive findings into clinically and empirically useful information.

Conclusions

In this analysis, we reported data from one of the few longitudinal studies of ASD to include the transition from preschool to school-age, replicating with sophisticated statistical modeling the general findings of previous studies examining the development of adaptive behavior. These findings illustrate that early delays in adaptive behavior are stable or worsen from the preschool to school-age periods for the majority of children enrolled in these research cohorts, characterized by growth in adaptive behavior skills that lags behind the change in chronological age. For some children with lower adaptive abilities, this slower-than-expected growth results in a decline in composite standard scores during childhood. These findings provide critical context for the interpretation of changes in adaptive behavior scores in clinical trials.

Abbreviations

ABC: Adaptive Behavior Composite; ADI-R: Autism Diagnostic Interview-Revised; ADOS: Autism Diagnostic Observation Scale; ASD: Autism spectrum disorder; CBCL: Child Behavior Checklist; DQ: Developmental quotient; GMM: Growth mixture model; IQ: Intelligence quotient; LCGA: Latent class growth analysis; PDD: Pervasive developmental disorder not otherwise specified; VABS: Vineland Adaptive Behavior Scales

Acknowledgements

We thank the participants and their families, as well as the study staff and Jill Leon, B.S., who contributed to the literature review and Asma Idriss and the Clinical Trials Database staff who provided data management support.

Funding
This work was supported by the Intramural Research Program of the National Institute of Mental Health (ZIAMH002868).

Authors' contributions
AT and SS conceived and designed the study. CF analyzed the data. AT, LS, and CF interpreted the data. All authors were involved in drafting or revising the manuscript, gave final approval for publication, and agreed to be accountable for all aspects of the work.

Competing interests
The authors declare that they have no competing interests.

Author details
[1]Pediatrics and Developmental Neuroscience Branch, National Institute of Mental Health, National Institutes of Health, Bethesda, MD 20892, USA. [2]Department of Speech and Hearing Sciences, Washington State University, Spokane, WA 99202, USA.

References
1. American Psychiatric Association. Diagnostic and statistical manual of mental disorders (4th ed., text rev.). Washington, DC: Author; 2000.
2. American Psychiatric Association. Diagnostic and statistical manual of mental disorders (5th ed.). Arlington: American Psychiatric Publishing; 2013.
3. Dykens E, Lense M. Intellectual disabilities and autism spectrum disorder: a cautionary note. In: Amaral D, Geschwind D, Dawson G, editors. Autism spectrum disorders. Oxford: Oxford University Press; 2011. p. 261–9.
4. Volkmar F, Sparrow S, Goudreau D, Cicchetti DV, Paul R, Cohen D. Social deficits in autism: an operational approach using the Vineland Adaptive Behavior Scales. J Am Acad Child Adolesc Psychiatry. 1987;26:156–61.
5. Kenworthy L, Case L, Harms MB, Martin A, Wallace GL. Adaptive behavior ratings correlate with symptomatology and IQ among individuals with high-functioning autism spectrum disorders. J Autism Dev Disord. 2010;40:416–23.
6. Zander E, Bolte S. The new DSM-5 impairment criterion: a challenge to early autism spectrum disorder diagnosis? J Autism Dev Disord. 2015;45:3634–43.
7. Scahill L. Diagnosis and evaluation of pervasive developmental disorders. J Clin Psychiatry. 2005;66(Suppl 10):19–25.
8. Magiati I, Tay XW, Howlin P. Cognitive, language, social and behavioural outcomes in adults with autism spectrum disorders: a systematic review of longitudinal follow-up studies in adulthood. Clin Psychol Rev. 2014;34:73–86.
9. Hedvall A, Westerlund J, Fernell E, Norrelgen F, Kjellmer L, Olsson MB, Carlsson LH, Eriksson MA, Billstedt E, Gillberg C. Preschoolers with autism spectrum disorder followed for 2 years: those who gained and those who lost the most in terms of adaptive functioning outcome. J Autism Dev Disord. 2015;45:3624–33.
10. Kraijer D. Review of adaptive behavior studies in mentally retarded persons with autism/pervasive developmental disorder. J Autism Dev Disord. 2000;30:39–47.
11. Green MF, Schooler NR, Kern RS, Frese FJ, Granberry W, Harvey PD, Karson CN, Peters N, Stewart M, Seidman LJ, et al. Evaluation of functionally meaningful measures for clinical trials of cognition enhancement in schizophrenia. Am J Psychiatry. 2011;168:400–7.
12. van der Lee JH, Morton J, Adams HR, Clarke L, Ebbink BJ, Escolar ML, Giugliani R, Harmatz P, Hogan M, Jones S, et al. Cognitive endpoints for therapy development for neuronopathic mucopolysaccharidoses: results of a consensus procedure. Mol Genet Metab. 2017;121:70–9.
13. Bal VH, Farmer C, Thurm A. Describing function in ASD: using the DSM-5 and other methods to improve precision. J Autism Dev Disord. 2017;47: 2938–41.
14. Anagnostou E, Jones N, Huerta M, Halladay AK, Wang P, Scahill L, Horrigan JP, Kasari C, Lord C, Choi D. Measuring social communication behaviors as a treatment endpoint in individuals with autism spectrum disorder. Autism. 2015;19:622–36.
15. Kanne SM, Gerber AJ, Quirmbach LM, Sparrow SS, Cicchetti DV, Saulnier CA. The role of adaptive behavior in autism spectrum disorders: implications for functional outcome. J Autism Dev Disord. 2011;41:1007–18.

16. Scahill L, Bearss K, Lecavalier L, Smith T, Swiezy N, Aman MG, Sukhodolsky DG, McCracken C, Minshawi N, Turner K, et al. Effect of parent training on adaptive behavior in children with autism spectrum disorder and disruptive behavior: results of a randomized trial. J Am Acad Child Adolesc Psychiatry. 2016;55:602–9. e603
17. Berry-Kravis E, Hagerman R, Visootsak J, Budimirovic D, Kaufmann WE, Cherubini M, Zarevics P, Walton-Bowen K, Wang P, Bear MF, Carpenter RL. Arbaclofen in fragile X syndrome: results of phase 3 trials. J Neurodev Disord. 2017;9:3.
18. Veenstra-VanderWeele J, Cook EH, King BH, Zarevics P, Cherubini M, Walton-Bowen K, Bear MF, Wang PP, Carpenter RL. Arbaclofen in children and adolescents with autism spectrum disorder: a randomized, controlled, phase 2 trial. Neuropsychopharmacology. 2017;42:1390–8.
19. Scahill L, McDougle CJ, Aman MG, Johnson C, Handen B, Bearss K, Dziura J, Butter E, Swiezy NG, Arnold LE, et al. Effects of risperidone and parent training on adaptive functioning in children with pervasive developmental disorders and serious behavioral problems. J Am Acad Child Adolesc Psychiatry. 2012;51:136–46.
20. Dawson G, Rogers S, Munson J, Smith M, Winter J, Greenson J, Donaldson A, Varley J. Randomized, controlled trial of an intervention for toddlers with autism: the Early Start Denver Model. Pediatrics. 2010;125:e17–23.
21. Hardan AY, Gengoux GW, Berquist KL, Libove RA, Ardel CM, Phillips J, Frazier TW, Minjarez MB. A randomized controlled trial of Pivotal Response Treatment Group for parents of children with autism. J Child Psychol Psychiatry. 2015;56:884–92.
22. Green J, Pickles A, Pasco G, Bedford R, Wan MW, Elsabbagh M, Slonims V, Gliga T, Jones EJ, Cheung CH, et al. Randomised trial of a parent-mediated intervention for infants at high risk for autism: longitudinal outcomes to age 3 years. J Child Psychol Psychiatry. 2017;58:1330–40.
23. Chatham CH, Taylor KI, Charman T, Liogier D'ardhuy X, Eule E, Fedele A, Hardan AY, Loth E, Murtagh L, Del Valle Rubido M, et al. Adaptive behavior in autism: minimal clinically important differences on the Vineland-II. Autism Res. 2017. https://doi.org/10.1002/aur.1874.
24. Bishop SL, Farmer C, Thurm A. Measurement of nonverbal IQ in autism spectrum disorder: scores in young adulthood compared to early childhood. J Autism Dev Disord. 2015;45:966–74.
25. Lord C, Bishop S, Anderson D. Developmental trajectories as autism phenotypes. Am J Med Genet C Semin Med Genet. 2015;169:198–208.
26. Bolte S, Poustka F. The relation between general cognitive level and adaptive behavior domains in individuals with autism with and without co-morbid mental retardation. Child Psychiatry Hum Dev. 2002; 33:165–72.
27. Jung T, Wickrama K. An introduction to latent class growth analysis and growth mixture modeling. Soc Personal Psychol Compass. 2008;2:302–17.
28. Baghdadli A, Assouline B, Sonié S, Pernon E, Darrou C, Michelon C, Picot M-C, Aussilloux C, Pry R. Developmental trajectories of adaptive behaviors from early childhood to adolescence in a cohort of 152 children with autism spectrum disorders. J Autism Dev Disord. 2012;42:1314–25.
29. Bal VH, Kim SH, Cheong D, Lord C. Daily living skills in individuals with autism spectrum disorder from 2 to 21 years of age. Autism. 2015;19:774–84.
30. Szatmari P, Georgiades S, Duku E, Bennett TA, Bryson S, Fombonne E, Mirenda P, Roberts W, Smith IM, Vaillancourt T, et al. Developmental trajectories of symptom severity and adaptive functioning in an inception cohort of preschool children with autism spectrum disorder. JAMA Psychiatry. 2015;72:276–83.
31. Rutter M, Le Couteur A, Lord C. Autism diagnostic interview-revised. Los Angeles: Western Psychological Services; 2003.
32. Lord C, Rutter M, DiLavore PC, Risi S. Autism Diagnostic Observation Schedule (ADOS). Los Angeles, California: Western Psychological Services; 1999.
33. Mullen EM. Mullen scales of early learning. Circle Pines: American Guidance Service; 1995.
34. Elliott CD, editor. Manual for the differential ability scales, second edition. San Antonio, TX: Harcourt Assessment; 2007.
35. Achenbach TM, Rescorla LA. Manual for the ASEBA School-Age Forms and Profiles. Burlington: University of Vermont, Research Center for Children, Youth and Families; 2001.
36. Sparrow SS, Cicchetti DV, Balla DA. Vineland Adaptive Behavior Scales, Second Edition. Circle Pines, MN: AGS Publishing; 2005.
37. Ram N, Grimm KJ. Methods and measures: growth mixture modeling: a method for identifying differences in longitudinal change among unobserved groups. Int J Behav Dev. 2009;33:565–76.

38. Masyn KE. Latent class analysis and finite mixture modeling. In: The Oxford handbook of quantitative methods in psychology: Vol 2; 2013.

39. Pugliese CE, Anthony LG, Strang JF, Dudley K, Wallace GL, Naiman DQ, Kenworthy L. Longitudinal examination of adaptive behavior in autism spectrum disorders: influence of executive function. J Autism Dev Disord. 2016;46:467–77.

40. Hill TL, Gray SA, Kamps JL, Enrique Varela R. Age and adaptive functioning in children and adolescents with ASD: the effects of intellectual functioning and ASD symptom severity. J Autism Dev Disord. 2015;45:4074–83.

41. Perry A, Flanagan HE, Dunn Geier J, Freeman NL. Brief report: the Vineland Adaptive Behavior Scales in young children with autism spectrum disorders at different cognitive levels. J Autism Dev Disord. 2009;39:1066–78.

42. Flanagan HE, Smith IM, Vaillancourt T, Duku E, Szatmari P, Bryson S, Fombonne E, Mirenda P, Roberts W, Volden J, et al. Stability and change in the cognitive and adaptive behaviour scores of preschoolers with autism spectrum disorder. J Autism Dev Disord. 2015;45:2691–703.

43. Klin A, Saulnier CA, Sparrow SS, Cicchetti DV, Volkmar FR, Lord C. Social and communication abilities and disabilities in higher functioning individuals with autism spectrum disorders: the Vineland and the ADOS. J Autism Dev Disord. 2007;37:748–59.

44. Budimirovic DB, Berry-Kravis E, Erickson CA, Hall SS, Hessl D, Reiss AL, King MK, Abbeduto L, Kaufmann WE. Updated report on tools to measure outcomes of clinical trials in fragile X syndrome. J Neurodev Disord. 2017;9:14.

45. McConachie H, Parr JR, Glod M, Hanratty J, Livingstone N, Oono IP, Robalino S, Baird G, Beresford B, Charman T, et al. Systematic review of tools to measure outcomes for young children with autism spectrum disorder. Health Technol Assess. 2015;19:1–506.

9

Development of fine motor skills is associated with expressive language outcomes in infants at high and low risk for autism spectrum disorder

Boin Choi[1,2]* iD, Kathryn A. Leech[1,3], Helen Tager-Flusberg[4] and Charles A. Nelson[1,2,5]

Abstract

Background: A growing body of research suggests that fine motor abilities are associated with skills in a variety of domains in both typical and atypical development. In this study, we investigated developmental trajectories of fine motor skills between 6 and 24 months in relation to expressive language outcomes at 36 months in infants at high and low familial risk for autism spectrum disorder (ASD).

Methods: Participants included 71 high-risk infants without ASD diagnoses, 30 high-risk infants later diagnosed with ASD, and 69 low-risk infants without ASD diagnoses. As part of a prospective, longitudinal study, fine motor skills were assessed at 6, 12, 18, and 24 months of age and expressive language outcomes at 36 months using the Mullen Scales of Early Learning. Diagnosis of ASD was determined at the infant's last visit to the lab (18, 24, or 36 months) using the Autism Diagnostic Observation Schedule.

Results: Hierarchical linear modeling revealed that high-risk infants who later developed ASD showed significantly slower growth in fine motor skills between 6 and 24 months, compared to their typically developing peers. In contrast to group differences in growth from age 6 months, cross-sectional group differences emerged only in the second year of life. Also, fine motor skills at 6 months predicted expressive language outcomes at 3 years of age.

Conclusions: These results highlight the importance of utilizing longitudinal approaches in measuring early fine motor skills to reveal subtle group differences in infancy between ASD high-risk and low-risk infant populations and to predict their subsequent language outcomes.

Keywords: Autism, Fine motor skills, Expressive language, Early development, Infant siblings

Background

Autism spectrum disorder (ASD) is characterized by deficits in social communication and interaction and repetitive and restricted behaviors [1]. While the hallmarks of ASD are impairments in social communication and interaction, a growing body of evidence suggests that the disorder is also associated with impaired motor development. For example, a meta-analysis reported that individuals with ASD show substantial impairments in motor coordination,

compared with typically developing control participants [2]. A comprehensive review on motor functioning in ASD suggested that children and adults with ASD exhibit persistent difficulties across a wide set of motor behaviors including fine and gross motor skills and postural control [3].

Fine motor skills are one specific domain for which deficits and delays are common in ASD [3, 4]. These skills refer to one's ability to make fine hand movements that often require sophisticated object manipulation and appear more vulnerable to delay in ASD relative to general gross motor behaviors such as walking [5]. In fact, children and adults with ASD show difficulties in fine motor skills ranging from grasping toys to handwriting [3]. Moreover, infants with an older sibling with ASD,

---
* Correspondence: boinchoi@g.harvard.edu
[1]Graduate School of Education, Harvard University, Cambridge, MA, USA
[2]Graduate School of Arts and Sciences, Harvard University, Cambridge, MA, USA
Full list of author information is available at the end of the article

who have an approximately 20% chance of developing the disorder themselves [6] (hereafter, "high-risk"), exhibit deficits and delays in fine motor skills in the first few years of life [4, 7–11]. A recent meta-analysis of 34 studies reported that high-risk infants as a group show significantly poorer fine motor skills measured on the Mullen Scales of Early Learning [12], compared to low-risk infants who do not have a family history of ASD [13]. Specifically, the study identified 12 months as the earliest point when differences in fine motor skills can be reliably detected between high- and low-risk groups. Relatedly, another study found that among high-risk infants, those who subsequently developed ASD exhibited more pronounced and persistent motor difficulties, relative to high-risk infants who were later typically developing [4].

Furthermore, a growing number of studies have suggested that motor abilities are associated with skills in other domains such as language in both typical and atypical development (for review, see [14, 15]). In children with ASD specifically, motor skills in the first 2 years predict expressive language at 4 years [16] and later speech fluency [17]. In high-risk infants, fine motor skills between 12 and 24 months significantly predict expressive language scores at 3 years [4]. And, more recently, early motor skills were found to be associated with the rate of expressive language development in high-risk infants who develop ASD [18]. These findings thus suggest that motor and language skills are interrelated in development.

One possible explanation for the relation between motor and language skills is that development of skills in one domain (i.e., motor) can extend across other domains (i.e., language) over time to influence an outcome—a concept known as *developmental cascades* [19]. Specifically, infants with new motor skills have new learning opportunities to interact with the environment and people, which may subsequently influence how others interact with them, which in turn facilitates child language development. For instance, a previous study found that 13-month-olds who could walk shared objects with their mothers more frequently than those who could only crawl [20]. Also, mothers of walking infants, in turn, were twice more likely to respond to their infants than mothers of crawling infants. Similarly, infants who can pick up objects such as a toy block are more likely to share it with their caregivers, who can then provide the label for the object (e.g., "do you want to build blocks?"). The response, in turn, helps the infant learn the word "block." In short, a change in fine motor skills can alter how infants interact with objects and people, which may facilitate their language learning.

Given evidence of the motor-language links in development, deficits in early fine motor skills may help identify children who are likely to have language difficulties at a later age. Examining this possibility seems particularly relevant to infants at high risk for ASD who also have an increased prevalence of language and communication delays [21–23]. Identifying children at risk for future language difficulties would be useful so that targeted intervention programs can be made available to them in a timely fashion.

Despite the promising research benefits of studying early fine motor skills in ASD, there are several limitations to previous work that must be acknowledged. First, although subtle group differences in early fine motor skills at single time points have been noted, growth trajectories of fine motor skills in infants at high and low risk for ASD have yet to be thoroughly studied across infancy (see [7, 22] for notable exceptions). Studying how children's fine motor skills develop over time may help depict a more complete picture of early development in infants at high and low risk for ASD than collecting a snapshot of their abilities at a single age. Relatedly, it remains unclear whether and to what extent growth trajectories of early fine motor skills are related to later language skills in infants at high and low risk for ASD. Previous research has pooled fine motor skill data across different time points (i.e., using composite scores of fine motor skills) to predict language outcomes (e.g., [4, 17]). Although useful, prior research thus leaves the open question of which specific growth parameters of fine motor skills (i.e., a child's status, velocity, and acceleration in fine motor skills) may help predict subsequent language skills.

In the current study, we studied growth, or change over time, in fine motor skills between 6 and 24 months in relation to expressive language scores at 36 months in infants at high and low familial risk for ASD. By examining growth, we investigated whether groups differ in their trajectories of fine motor skills and determined which growth parameters of fine motor skills are linked to later language outcomes. First, we employed a unique growth modeling approach to ask whether growth in fine motor skills may differentiate three diagnostic groups: high-risk infants who were later diagnosed with ASD (HRA+), high-risk infants with no ASD diagnosis (HRA−), and low-risk control (LRC) infants with no diagnosis. We then used individual growth parameters of fine motor skills to predict expressive language at 36 months. Our specific research questions were as follows:

1. Do HRA+, HRA−, and LRC infants differ in their growth trajectories of fine motor skills between 6 and 24 months of age?
2. Do growth parameters of early fine motor skills (i.e., a child's status, velocity, and acceleration in

fine motor skills) predict expressive language at 36 months?

Methods

Participants

Participants were drawn from a prospective, longitudinal study of infants at high and low risk for ASD across the first 3 years of life. Eligibility criteria for all infants included a gestational age of at least 36 weeks, no known prenatal or perinatal complications, and no known genetic disorders. For the present study, the sample included infants who had fine motor skill data available for at least one time point at 6, 12, 18, and/or 24 months and an ASD evaluation at their last visit to the lab (either at 18, 24, or 36 months). The final analysis sample included 170 infants.

Of the 170 infants, 101 infants were classified as high risk for autism (HRA) because they had an older sibling with a community diagnosis of ASD. To verify older siblings' ASD diagnoses, we used the Autism Diagnostic Observation Schedule (ADOS) [24] and/or age-appropriate screeners including the Social Communication Questionnaire (SCQ), for probands older than four, [25] and the Pervasive Developmental Disorders Screening Test-II (PDDST-II) [26], for probands younger than four, with the best clinical judgment by a psychologist, where required.

ASD diagnoses in 52 older siblings of HRA infants (51% of the HRA sample in the current study) were verified using both the ADOS and SCQ. Four HRA older siblings (4%) had the ADOS. Thirty-seven older siblings (37%) had their diagnosis verified using the SCQ, and three older siblings (3%) had the PDDST-II, as they did not have the ADOS. Five older siblings (5%) did not have an ADOS, SCQ, or PDDST-II and therefore were unable to have their diagnoses verified; however, all five of them had received their ASD diagnoses in specialist clinics, and data from their younger siblings were included in the current study.

Sixty-nine infants were classified as low-risk control infants (LRC) if they had a typically developing older sibling and no first- or second-degree family members with ASD. ASD diagnoses in 48 older siblings of LRC infants (70% of the LRC sample) were verified using both the ADOS and SCQ. Three older siblings (4%) had the ADOS. Thirteen older siblings (19%) had the SCQ and one sibling (1%) had the PDDST-II, as they did not have the ADOS. Finally, four LRC older siblings (6%) did not have an ADOS, SCQ, or PDDST-II; however, data from their younger siblings were included in the study, as their parents reported no clinical concerns in the older siblings.

For purposes of analyses, infants were further categorized into three groups based on their risk status (high-vs. low-risk) and an eventual ASD diagnosis (ASD vs. no

ASD). Of the 101 HRA infants, 30 later met criteria for ASD (HRA+) and 71 did not meet criteria for ASD (HRA−). Of the 69 LRC infants, none met criteria for ASD (LRC).

Demographic characteristics for participants were collected at the first laboratory visit and are shown in Table 1, broken down by three groups and age. Infants in the three groups did not differ significantly on their race/ethnicity, sex distributions, and household income. However, there was a significant group difference in maternal education.[1] For data analysis, a composite score for socioeconomic status (SES) was generated by combining household income and maternal education using principal component analysis, as the two variables were significantly and positively related to each other ($r = .29$, $p = .0004$). The first principal component weighted maternal education and income positively and equally and explained about 64% of the original variance ($M = 0$, $SD = 1.14$). The group difference remained significant in the SES composite such that HRA+ infants had the lowest level of SES.

Procedures

This study was approved by the Institutional Review Boards (IRBs) at Boston Children's Hospital and Boston University. Written, informed consent was obtained from all caregivers prior to their infants' participation in the study. Infants were recruited and allowed to enter the study at different ages (e.g., 6 or 12 months) as long as their first visit took place no later than 12 months of age.

At 6, 12, 18, 24, and 36 months of age, trained examiners administered the Mullen Scales of Early Learning (MSEL) [12] to children who visited the laboratory. ASD diagnoses were made at 18, 24, and 36 months. At the child's last visit (either 18, 24, or 36 months), final ASD diagnoses for children were determined on the basis of the ADOS using the revised algorithm, with the best clinical judgment by a psychologist, where required. If there were multiple diagnostic evaluations (e.g., children completed ASD evaluations at 18, 24, and 36 months), the ultimate categorization was made at the last visit (e. g., 36 months) by a licensed psychologist. Depending on the child's last visit, ASD outcome classifications were made at 18 months for 13 children (8% of the sample in the present study; $n_{HRA+} = 3$; $n_{HRA-} = 4$; $n_{LRC} = 6$), at 24 months for 24 children (14%; $n_{HRA+} = 3$; $n_{HRA-} = 13$; $n_{LRC} = 8$), or at 36 months for 133 children (78%; $n_{HRA+} = 24$; $n_{HRA-} = 54$; $n_{LRC} = 55$). Although the majority of our children had their ASD outcome classifications made at 36 months, the rest of the children had their ASD outcomes made at earlier age points (18 or 24 months) due to sample attrition. As prior research suggests the high diagnostic stability of ASD at 18 and

Table 1 Sample characteristics, by age and group

	HRA+	HRA−	LRC	[c] p (3-group)
Sex (% female)	30.0	53.5	44.9	.09
	$n = 30$	$n = 71$	$n = 69$	
Race/ethnicity (% White)	83.3	95.7	88.4	.08
	$n = 30$	$n = 71$	$n = 69$	
[a] Household income	7.08 (2.02)	7.69 (0.91)	7.52 (1.38)	.79
	$n = 24$	$n = 67$	$n = 58$	
[b] Mother's level of education	5.04 (1.72)	5.74 (1.65)	6.65 (1.22)	.0002[***]
	$n = 25$	$n = 68$	$n = 62$	
Actual age at visits (month)				
6 months	5.91 (0.43)	5.96 (0.28)	5.97 (0.36)	.79
	$n = 22$	$n = 50$	$n = 61$	
12 months	11.93 (0.45)	11.94 (0.38)	11.87 (0.42)	.54
	$n = 30$	$n = 67$	$n = 67$	
18 months	18.12 (0.78)	17.91 (0.42)	18.01 (0.27)	.11
	$n = 25$	$n = 67$	$n = 67$	
24 months	24.16 (0.55)	24.03 (0.55)	24.10 (0.56)	.60
	$n = 25$	$n = 61$	$n = 63$	
36 months	36.09 (0.68)	36.57 (1.50)	36.33 (0.64)	.20
	$n = 22$	$n = 51$	$n = 54$	

Data are reported as group means with standard deviations in parentheses

[a]Income was reported on an 8-point scale: (1) less than $15,000, (2) $15,000–$25,000, (3) $25,000–$35,000, (4) $35,000–$45,000, (5) $45,000–$55,000, (6) $55,000–$65,000, (7) $65,000–$75,000, (8) more than $75,000

[b]Education was reported as the highest level attained on a 9-point scale: (1) some high school, (2) high school graduate, (3) some college, (4) community college/two-year degree, (5) four-year college degree, (6) some graduate school, (7) master's degree, (8) doctoral degree, (9) professional degree

[c]Fisher's exact tests were used to determine p values for group differences in sex and race/ethnicity. Kruskal-Wallis tests were used to determine p values for group differences in income and maternal education. One-way ANOVA tests were used to determine p values for group differences in age

[***]$p < .001$

24 months [27, 28], infants with ASD diagnoses made between 18 and 36 months were included in the current study, similar to previous studies [29, 30].

Measures

Mullen Scales of Early Learning (MSEL) [12]

The MSEL is a standardized, normed, developmental assessment for children from 0 to 68 months and provides an overall index of cognitive ability and potential delay. The MSEL consists of five scales: Gross Motor, Visual Reception, Fine Motor, Expressive Language, and Receptive Language. In this study, we used the MSEL Fine Motor, Expressive Language, and Visual Reception scales. More specifically, we used raw scores from the Fine Motor scale at 6, 12, 18, and 24 months to study longitudinal trajectories of children's fine motor skills development. We used children's raw scores from the Expressive Language scale at 36 months to assess children's expressive language outcomes. Raw scores from the Visual Reception scale at 6 months were used as a covariate to control for nonverbal cognition in regression analyses of fine motor and expressive language relations, as variation in children's early fine motor skills may arise from differences in general nonverbal skill [4]. The possible ranges of raw scores for the Fine Motor scale are 0 to 49 and 0 to 50 for the Expressive Language and Visual Reception

scales. We used raw scores rather than standardized scores (i.e., T scores), as raw scores allowed us to better capture individual differences in skills across time. Relatedly, we used child exact age at each visit as our measure of time to control for differences in age of testing (Table 1), which might affect children's raw scores on MSEL.

Autism Diagnostic Observation Schedule (ADOS) [24]

The ADOS is a semi-structured play assessment of social interaction, communication, and restricted interests/repetitive behavior. Research staff with extensive experience in testing children with developmental disorders administered and scored children's ADOS. In addition, an ADOS-reliable researcher co-scored the ADOS via video recording. When children met the criteria for ASD on the ADOS or came within three points of cutoffs, a licensed clinical psychologist reviewed the ADOS scores and behavioral assessment videos to determine final clinical judgment: ASD or no ASD.

Data reduction and analysis

Because of data attrition associated with longitudinal design (e.g., infants not yet enrolled in study, visits missed by families), 6-month fine motor skill data were available for $n = 133$, 12-month data for $n = 164$, 18-month data for $n = 159$, and 24-month data for $n = 149$ children. Of note, 110 of 170 infants contributed fine motor skills data at all four time points.

In order to address our research goals, we carried out analyses in two stages. In the first step, to explore group differences, we used hierarchical linear modeling (HLM) to best characterize each group's fine motor skills growth between 6 and 24 months (see Additional file 1). HLM allowed us to model developmental trajectories of each individual and accommodate the nested, hierarchical nature of the data (i.e., multiple measurements within infants) and missing data in our longitudinal design. Applications of HLM for growth involved a two-level hierarchical structure, where we first modeled each child's change over time in fine motor skills (Level 1) and then determined whether fine motor skills among the groups showed differences in growth parameters (Level 2). Specifically, at Level 1 (within children), we included time-variant predictors such as a linear age variable (*age*) and a quadratic age variable (*age*^{2}). We centered age at the earliest data collection point, 6 months or 0.5 years, so that parameters are more interpretable [31] and reflect children's fine motor skills and rate of growth at 6 months. In addition, we performed post hoc analyses by re-centering time so that the trajectories' intercept systematically varied by age (i. e., $age_{ti}-12$, $age_{ti}-18$, $age_{ti}-24$). Re-centering time allowed us to examine the point at which the divergence of developmental trajectories between outcome groups became statistically significant. If we did not center age, the model would estimate growth rates when children are at birth (i.e., 0 months), for which we would expect no measureable fine motor skill or growth. The quadratic age variable (*age*^{2}) represents the acceleration (or deceleration) in the rate of change and was calculated by squaring the centered linear age variable. At Level 2 (between children), time-invariant predictors included groups (*group*; HRA+, HRA−, LRC). The fully specified equation for our model is summarized in Additional file 1.

In the second step, our goal was to determine which growth parameters of early fine motor skills (i.e., status, velocity, and acceleration) between 6 and 24 months explain significant variance in children's expressive language outcomes at 36 months. Thus, we employed individual growth rates of fine motor skills from our Level-1 HLM model as independent variables to predict later expressive language skills in regression analyses (see Additional file 2). That is, we used a prediction model, in which we calculated individual growth rates, or Empirical Bayes' posterior means [32], using the random effects and fixed effects coefficients from our HLM model that includes only Level 1 predictors. An estimate was created for each child computed from a weighted combination of the individual child's growth trajectory (the random effect coefficient) as well as the average trajectory of the entire sample (the fixed effect coefficient). The rationale for using the method of Empirical Bayes stems from prior work that shows these Empirical Bayes' predictions from models are unbiased and precise (i.e., more similar to true values) than the predictions generated from a standard ordinary least squares (OLS) regression [32]. Similar to previous work employing the same analytic strategy [33], we found that the three predictors were too collinear to include simultaneously into one regression model. Thus, we fit three separate models for each predictor. All analyses were conducted using Stata and R, and HLM models were fit with the lmer package within R [34].

Results

Modeling fine motor skills growth

Descriptive data on cross-sectional fine motor skills, as measured on MSEL, between 6 and 24 months are presented in Table 2. Of note, although HRA+ infants as a group demonstrated lower raw scores on the MSEL Fine Motor scale, compared to HRA− and LRC infants, the scores of all groups were within the range of typical development.

To best characterize the developmental trajectories of fine motor skills between 6 and 24 months in HRA+, HRA−, and LRC infants, we used the following model building strategies. Preliminary visual inspection of the raw data suggested fine motor skills followed a curvilinear trajectory between 6 and 24 months. Statistical analyses confirmed this pattern: the best fitting model to

Table 2 Means, standard deviations, ranges, and sample sizes of cross-sectional data from the MSEL Fine Motor scale, by age and group

Age	HRA+	HRA−	LRC	p (3-group)	d (HRA+ vs. HRA−)	d (HRA+ vs. LRC)	d (HRA− vs. LRC)
6 months	7.86 (1.21) 6–11 $n = 22$	8.42 (1.28) 6–12 $n = 50$	8.13 (1.27) 6–12 $n = 61$	0.20	− 0.44	− 0.22	0.23
12 months	16.5 (2.08) 12–21 $n = 30$	17.27 (1.80) 12–20 $n = 67$	16.58 (1.63) 12–20 $n = 67$	0.04	− 0.41	− 0.05	0.40
18 months	20.36 (1.66) 16–24 $n = 25$	21.03 (1.64) 17–24 $n = 67$	20.96 (1.54) 19–25 $n = 67$	0.19	−0.41	− 0.38	0.04
24 months	24.12 (2.42) 19–28 $n = 25$	25.13 (2.12) 20–29 $n = 61$	25.56 (2.59) 20–32 $n = 63$	0.04	−0.46	− 0.57	−0.18

the data contained both a linear and quadratic growth term, $-2\ Log\ Likelihood = -1231$, $\chi^2\ (7) = 1481$, $p < .001$. Next, we added the interaction between group (HRA+, HRA−, LRC) and age (both linear and quadratic) to determine whether change in fine motor skills differed between groups. Results revealed that the groups differed significantly from one another in the linear growth only, $\hat{\beta}_{HRA+ \times AGE} = -0.83$, $SE_{HRA+ \times AGE} = 0.39$, $p = .04$; $\hat{\beta}_{HRA- \times AGE} = -0.51$, $SE_{HRA- \times AGE} = 0.30$, $p = .09$. A model with a *group × quadratic age* interaction fit the data no better than a model without it. As such, we removed this term and retained only the *group × linear age* interaction in subsequent models. We completed our model building process by adding demographic covariates (i.e., sex and SES). Neither of the covariates significantly predicted fine motor skills and were thus not included in the final model.

Our final HLM model summaries are presented in Table 3. The final model considered between-child associations of groups with status (intercept), velocity (linear growth), and acceleration (quadratic growth) in fine motor skills and an interaction effect between groups and linear growth at 6 months. Note that we entered the LRC group into all models as a reference group; therefore, the coefficients generated for HRA+ and HRA− groups reflected deviations in intercept, slope, and acceleration from the LRC group. The final model shows that, on average, LRC infants at 6 months had estimated fine motor skills of approximately 8 points, with an increase in fine motor skills at this age at a rate of 17.71 points per year. Of note, after studying how high-risk infants differed in their fine motor skills development from those of low-risk infants (i.e., LRC as a reference

group), we systematically rotated which group served as the comparison to examine potential differences in growth trajectories among three groups.

Estimated growth trajectories of fine motor skills from 6 to 24 months are presented for all three groups in Fig. 1.

As can be seen in the figure, when we compared *status* of fine motor skills (i.e., intercept) among three groups, HRA+ infants did not significantly differ from their typically developing peers (both HRA− and LRC) at 6 months, indicating that the three groups were indistinguishable by their fine motor skills at 6 months. However, when age was re-centered at 12, 18, and 24 months to identify points of divergence in developmental trajectories of fine motor skills, HRA+ infants showed significantly lower fine motor skills than HRA− infants starting at 12 months ($t = 2.45$, $p = .015$) and LRC infants at 18 months ($t = -2.34$, $p = .02$). Thus, these results indicate that infants later diagnosed with ASD began to diverge from their typically developing peers by their first birthday, although when these groups diverged depended on whether they were infants at high or low risk for autism. Interestingly, at 6 months, HRA− infants had significantly stronger fine motor scores compared to LRC infants, $t = 2.19$, $p = .03$, but this difference no longer reached significance beginning at 12 months.

When we compared *velocity* in fine motor skills (i.e., linear growth) among the three groups, HRA+ infants had significantly slower growth rates than LRC infants at 6 through 24 months, $t = -2.11$, $p = .036$. Specifically, the average growth rate for the HRA+ group ($M = 16.88$, $SE = 0.39$) was approximately two standard errors below the mean of the LRC group ($M = 17.71$, $SE = 0.44$). The HRA− infants also had slower growth rates than the

Table 3 Final growth model of group predicting growth trajectories for fine motor skills (age centered at 6 months; $N = 170$)

	Coefficient	SE
Intercept	8.38***	0.19
Linear growth	17.71***	0.44
Quadratic growth	−4.38***	0.27
HRA+	0.08	0.34
HRA−	0.58*	0.26
Linear × HRA+	−0.83*	0.39
Linear × HRA−	−0.51	0.30
Variance components		
Goodness of fit (− 2 Log Likelihood)	− 1226.94	
Variance in intercept	0.27	
Variance in growth rate	1.70	
Variance in acceleration	1.72	

***$p < .001$, *$p < .05$

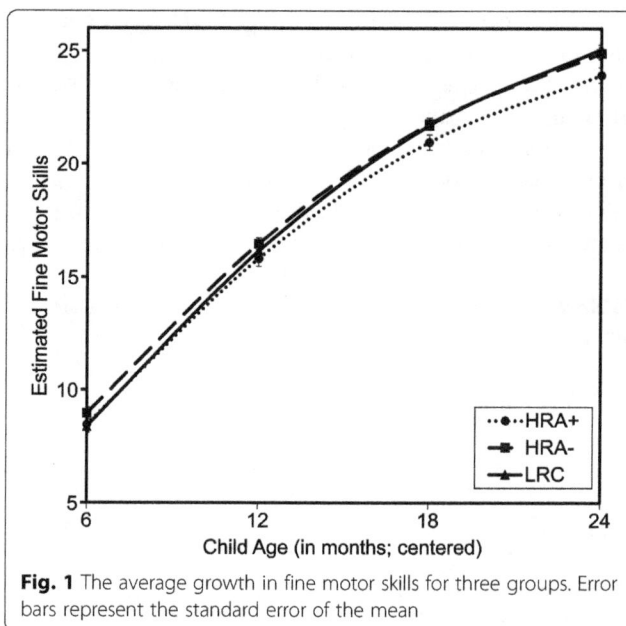

Fig. 1 The average growth in fine motor skills for three groups. Error bars represent the standard error of the mean

LRC group between 6 and 24 months, but this difference did not reach statistical significance, $t = -1.68$, $p = .094$. Thus, while the groups demonstrated comparable status of fine motor skills at 6 months, HLM revealed subtle group differences in growth in fine motor skills from 6 months.

Using growth parameters of fine motor skills to predict expressive language outcomes

To investigate which growth parameters of fine motor skills between 6 and 24 months predict expressive language outcomes at 36 months, we first examined descriptive statistics on the language outcomes (Table 4) and found significant group differences on 36-month expressive language scores. Specifically, high-risk infants scored significantly lower on the MSEL Expressive Language scale at 36 months, compared to low-risk infants.

Next, we fitted a series of regression models with each of the growth parameters as the independent variable and expressive language scores as the dependent variable. In regression analyses, we controlled for children's nonverbal cognition, as indexed by MSEL visual reception scores at 6 months, to evaluate whether variance in expressive language skills was accounted for by the fine motor growth parameters above and beyond any variance accounted for by children's general nonverbal skill. The visual reception scores, assessed independently of children's motor abilities, did not differ across groups at 6 months (Table 4). In addition, child sex and SES, which significantly differed across groups and also are identified as related to children's language skills in previous research [35, 36], were included as covariates.

Table 5 shows the results of regression analyses. Specifically, the status of fine motor skills at 6 months (Model 1) was a significant, positive predictor of 36-month expressive language scores, when controlling for 6-month visual reception scores, sex, and SES. In other words, these results illustrate that when accounting for children's general nonverbal cognition, sex, and SES, a child whose 6-month fine motor skills scored at the sample mean had an expressive language score of 35 points at 36 months, and every one unit increment in fine motor skills at 6 months was associated with approximately four-point difference ($SE = 1.22$) in 36-month language scores, $t = 3.64$, $p < .001$, $R^2 = 23.6\%$, 95% CI = [2.02, 6.88]. When

Table 5 Growth models predicting 36-month Expressive Language skills, when controlling for nonverbal cognition, SES, and sex

	Model 1	Model 2	Model 3
Intercept	34.89***	33.28***	31.82***
Predicted status at 6 months	4.45***		
Predicted velocity at 6 months		1.14~	
Predicted acceleration at 6 months			−0.02
Nonverbal cognition at 6 months	0.07	0.25	0.39
SES	1.45**	1.54**	1.50**
Sex	0.08	0.63	0.97
R^2	23.6%	14.4%	10.9%
BIC	510	520	523

*** $p < .001$, ** $p < .01$

accounting for the covariates, the velocity in fine motor skills (Model 2) was marginally significant in predicting later expressive language scores, $t = 1.81$, $p = .07$, $R^2 = 14.4\%$. The acceleration (Model 3) did not result in significant variance explained in later language skills, $t = -.03$, $p = .98$, $R^2 = 10.9\%$. As the models were not nested, we compared Bayesian Information Criterion (BIC) estimates to determine which growth parameter best accounted for variance in the language outcomes. This comparison suggests that the model with the status of fine motor skills had the lowest BIC (510) value, relative to the models with the velocity or acceleration parameters ($BICs = 520$, 523, respectively). Altogether, a child's 6-month fine motor skills provided the most helpful information to estimate the child's expressive language at 3 years of age.

Finally, we included interaction terms between each of the growth parameters and groups (e.g., *linear x group*) to determine whether the relations between growth parameters of fine motor skills and expressive language outcomes differ across groups. A model resulted in no significant interactions between growth parameters and groups, suggesting that the effect of fine motor skills on later expressive language outcomes did not differ for HRA+, HRA−, and LRC infants.

Discussion

In the current study, we examined growth trajectories of fine motor skills between 6 and 24 months and

Table 4 Means and standard deviations for MSEL Expressive Language scale raw scores at 36 months and MSEL Visual Reception scale raw scores at 6 months

	HRA+	HRA−	LRC	p (3-group)
MSEL Expressive Language at 36 months	31.32 (4.28) $n = 22$	35.02 (4.53) $n = 51$	37.26 (3.89) $n = 54$	< .0001***
MSEL Visual Reception at 6 months	8.41 (1.74) $n = 22$	8.6 (1.54) $n = 50$	8.44 (1.65) $n = 61$	.85

*** $p < .001$

determined which growth parameters of fine motor skills predict language outcomes at 36 months in high-risk infants later diagnosed with ASD, high-risk infants with no ASD diagnosis, and low-risk infants with no ASD diagnosis. Our key findings were that the development of fine motor skills was slower between 6 and 24 months in high-risk infants later diagnosed with ASD, compared to that of their typically developing peers, and that early fine motor skills were associated with subsequent expressive language skills at 36 months in all three groups.

Growth trajectories of early fine motor skills

HLM revealed that infants at high risk for ASD who themselves later developed ASD had slower *growth* in fine motor skills between 6 and 24 months of age, compared to infants at low risk for ASD. This finding is consistent with those of previous studies that also employed longitudinal approaches and examined infants' performance on the MSEL. Specifically, a prior study reported that high-risk infants later diagnosed with ASD deviated from unaffected infants at around 14 months and developed more slowly through 24 months on the MSEL Fine Motor scale [8]. Similarly, another study using latent class analysis identified slower developmental trajectories of fine motor skills in children with ASD between 6 and 36 months, compared to children without ASD [37]. This study thus adds to the existing research suggesting slower development in infancy in children with ASD. However, while these group differences between high-risk infants with ASD diagnoses and low-risk infants without ASD diagnoses were statistically significant, they were subtle and small (Fig. 1; Table 2). Moreover, fine motor scores for all groups were within the range of typical development, indicating that these modest group differences may not rise to the level of detection by parents or clinicians in many cases.

Our data indicated that although high-risk infants later diagnosed with ASD showed slower growth in fine motor skills between the 6- and 24-month periods, relative to that of high-risk infants without ASD diagnoses, this difference was not statistically significant. This nonsignificant difference between the two high-risk groups suggests that slower fine motor growth may not be specific to ASD. Our finding is consistent with those from prior research indicating that fine motor differences may be a characteristic of infants at high risk for ASD, rather than a core characteristic of the disorder [10].

With regard to the *status* of fine motor skills at 6 months, there was no statistically significant difference between high-risk infants who later developed ASD and typically developing high- and low-risk infants. Only beginning in the second year of life, did high-risk infants who were later diagnosed with ASD score significantly lower on the MSEL Fine Motor scale than high- and

low-risk infants without eventual diagnosis. The nonsignificant group difference in status of fine motor skills at 6 months stands in contrast to some of the prior findings that reported high-risk infants tend to show differences in fine motor skills, relative to their low-risk peers as early as 6 months [10]. Given mixed evidence of fine motor differences in infancy (i.e., 6–7 months), future research is needed to replicate the examination of fine motor skill development with larger samples, particularly within the first year of life in ASD risk populations.

To our surprise, high-risk infants who did not develop ASD showed stronger fine motor scores than low-risk infants at 6 months, but the difference was transient, with these infants showing comparable fine motor scores from 12 months onward. This difference may reflect a random sampling error. Alternatively, strong early fine motor skills may function as a protective factor, rather than a risk factor, for some high-risk infants. That is, while all high-risk infants presumably carry genetic risk factors for ASD, those with stronger fine motor skills may require greater familial etiologic load to manifest the ASD phenotype [38]. Examining the extent to which fine motor skills may act as a protective or risk factor for high-risk infants will be an important avenue for future research.

The results of the first part of our study highlight the importance of investigating the course of developmental change in skills over time. Studies of other behavioral domains lend support for this need to focus on developmental change [39]. For example, an eye-tracking study reported that infants later diagnosed with ASD showed a decline in fixation to the eye region of the face from 2 to 6 months and were distinguishable from their typically developing peers by change over time; however, cross-sectional group differences in eye fixation emerged only later in the first year [40]. Thus, while cross-sectional research identifies group differences at individual time points, longitudinal approaches can capture developmental change over time and depict a more complete and nuanced picture of early development in infants at high and low risk for ASD.

Fine motor growth trajectories predict expressive language outcomes

In our analysis to determine which growth parameters of early fine motor skills predict subsequent expressive language outcomes at 36 months, we found that the status of fine motor skills from the 6- to 24-month growth model was a significant, positive predictor of later expressive language outcomes, even after controlling for nonverbal cognition scores, sex, and SES. In other words, infants with poorer fine motor skills across the first 2 years of life scored significantly lower on expressive language at 36 months, even when the covariates were taken into account. On the other hand, the velocity in fine motor skills was marginally associated with subsequent expressive language outcomes, and the acceleration was not significantly associated with the outcomes, when controlling for the covariates. Thus, it appears that status of early fine motor skills may provide the most useful information about later expressive language skills among the growth parameters (i.e., status, velocity, and acceleration).

Also, the significant, positive associations between early fine motor skills and subsequent expressive language outcomes did not differ across all three groups, suggesting that differences in fine motor skills over time can have cascading effects on language outcomes for both high-risk infants who later developed ASD and typically developing high- and low-risk infants. These findings align with prior work on developmental motor-language cascades [4, 41] demonstrating that children's early motor skills are significantly and positively related to later expressive language skills in both typical and atypical development.

Finally, the associations between early fine motor skills and later language abilities highlight a potential avenue for early intervention practices. Given that the findings of this study suggest that fine motor skills in infancy may influence subsequent expressive language outcomes, an assessment of early fine motor skills holds promise for early identification of difficulties in language which emerge later in life in high-risk infants [21, 22]. By identifying and addressing infants' difficulties in fine motor skills in a timely fashion, we may then prevent cascading effects of motor impairments on children's language development. In fact, a growing body of literature suggests promising effects of early motor training on other domains of development. For example, "sticky mittens" with Velcro strips are associated with increased object exploration behaviors in infants that are shown positively related to subsequent language development [42, 43].

Our findings should be interpreted in light of key limitations, however. First, due to the high levels of maternal education, our sample may not be a nationally representative sample of infants at high and low risk for ASD. Therefore, findings may not be generalizable to the larger population of infants at high and low risk for ASD. Second, our study focused on examining the relations between early fine motor skill development and later expressive language outcomes in infants at risk for ASD. More studies are needed to closely investigate the motor-language relations in other neurodevelopmental disorders such as developmental language disorders and dyslexia. Third, ASD outcomes of 22% of our participants were made at 18 or 24 months instead of at 36 months, when diagnosis can be reliably made [44]. Therefore, it is possible that those diagnosed at 18 or 24 months would or would not have met criteria for ASD at 36 months. However, the best clinical judgment was made by an expert clinician for those children using comprehensive data including developmental history and standardized tools. In addition, recent studies suggest high diagnostic stability for infants at high familial risk at this age [27, 28]. While we made a decision to include those with ASD outcomes made at 18–36 months to maximize our sample size, future research could minimize the variation in age of diagnosis until there is more evidence for stable diagnosis as early as 18 months of age. Despite these limitations, our findings have the potential to promote longitudinal examinations of infants at increased risk for ASD and influence how we intervene to promote their optimal language outcomes.

Conclusions

Overall, our results suggest that fine motor skills growth between 6 and 24 months is significantly slower in high-risk infants with eventual ASD diagnosis, compared to high- and low-risk peers without eventual diagnosis, and predicts expressive language skills at 3 years of age. This work highlights the importance of studying children's skills within the context of developmental trajectories. Specifically, examining children's developmental change over time may create a more complete picture than collecting a snapshot of their abilities at a single age. Finally, poor performance on early fine motor skills may indicate an increased risk for language difficulties in children and be addressed early in life to promote children's optimal language outcomes. Targeting early fine motor skills in infancy seems promising, considering that these skills seem amenable to intervention [42, 43] and that children can have the most gains during sensitive periods when their brains are receptive to the environment [45]. Altogether, our results suggest that closer attention to developmental trajectories of fine motor skills in relation to later developmental outcomes may be warranted in infants at high familial risk for ASD.

Endnotes

[1]LRC mothers demonstrated the highest levels of maternal education. Although our sample as a whole was recruited from a relatively high socioeconomic area of greater New England area, our LRC families, in particular, had unusually high levels of maternal education. Specifically, the majority of mothers of LRC infants (60 out of 62 families; 97%) had at least four-year college degree, and the remaining two families (3%) indicated community college/two-year degree as the highest education level attained.

Abbreviations

ADOS: Autism Diagnostic Observation Schedule; ASD: Autism spectrum disorder; HLM: Hierarchical linear modeling; HRA: High risk for autism; HRA +: High-risk infants with autism; HRA−: High-risk infants without autism; IRB: Institutional Review Board; LRC: Low-risk control; MSEL: Mullen Scales of Early Learning; OLS: Ordinary least squares; PDDST-II: Pervasive Developmental Disorders Screening Test-II; SCQ: Social Communication Questionnaire; SES: Socioeconomic status

Acknowledgements

The authors would like to thank all the children and families who participated in this study as well as the former and current Infant Sibling Project team members for their help in the data collection. BC is also grateful to Dr. Meredith Rowe and Dr. Heather Hill for comments and revisions on an earlier draft of this manuscript.

Funding

This work was supported by the grants from the National Institutes of Health (R01-DC010290 to HTF and CAN; R21-DC08637 to HTF), Autism Speaks (1323 to HTF), and Simons Foundation (137186 to CAN). The funding bodies did not have any role in the design, collection, analyses, and interpretation of data or in writing the manuscript.

Authors' contributions

BC performed data analysis and manuscript writing. KL contributed to data analysis and manuscript revisions. HTF and CAN were the principal investigators of the larger Infant Sibling Project and critically revised the manuscript for important intellectual content. All authors read and approved the final manuscript.

Competing interests

The authors declare that they have no competing interests.

Author details

[1]Graduate School of Education, Harvard University, Cambridge, MA, USA. [2]Graduate School of Arts and Sciences, Harvard University, Cambridge, MA, USA. [3]Boston University School of Education, Boston, MA, USA. [4]Department of Psychological and Brain Sciences, Boston University, Boston, MA, USA. [5]Laboratories of Cognitive Neuroscience, Division of Developmental Medicine, Boston Children's Hospital, Harvard Medical School, Boston, MA, USA.

References

1. American Psychiatric Association. Diagnostic and statistical manual of mental disorders. 5th ed. Arlington: American Psychiatric Publishing, Inc.; 2013.

2. Fournier KA, Hass CJ, Naik SK, Lodha N, Cauraugh JH. Motor coordination in autism spectrum disorders: a synthesis and meta-analysis. J Autism Dev Disord. 2010;40:1227–40.

3. Bhat AN, Landa RJ, Galloway JC. Current perspectives on motor functioning in infants, children, and adults with autism spectrum disorders. Phys Ther. 2011;91:1116–29.

4. LeBarton ES, Iverson JM. Fine motor skill predicts expressive language in infant siblings of children with autism. Dev Sci. 2013;16 https://doi.org/10.1111/desc.12069.

5. Landa R, Gross AL, Stuart EA, Bauman M. Latent class analysis of early developmental trajectory in baby siblings of children with autism. J Child Psychol Psychiatry. 2012;53:986–96.

6. Ozonoff S, Young GS, Carter A, Messinger D, Yirmiya N, Zwaigenbaum L, et al. Recurrence risk for autism spectrum disorders: a baby siblings research consortium study. Pediatrics. 2011;128:e1–8.

7. Estes A, Zwaigenbaum L, Gu H, St. John T, Paterson S, Elison JT, et al. Behavioral, cognitive, and adaptive development in infants with autism spectrum disorder in the first 2 years of life. J Neurodev Disord. 2015;7 https://doi.org/10.1186/s11689-015-9117-6.

8. Landa R, Garrett-Mayer E. Development in infants with autism spectrum disorders: a prospective study. J Child Psychol Psychiatry. 2006;47:629–38.

9. Leonard HC, Bedford R, Charman T, Elsabbagh M, Johnson MH, Hill EL, et al. Motor development in children at risk of autism: a follow-up study of infant siblings. Autism Int J Res Pract. 2014;18:281–91.

10. Libertus K, Sheperd KA, Ross SW, Landa RJ. Limited fine motor and grasping skills in 6-month-old infants at high risk for autism. Child Dev. 2014;85:2218–31.

11. Toth K, Dawson G, Meltzoff AN, Greenson J, Fein D. Early social, imitation, play, and language abilities of young non-autistic siblings of children with autism. J Autism Dev Disord. 2007;37:145–57.

12. Mullen EM. Mullen Scales of Early Learning. AGS. Circle Pines: American Guidance Service; 1995.

13. Garrido D, Petrova D, Watson LR, Garcia-Retamero R, Carballo G. Language and motor skills in siblings of children with autism spectrum disorder: a meta-analytic review. Autism Res Off J Int Soc Autism Res. 2017;10:1737–50.

14. Leonard HC, Hill EL. Review: the impact of motor development on typical and atypical social cognition and language: a systematic review. Child Adolesc Ment Health. 2014;19:163–70.

15. Iverson JM. Developing language in a developing body: the relationship between motor development and language development. J Child Lang. 2010;37:229–61.

16. Stone WL, Yoder PJ. Predicting spoken language level in children with autism spectrum disorders. Autism Int J Res Pract. 2001;5:341–61.

17. Gernsbacher MA, Sauer EA, Geye HM, Schweigert EK, Goldsmith H. Infant and toddler oral- and manual-motor skills predict later speech fluency in autism. J Child Psychol Psychiatry. 2008;49:43–50.

18. Leonard HC, Bedford R, Pickles A, Hill EL. Predicting the rate of language development from early motor skills in at-risk infants who develop autism spectrum disorder. Res Autism Spectr Disord. 2015;13(Supplement C):15–24.

19. Masten AS, Cicchetti D. Developmental cascades. Dev Psychopathol. 2010;22:491–5.

20. Karasik LB, Tamis-LeMonda CS, Adolph KE. Crawling and walking infants elicit different verbal responses from mothers. Dev Sci. 2014;17:388–95.

21. Mitchell S, Brian J, Zwaigenbaum L, Roberts W, Szatmari P, Smith I, et al. Early language and communication development of infants later diagnosed with autism spectrum disorder. J Dev Behav Pediatr JDBP. 2006;27(2 Suppl):S69–78.

22. Iverson JM, Wozniak RH. Variation in vocal-motor development in infant siblings of children with autism. J Autism Dev Disord. 2007;37:158–70.

23. Messinger D, Young GS, Ozonoff S, Dobkins K, Carter A, Zwaigenbaum L, et al. Beyond autism: a baby siblings research consortium study of high-risk children at three years of age. J Am Acad Child Adolesc Psychiatry. 2013;52:300–8.

24. Lord C, Risi S, Lambrecht L, Cook EH, Leventhal BL, DiLavore PC, et al. The autism diagnostic observation schedule-generic: a standard measure of social and communication deficits associated with the spectrum of autism. J Autism Dev Disord. 2000;30:205–23.

25. Rutter M, Bailey A, Lord C. The Social Communication Questionnaire. Los Angeles: Western Psychological Services; 2003.

26. Siegel B. Pervasive Developmental Disorder Screening Test-II (PDDST-II). San Antonio: Harcourt; 2004.

27. Ozonoff S, Young GS, Landa RJ, Brian J, Bryson S, Charman T, et al. Diagnostic stability in young children at risk for autism spectrum disorder: a baby siblings research consortium study. J Child Psychol Psychiatry. 2015;56:988–98.

28. Zwaigenbaum L, Bryson SE, Brian J, Smith IM, Roberts W, Szatmari P, et al. Stability of diagnostic assessment for autism spectrum disorder between 18 and 36 months in a high-risk cohort. Autism Res Off J Int Soc Autism Res. 2016;9:790–800.

29. Levin AR, Varcin KJ, O'Leary HM, Tager-Flusberg H, Nelson CA. EEG power at 3 months in infants at high familial risk for autism. J Neurodev Disord. 2017;9:34.

30. Talbott MR, Nelson CA, Tager-Flusberg H. Maternal vocal feedback to 9-month-old infant siblings of children with ASD. Autism Res. 2016;9:460–70.

31. Singer J, Willett J. Applied longitudinal data analysis: modeling change and event occurrence. New York: Oxford University Press; 2003.

32. Raudenbush SW, Bryk AS. Hierarchical linear models: applications and data analysis methods. 2nd ed. Thousand Oaks: SAGE Publications, Inc; 2002.

33. Rowe ML, Raudenbush SW, Goldin-Meadow S. The pace of vocabulary growth helps predict later vocabulary skill. Child Dev. 2012;83:508 25.

34. Bates D, Mächler M, Bolker B, Walker S. Fitting linear mixed-effects models using lme4. J Stat Softw. 2015;67. https://www.jstatsoft.org/article/view/v067i01/0.

35. Fernald A, Marchman VA, Weisleder A. SES differences in language processing skill and vocabulary are evident at 18 months. Dev Sci. 2013;16:234–48.

36. Hart B, Risley T. American parenting of language-learning children: persisting differences in family-child interactions observed in natural home environments. Dev Psychol. 1992;28:1096–105.

37. Landa RJ, Gross AL, Stuart EA, Faherty A. Developmental trajectories in children with and without autism spectrum disorders: the first 3 years. Child Dev. 2013;84:429–42.

38. Szatmari P. Risk and resilience in autism spectrum disorder: a missed translational opportunity? Dev Med Child Neurol. 2017;60:225–9.

39. Zwaigenbaum L, Bauman ML, Stone WL, Yirmiya N, Estes A, Hansen RL, et al. Early identification of autism spectrum disorder: recommendations for practice and research. Pediatrics. 2015;136(Supplement 1):S10–40.

40. Jones W, Klin A. Attention to eyes is present but in decline in 2–6 month-olds later diagnosed with autism. Nature. 2013;504:427–31.

41. Libertus K, Violi DA. Sit to talk: relation between motor skills and language development in infancy. Front Psychol. 2016;7 https://doi.org/10.3389/fpsyg.2016.00475.

42. Koterba EA, Leezenbaum NB, Iverson JM. Object exploration at 6 and 9 months in infants with and without risk for autism. Autism Int J Res Pract. 2014;18:97–105.

43. Libertus K, Joh AS, Needham AW. Motor training at 3 months affects object exploration 12 months later. Dev Sci. 2015;19:1–9.

44. Chawarska K, Klin A, Paul R, Volkmar F. Autism spectrum disorder in the second year: stability and change in syndrome expression. J Child Psychol Psychiatry. 2007;48:128–38.

45. Fox SE, Levitt P, Nelson CA. How the timing and quality of early experiences influence the development of brain architecture. Child Dev. 2010;81:28–40.

10

Neural patterns elicited by sentence processing uniquely characterize typical development, SLI recovery, and SLI persistence

Eileen Haebig[1]* (iD), Christine Weber[1], Laurence B. Leonard[1], Patricia Deevy[1] and J. Bruce Tomblin[2]

Abstract

Background: A substantial amount of work has examined language abilities in young children with specific language impairment (SLI); however, our understanding of the developmental trajectory of language impairment is limited. Along with studying the behavioral changes that occur across development, it is important to examine the neural indices of language processing for children with different language trajectories. The current study sought to examine behavioral and neural bases of language processing in adolescents showing three different trajectories: those with normal language development (NL), those exhibiting persistent SLI (SLI-Persistent), and those with a history of SLI who appear to have recovered (SLI-Recovered).

Methods: Through a sentence judgment task, we examined semantic and syntactic processing. Adolescents judged whether or not each sentence was semantically and syntactically correct. Stimuli consisted of naturally spoken sentences that were either correct, contained a semantic verb error, or contained a syntactic verb agreement error. Verb agreement errors consisted of omission and commission violations of the third-person singular -s. Behavioral button-press responses and electroencephalographic recordings were collected. Behavioral judgments and mean amplitude of the N400 and P600 components were examined.

Results: Adolescents in the SLI-Persistent group had lower sentence judgment accuracy overall, relative to the NL and SLI-Recovered groups. Accuracy in judging omission and commission syntactic errors were marginally different, with marginally lower accuracy for commission errors. All groups demonstrated an N400 component elicited by semantic violations. However, adolescents in the SLI-Persistent group demonstrated a less robust P600 component for syntactic violations. Furthermore, adolescents in the SLI-Recovered group exhibited a similar neural profile to the NL group for the semantic and syntactic omission violations. However, a unique profile with initial negativity was observed in the SLI-Recovered group in the commission violation condition.

Conclusions: Adolescents with persistent language impairment continue to demonstrate delays in language processing at the behavioral and neural levels. Conversely, the adolescents in the SLI-Recovered group appear to have made gains in language processing skills to overcome their initial impairments. However, our findings suggest that the adolescents in the SLI-Recovered group may have compensatory processing strategies for some aspects of language, as evidenced by a unique event-related potential profile.

Keywords: Specific language impairment, Language trajectories, Sentence processing, Event-related brain potentials, N400, P600

* Correspondence: ehaebig1@lsu.edu
[1]Purdue University, West Lafayette, IN, USA
Full list of author information is available at the end of the article

Background

With some exceptions, studies of children with specific language impairment (SLI) have focused on earlier stages of development. Consequently, we have limited knowledge of how the language abilities of these children change over time [7, 80]. As such, it is important to examine later developmental periods to enhance our understanding of the trajectory of SLI. This seems especially crucial because some children initially diagnosed with SLI appear to achieve close-to-normal language skills at a later age, whereas others continue to exhibit a significant language deficit.

Beyond behavioral changes, it is important to study neural modifications throughout development. We have limited understanding of the link between the brain and behavior, especially in individuals with atypical development. Karmiloff-Smith [28] suggested that children with disorders may demonstrate behaviors that resemble those of typically developing children; however, despite overlap in behavioral performance, the underlying neural correlates may differ. In addition, it is possible that children with SLI demonstrate delays in early neuromaturation that could lead to delayed language development [39]. Therefore, it is important to examine whether there is neural evidence of language deficits or delays later in development [80]. This study examined behavioral and neural bases of language processing in adolescents with SLI who demonstrate persistent language impairment and those who appear to have recovered.

SLI across development

Children with SLI have a core deficit in language in the absence of frank neurological or genetic disorders, intellectual disability, or hearing impairment [32, 75]. Both lexical-semantic deficits and grammatical deficits in the expressive and receptive domains have been documented in these children [34, 62, 63, 70]. In addition to linguistic deficits, however, children with SLI have nonlinguistic impairments such as working memory deficits and limitations in processing speed [12, 35, 45, 54].

As children with SLI age, hallmark features of grammatical deficits become less apparent. Some children with SLI no longer meet diagnostic criteria for an SLI classification by late childhood or adolescence; however, language deficits in others can persist [7, 63]. In addition to changes in diagnostic classifications across development, it has been suggested that the pattern of language difficulties may shift with maturation [23]. It is therefore important to explore language profiles in children with persistent language impairment and children with a history of language impairment who appear to have overcome their deficits in language.

Children with a history of SLI

Careful examination of abilities in children with a history of SLI is particularly important given that, despite growth in language abilities, many children continue to experience academic struggles including reading and math difficulties [5, 6, 13]. In fact, it has been suggested that children who have a history of SLI but no longer meet diagnostic criteria often fit into an "illusory recovered" group [66]. Thus, additional research is needed to identify areas of processing in which adolescents with a history of SLI demonstrate subclinical residual vulnerability.

Some initial work has been devoted to the study of children with a history of SLI. Hesketh and Conti-Ramsden [23] examined predictive profiles of sentence repetition abilities. Grammatical and phonological working memory abilities were found to predict sentence repetition in children with a history of SLI; however, for typically developing children, only grammatical abilities were predictive. Hesketh and Conti-Ramsden suggested that children with a history of SLI may not have sufficiently secure language knowledge (i.e., word representations, knowledge of predictable sentence structures) to facilitate chunking linguistic information for sentence repetition. As such, these children also must rely on phonological working memory abilities. Borovsky and colleagues [4] also found subtle language weaknesses in adolescents with a history of SLI, relative to typically developing adolescents. Using an eye-gaze study to examine real-time lexical processing at the sentence level, Borovsky and colleagues found that adolescents with a history of SLI were less likely to look at images that could be relevant with an alternative sentence interpretation (e.g., action-related images), suggesting difficulties with lexical integration [4].

Lastly, Purdy and colleagues found that children with a history of SLI were able to identify verb agreement violations in simple, local-dependency sentences [57]. However, when sentences were more taxing, with long-distance finiteness errors, children with a history of SLI had lower grammaticality judgment accuracy and less robust event-related potential (ERP) components indexing grammatical language processing. Therefore, although children with a history of SLI have gained linguistic skills, the current literature suggests that language processing remains divergent from typically developing peers at the behavioral and neural levels. The current study aims to contribute additional information about the neural and behavioral profiles of language processing in children with a history of SLI who appear to recover, and to compare these profiles with children who continue to meet the diagnostic criteria for SLI.

Lexical processing and the importance of examining verbs

In addition to syntactic deficits, previous work has identified lexical-semantic deficits in children with SLI [64, 70]. These children are believed to have a reduced breadth and depth of word knowledge [59, 70]. Importantly, findings of lexical-semantic weakness align with accounts indicating that children with SLI have difficulties processing verbs [2, 4, 32]. Despite this, there is limited research examining the lexical-semantic processing of verbs by children with SLI; thus, additional work specifically examining lexical-semantic processing of verbs is needed.

Furthermore, relatively little is known about online lexical processing at the sentence level [4]. Although several studies have examined sentence processing in children with SLI, the majority of this work has examined morphosyntactic aspects of sentence processing rather than semantic (e.g., [61, 83]). Additionally, many of these studies have relied on button-press responses that reflect behavioral indices of language processing that typically occur at the end of a sentence, after the majority of the information in the sentence has been presented. Conflicts in semantic processing may resolve quickly and therefore may not be identified on behavioral tasks. A benefit of using electrophysiological data is that it can capture indices of lexical integration at or shortly after lexical-semantic verb violations.

ERP components of lexical processing

When examining neural indices of language processing, the N400 component has been widely used as a means of assessing lexical integration [30, 31]. The N400 is associated with an increase in negative polarity that typically peaks around 400 ms after a semantically anomalous word is presented (e.g., "I like my coffee with cream and *turtle*."). This component is typically observed at electrode sites over centroparietal regions of the brain [42].

In a sentence-level semantic processing task, Neville and colleagues measured the N400 component in 8- to 10-year-old children [46]. Neville and colleagues found that children with SLI displayed larger N400s over the occipital regions when reading open-class words (e.g., nouns, adjectives, verbs). It was suggested that the larger N400 amplitudes indicated greater effort to integrate semantically rich word classes, relative to typically developing peers. Importantly, Neville et al. [46] also measured responses to anomalous nouns at the end of the printed sentences. They found that not only did children with SLI have reduced behavioral accuracy in identifying anomalous words, but they also displayed larger amplitudes for the N400 elicited by anomalous nouns, relative to the typically developing peers. Overall, Neville and colleagues proposed that the relatively larger N400 amplitudes in the children with SLI indexed greater effort for lexical integration and increased reliance on context for word recognition. In contrast, Fonteneau and van der Lely [15] examined the N400 elicited by anomalous nouns in the middle of sentences that were presented auditorily (e.g., "Sally cooks the *car* in the kitchen.") to children between the ages of 10 and 21 years.

Children with SLI, with particularly weak grammatical skills, were found to show similar N400 responses to age-matched controls. The authors concluded that, in this older and more specific sample of children with SLI, ERP findings suggested that semantic processing is relatively intact.

Lastly, two studies have examined semantic violations of verbs using ERPs. Sabisch and colleagues [64] played recorded sentences with sentence final verbs that were anomalous or semantically correct to German-speaking children between 9 and 10 years of age. Typically developing children exhibited larger N400 amplitudes for anomalous verbs relative to control verbs. In contrast, children with SLI did not have differences between the conditions. However, the children with SLI had relatively large N400 amplitudes for both correct and anomalous verbs, which indicated that children with SLI have weak representations of verbs and as a result have difficulties integrating verb meanings within the context of the broader sentence. Weber-Fox and colleagues [80] also examined verb processing in adolescents with typical language abilities or with SLI. Adolescents with SLI had lower accuracy in identifying anomalous verbs, relative to their peers, aligning with previous research that children with SLI may have weak semantic representations of verbs [32, 64]. However, there were no group differences in the mean amplitude of the N400 component; both groups demonstrated larger N400 effects in response to anomalous verbs than to control verbs. Weber-Fox and colleagues suggested that more robust N400 effects and possibly group differences may have been seen had they used more frank semantic violations instead of open-class semantic violations that may be more easily integrated into a sentence. Therefore, given the mixed findings in the current literature, additional work is needed to examine verb processing in children with different language trajectories using both behavioral and neural measures. In addition to providing a careful examination of semantic processing of verbs, the current study provides unique insight into processing in adolescents with a history of SLI who appear to have recovered.

Verb agreement

As previously noted, it is well documented that children with SLI have hallmark deficits in verb agreement (e.g., [33, 60]). With age, language deficits become more subtle across a range of language areas and deficits in grammatical morphology become less salient. Nevertheless, studies have demonstrated that school-age children and adolescents with SLI continue to have poorer performance relative to their age-matched peers on grammaticality judgment tasks that include verb agreement errors [45, 58, 61]. Two types of verb agreement violations that have been studied are errors of omission and errors of commission. In omission errors, a necessary bound morpheme is omitted (e.g., dog play vs. dog plays). Conversely, a bound morpheme is inappropriately inserted during commission errors (e.g., babies cries vs. babies cry). Although commission errors are rarely produced in spoken language in children with SLI, Redmond and Rice [58] found that school-age children with SLI accepted commission errors within complex sentences in a sentence judgment task more often than typically developing children.

Leonard et al. [36] also explored effects of omission and commission errors on sentence processing in adolescents with SLI. Leonard et al. carefully controlled for potential confounds of high metalinguistic and working memory demands by creating a word monitoring task. In this task, adolescents were asked to identify a target word as soon as they heard it in a sentence. Importantly, some of the sentences were grammatically correct, but other sentences contained an omission or commission error in the word preceding the target. If the omission or commission error was detected, the response to the subsequent target word was expected to be slower. As predicted, the typically developing children had slower reaction times when identifying the target word if a grammatical commission or omission error occurred before the target word. However, children with SLI did not have slower reaction times when an omission error preceded the target; this pattern was more apparent for past tense -ed omissions, relative to third-person singular -s omissions. Leonard and colleagues suggested that adolescents with language impairment may continue to have subtle difficulties with verb agreement in later points of development.

ERP components of syntactic processing

Syntactic violations are associated with a late positivity, the P600 component, which is thought to indicate syntactic reanalysis that occurs after identifying a syntactic violation or ambiguity [18, 50, 51]. Friederici [16] also suggested that an earlier component generally referred to as an anterior negativity (AN; sometimes also referred to as the left anterior negativity (LAN) or the early left anterior negativity (ELAN)) marks the initial detection of a morphosyntactic error between 100 and 500 ms after the violation. However, the anterior negativity has not been consistently elicited [72]. It also has been proposed that earlier negativities observed in stimuli with long-distance dependencies may reflect the increased memory load associated with holding incomplete syntactic dependencies in memory [55].

Studies examining neural components associated with syntactic errors in children with SLI have reported mixed findings. Fonteneau and van der Lely [15] found that violations of syntactic dependencies, for example in wh- questions, elicited a P600 response in children with

typical development and SLI. However, children with SLI with particularly weak syntactic skills did not display the AN component. Instead, the children with SLI had a later posterior negativity that was similar to the N400 component. In contrast, Sabisch and colleagues observed the P600 component but also the AN component when children were presented with word category violations and prosodic incongruities [65].

Weber-Fox and colleagues [80] specifically examined neural components following verb agreement violations that included omission and commission errors of the third-person singular -s. They found that verb agreement violations elicited the AN component in adolescents with typical development and adolescents with SLI. However, the P600 component was only observed in the typically developing group. In addition, as previously noted, Purdy and colleagues [57] found that local third-person singular -s commission violations elicited the AN and P600 components in school-age typically developing children and children with a history of SLI. Long-distance commission violations elicited a robust mean amplitude of the P600 for the typically developing group. The children with a history of SLI, however, displayed a P600 that was delayed, was shortened in duration, and had reduced amplitude. The AN component was not observed for the long-distance commission violations for either group. Additional work is required to form a more complete understanding of ERP components elicited by verb agreement violations in children with varying trajectories of language development. Furthermore, it is important to examine whether the neural profiles differ for omission and commission verb agreement errors, given that only omission errors are commonly seen in the productions of children with SLI.

The current study

The current study examined the neural indices of lexical-semantic and syntactic processing in adolescents with different language trajectories. This work contributes information about language processing in children with language impairment at later points of development to provide a more complete picture of the developmental course of language impairments. Additionally, this work contributes insights into the ways in which children with atypical language development potentially rely on compensatory processing strategies to overcome early language deficits. In addition to examining semantic processing of verbs, we specifically examined two types of verb agreement errors (i.e., omission and commission violations) during language processing using behavioral and neural methods, which can allow for direct comparisons of linguistic forms that are more apparent in language impairments than others. Furthermore, this study contributes needed information about the neural profiles of adolescents with normal language development, a history of language impairment, and persistent language impairment, providing a more comprehensive picture of language trajectories. As such, the current study has the potential to provide insight into the underlying neural processes that mediate recovery of language impairments. Our specific research questions were:

1. Does behavioral performance on sentence processing differ across adolescents with different language trajectories?
2. Do neural signals differentiate adolescents with different language trajectories during a sentence processing task?
3. Does verb agreement error type influence group differences?

Given previous findings, we predicted that adolescents with persistent SLI (SLI-Persistent) and adolescents with a history of SLI who had normal language abilities later in development (SLI-Recovered) would have lower accuracy on the sentence judgment task than adolescents with no history of language impairment. Additionally, we predicted that some neural profiles would differentiate the groups. First, given the age of our participants, we predicted that all three groups would demonstrate an N400 effect in response to lexical-semantic verb violations. However, if differences were observed, we would predict that the adolescents in the SLI-Persistent group may present with a less mature neural response to the lexical-semantic violations, following Locke's [39] suggestion that children with SLI experience a persistent lag in neuromaturation. We also predicted that adolescents with SLI would demonstrate a less robust P600 component following syntactic violations (commission and omission violations). Furthermore, if the sentence judgment task was sufficiently difficult, we predicted that adolescents in the SLI-Recovered group would also demonstrate a different neural profile relative to adolescents with typical language development in response to verb agreement violations. Lastly, we expected to see differences in judgment accuracy for errors of omission and errors of commission. Specifically, we expected accuracy to be higher for commission errors than for omission errors. Given the limited previous work examining omission and commission errors separately, our predictions were tentative, but we expected the commission verb agreement violations to elicit a robust P600 component because it is not a common error that individuals produce and therefore may be more salient.

Methods
Participants
Participants were 52 adolescents who participated in a larger longitudinal study on the prevalence of SLI [75].

In the Tomblin et al. study, children completed standardized cognitive and language tests in kindergarten, second grade, fourth grade, and eighth grade. Test scores determined group classification for each visit. The group classifications from the parent grant were used to assign participants in the current study to one of three categories: Normal Language (NL), SLI-Recovered (SLI-R), and SLI-Persistent (SLI-P).

Adolescents in the NL group ($n = 18$) had no history of language impairment across the larger study's four time points. Adolescents in the SLI-Recovered group ($n = 15$) had a history of SLI in kindergarten and/or second grade, but normal language abilities in fourth and eighth grades. Lastly, adolescents in the SLI-Persistent group ($n = 19$) received a classification of SLI in eighth grade and a status of SLI or nonspecific language impairment during at least two of the three previous grades. Across the four visits during the longitudinal study, the children in the NL had significantly higher language composite scores than the SLI-Recovered and SLI-Persistent groups. Additionally, the children in the SLI-Recovered group had significantly higher language composite scores relative to the SLI-Persistent group. However, as would be expected given the group classifications, the difference in language abilities between the SLI-Recovered and SLI-Persistent groups grew across the longitudinal study (kindergarten Cohen's $d = -1.42$, eighth grade Cohen's $d = -3.38$). The adolescents who participated in the current study were matched on chronological age. See Table 1 for participant characteristics.

Ethics, consent, and permission
This study was approved by the institutional review board. All participants provided informed written assent or consent, and when necessary, parents or legal guardians provided informed written consent.

Standardized assessments
Test batteries differed across the four visits in the longitudinal study in order to be developmentally appropriate. The eighth grade test battery included the Peabody Picture Vocabulary Test—Revised (PPVT-R; [11]) to assess receptive vocabulary knowledge and the Comprehensive Receptive and Expressive Vocabulary Test (CREVT; [78]) to assess expressive vocabulary. In addition, the Concepts and Following Directions and the Recalling Sentences subtests from the Clinical Evaluation of Language Fundamentals—Third Edition (CELF-3; [68]) were used to evaluate receptive and expressive grammatical skills. Lastly, the Qualitative Reading Inventory—Third Edition (QRI-3; [37]) tested narrative comprehension and production skills. Previous visits also included the Test of Language Development—Primary, 2nd edition (TOLD-P2; [47]) and a receptive and expressive narrative story task [9]. Scores from

Table 1 Participant characteristics

	Normal Language $n = 18$ (10 females)		SLI-Recovered $n = 15$ (7 females)		SLI-Persistent $n = 19$ (7 females)	
	Mean	SD	Mean	SD	Mean	SD
Chronological age	15.82	1.21	15.87	1.21	16.50	1.46
Cognitive standard score[a]	103.22	9.81	99.53	6.90	94.79	8.80
8th grade language composite Z-score	0.38	0.72	−0.47	0.38	−1.84	0.43
4th grade language composite Z-score	0.59	0.96	−0.62	0.47	−1.66	0.75
2nd grade language composite Z-score	0.52	0.95	−0.95	0.52	−1.85	0.48
Kindergarten language composite Z-score	0.67	0.98	−1.05	0.44	−1.69	0.46
Race	18 White		14 White 1 Black		16 White 3 Black	
Ethnicity	0 Hispanic		0 Hispanic		1 Hispanic	

Note. Chronological age at the time the ERP experiment was completed
[a]Performance IQ on the Wechsler Intelligence Scale for Children—Third Edition during the 8th grade visit. SLI classification for each visit followed the EpiSLI standard [74]

the battery of tests for each visit were used to create five composite scores, which were converted into Z-scores based on the entire dataset of the parent study [74]. Children were identified as having a language impairment if two or more language composite scores were 1.25 SD below the mean for the child's chronological age group. The Z-scores were corrected to account for the disproportionate number of children with SLI in the sample relative to the prevalence in the general population. Additional details about diagnostic testing and the diagnostic EpiSLI standard is provided in Tomblin et al. [74].

Nonverbal intelligence was tested using the Performance Scale subtests in the Wechsler Intelligence Scale for Children—Third Edition (WISC-III; [81]). Handedness was measured by the Edinburgh Inventory for Assessment of Handedness [49]. All adolescents were right-handed, except for one adolescent in the SLI-Persistent group who was ambidextrous. Lastly, we confirmed that all adolescents had normal hearing with a hearing screening at a level of 20 dB HL at 500, 1000, and 2000 Hz, presented through headphones.

Experimental task

Adolescents participated in a sentence judgment task that required them to judge whether or not each sentence was semantically and syntactically correct. Data from some of the current participants were presented in a previous study by Weber-Fox and colleagues [80]. The task contained 30 trials with a third-person singular subject and a verb correctly marked for agreement (i.e., third-person singular -*s*), 30 trials with a plural subject and a verb correctly marked for agreement, 30 trials with a third-person singular subject and a verb with an agreement omission error, 30 trials with a plural noun and a verb with an agreement commission error, 30 trials with a third-person singular subject and

a semantically anomalous verb that is correctly marked for agreement, and 30 trials with a plural subject and a semantically anomalous verb that is correctly marked for agreement. A complete list of the stimuli appears in the Appendix. To enhance ecological validity, a female voice was recorded reading the stimuli sentences using normal prosody. The natural speech sentence stimuli were digitized at a rate of 16 kHz [79]. The auditory waveforms of the stimuli were visualized and the onset and offsets were identified using visual and auditory inspection to prevent clipping (using Cool Edit Pro software). The wave files of each word were saved as sound files. During the task, the sound file for each word was presented (using the Neuroscan STIM program) and followed by a 50-ms interstimulus interval. The sentences were approximately 3.5 s in duration (ranging from 2.7 to 4.9 s). The critical words (the verbs) were approximately 0.531 s in duration (ranging from 0.322 to 0.764 s). Codes for each word were inserted into the online EEG data recordings using Neuroscan, to allow for off-line data analysis of neural responses to the critical verbs of interest. The onsets of each word were clearly discernable, and the sentences maintained a natural-sounding rate, rhythm, and prosody.

The sentence stimuli were designed so that all of the words leading up to the critical word (the verb) were identical across the three conditions, which therefore allowed the ERPs elicited by the verbs in each condition to be directly compared. The sentences were presented in a counterbalanced manner in the following ways: (1) half of the noun subjects were singular and the other half were plural, and (2) each word that served as a control verb also served as a semantically anomalous verb in another sentence. The semantically anomalous verbs did not produce a frank anomaly in many cases, but were unexpected verbs given the preceding sentential context. This feature is an attribute of verbs given that verbs, unlike nouns, are quite flexible in use. Despite this, the anomalous verbs were apparent as the sentence continued (e.g., "Every day the ballerina submerges on her pointed toe shoes."). The ERP components were measured at the point of the critical verb; therefore, the ERP data do not reflect the additional semantic information provided by the completion of the sentence. As such, the ERPs elicited by the verbs across the three conditions reflect processing of identical information leading up to the verb, and the additional information that follows the verb does not confound a comparison of the ERP measures across the three conditions.

Electroencephalographic recordings

We measured electrical activity at the scalp using electrodes that were secured in an elastic cap (Quik-Cap, Compumedics Neuroscan). There were 28 electrodes (Ag-AgCl) that were positioned over homologous hemisphere locations according to the International 10-10 system [27]. Locations were as follows: lateral sites F7/F8, FT7/FT8, T7/T8, TP7/TP8, P7/P8; mid-lateral sites FP1/FP2, F3/F4, FC3/FC4, CP3/CP4, P3/P4, O1/O2; and midline sites FZ, FCZ, CZ, CPZ, PZ, OZ (see Fig. 1). Electrodes on the left and right mastoids served as the reference to the electrical recordings during data collection. Electrodes placed over the left and right outer canthi recorded horizontal eye movements. Vertical eye movement was monitored through recordings from electrodes placed over the left inferior and superior orbital ridges. We also adjusted all electrode impedances to 5 kΩ

or less, amplified electrical signals within a bandpass of 0.1 and 100 Hz, and digitized online electrical signals (Neuroscan 4.0) at a rate of 500 Hz.

Procedures

After appropriate impedance levels were obtained, the participants sat in a sound-attenuating room and positioned 160 cm from a 47.5-cm monitor. The participants were instructed to listen to each sentence and then judge whether the sentence was semantically and syntactically correct. A fixation cross appeared on the screen, and, after a delay of 1000 ms, the sentence was presented binaurally through headphones at 70 to 75 dB SPL. The participants were asked to refrain from blinking during trials. After the presentation of each sentence, there was a 500-ms delay, followed by a "Yes/No?" prompt on the screen to cue the participant to press the "Yes" button if the sentence was semantically and syntactically correct or the "No" button if there was an error in the sentence. The response hands corresponding to the "Yes" and "No" buttons were counterbalanced across participants and sex. The sentence stimuli were presented in 5 blocks with 36 sentences in each block. Within each block, the sentences were pseudorandomized so that each condition was represented equally in each block.

ERP measures

The neural data were processed using EEGLAB, version 12-0-2-6b [10], and ERPLAB, version 5.0.0.0 [41, 40], which are MATLAB© toolboxes (MathWorks, Natick, MA, USA). We used independent component analysis (ICA; EEGLAB [26]) to remove eye artifact. Specifically,

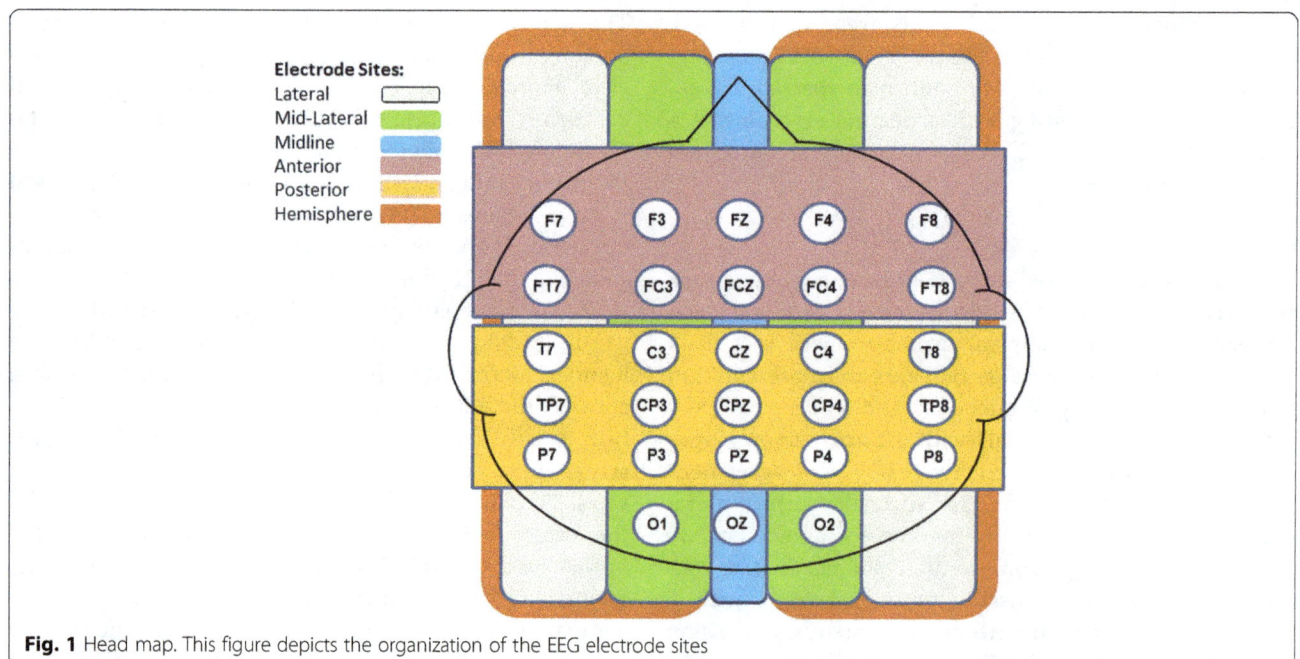

Fig. 1 Head map. This figure depicts the organization of the EEG electrode sites

ICA identifies independent sources of EEG signals. Components represent patterns from the EEG signal. Components that represent artifact, such as blinks, horizontal eye movements, and voltage drifts, were identified by two independent trained research assistants. Discrepancies were resolved by a third research assistant. Next, the EEG signals were low-pass filtered at 30 Hz with a 12-dB roll-off to remove high-frequency noise. After filtering, the data were epoched from 200 ms prior to the onset of the verb to 2500 ms post-stimulus to allow for averaging and ERP component measures. All of the EEG channels underwent automatic voltage-dependent thresholds to remove any trials that still contained artifact. The voltage-dependent thresholds were adjusted to take into account individual differences in EEG artifact amplitudes (e.g., size of blinks) to reliably reject true artifact without rejecting usable trials. The average voltage-dependent threshold for eye movement artifacts was 114 μV, and the average for the remaining artifacts (e.g., drift) at the remaining electrode sites was 209 μV. Each participant was required to contribute at least 20 artifact-free trials within each condition. The average number of usable trials in each sentence condition for each group was slightly higher than previous studies of auditory sentence processing in children and adolescents [21, 64]. Additionally, the number of artifact-free trials did not significantly differ across the groups, $F(2, 49) = 3.07$, $p = .055$. Finally, the EEG epochs of each individual were averaged for analysis of ERPs that were elicited by each task condition. Specifically, the ERP averages were triggered 200 ms prior to the verb onset in each sentence and included 2000 ms post-stimulus onset. The 200-ms interval preceding the onset of the critical verbs served as the baseline activity.

Adolescents' brains are still undergoing neural maturation. Although the ERP components that were selected typically are most robust in the centroparietal regions, immature neural profiles often demonstrate a more distributed topography [24]. Therefore, of the 28 electrodes (Ag-AgCl) that were positioned over homologous hemisphere locations, we conducted omnibus analyses including the following electrodes: lateral sites F7/F8, FT7/FT8, T7/T8, TP7/TP8, P7/P8 and mid-lateral sites FP1/FP2, F3/F4, FC3/FC4, CP3/CP4, P3/P4.

Temporal windows for measuring the ERP mean amplitudes were selected after the grand averages were examined for each group. The windows were centered around the regions of maximal activity. In the current dataset, the same temporal windows were appropriate for each group's grand averages. As a second step in the window selecting procedures, we examined each individual record to ensure the windows captured the components of interest (if present). The mean amplitudes of the N400 were measured within the temporal window of 370–570 ms, and the mean amplitudes of the P600 were measured within the

temporal window of 800–1200 ms. The windows selected in these analyses are within the range of windows used to measure the N400 and P600 in children and adolescents and for stimuli that use connected speech (e.g., [46, 57, 65, 80]).

Analysis procedures

A repeated measures ANOVA tested whether behavioral performance differed according to condition (semantic vs. syntactic violations) and group and whether there was an interaction of condition and group. In order to control for response bias, A' scores served as the dependent variable [19, 61]. Briefly, A' scores serve as a measure of the proportion of correct responses in a two-alternative forced-choice task. The A' value consists of scores from a control condition and an experimental condition (e.g., correct sentences and sentences with syntactic violations). The formula was $A' = 0.5 + (y - x)(1 + y - x) / 4y(1 - x)$, where y represents correct identifications (hits) and x represents incorrect identifications (false alarms; [38]). An A' value of 1.00 represents perfect discrimination of correct and incorrect sentences. An A' value of .50 indicates chance performance, for example, a "yes" response to 50% of the correct sentences and to 50% of the semantically anomalous sentences.

The ERP data were analyzed using a series of repeated measures ANOVAs. The omnibus models included condition (correct sentences vs. semantic/syntactic violation), hemisphere (right vs. left), laterality (lateral and mid-lateral), anterior-posterior (AP) order, and interactions across the predictor variables. When there was more than 1° of freedom in the numerator, the Huynh-Feldt (H-F) adjusted p value was used to determine significance [22].

In order to succinctly present the results, we report outcomes from the ERP measures recorded from the lateral and mid-lateral sites. Results from the midline electrode sites are also provided if they contribute additional information. Furthermore, given that the aim of the current study was to identify differences across language trajectory (i.e., group membership) and error type on behavioral and ERP data, we report significant results only for the group and error type factors and interactions between group and error type with each other, or other factors. Significant interactions among group, condition, and other predictor variables were followed up with step-down ANOVAs to better understand the significant effects.

Lastly, because high temporal resolution is a strength of ERPs, we conducted additional analyses that highlight time as a factor. To do so, we conducted sequential temporal analyses that examined three 50-ms temporal windows that lead up to and continued throughout the N400 and P600 time windows. Given that this approach increased the number of analyses that were conducted, we reduced the complexity of the statistical models by only examining the mean amplitudes of polarity shifts that came from electrodes in prespecified regions of interest. The regions of interest for the N400 effect were centroparietal electrode sites: C3, CZ, C4, CP3, CPZ, CP4, aligning with previous work examining the N400 [30] and visual inspection of the current data. The regions of interest for the P600 component were electrode sites: CP3, CPZ, CP4, P3, PZ, P4, aligning with previous work examining the P600 [18, 51] and visual inspection of the current data. The repeated measures ANOVAs contained the following factors: condition (correct vs. semantic/syntactic violation), group, electrodes, and interactions of group by condition, group by condition by electrodes, and condition by electrodes. In these analyses, we were most interested in whether there were interactions between group and condition, which had the potential to identify whether one group demonstrated earlier-onset ERP components elicited by the task stimuli. When appropriate, we conducted step-down analyses within each group to more accurately describe the nature of the group by condition interaction.

Results

Behavioral performance

Behavioral performance across the conditions was examined first (see Table 2). When comparing A' scores for the syntactic violation condition relative to the semantic violation condition, we found that there was no main effect of condition, $F(1, 49) = 0.069$, $p = .793$, indicating that performance was similar for the semantic violation and syntactic violation conditions. However, there was a main effect of group, $F(2, 49) = 25.052$, $p < .001$, $\eta_p^2 = 0.506$. Follow-up comparisons revealed that the NL and SLI-Recovered groups did not have significantly different A' scores, $p = .153$, but the NL and SLI-Recovered groups had significantly higher A' scores than the SLI-Persistent group, $ps < .001$. There was no interaction between condition and group, $F(2, 49) = 1.209$, $p = .307$ (see Fig. 2).

Next, we compared behavioral performance on the omission and commission trials. A repeated measures ANOVA tested whether there was a difference between omission and commission A' scores, a difference between groups, and whether there was an interaction of error type and group. The difference between error type did not reach significance, $F(1, 49) = 3.879$, $p = .055$, $\eta_p^2 = 0.073$; omission A' scores were only slightly higher than commission A' scores. There was a significant effect of group, $F(2, 49) = 21.399$, $p < .001$, $\eta_p^2 = 0.466$. Post hoc comparisons revealed that the NL and SLI-Recovered groups had significantly higher A' scores than the SLI-Persistent group, $ps < .001$, but differences between the NL and SLI-Recovered groups did not reach significance, $p = .079$. Lastly, there was no interaction of error type and group, $F(2, 49) = 0.356$, $p = .702$ (see Fig. 3).

ERP patterns elicited by sentence processing

Our second research question asked whether ERPs elicited from the sentence processing task differentiated the three groups. Below, we present our findings for each violation type.

Semantic violation N400 results

The mean amplitude in the N400 window (370–570 ms following the onset of the verb) was analyzed to examine lexical processing during correct sentences and sentences with semantic errors. There was a significant effect of condition, $F(1, 49) = 11.318$, $p < .001$, $\eta_p^2 = 0.188$, with an N400 effect appearing in the semantic violation condition. There was no group or group by condition effect, $ps > .35$. However, there was a significant interaction between condition and laterality, $F(1, 49) = 44.099$, $p < .001$, $\eta_p^2 = 0.241$, identifying a larger amplitude distribution over mid-lateral compared to lateral electrode sites. Additionally, there was a significant interaction across condition, hemisphere, laterality, and group, $F(2, 49) = 3.613$, $p = .003$, $\eta_p^2 = 0.210$. Figure 4 depicts the ERPs elicited by verbs in the correct sentences and sentences with a semantic violation for each group.

Table 2 Sentence judgment behavioral performance

	Normal Language		SLI-Recovered		SLI-Persistent	
	Mean	SD	Mean	SD	Mean	SD
Correct condition proportion correct	0.863	0.216	0.864	0.077	0.771	0.128
Semantic violation proportion correct	0.706	0.251	0.759	0.151	0.552	0.228
Syntactic violation proportion correct	0.781	0.195	0.715	0.244	0.443	0.168
Semantic violation A'	0.705	0.124	0.688	0.098	0.565	0.060
Syntactic violation A'	0.734	0.111	0.674	0.108	0.538	0.052
Omission violation A'	0.744	0.121	0.681	0.108	0.555	0.067
Commission violation A'	0.726	0.109	0.673	0.119	0.528	0.046

Note. A' scores of .5 indicate chance performance

Comparison of Sentence Judgment Accuracy for Semantic and Syntactic Violations

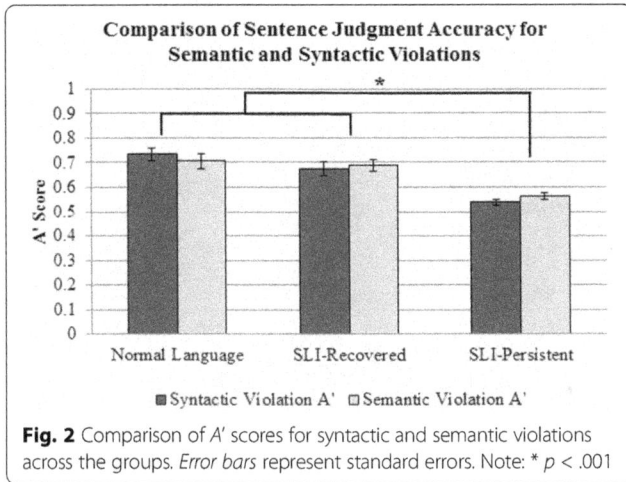

Fig. 2 Comparison of A' scores for syntactic and semantic violations across the groups. *Error bars* represent standard errors. Note: * *p* < .001

N400 sequential temporal analysis In order to examine additional information about the timing of the emergence of the N400 across the groups, we conducted a series of sequential temporal analyses on 50-ms temporal windows leading up to and comprising the N400 time window. Within our region of interest (C3, CZ, C4, CP3, CPZ, CP4), there were no main effects or interactions in the three 50-ms temporal windows preceding the N400 time window. During the 50-ms temporal windows that made up the N400 time window, each of the analyses yielded a main effect of condition, indexing the negative polarity shift that was elicited by the semantically anomalous verb. However, there was not a significant interaction of group by condition or group by condition by electrodes ($ps > .45$). There also were no group differences ($ps > .20$), but there was a main effect for electrodes ($ps < .02$), indicating that the N400 component was left-lateralized.

Omission violation P600 results
The mean amplitude in the P600 window (800–1200 ms following the onset of the verb) was examined to test

Comparison of Detection of Omission and Commission Violations

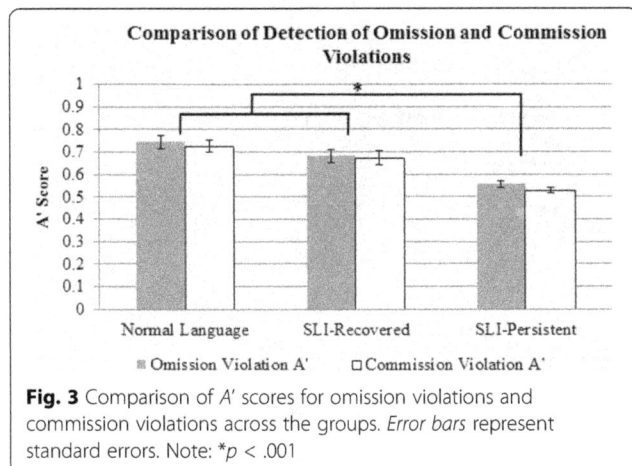

Fig. 3 Comparison of A' scores for omission violations and commission violations across the groups. *Error bars* represent standard errors. Note: **p* < .001

the singular sentences with the third-person singular -*s* correctly marked and the sentences with omission violations. As depicted in Fig. 5, there was a larger P600 component elicited by omission violations compared to correctly marked verbs, $F(1, 49) = 11.596$, $p < .001$, $\eta_p^2 = 0.191$. There was no group effect, $p = .442$; however, there was a marginal interaction between condition and group, $F(2, 49) = 2.715$, $p = .076$, $\eta_p^2 = 0.100$. In addition, there was a significant interaction between condition and laterality, $F(1, 49) = 14.626$, $p < .001$, $\eta_p^2 = 0.230$, indicating that there was larger amplitude distribution in the mid-lateral electrode sites for the omission condition. There also was a significant interaction between condition and AP, $F(4, 196) = 3.345$, $p = .011$, $\eta_p^2 = 0.064$, with greater positivity in the posterior electrode sites during the omission condition. A three-way interaction across condition, AP, and hemisphere, $F(4, 196) = 3.425$, $p = .019$, $\eta_p^2 = 0.065$, indicated that greater positivity appeared during the omission condition in the posterior electrodes in the left hemisphere. Lastly, there was a significant interaction between group and laterality, $F(2, 49) = 6.072$, $p = .004$, $\eta_p^2 = 0.199$, indicating that there was larger amplitude distribution in the mid-lateral electrode sites than the lateral electrode sites for the NL and SLI-Recovered groups, relative to the SLI-Persistent group.

Because the marginal interaction between group and condition may provide further insight into the neural processing of omission violation errors, we conducted a series of step-down repeated measures ANOVAs within each group. The ANOVA in the NL group revealed a significant effect of condition, $F(1, 17) = 8.566$, $p = .009$, $\eta_p^2 = 0.335$. There also was a significant interaction of condition and laterality, indicating a stronger positivity elicited by the omission condition on the mid-lateral electrode sites, $F(1, 17) = 7.039$, $p = .017$, $\eta_p^2 = 0.293$. The SLI-Recovered group also demonstrated a significant effect of condition, $F(1, 14) = 8.798$, $p = .010$, $\eta_p^2 = 0.386$. Conversely, the SLI-Persistent group did not demonstrate a condition effect, $F(1, 18) = 0.013$, $p = .911$, $\eta_p^2 = 0.001$. However, there was a significant three-way interaction of condition, hemisphere, and AP, $F(4, 72) = 2.935$, $p = .048$, $\eta_p^2 = 0.140$, indicating that there was greater positivity in the omission condition relative to the correct condition in the posterior electrode sites in the left hemisphere. The SLI-Persistent group demonstrated a marginally more restricted P600, relative to the NL and SLI-Recovered groups.

P600 omission violation sequential temporal analysis Next, we conducted a series of sequential temporal analyses on 50-ms temporal windows leading up to and comprising the P600 time window. Within our region of interest (CP3, CPZ, CP4, P3, PZ, P4), there were no main effects or interactions of group, condition, or group

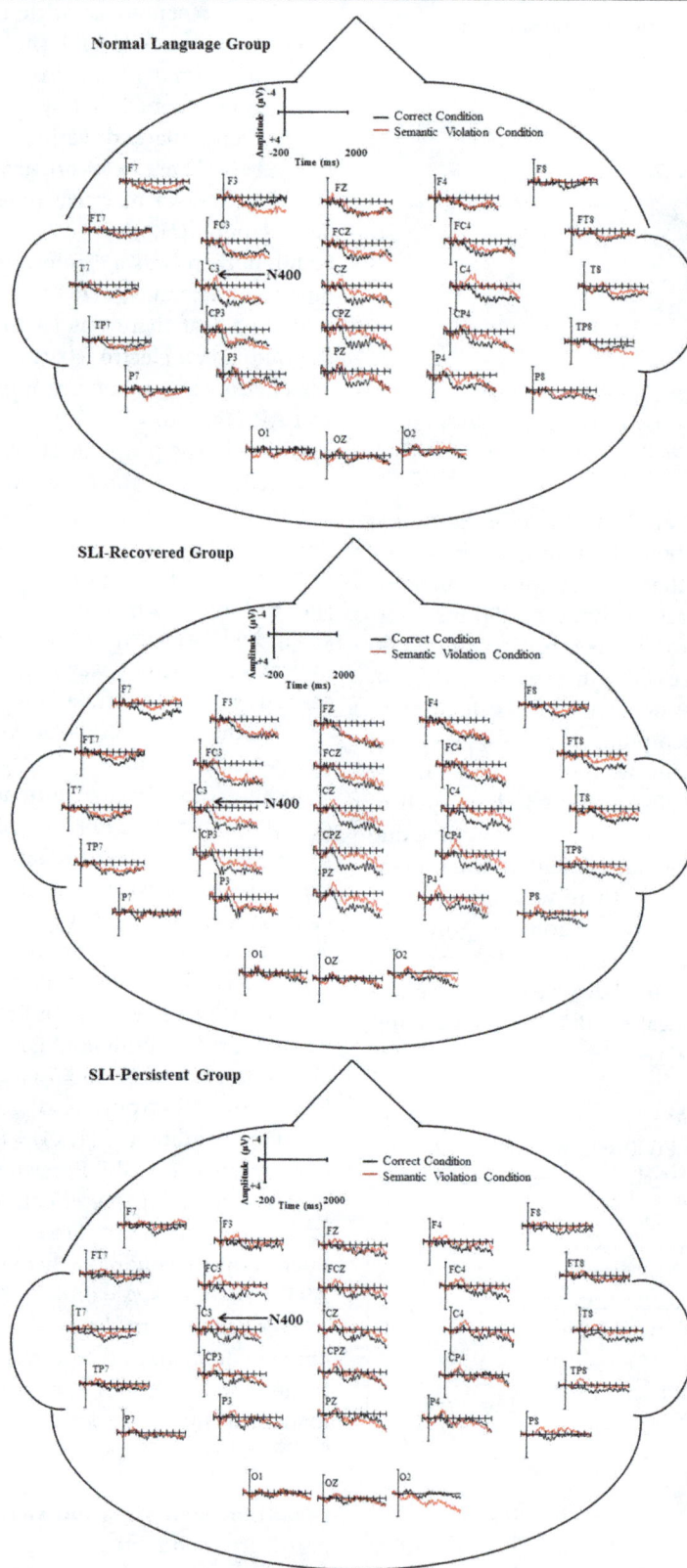

Fig. 4 Head maps by group for correct and semantic violation conditions

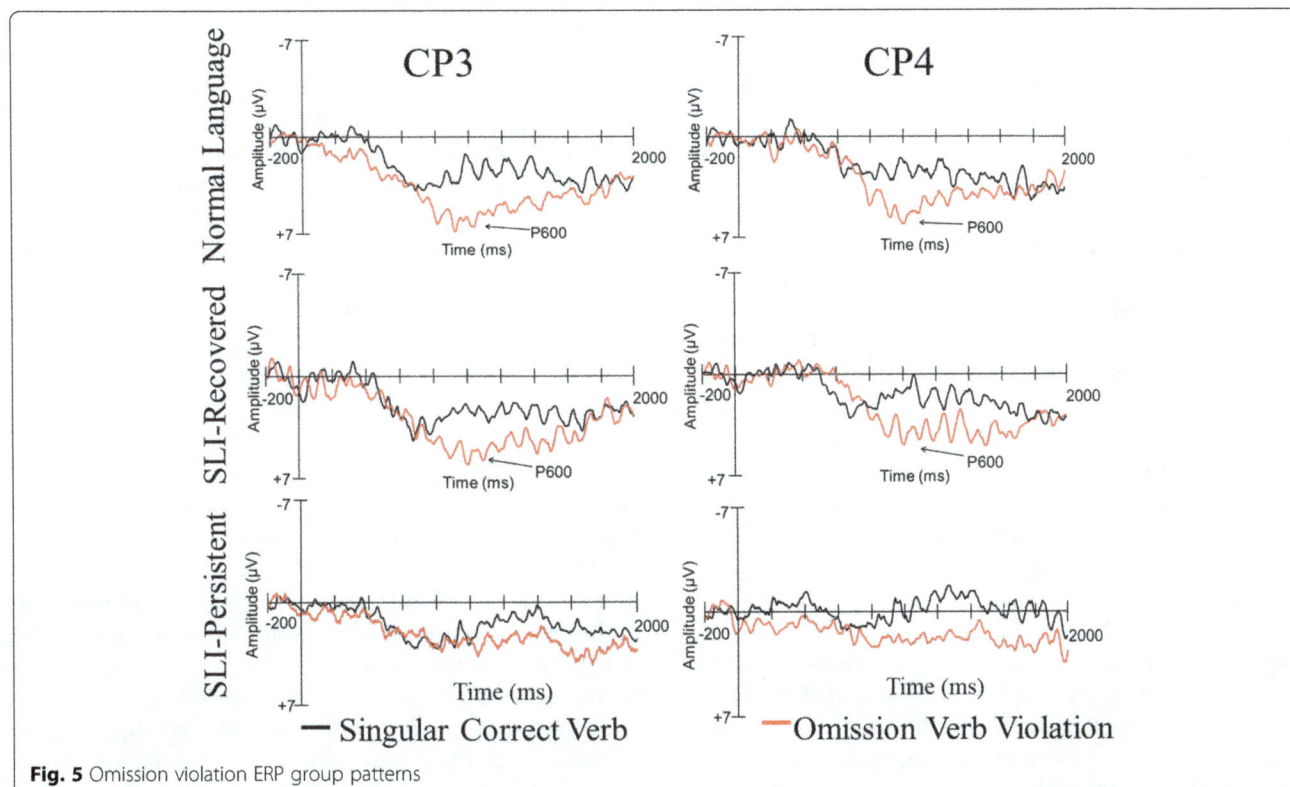

Fig. 5 Omission violation ERP group patterns

by condition in the three 50-ms temporal windows preceding the P600 time window. When examining each 50-ms time bin within the P600 time window, we found that the 800- to 850-ms temporal window yielded a significant effect of condition ($p = .033$) and electrodes ($p = .033$) and, importantly, a significant interaction across group, condition, and electrodes ($p = .043$). There was no main effect of group ($p = .059$), and no interaction of group by condition or electrodes by group ($ps > .65$). Within-group analyses were conducted to more accurately describe the interaction across group, condition, and electrodes. None of the within-group analyses yielded a main effect of condition ($ps > .10$); however, the SLI-Recovered group had a significant interaction between condition and electrodes ($p = .041$). This indicates that the SLI-Recovered group had an earlier neural response in the medial and left electrode sites that differentiated the correct verbs and the verbs with omission violations.

In the remaining 50-ms temporal windows (ranging from 850 to 1200 ms), there was a consistent effect of condition ($ps < .003$), indicating that the omission violations elicited a P600, and an effect of electrodes ($ps < .001$), indicating that larger amplitudes were observed in the left and medial electrode sites. In addition, the 900- to 950-ms temporal window analysis yielded a significant effect of group ($p = .003$), with the NL and SLI-Recovered groups having

significantly higher positivity relative to the SLI-Persistent group. The 50-ms temporal window analyses starting at 950, 1050, and 1150 ms also yielded significant effects of group ($ps < .05$), with the NL group demonstrating significantly larger amplitude P600 relative to the SLI-Persistent group.

Commission violation P600 results

Following our analyses of the omission violations, we examined the mean amplitude in the P600 window (800–1200 ms following the onset of the verb) for the plural sentences with correct verb agreement and plural sentences with commission violations. Unlike the omission condition, there was no main effect of the commission violation condition, relative to the correct sentences with plural subjects, $p = .629$. However, there was a significant three-way interaction of condition, AP, and laterality, $F(4, 196) = 2.592$, $p = .049$, $\eta_p^2 = 0.050$, indicating that there was greater positivity in the posterior mid-lateral electrodes in the commission condition. Moreover, there was a significant effect of group, $F(2, 49) = 4.952$, $p = .011$, $\eta_p^2 = 0.168$, with the NL and SLI-Recovered groups having overall significantly greater positivity than the SLI-Persistent group ($ps < .03$), but similar positivity in the NL and SLI-Recovered groups ($p = .561$). Lastly, there was not a significant interaction between group and condition, $p = .180$.

After visualizing the waveforms in the plural control and commission conditions (see Fig. 6), it was apparent that each group presented with a unique pattern of neural activity. Specifically, children in the NL group demonstrated a robust P600 in the commission condition at electrode sites over more medial and posterior brain regions. In contrast, the SLI-Recovered group demonstrated a differing profile with an earlier N400-like negativity that was followed by a positive-moving polarity shift, which did not exceed the positivity that was also elicited in the correct plural sentences. Although the positivity observed in the commission agreement errors and correct plural sentences was mostly overlapping, there was a greater overall change in polarity elicited by the commission agreement errors given the morphology of the ERP waveforms. Lastly, the SLI-Persistent group portrayed a restricted P600 amplitude over the left centroparietal sites for the commission violation condition.

Negativity related to commission violations To further examine the negativity in the SLI-Recovered group, we conducted a repeated measures ANOVA on the mean amplitude of the waves between 600 and 800 ms after the onset of the verb. This temporal window was centered around the negativity elicited in the SLI-Recovered group. There was no significant effect of condition; however, there was an interaction between group and condition, $F(2, 49) = 4.452$, $p = .017$, $\eta_p^2 = 0.154$.

Therefore, we conducted step-down ANOVAs within each group to examine the patterns associated with the commission violations. There were no significant findings in the NL group analyses. Within the SLI-Recovered group analysis, there was a main effect of condition, $F(1, 14) = 11.516$, $p = .004$, $\eta_p^2 = 0.451$, with larger amplitude negativity elicited by the commission violation relative to the correct condition. Lastly, the SLI-Persistent group analyses revealed a marginal interaction across condition, hemisphere, and AP, $F(4, 72) = 2.480$, $p = .078$, $\eta_p^2 = 0.121$, with greater amplitude positivity observed in the posterior electrodes in the left hemisphere during the commission condition. There also was a marginal interaction across condition, AP, and laterality, $F(4, 72) = 2.098$, $p = .096$, $\eta_p^2 = 0.104$, indicating that there was slightly greater amplitude positivity distributed over the mid-lateral posterior electrode sites.

Sequential temporal analyses for the commission violation As in the previously discussed conditions, we conducted a series of sequential temporal analyses on 50-ms temporal windows that preceded the negativity window and 50-ms temporal windows that captured the negativity and P600 time windows. Our region of interest included electrode sites CP3, CPZ, CP4, P3, PZ, and P4. Our results are presented in Fig. 7. Briefly, the sequential temporal analyses revealed several group by condition interactions. Most of the findings highlighted the different profiles in the negativity window,

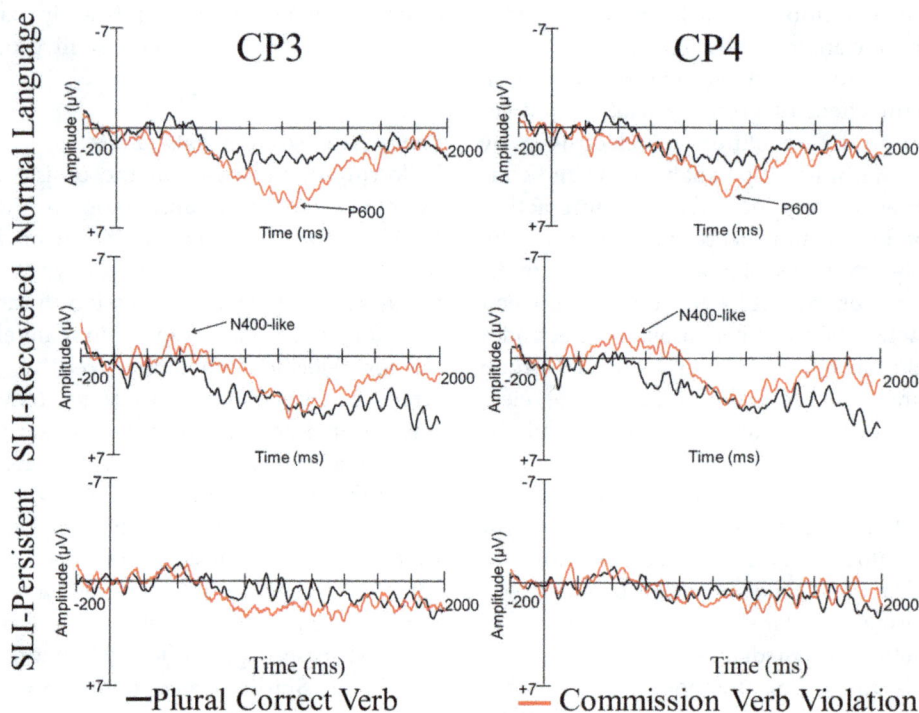

Fig. 6 Commission violation ERP group patterns

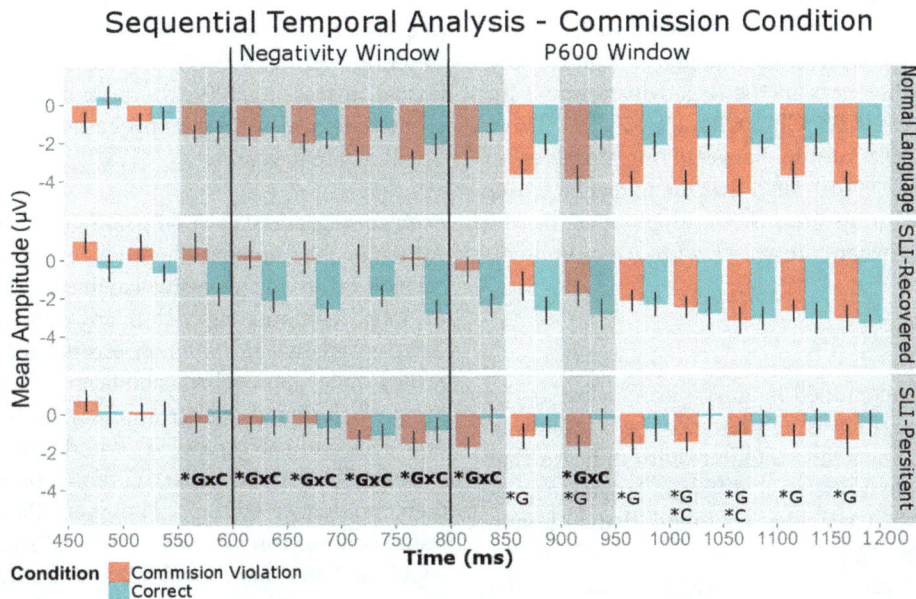

Fig. 7 *p < .05 for the repeated measures ANOVAs that included condition, electrodes, group, and interactions across condition, electrodes, and group. All repeated measures ANOVAs had significant main effects of electrodes. G main effect of group, C main effect of condition, GxC group by condition interaction. At 850–900, 900–950, and 950–1000 ms, the NL group had a larger positive amplitude relative to the SLI-Persistent group. At 1000-1050, 1050–1100, 1100–1150, and 1150–1200 ms, the mean amplitude across the conditions in the NL and SLI-Recovered groups was larger than that in the SLI-Persistent group, supporting the omnibus P600 finding that the NL and SLI-Recovered groups had overall significantly greater positivity than the SLI-Persistent group. The interactions between group and condition highlighted the different profiles in the negativity window, contributing to the SLI-Recovered group's unique neural profile. The NL group had an earlier-emerging P600 component elicited by the commission violation relative to the other groups (highlighted in the 900–950-ms temporal window)

highlighting the SLI-Recovered group's unique neural profile. Our findings also revealed a significant interaction of group by condition in the 900- to 950-ms temporal window. The follow-up analyses conducted within the groups revealed that there was a significant condition effect in the NL group, but not the SLI-Recovered or SLI-Persistent groups, indicating that the NL group may have had an earlier-emerging P600 component that was elicited by the commission violation condition relative to the other groups.

Exploration of individual differences

Lastly, we explored the individual differences within our participants. Figure 8 depicts the individual variability of the neural correlates of processing sentences with commission violations, relative to the sentences with correct verbs and plural subjects, within and across the groups. Specifically, we explored the relationship between the mean amplitude of the negativity window and the behavioral A' accuracy scores. As such, Fig. 8 depicts five adolescents in the Normal Language and SLI-Recovered groups who had the lowest A' scores for the commission condition (depicted in red; Normal Language range .499–.668, SLI-Recovered range .502–.602) and five adolescents in the SLI-Recovered and SLI-Persistent groups with the highest behavioral performance (depicted

in blue; SLI-Recovered range .830–.800, SLI-Persistent range .683–.541). Furthermore, to provide insight into whether the early negativity may have indicated a compensatory route to support performance on our language processing task in our adolescents with a history of SLI

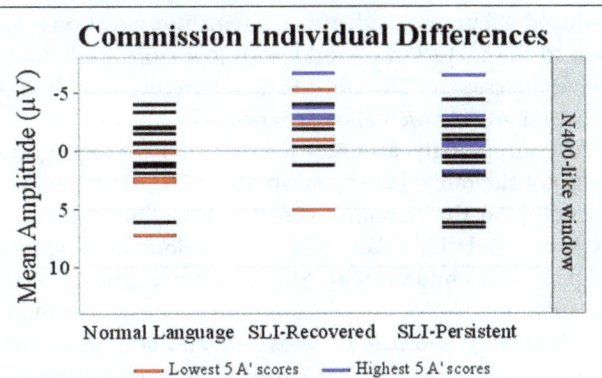

Fig. 8 Commission individual differences. This scatterplot depicts the individual differences in mean amplitude differences (sentences with commission violations minus sentences with correct verbs with plural subjects) for our regions of interest (CP3, CPZ, CP4, P3, PZ, P4) for the negativity time window. *Blue lines* highlight five participants within the SLI-Recovered and SLI-Persistent groups who had the highest behavioral accuracy scores (A'). The *red lines* depict the five lowest scoring adolescents in the Normal Language and SLI-Recovered groups. See text (individual differences) for the corresponding ranges of A' scores

and persistent SLI, we conducted a bivariate correlation analysis. We tested for a correlation between the A' accuracy scores for the commission violation condition and mean amplitude differences in the negativity window for our region of interest (CP3, CPZ, CP4, P3, PZ, P4). There was a significant relationship between our variables of interest, $r = -0.438$, $p = .010$, such that the higher A' scores were associated with greater mean amplitudes in the negativity window, when presented with a commission violation sentence.

Discussion

The current study examined language processing at the behavioral and neural levels in adolescents who followed different language trajectories. Our results indicate that the three groups demonstrated different language processing profiles. Most notably, we found that although adolescents in the SLI-Recovered group had similar behavioral performance to their typically developing peers, they appear to have processed some aspects of the language stimuli in a different manner. We discuss our specific findings below.

Sentence processing behavioral accuracy

The sentence processing task yielded a rich dataset that tested both semantic and syntactic processing of verbs. Although it is informative to examine both semantic and syntactic features of verb processing, including both types of judgments (semantic and syntactic accuracy) in the same task likely placed high metalinguistic demands and contributed to the relatively lower A' scores for all of the groups compared to scores seen in previous studies with semantic violations [46, 64]. It is also likely that the reduced accuracy in identifying semantic violations was due to the inclusion of verbs with low cloze probability. Nevertheless, the NL and SLI-Recovered groups had A' scores that were well above chance.

Not surprisingly, accuracy for the SLI-Persistent group was considerably lower (mean $A' = .575$). The reduced accuracy on the semantic violation trials, in addition to syntactic violation trials, supports previous findings that suggest that children with SLI have weak semantic representations [1, 65, 70]. Furthermore, poor performance in identifying anomalous verbs provides additional support that children with SLI have difficulties processing verbs [2, 4, 32]. The lexical-semantic difficulties in the SLI-Persistent group may have become more apparent in the current study given the coupling of the additional metalinguistic task demands and nonverbal processing difficulties that many children with SLI experience [32, 35]. In fact, the dual monitoring nature of the task likely increased the processing demands that are associated with executive function abilities. Given that children

with SLI have been found to have weaknesses in executive function abilities [43, 44, 82] and that executive function abilities have been found to be associated with lexical processing [20], the task design may have exacerbated lexical-semantic processing weaknesses in the SLI-Persistent group.

Behavioral processing of omission and commission errors

Although children typically produce omission and not commission errors in expressive language, contrary to our predictions, commission violations were not more easily detected relative to omission errors. In fact, although our results only approached significance, adolescents in our sample had slightly higher accuracy in the omission condition. Rice and colleagues [61] found that children with and without SLI correctly reject commission errors, paralleling their productive speech. However, Rice and colleagues tested commission errors that differed from ours, including copula and auxiliary *be* and third-person singular *-s* in combination with first-person singular subjects (e.g., "He *are* sad.", "I *likes* cake."). It is possible that some types of agreement errors may have disproportionally influenced child accuracy. It is unclear whether Rice and colleagues would have observed similar results if they tested the particular commission errors used within the present study.

In contrast to the Rice et al. [61] study, Redmond and Rice [58] focused on one category of finiteness markers, the irregular past tense. Redmond and Rice found that 8-year-old children with SLI or a history of SLI were more likely than age-matched peers to accept omission and commission errors, even when their productive language did not include commission errors. Although not directly tested, children with SLI had lower accuracy in detecting omission errors than commission errors; age-mates correctly identified both errors with similarly high accuracy [58]. Miller and colleagues [45] also found that identifying past tense *-ed* omission errors was particularly challenging in adolescents with typical language and language impairment. However, the children performed equally well at identifying commission and omission errors of the third-person singular *-s*.

Lastly, Leonard and colleagues [36] found that, in a less metalinguistically demanding word detection task, adolescents with SLI, nonspecific language impairment (NLI), and typical development were slower to respond to target words during the commission condition, relative to the grammatical condition. Reduced sensitivity to finiteness marking errors was only observed in the SLI and NLI groups during the omission condition. However, the omission and commission conditions contained errors of past tense *-ed* and third-person singular *-s*. Leonard et al. [36] also found that adolescents responded more quickly during past tense *-ed* items than third-person singular *-s* items, but could only speculate as to why this was the case.

Therefore, processing of omission and commission errors may differ according to the specific grammatical marker.

Neural profiles of language processing
Semantic violation processing

Despite the below-ceiling behavioral accuracy on judging correct sentences and sentences with an anomalous verb, all groups displayed an N400 in the semantic violation condition and there were no differences in the onset of the N400 across the groups, as indicated by our sequential temporal analysis of the N400. As previously noted, the anomalous verbs used in the current study were not frank violations, which may have allowed for the open-class anomalous verbs to be more easily integrated into the sentences than frank violations of high cloze class probability words. Previous studies have used more frank semantic violations and therefore demonstrated more robust N400s than the current study. This example with open-class semantic verb violations may demonstrate adolescents' abilities to gather the gestalt of the sentence despite the presence of subtle infelicities [14, 71].

Regardless, our findings are in line with results from a subset of these data presented by Weber-Fox et al. [80] and extend it to including information on lexical integration in adolescents with a history of SLI (i.e., SLI-Recovered group). In addition, our results mirror findings presented by Fonteneau and van der Lely [15] in suggesting that, at least in older children and adolescents with SLI, neural profiles of lexical integration do not seem to robustly differ from typically developing peers (but see studies of lexical integration in earlier developmental periods, e.g., [17, 64]).

Although we did not observe a significant group effect or interaction of group and condition, there was a significant interaction across condition, hemisphere, laterality, and group. Complex interactions like these can be difficult to interpret without numerous post hoc analyses. However, one potential implication of this interaction is that the SLI-Persistent group had a broader distribution of the N400 component, relative to the NL and SLI-Recovered groups. The broader distribution of the N400 component resembles a less mature neural profile of lexical integration [3, 25]. However, additional work is needed to explore potential differences in neuromaturational profiles in children with typical and atypical language development. In addition, it is possible that adolescents in the SLI-Recovered group were able to overcome early neuromaturational delays, whereas the adolescents in the SLI-Persistent group experienced a persistent lag in neuromaturation [39]. Therefore, slight variations in semantic processing at the neural level may persist in adolescents across a continuum of language abilities [56]. This interaction, combined with the differences in behavioral performance, suggests that semantic processing of verbs within sentences may still pose slight challenges for some adolescents with SLI or a history of SLI.

Omission violations

The typical ERP profile of syntactic violations, with a P600 component, was observed for the NL and SLI-Recovered groups. Despite early language impairments, adolescents in the SLI-Recovered group demonstrated similar behavioral performance and neural profiles to adolescents with no history of language impairments. Although differences may have been detected at earlier points in development, the adolescents in the SLI-Recovered group may have made sufficient language proficiency gains and maturational changes to demonstrate a more typical neural profile while processing sentences with omission errors.

In contrast, there was a marginal difference in the P600 component elicited from omission violations in adolescents in the SLI-Persistent group. They demonstrated a marginally more restricted distribution of the P600 in the posterior region of the left hemisphere, as evidenced by the interaction across condition, hemisphere, and AP. Previous work designed to use the P600 component to examine the processes related to verb agreement errors in children with SLI is lacking. In one study using an overlapping dataset with the current study, Weber-Fox and colleagues [80] also found that adolescents with SLI did not demonstrate a P600 component after listening to verb agreement violations of the third-person singular -s marker, but typically developing adolescents did. These results differ from studies examining other types of syntactic errors, such as wh- dependencies and word category violations [15, 65]. Although adolescents with persistent language impairment no longer produce consistent omission errors in their expressive language, difficulties in processing verb agreement omission errors may persist at both the behavioral and neural levels.

Commission violations

The current study extended previous work by separately examining omission and commission errors of the third-person singular -s tense marker. We found that, when examining plural correct sentences and sentences with commission errors, the adolescents in the NL and SLI-Recovered groups demonstrated overall significantly greater positivity in the P600 window than the adolescents in the SLI-Persistent group. In addition, the sequential temporal analyses indicated that the NL group demonstrated an earlier onset of the P600 component relative to the other groups. Purdy and colleagues [57] observed a P600 component after hearing a local verb agreement commission error and a negative polarity shift in the anterior regions of the brain (i.e., anterior negativity) in both children with typical development and children with a history of SLI. In the current study, visual inspection of the group waveforms revealed that the adolescents in the SLI-Recovered group also demonstrated a negative polarity shift after a commission error, which was followed by similar positive mean amplitudes for the plural correct sentences and the sentences with commission errors. The negativity observed in the current SLI-Recovered group, however, was observed more globally and temporally later, causing it to be more characteristic of an N400 than the AN component.

The unique neural profile, indexed by the N400-like negativity, observed in the SLI-Recovered group was one of the most important and novel findings in the current study. Although syntactic deficits are more often associated with the AN component, later-occurring negativities resembling the N400 component have been found for morphosyntactic violations (e.g., [48, 69]). As such, recent work has suggested that the dominance of the N400 or the P600 component provides insight into the competition between two interactive processing "streams" [29, 52, 77]. One stream is associated with the N400, indexing lexically or memory-based processing, and the other is associated with the P600 and thought to indicate combinatorial, algorithmic processing that often relies on linguistic constraints such as morphosyntactic rules [29, 30, 52]. Furthermore, it is thought that the robustness of the N400 and P600 may provide insight into the processing stream that is engaged during language processing.

Along this line, recent studies have begun to explore individual differences in relation to neural profiles during language processing. For example, Pakulak and Neville [53] observed that monolingual adults with high language proficiency demonstrated the well-documented AN and P600 waveforms following phrase structure violations. In contrast, adults with relatively low language proficiency demonstrated a later negativity waveform that was N400-like, in addition to a smaller P600 component. Additional work has documented individual differences in neural profiles that appeared to be associated with language proficiency [73] and chronological age [67]. These findings, along with our findings, suggest that there are several neurocognitive routes to grammatical comprehension.

Our sample of adolescents in the SLI-Recovered group resembled the NL group in their behavioral accuracy in the language processing task; it is possible that these individuals developed compensatory routes to successfully process language despite early language weaknesses. In fact, the Procedural Deficit Hypothesis predicts that individuals with SLI may rely on declarative memory to compensate for procedural memory weaknesses [76]. Behavioral work also has demonstrated that declarative

memory predicts syntactic abilities in children with SLI [8]. In the current study, across adolescents in the SLI-Recovered and SLI-Persistent groups, we found a significant correlation between the A' accuracy scores for the commission violation condition and mean amplitude differences in the negativity window. An alternative explanation may be that the N400-like pattern observed in the SLI-Recovered group may have emerged because the task required monitoring of both semantic and syntactic aspects of sentences; however, it is unclear why the task demands would elicit this robust neural profile for only the SLI-Recovered group. Additional work examining individual differences that measure behavioral and neural indices of language processing is needed.

Limitations

Despite the unique insights the current study provides, there are limitations that we would like to address. First, we were unable to limit our analyses to examining correct trials only. We required the adolescents to contribute at least 20 artifact-free trials within each condition. Given the challenging nature of the task and given that we were examining language processing in adolescents who have language impairments, we would have had to drastically reduce the number of participants in each group if we had required 20 artifact-free correct trials. Despite this limitation, we explored the waveforms for the correct trials only for each group and found that the neural profiles were similar to the waveforms that included all trials regardless of accuracy. This leads us to believe that we would have found similar results had we been able to analyze correct trials only. Relatedly, although our task yielded a rich dataset, it would have been more ideal to have been able to have an equal number of (semantically or syntactically) correct and incorrect sentences. To do so, we would have had to increase the number of trials in the task, which may have fatigued our participants and increased data loss associated with fatigue.

Conclusions

The current study expanded on previous studies to contribute needed information about the trajectory of language impairments. We observed that adolescents in the SLI-Persistent group had lower accuracy on the sentence judgment task than the NL and SLI-Recovered groups. In addition, the SLI-Persistent group demonstrated a restricted P600 after listening to syntactic violations. Furthermore, although sentence processing accuracy was slightly lower in the SLI-Recovered group relative to the NL group, differences did not reach significance. This suggests that adolescents who had a history of SLI but later scored in the normal range of language assessments may have experienced sufficient language gains through therapy and/or development to enhance language processing abilities. Although subtle weaknesses may still be present, on the whole, they did not appear to fit under an "illusory recovery" classification. More interesting, though, is the way in which adolescents in the SLI-Recovered group processed language. The ERP data from the commission condition indicated that ERPs from adolescents in the SLI-Recovered group may have reflected compensatory strategies to facilitate some aspects of language processing during the task. Specifically, they appear to have recruited lexical processing streams to support syntactic processing. Additional work examining underlying neural indices of language processing in children with a history of SLI is greatly needed. Furthermore, future work should strive to collect neural data longitudinally to contribute much needed information about the trajectory of language impairments and the neural mechanisms that underlie developmental changes.

Appendix
Correct verb (verb agreement violation, semantic violation)

1. Every day, the horses *gallop* (*gallops, sing*) to the top of the hill.

2. Every day, the canaries *sing* (*sings, gallop*) at the top of their lungs.

3. Every day, the cow *grazes* (*graze, types*) to the top of the hill.

4. Every day, the secretary *types* (*type, grazes*) many legal documents.

5. Every day, the ballerina *dances* (*dance, submerges*) on her pointed toe shoes.

6. Every day, the submarine *submerges* (*submerge, dances*) to a depth of five hundred feet.

7. Every day, the beautician *style* (*styles, slither*) at least 30 heads.

8. Every day, the snakes *slither* (*slithers, style*) through the fallen leaves.

9. Every day, the lieutenant *salutes* (*salute, meows*) his captain during routine inspections.

10. Every day, the cat *meows* (*meow, salutes*) when he thinks he is going to be fed.

11. Every day, the grandmothers *knit* (*knits, peck*) scarves and sweaters for their friends and families.

12. Every day, the chickens *peck* (pecks, *knit*) at the dirt for bits of dried corn.

13. Every day, the earrings *dangle* (*dangles, cry*) from her earlobes.

14. Every day, the babies *cry* (*cries, dangle*) when they are hungry.

15. Every day, the customers *gossip* (*gossips, swoop*) about the hot news in town.

16. Every day, the eagles *swoop* (*swoops, gossip*) down to hunt for their food.

17. Every day, the mailman *delivers* (*deliver, growls*) our letters and packages with care.

18. Every day, the dog *growls* (*growl, delivers*) when someone passes his yard.

19. Every day, the teachers *assign* (*assigns, gnaw*) on the old boxes stored there.

20. Every day, the mice *gnaw* (*gnaws, assign*) on the old boxes stored there.

21. Every day, the children *pretend* (*pretends, rust*) to be superheroes.

22. Every day, the cars *rust* (*rusts, pretend*) a little bit more.

23. Every day, the senator *votes* (*vote, perches*) on important issues.

24. Every day, the bird *perches* (*perch, votes*) at the top of our tree.

25. Every day, the owner *rents* (*rent, backfires*) his rooms for reasonable rates.

26. Every day, the engine *backfires* (*backfire, rents*) on my way to work.

27. Every day, the farms *plow* (*plows, buzz*) their corn and soybean fields.

28. Every day, the bees *buzz* (*buzzes, plow*) happily as they make honey.

29. Every day, the president *plans* (*plan, blasts*) his next course of action.

30. Every day, the wind *blasts* (*blast, plans*) the lakefront residents.

31. Every day, the officers *arrest* (*arrests, shimmer*) people who break the law.

32. Every day, the pennies *shimmer* (*shimmers, arrest*) in the sunlight.

33. Every day, the sirens *blare* (*blares, sew*) to signal emergencies.

34. Every day, the seamstresses *sew* (*sews, blare*) custom designed gowns.

35. Every day, the telephones *ring* (*rings, scurry*) constantly until closing time.

36. Every day, the squirrels *scurry* (*scurries, ring*) under the rose bushes.

37. Every day, the tree *grows* (*grow, plays*) taller and more beautiful.

38. Every day, the theater *plays* (*play, grows*) seven different movies.

39. Every day, the hikers *climb* (*climbs, sparkle*) closer to the mountain's peak.

40. Every day, the minerals *sparkle* (*sparkles, climb*) in the midday sun.

41. Every day, the girls *giggle* (*giggles, roar*) about the funny cartoons.

42. Every day, the lions *roar* (*roars, giggle*) around dinner time.

43. Every day, the seagull *flies* (*fly, melts*) over the waves.

44. Every day, the wax *melts* (*melt, flies*) onto the table.

45. Every day, the boys *plan* (*plans, overflow*) the next football game.

46. Every day, the rivers *overflow* (*overflows, plan*) the low lands.

47. Every day, the lifeguard *watches* (*watch, sprouts*) the swimmers.

48. Every day, the plant *sprouts* (*sprout, watches*) new leaves.

49. Every day, the gardener *digs* (*dig, drips*) in the flower bed.

50. Every day, the water *drips* (*drip, digs*) into the sink.

51. Every day, the pen *leaks* (*leak, wrinkles*) in my pocket.

52. Every day, the shirt *wrinkles* (*wrinkle, leaks*) in the dryer.

53. Every day, the musicians *tune* (*tunes, rumble*) their instruments.

54. Every day, the trucks *rumble* (*rumbles, tune*) down the highway.

55. Every day, the tooth *aches* (*ache, sing*) when I eat sweets.

56. Every day, the tire *deflates* (*deflate, aches*) a little bit more.

57. Every day, the rose *wilts* (*wilt, swings*) in the hot sunshine.

58. Every day, the door *swings* (*swing, wilts*) shut by the draft.

59. Every day, the chefs *prepare* (*prepares, flicker*) hundreds of meals.

60. Every day, the lights *flicker* (*flickers, prepare*) in the window.

Abbreviations

AN: Anterior negativity; ERP: Event-related potential; NL: Normal Language; SLI: Specific language impairment; SLI-Persistent, SLI-P: Specific Language Impairment-Persistent; SLI-Recovered, SLI-R: Specific Language Impairment-Recovered

Acknowledgments

We thank the families who participated in the study. Also, we thank Wendy Fick for the ERP data collection and Marlea O'Brien for recruiting the participants. In addition, we thank John Spruill for the help with stimulus development and piloting and Amanda Hampton Wray for the preliminary data processing.

Funding

This research was funded by the National Institute of Deafness and Other Communication Disorders, National Institutes of Health, P50 DC02746 and T32 DC00030.

Authors' contributions

EH processed, analyzed, and interpreted the data and drafted the manuscript. CW conceived of the study; designed the experiment; oversaw the data collection, processing, and analysis; assisted with the interpretation of the findings; and provided critical feedback on the manuscript. LBL assisted with the interpretation of the findings and provided critical feedback on the manuscript. PD provided critical feedback on the manuscript. JBT wrote the grant application that funded this research, oversaw the parent project, and provided critical feedback on the manuscript. All authors have read and approved the final manuscript.

Competing interests

The authors declare that they have no competing interests.

Author details

[1]Purdue University, West Lafayette, IN, USA. [2]University of Iowa, Iowa City, IA, USA.

References

1. Alt M, Meyers C, Alt PM. Using ratings to gain insight into conceptual development. J Speech Lang Hear Res. 2013;56:1650–61.
2. Andreu L, Sanz-Torrent M, Guàrdia-Olmos J. Auditory word recognition of nouns and verbs in children with Specific Language Impairment (SLI). J Commun Disord. 2012;45:20–34.
3. Atchley RA, Rice ML, Betz SK, Kwasny KM, Sereno JA, Jongman A. A comparison of semantic and syntactic event related potentials generated by children and adults. Brain Lang. 2006;99:236–46.
4. Borovsky A, Burns E, Elman JL, Evans JL. Lexical activation during sentence comprehension in adolescents with history of specific language impairment. J Commun Disord. 2013;46:413–27.
5. Catts HW, Fey ME, Tomblin JB, Zhang X. A longitudinal investigation of reading outcomes in children with language impairments. J Speech Lang Hear Res. 2002;45:1142–57.
6. Conti-Ramsden G, Durkin K, Simkin Z, Knox E. Specific language impairment and school outcomes. I: identifying and explaining variability at the end of compulsory education. Int J Lang Commun Disord. 2009;44:15–35.
7. Conti-Ramsden G, Clair CS, Pickles A, Durkin K. Developmental trajectories of verbal and nonverbal skills in individuals with a history of specific language impairment: from childhood to adolescence. J Speech Lang Hear Res. 2012; 55:1716–35.
8. Conti-Ramsden G, Ullman MT, Lum JAG. The relation between receptive grammar and procedural, declarative, and working memory in specific language impairment. Front Psychol. 2015;6:1–11.
9. Culatta B, Page J, Ellis J. Story retelling as a communicative performance screening tool. Lang Speech Hear Serv Sch. 1983;14:66–74.
10. Delorme A, Makeig S. EEGLAB: an open source toolbox for analysis of single-trial EEG dynamics including independent component analysis. J Neurosci Methods. 2004;134:9–21.
11. Dunn LM, Dunn LM. Peabody Picture Vocabulary Test—Revised. 2nd ed. Circle Pines: American Guidance Service; 1981.
12. Ellis Weismer S, Evans J, Hesketh LJ. An examination of verbal working memory capacity in children with specific language impairment. J Speech Lang Hear Res. 1999;42:1249–60.
13. Fazio BB. Arithmetic calculation, short-term memory, and language performance in children with specific language impairment: a 5-year follow-up. J Speech Lang Hear Res. 1999;42:420–32.
14. Ferreira F, Bailey KGD, Ferraro V. Good-enough representations in language comprehension. Curr Dir Psychol Sci. 2002;11:11–5.
15. Fonteneau E, van der Lely HKJ. Electrical brain responses in language-impaired children reveal grammar-specific deficits. Plos One. 2008;3:1–6.
16. Friederici AD. Towards a neural basis of auditory sentence processing. Trends Cogn Sci. 2002;6:78–84.
17. Friedrich M, Friederici AD. Maturing brain mechanisms and developing behavioral language skills. Brain Lang. 2010;114:66–71.
18. Gouvea AC, Phillips C, Kazanina N, Poeppel D. The linguistic processes underlying the P600. Lang Cogn Process. 2010;25:149–88.
19. Grier JB. Nonparametric indexes for sensitivity and bias: computing formulas. Psychol Bull. 1971;75:424–9.
20. Haebig E, Kaushanskaya M, Ellis Weismer S. Lexical processing in school-age children with autism spectrum disorder and children with specific language impairment: the role of semantics. J Autism Dev Disord. 2015;45:4109–23.
21. Hahne A, Eckstein K, Friederici AD. Brain signatures of syntactic and semantic processes during children's language development. J Cogn Neurosci. 2004;16:1302–18.

22. Hays WL. Inferences about population means. Statistics. 1994;5:311–42.

23. Hesketh A, Conti-Ramsden G. Memory and language in middle childhood in individuals with a history of specific language impairment. Plos One. 2013;8:1–7.

24. Holcomb PJ, Coffey S a, Neville H. Visual and auditory sentence processing: a developmental analysis using event-related brain potentials. Dev Neuropsychol. 1992;8:203–41.

25. Holcomb PJ, Coffey SA, Neville HJ. Visual and auditory sentence processing: a developmental analysis using event-related brain potentials. Dev Neuropsychol. 1992;8:203–41.

26. Jung TP, Makeig S, Westerfield M, Townsend J, Courchesne E, Sejnowski TJ. Removal of eye activity artifacts from visual event-related potentials in normal and clinical subjects. Clin Neurophysiol. 2000;111:1745–58.

27. Jurcak V, Tsuzuki D, Dan I. 10/20, 10/10, and 10/5 systems revisited: their validity as relative head-surface-based positioning systems. Neuroimage. 2007;34:1600–11.

28. Karmiloff-Smith A. Nativism versus neuroconstructivism: rethinking the study of developmental disorders. Dev Psychol. 2009;45:56–63.

29. Kim A, Osterhout L. The independence of combinatory semantic processing: evidence from event-related potentials. J Mem Lang. 2005;52:205–25.

30. Kutas M, Federmeier KD. Thirty years and counting: finding meaning in the N400 component of the event-related brain potential (ERP). Annu Rev Psychol. 2011;62:621–47.

31. Kutas M, Hillyard SA. Reading senseless sentences: brain potentials reflect semantic incongruity. Science. 1980;207:203–5.

32. Leonard LB. Children with specific language impairment. 2nd ed. Cambridge: MIT Press; 2014.

33. Leonard LB, Eyer JA, Bedore LM, Grela BG. Three accounts of the grammatical morpheme difficulties of English-speaking children with specific language impairment. J Speech Lang Hear Res. 1997;40:741–53.

34. Leonard LB, Camarata SM, Brown B, Camarata MN. Tense and agreement in the speech of children with specific language impairment: patterns of generalization through intervention. J Speech Lang Hear Res. 2004;47:1363–79.

35. Leonard LB, Ellis Weismer S, Miller CA, Francis DJ, Tomblin JB, Kail RV. Speed of processing, working memory, and language impairment in children. J Speech Lang Hear Res. 2007;50:408–28.

36. Leonard LB, Miller CA, Finneran DA. Grammatical morpheme effects on sentence processing by school-aged adolescents with specific language impairment. Lang Cogn Process. 2009;24:450–78.

37. Leslie L, Cladwell J. Qualitative Reading Inventory-3. 3rd ed. Boston: Allyn & Bacon; 2000.

38. Linebarger MC, Schwartz MF, Saffran EM. Sensitivity to grammatical structure in so-called agrammatic aphasics. Cognition. 1983;13:361–92.

39. Locke JL. Gradual emergence of developmental language disorders. J Speech Lang Hear Res. 1994;37:608–16.

40. Lopez-Calderon J, Luck SJ. ERPLAB: an open-source toolbox for the analysis of event-related potentials. Front Hum Neurosci. 2014;8:1–14.

41. Lopez-Calderon, J., & Luck, S. J. ERPLAB Toolbox (1.1.0). (2010). Retrieved from http://erpinfo.org/erplab. Accessed 10 Sept 2015.

42. Luck SJ. An introduction to the event-related potential technique. 2nd ed. Boston: MIT Press; 2014.

43. Marton K. Visuo-spatial processing and executive functions in children with specific language impairment. Int J Lang Commun Disord. 2008;43:181–200.

44. Marton K, Eichorn N. Interaction between working memory and long-term memory. Zeitschrift Für Psychologie. 2014;222:90–9.

45. Miller CA, Leonard LB, Finneran D. Grammaticality judgements in adolescents with and without language impairment. Int J Lang Commun Disord. 2008;43:346–60.

46. Neville H, Coffey S a, Holcomb PJ, Tallal P. The neurobiology of sensory and language processing in language-impaired children. J Cogn Neurosci. 1993;5:235–53.

47. Newcomer P, Hammill D. Test of Language Development-Primary. 2nd ed. Austin: Pro-Ed; 1988.

48. Nieuwland MS, Martin AE, Carreiras M. Event-related brain potential evidence for animacy processing asymmetries during sentence comprehension. Brain Lang. 2013;126:151–8.

49. Oldfield RC. The assessment and analysis of handedness: the Edinburgh inventory. Neuropsychologia. 1971;9:97–113.

50. Osterhout L, Holcomb PJ. Event-related brain potentials elicited by syntactic anomaly. J Mem Lang. 1992;31:785–806.

51. Osterhout L, Holcomb PJ, Swinney DA. Brain potentials elicited by garden-path sentences: evidence of the application of verb information during parsing. J Exp Psychol Learn Mem Cogn. 1994;20:786–803.

52. Osterhout L, Kim A, Kuperberg G. The neurobiology of sentence comprehension. In: Spivey M, Joannisse M, McRae K, editors. Cambridge handbook of psycholinguistics. Cambridge: Cambridge University Press; 2012. p. 365–89.

53. Pakulak E, Neville H. Proficiency differences in syntactic processing of monolingual native speakers indexed by event-related potentials. J Cogn Neurosci. 2010;22:2728–44.

54. Park J, Miller CA, Mainela-Arnold E. Processing speed measures as clinical markers for children with language impairment. J Speech Lang Hear Res. 2015;58:954–60.

55. Phillips C, Kazanina N, Abada SH. ERP effects of the processing of syntactic long-distance dependencies. Cogn Brain Res. 2005;22:407–28.

56. Plante E, Van Petten C, Senkfor AJ. Electrophysiological dissociation between verbal and nonverbal semantic processing in learning disabled adults. Neuropsychologia. 2000;38:1669–84.

57. Purdy JD, Leonard LB, Weber-Fox C, Kaganovich N. Decreased sensitivity to long-distance dependencies in children with a history of specific language impairment: electrophysiological evidence. J Speech Lang Hear Res. 2014;57:1040–59.

58. Redmond SM, Rice ML. Detection of irregular verb violations by children with and without SLI. J Speech Lang Hear Res. 2001;44:655–69.

59. Rice ML, Hoffman L. Predicting vocabulary growth in children with and without specific language impairment: a longitudinal study from 2;6 to 21 years of age. J Speech Lang Hear Res. 2015;58:345–59.

60. Rice ML, Wexler K. Toward tense as a clinical marker of specific language impairment in English-speaking children. J Speech Lang Hear Res. 1996;39:1239–57.

61. Rice ML, Wexler K, Redmond SM. Grammaticality judgements of extended optional infinitive grammar: evidence from English-speaking children with specific language impairment. J Speech Lang Hear Res. 1999;42:943–61.

62. Rice ML, Redmond SM, Hoffman L. Mean length of utterance in children with specific language impairment and in younger control children shows concurrent validity and stable and parallel growth trajectories mean length of utterance in children and parallel growth trajectories. J Speech Lang Hear Res. 2006;49:793–808.

63. Rice ML, Hoffman L, Wexler K. Judgments of omitted BE and DO in questions as extended finiteness clinical markers of specific language impairment (SLI) to 15 years: a study of growth and asymptote. J Speech Lang Hear Res. 2009;52:1417–33.

64. Sabisch B, Hahne A, Glass E, von Suchodoletz W, Friederici AD. Lexical-semantic processes in children with specific language impairment. Neuroreport. 2006;17:1511–4.

65. Sabisch B, Hahne CA, Glass E, von Suchodoletz W, Friederici AD. Children with specific language impairment: the role of prosodic processes in explaining difficulties in processing syntactic information. Brain Res. 2009;1261:37–44.

66. Scarborough HS, Dobrich W. Development of children with early language delay. J Speech Lang Hear Res. 1990;33:70–83.

67. Schneider JM, Abel AD, Ogiela DA, Middleton A, Maguire MJ. Developmental differences in beta and theta power during sentence processing. Dev Cogn Neurosci. 2016;19:19–30.

68. Semel E, Wiig EH, Secord W. Clinical evaluation of language fundamentals. (T. P. Corporation, Ed.). 3rd ed. San Antonio: Harcourt Brace & Co.; 1995.

69. Severens E, Jansma BM, Hartsuiker RJ. Morphophonological influences on the comprehension of subject-verb agreement: an ERP study. Brain Res. 2008;1228:135–44.

70. Sheng L, McGregor KK. Lexical-semantic organization in children with specific language impairment. J Speech Lang Hear Res. 2010;53:146–59.

71. Sitnikova T, Holcomb PJ, Kuperberg GR. Neurocognitive mechanisms of human comprehension. In: Shipley TF, Zacks JM, editors. Understanding events: how humans see, represent, and act on events. Oxford: Oxford University Press; 2008. p. 639–83.

72. Steinhauer K, Drury JE. On the early left-anterior negativity (ELAN) in syntax studies. Brain Lang. 2012;120:135–62.

73. Tanner D, Van Hell JG. ERPs reveal individual differences in morphosyntactic processing. Neuropsychologia. 2014;56:289–301.

74. Tomblin JB, Records NL, Zhang X. A system for the diagnosis of specific language impairment in kindergarten children. J Speech Lang Hear Res. 1996;39:1284–94.

75. Tomblin JB, Records NL, Buckwalter P, Zhang X, Smith E, O'Brien M. Prevalence of specific language impairment in kindergarten children. J Speech Lang Hear Res. 1997;40:1245–60.

76. Ullman MT, Pierpont EI. Specific language impairment is not specific to language: the procedural deficit hypothesis. Cortex. 2005;41:399–433.

77. van de Meerendonk N, Kolk HHJ, Vissers CTWM, Chwilla DJ. Monitoring in language perception: mild and strong conflicts elicit different ERP patterns. J Cogn Neurosci. 2010;22:67–82.

78. Wallace GL, Hammill D. Comprehensive receptive and expressive vocabulary test. Austin: Pro-Ed; 1994.

79. Weber-Fox C, Hampton A. Stuttering and natural speech processing of semantic and syntactic constraints on verbs. J Speech Lang Hear Res. 2008; 51:1058–71.

80. Weber-Fox C, Leonard LB, Hampton Wray A, Tomblin JB. Electrophysiological correlates of rapid auditory and linguistic processing in adolescents with specific language impairment. Brain Lang. 2010;115:162–81.

81. Wechsler D. Wechsler Intelligence Scale for Children—Third Edition. 3rd ed. San Antonio: The Psychological Corporation; 1991.

82. Wittke K, Spaulding TJ, Schechtman CJ. Specific language impairment and executive functioning: parent and teacher ratings of behavior. Am J Speech Lang Pathol. 2013;22:161–72.

83. Wulfeck B, Bates E, Krupa-Kwiatkowski M, Saltzman D. Grammaticality sensitivity in children with early focal brain injury and children with specific language impairment. Brain Lang. 2004;88:215–28.

11

A resting EEG study of neocortical hyperexcitability and altered functional connectivity in fragile X syndrome

Jun Wang[1*], Lauren E. Ethridge[2,3], Matthew W. Mosconi[4], Stormi P. White[5], Devin K. Binder[6], Ernest V. Pedapati[7], Craig A. Erickson[7], Matthew J. Byerly[8] and John A. Sweeney[9]

Abstract

Background: Cortical hyperexcitability due to abnormal fast-spiking inhibitory interneuron function has been documented in *fmr1* KO mice, a mouse model of the fragile X syndrome which is the most common single gene cause of autism and intellectual disability.

Methods: We collected resting state dense-array electroencephalography data from 21 fragile X syndrome (FXS) patients and 21 age-matched healthy participants.

Results: FXS patients exhibited greater gamma frequency band power, which was correlated with social and sensory processing difficulties. Second, FXS patients showed increased spatial spreading of phase-synchronized high frequency neural activity in the gamma band. Third, we observed increased negative theta-to-gamma but decreased alpha-to-gamma band amplitude coupling, and the level of increased theta power was inversely related to the level of resting gamma power in FXS.

Conclusions: Increased theta band power and coupling from frontal sources may represent a mechanism providing compensatory inhibition of high-frequency gamma band activity, potentially contributing to the widely varying level of neurophysiological and behavioral abnormalities and treatment response seen in full-mutation FXS patients. These findings extend preclinical observations and provide new mechanistic insights into brain alterations and their variability across FXS patients. Electrophysiological measures may provide useful translational biomarkers for advancing drug development and individualizing treatments for neurodevelopmental disorders with associated neuronal hyperexcitability.

Keywords: Fragile X syndrome, EEG, Hyperexcitability, Gamma, Cross-frequency coupling, Top-down modulation

Background

Fragile X syndrome (FXS) is a neurodevelopmental disorder resulting from silencing of the fragile X mental retardation gene (*FMR1*) on the X chromosome, leading to reduced production of Fragile X Mental Retardation Protein (FMRP) [1] that causes atypical brain development and function. Studies in *fmr1* knockout (KO) mice have shown enhanced activity of metabotropic glutamate receptors [2] and reduced GABAergic transmission [3]. These alterations are believed to cause an imbalance favoring excitation over inhibition in brain neurophysiology [3–5].

Neurophysiological studies can clarify the functional brain consequences of neurochemical and neuroanatomic changes in FXS. *fmr1* KO mice have abnormally high synchrony of neocortical network activity and a threefold higher neuronal firing rate during Up states [6, 7]. *fmr1* KO mice have also shown increased EEG responses to auditory stimuli via in vivo recordings [8–10]. Similarly, enhanced auditory event-related potential (ERP) responses (e.g. N1, P2) and reduced response habituation have been reported in FXS patients [11–14].

Given the model of a neurophysiological imbalance leading to heightened neural excitability and the increased

* Correspondence: jun.wang@zjnu.edu.cn
[1]Department of Psychology, Zhejiang Normal University, 688 Yingbin Road, Jinhua, Zhejiang, China 321004
Full list of author information is available at the end of the article

prevalence of seizures in FXS patients and *fmr1* KO mice, and with due consideration of the challenges integrating knowledge from intracranial recordings and clinical data, it is noteworthy that few EEG studies of resting brain function have yet been conducted with FXS patients. To our knowledge there has only been one quantitative study of resting state EEG in FXS presented in two reports [15, 16]. Excessive resting state theta and reduced alpha power in FXS were reported, as well as decreased connectivity in alpha and beta bands but increased connectivity in the theta band. While informative, there were certain limitations to that study. First, the sample size was small (8 FXS patients). Second, the study investigated activity under 50 Hz, which excludes a significant component of the gamma frequency band (30–80 Hz) [17–19]. This limitation is important because gamma band power reflects the level of high frequency spontaneous neural activity and is of special interest for FXS in light of *fmr1* KO mouse studies that have identified abnormalities in fast-spiking inhibitory GABAergic interneurons [7, 20] which are critical generators of gamma power in cell populations [21]. Third, functional connectivity analysis was done using only 28 electrodes; a dense electrode montage can better capture the full pattern of functional connectivity across the neocortex. Fourth, the study was insufficiently powered to identify correlations between resting state oscillatory abnormalities in FXS and measures of clinical symptom severity.

Alpha rhythms are the most dominant oscillation during the resting state and play an inhibitory role in information processing systems [22]. Theta rhythms also reflect topdown inhibitory and organizational influences especially during higher cognitive activity [23], and altered thetagamma coupling has been linked with cognitive dysfunction in *fmr1* KO mice [24]. As increased gamma activity is believed to be linked to increased neural excitability, examining the relationship of alpha and theta band activity with gamma band activity might provide mechanistic system-level understanding about the altered balance between excitatory and inhibitory activity.

The aim of the present study was to investigate resting state EEG activity in FXS patients focusing on resting EEG power—specifically gamma band power, functional connectivity, and gamma coupling. We hypothesized that resting state EEG power in FXS would be enhanced in both low- and high-frequency bands (theta and gamma) but reduced in middle range frequencies (alpha) relative to healthy controls. Second, we predicted that functional connectivity in FXS would be reduced in long-range connections but increased in short-range connections dominated by gamma band oscillations relative to controls. Third, we predicted that FXS patients would show reduced alpha-to-gamma coupling consistent with reduced top-down alpha-related inhibition on local cortical excitability in sensory systems. Fourth, we hypothesized that altered resting EEG power spectra in FXS individuals would be correlated with social and sensory processing difficulties.

Methods

Participants

Twenty-one FXS participants with a full mutation (greater than 200 CGG repeats) (six females, 15 males, mean age = 25.6 years, SD = 11.1, range 12–57) and 21 healthy agematched controls (six females, 15 males, mean age = 26.4 years, SD = 10.5, range 10–55) participated in this study (Table 1). None had a history of nonfebrile seizures or treatment with anticonvulsant medication. Healthy controls had no known prior diagnosis or treatment for a psychiatric or neurological illness or history of developmental delay in educational achievement. FXS participants taking psychiatric medications were receiving a stable dose for at least 4 weeks prior to participation. Nine FXS participants were receiving one or more psychiatric medications: 5 on antipsychotics, 5 on antidepressants, and 2 on psychostimulants. Treated patients did not differ on reported EEG measures (see Additional file 1: Table S1). Primary analyses were done with the whole sample, with confirmatory analyses done with the male participants.

The Adolescent and Adult Sensory Profile [25] and the Social Communication Questionnaire (SCQ) [26] were completed for FXS participants by their primary caregiver or close family member. IQ of FXS participants was

Table 1 Demographic, intellectual, and clinical characteristics of study participants

	FXS *n* = 21				Healthy controls *n* = 21			
	Mean	Std dev	Range		Mean	Std dev	Range	*t* statistic (*df*)
Age	25.6	11.1	12–57	Age	26.4	10.5	10–55	0.24 (40) *p* = 0.809
Full scale IQ	55.1	14.8	47–94	Full scale IQ	106.3	10.7	82–123	12.8 (40) *p* < 0.001
Verbal	2.9	3.2	1–11	Verbal	107.7	11.7	82–124	
Nonverbal	2.0	1.9	1–7	Performance	103.2	11.8	82–125	
SCQ scores	17.7	8.6	2–31					
Sensory Profile	31.6	4.7	24–40					

IQ assessed by Stanford Binet in FXS and estimated using the Wechsler Adult Scale of Intelligence in healthy controls
SCQ Social and Communication Questionnaire

assessed using the Stanford-Binet Intelligence Scale 5th Ed. [27] which characterizes intellectual ability across a broad ability and age range. IQ of healthy controls was estimated using the briefer Wechsler Abbreviated Scale of Intelligence (WASI) [28] (Table 1). The project was approved by the University of Texas Southwestern Institutional Review Board, and informed consent was obtained from all participants, except when appropriate from a parent with participant assent.

EEG recordings and preprocessing

Five minutes of continuous EEG data was collected. Participants were comfortably seated while watching a silent video (cartoon movie, standardized across participants), done to facilitate cooperation in the FXS patients as in previous studies [29]. EEG data were recorded with a 128-electrode Biosemi Active Two system at a sampling rate of 512 Hz. Two additional electrodes, positioned near to the electrode POz of the international 10-20 system [30], served as recording reference [common mode sense (CMS) active electrode] and ground. The initial 10 s of recordings were excluded from processing to minimize movement artifacts. Raw EEG data were filtered and transformed to an average reference using the EEGLAB toolbox [31]. High- and low-pass cutoff frequencies were set at 0.5 and 100 Hz; a 60-Hz notch filter was used for removal of power-line noise. Then, EEG data were subjected to Fully Automated Statistical Thresholding for segmentation with 2 s each and EEG Artifact Rejection (FASTER) [32], and artifacts including eye blink, muscle activity, and cardiac activity were removed. This process included 5 steps: (1) outlier channels were identified and replaced with interpolated values in continuous data; (2) continuous data was segmented into 2-s epochs; (3) outlier epochs were removed from participants' epoch set; (4) spatial independent components analysis was applied to remaining epochs, outlier components were identified (including components that correlated with EOG activity), and data were backprojected without these components; and (5) within an epoch, outlier channels were interpolated.

EEG power

There was no significant group difference in the number of artifact-free epochs (Epochs$_{control}$ = 138, SD = 5.8; Epochs$_{FXS}$ = 139, SD = 4.7, $p > 0.05$) or number of interpolated channels (Interplolated_channel$_{control}$ = 2.33, SD = 1.2; Interplolated_channel$_{FXS}$ = 2.81, SD = 2.06, $p > 0.05$). For each channel, every 2-s epoch was detrended, tapered with a Hanning window, and transformed in Matlab using a Fourier (FFT) algorithm, yielding Fourier coefficients in 0.5 Hz frequency steps. The Fourier coefficients were then squared to yield power values (uV^2). To be comparable with previous resting-state EEG reports on FXS [16], we divided our frequencies into six frequency bands of interest as follows: delta (1–3 Hz), theta (4–7 Hz), lower alpha (8–10 Hz), upper alpha (10–12 Hz), beta (13–30 Hz), and gamma (30–80 Hz). Alpha band activity was separated into higher and lower bands because previous studies showed that higher alpha is state dependent and sensitive to arousal while lower alpha is not [33], as well as to permit direct comparison with the previous resting EEG study of FXS [15, 16]. To minimize effects of interindividual variability in total power, relative power was obtained by computing the fraction of power in each frequency band divided by the sum of power measurements across 1–80 Hz for each frequency band in each of the 128 channels. Group comparisons in relative power (power at specific frequency/total power) between healthy and FXS individuals were performed at every channel. To correct for multiple comparisons and identify significant clusters among channels with group differences in a frequency band, a cluster-based permutation test in the Mass Univariate ERP Toolbox was used for statistical comparisons (5000 permutations [34]).

Connectivity analysis

Functional connectivity among all electrode pairs was examined separately in each of the six frequency bands of interest using the debiased weighted phase lag index (dbWPLI) [35]. This method minimizes artifacts resulting from spurious inflation of scalp EEG connectivity caused by volume conduction. The dbWPLI calculates an unbiased index of phase synchronization between two time series, weighted by the magnitude of the imaginary component of the cross-spectrum. Compared to a direct phase lag index (PLI), the dbWPLI has minimum sample-size bias and improved ability to detect phase synchronization patterns. The dbWPLI value ranges from 0 to 1, with zero indicating the absence of phase-lagged coupling and one indicating the strongest possible coupling.

EEG data were imported to FieldTrip (Donders Institute for Brain, Cognition and Behaviour, Radboud University, Nijmegen, The Netherlands: http://www.ru.nl/neuroimaging/fieldtrip/) for calculating dbWPLI among all electrode pairs (8128 pairs) at each of the six frequency bands of interest. Then, at each frequency band, the obtained dbWPLI difference between FXS and control groups at each electrode pair was tested using a permutation approach [36]. At each electrode pair, dbWPLI from the 21 FXS and 21 control participants were shuffled and randomly separated into two groups in order to calculate the difference in group-mean dbWPLI for each permutation. This was repeated 5000 times, providing a distribution of dbWPLI values for each electrode pair for comparison with actual group differences, which were considered statistically significant if they exceeded the 95% confidence interval of the distribution of dbWPLI differences at the corresponding electrode pair (two-tailed test). A false discovery rate (FDR) approach was implemented in EEGLAB [31] to control the Type I error rate given the multiple comparisons.

We then evaluated the channel pair distribution for each frequency band showing group differences (Fig. 1) by calculating Euclidean distances between channel pairs based on the 3D position coordinates of electrodes for BioSemi headcaps (Biosemi Instrumentations, Amsterdam, Netherlands), with distances normalized (maximum distance was set to 1). This was done to determine if there was a pattern of altered connectivity between groups specific to short- or long-range connections.

Cross-frequency amplitude coupling

To investigate potential associations of alpha and theta activity with gamma activity, we evaluated cross-frequency amplitude coupling over time. Cross-frequency coupling refers to dependence between electrophysiological activities in different frequency bands [37]. Time series in each electrode were segmented into 2-s epochs. Relative lower and upper alpha, theta, and gamma power were calculated for each epoch. After that, two kinds of correlations were computed

between the epoch-by-epoch gamma power with alpha (lower and upper) and theta power [38]. First, correlations were computed in data from every electrode to investigate the local interaction among frequency bands, which we referred as "local coupling" (Additional file 2: Figure S1). Second, correlations were computed between mean power of electrode clusters at the anterior locus showing maximum relative theta power and at the posterior locus showing maximum relative alpha power based on topographies of EEG power (Fig. 2) with gamma power in all other electrodes, which we refer to as "global coupling". This was done to investigate the association of gamma power in an electrode with activity in alpha and theta bands in other electrodes, the latter both being believed to exert inhibitory modulation over distant brain regions [22]. To correct for multiple comparisons and evaluate differences between control and FXS groups, the correlation coefficients in each electrode and for each subject were transformed to Z scores via Fisher's Z-transform and then evaluated with a cluster-based permutation test in the Mass Univariate ERP Toolbox for statistical comparisons (5000 permutations [34]).

For correlations showing significant differences between controls and FXS patients (Fig. 3a, Additional file 2: Figure S1A), we also tested whether they were significantly

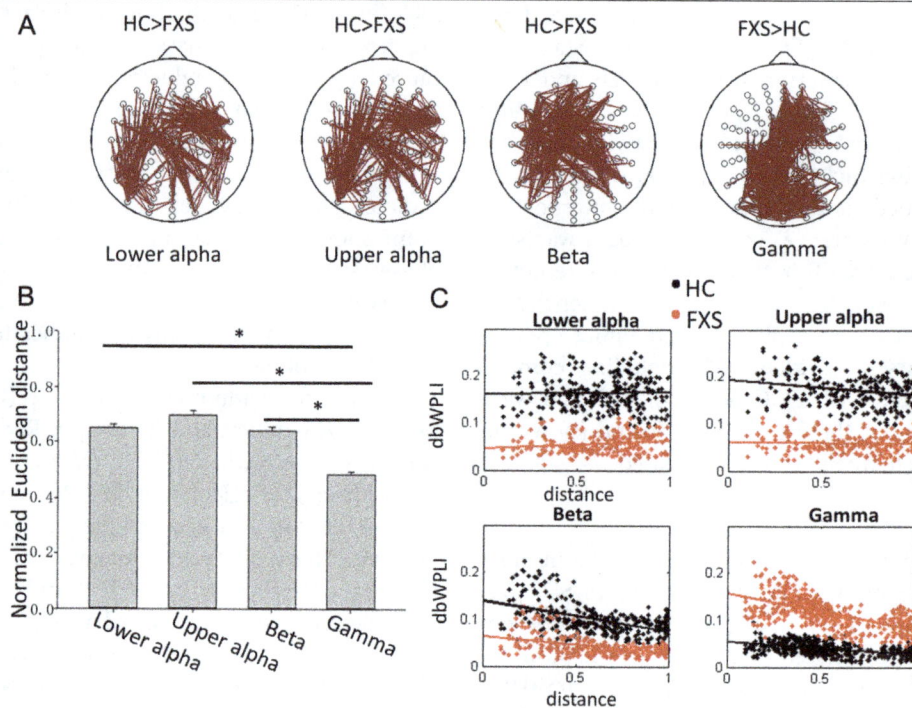

Fig. 1 a Significant group differences in connectivity strength between FXS and healthy control participants based on permutation tests (p < 0.05) show increased connectivity in FXS in the gamma band across electrodes but reduced within-band connectivity in the alpha (lower and upper) and beta range. b Mean and standard error of between-electrode distances for electrode pairs showing group differences (plotted in a) in lower alpha, upper alpha, beta and gamma bands. Asterisk denotes significant differences in connectivity distances with significant group differences between bands at p < 0.05. c Bivariate scatter plots depicting the relationship between average connectivity strength (dbWPLI) and average between-electrode distance for FXS (red dots) and healthy control participants (black dots)

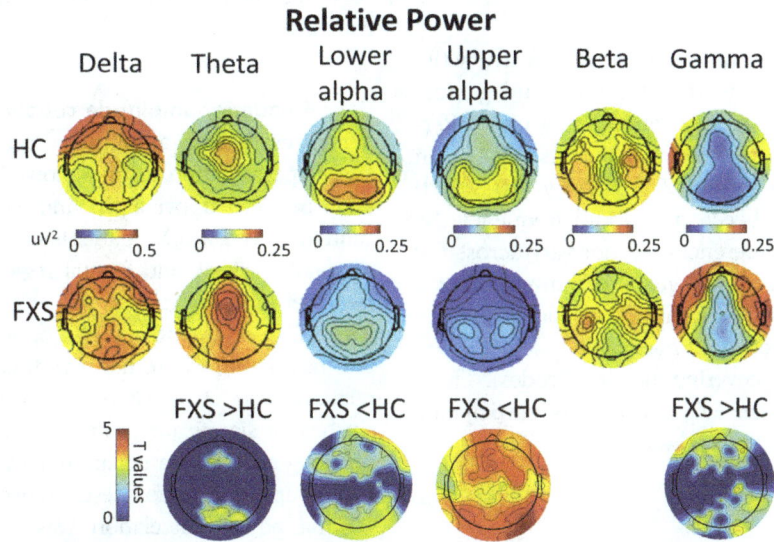

Fig. 2 Scalp topographies of relative power spectrum for FXS and healthy control participants per frequency band, with significant group differences presented in the bottom row ($p < 0.05$, corrected). Relative power represents the percentage of power in each frequency band divided by total power across 1–80 Hz

different from zero using a non-parametric permutation approach. To obtain a null distribution for these exploratory correlational analyses, epoch order of gamma power was shuffled while keeping the same epoch order for alpha and theta power. Correlations between alpha and gamma and between theta and gamma were computed for each permutation and repeated 2000 times providing a distribution of correlation values. The correlation for each subject was considered statistically significant if it was beyond the 95th percentile of this distribution.

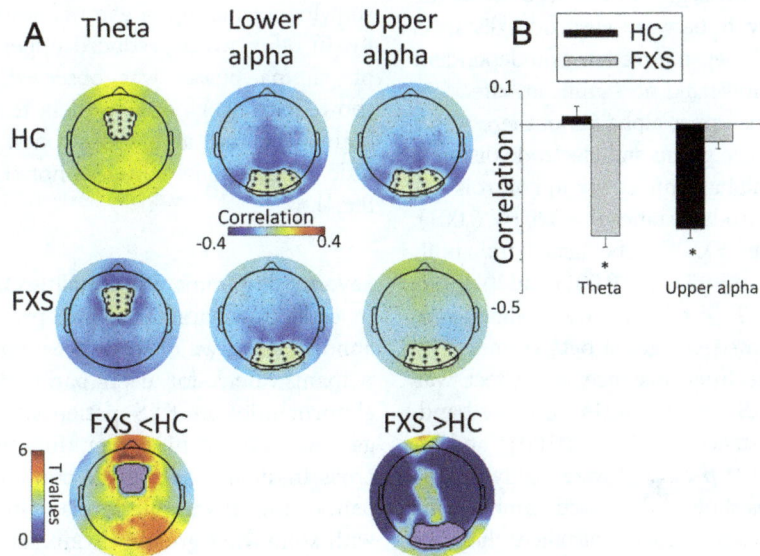

Fig. 3 a Scalp topographies of "global coupling" showing correlations between activity in the region showing the maximum relative power of activity in the theta, and lower and upper alpha power bands defined as the average of the power in that region of electrodes clusters (marked with *) and gamma power in all other electrodes for FXS and healthy control participants. Significant group differences are presented in the bottom row ($p < 0.05$, corrected), with dark blue reflecting no group difference. **b** Mean and standard error of correlations for all electrodes showing group differences as are plotted in A. *Asterisk* denotes correlations of spectral power in theta and upper alpha bands with gamma band power that are significantly different from zero based on the results of permutation analyses at $p < 0.05$

Results

EEG power

Cluster-permutation testing showed stronger relative activity in FXS compared to controls in the theta and gamma frequency bands, with clusters of significant group differences seen in the frontal and occipital regions (Fig. 2). In addition, two way anova (group X frequency [30-80Hz]) showed no interaction between group and frequency. So the magnitude of group differences did not vary across the gamma band (30-80Hz). FXS patients also showed reduced lower alpha band activity than controls in frontal and occipital regions, while reduced upper alpha activity was widely distributed (cluster covering most electrodes). There were no differences between FXS and control participants in delta or beta frequency band power.

Functional connectivity

The pattern of resting state functional connectivity results is illustrated in Fig. 1. The FXS group showed reduced connectivity in lower alpha, upper alpha, and beta frequency bands, but increased connectivity in the gamma frequency band (Fig. 1a). There were no group differences in within frequency band connectivity for delta or theta band activity.

Paired t tests (Fig. 1b) showed that distances between electrode pairs with significant group differences in phase synchronized connectivity were significantly shorter in the gamma band where connectivity was increased in FXS than in lower alpha, upper alpha, and beta bands where connectivity in FXS was reduced. In each frequency band, a linear regression was computed with degree of connectivity as the dependent variable and with between-electrode distance, group (FXS, Controls), and their interaction as independent variables (Fig. 1c). Results indicated no significant effects in the lower alpha band. In the upper alpha band, there was a significant interaction between group and electrode distance ($t = 3.0$, $p = 0.003$). Upper alpha connectivity in controls decreased with increased electrode distance ($t = 3.6$, $p < 0.001$); this effect was not seen in FXS. In the beta band, both between-electrode distance ($t = 12.0$, $p < 0.001$) and its interaction with group ($t = 3.8$, $p < 0.001$) were significant. Although both groups showed decreased beta connectivity with increased between-electrode distance, the effect was significantly reduced in FXS patients. In the gamma band, both between-electrode distance ($t = 7.9$, $p < 0.001$) and its interaction with group ($t = 9.9$, $p < 0.001$) were highly significant. Although both groups showed decreased gamma connectivity with greater between-electrode distance, the FXS group showed stronger effects. Because connectivity at a scale on the order of even short electrode distances is well beyond the scale maintained by individual PV positive inhibitory neurons, the observation of increased functional connectivity of gamma band activity in FXS across a variety of inter-electrode distances indicates a greater spread of coherent high frequency neural activity in FXS than in controls.

Cross-frequency amplitude coupling

When evaluating amplitude coupling across electrodes, cluster-permutation testing showed that the inverse correlation between upper alpha and gamma power was significantly reduced in FXS patients compared to controls in the occipital, parietal, and frontal regions (Fig. 3a). There were no lower alpha to gamma power correlation differences between FXS and controls. The opposite pattern was seen in the theta band, where negative theta to gamma power correlations were stronger in FXS compared to controls, with clusters of significant group differences in cross-frequency coupling seen in the occipital, parietal, and frontal regions. Follow-up permutation tests showed that negative theta to gamma power correlation was significantly greater than zero only in FXS participants, while the negative upper alpha to gamma power correlation was significant only in controls (Fig. 3b). For amplitude coupling within individual electrodes, performed to examine local circuitry effects, cluster-permutation testing showed a similar pattern with stronger negative theta to gamma power correlation, but reduced upper alpha to gamma power correlation in FXS compared to controls (Additional file 2: Figure S1 and Additional file 3: Figure S2).

These results suggest that while upper alpha power negatively coupled with gamma power both within and across electrodes in controls, FXS patients displayed excessive gamma activity and reduced upper alpha power without showing a coupling of gamma and upper alpha band activity. In other words, reduced upper alpha-related inhibition of gamma power was observed in FXS. Instead, FXS showed stronger negative theta to gamma power coupling both within and across electrodes. Follow-up phase amplitude coupling analyses were not significant (see Additional file 4).

Severity of gamma abnormalities in FXS patients

In order to characterize the prevalence of the different abnormalities we observed, we computed individual participant values for each parameter showing significant abnormalities in FXS patients, including alterations in gamma activity in power, functional connectivity, and cross-frequency amplitude coupling (Fig. 4). FXS participants showed variable levels of increased gamma power, with somewhat greater group separation in gamma connectivity indices. Amplitude coupling measurements more robustly and consistently separated FXS and healthy study participants. For example, while only approximately 50% of FXS patients had gamma power levels increased more than 1 SD beyond healthy controls, almost every FXS participant had altered long distance

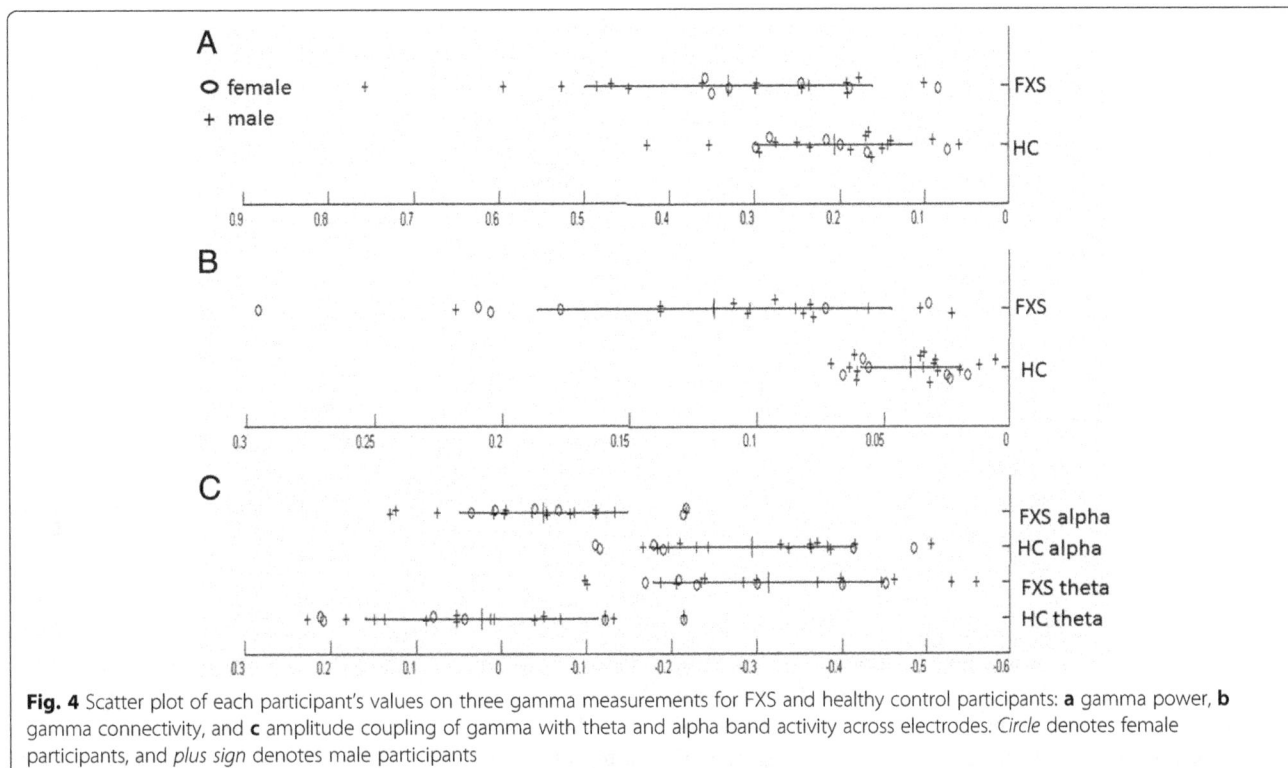

Fig. 4 Scatter plot of each participant's values on three gamma measurements for FXS and healthy control participants: **a** gamma power, **b** gamma connectivity, and **c** amplitude coupling of gamma with theta and alpha band activity across electrodes. *Circle* denotes female participants, and *plus sign* denotes male participants

coupling (outside the range of normal values) of local gamma with local and global upper alpha and theta activity. The heterogeneity in gamma power is noteworthy since all FXS participants had documented full mutations. The findings of altered long distance functional connectivity suggest that different patterns of cortico-cortical connectivity may be an important factor contributing to neural hyperexcitability reflected in increased gamma power in FXS.

Correlations with demographic and clinical variables

Exploratory correlational analyses were performed between EEG measurements showing significant alteration in FXS and SCQ and Adolescent/Adult Sensory Profile scores in FXS participants. Increased resting gamma power was significantly correlated with social-communication abnormalities as assessed with the SCQ ($r = 0.56$, $p = 0.03$). Lower alpha power was significantly correlated with greater social impairment in SCQ scores ($r = -0.58$, $p = 0.02$) and with hypersensitivity to sensory stimuli on the Sensory Profile scale ($r = -0.51$, $p = 0.03$). For functional connectivity and cross-frequency coupling measurements, no correlations with clinical variables were significant. Within each group, no significant correlations for EEG parameters were observed with age or gender. The consistent and marked reductions in IQ, especially in male FXS patients (all with IQ between 40

and 50), made correlations with electrophysiological parameters difficult to meaningfully evaluate.

Sex differences in FXS

The FXS full mutation in males is typically associated with a more severe profile of intellectual and behavioral deficits due to females having a compensatory functional FMR1 gene on their typically unaffected X chromosome. Therefore, it is important to consider gender effects in our analyses. We repeated all of the above analyses in two ways. First, we analyzed the male only group and all reported effects remained significant (see Additional file 5: Figure S3, Additional file 6: Figure S4, Additional file 7: Figure S5, and Additional file 8: Figure S6). Second, we compared male and female participants and did not find significant sex differences (see Additional file 9: Figure S7, though power to detect such effects was not high).

Discussion

This case-control study investigated multiple aspects of brain system function in the largest sample of non-epileptic, full mutation FXS patients studied to date with quantitative dense-array resting-state EEG. Abnormalities were evident across measures of spectral power, functional connectivity, and cross-frequency amplitude coupling and were consistent with predictions based on the *fmr1* KO mouse electrophysiology [7, 20, 24]. First, alterations in gamma band activity involved increased relative gamma power and an increased coherence of gamma band activity across nearby electrodes. This pattern is consistent with an imbalance of excitatory over inhibitory activity in FXS. The associations of electrophysiological alterations with abnormalities in social function and sensory sensitivities provide the first evidence of the clinical relevance of quantitative EEG findings in this population. Secondly, relative to controls, individuals with FXS showed reduced gamma amplitude coupling with upper alpha band activity but increased coupling with theta activity. As alpha and theta band activity are believed to exert top down inhibitory and regulatory modulation of sensory systems, these observations provide novel evidence that hyperexcitability in sensory cortex involves not only altered local circuit dysfunction in the interaction of interneurons and pyramidal cells as demonstrated in the fmr1 KO mouse [7], but also alterations in the long distance functional connectivity from association cortex and thalamus to sensory cortex known to regulate local circuit excitability. While there was better group separation on the amplitude coupling indices, clinical correlations were significant only with the power of resting gamma alterations. This pattern of findings suggests that variable disease-related disturbances and compensatory adaptations may leave FXS patients with a net level of residual neural hyperexcitability reflected in elevated gamma power that determines important aspects of their level of neurological and functional disability. These findings provide new mechanistic understanding of cortical hyperexcitability in FXS, involving increased high-frequency local circuit activity that varied in relation to what appear to be abnormal and compensatory long-distance functional connectivity. They also suggest a potential utility of resting state EEG alterations as translational biomarkers for clinically relevant aspects of FXS biology for identifying individual FXS patients likely to benefit from treatments aimed at reducing neocortical hyperexcitability and for tracking those effects.

The U-shaped pattern of relative EEG power in individuals with FXS (Fig. 2) is similar in form to one we described previously in autism [39]. Compared to healthy age-matched control participants, FXS patients showed enhanced power in lower (theta) and higher (gamma) bands, but reduced power in intermediate low and high alpha bands. Elevated theta and reduced alpha power have been reported previously in FXS [15], but the enhanced power in the gamma band and its clinical relevance have not been previously described. This enhanced gamma power is consistent with studies of fmr1 knockout mice demonstrating heightened neuronal excitability related to alterations in input to fast-spiking inhibitory interneurons that synchronize and control high-frequency gamma band neural activity [4, 40]. A recent study in wild-type rats showed that enhanced

gamma oscillation was observed when NMDA-receptor blockade was established [41]. NMDA-receptor hypofunction has been reported in several studies with fmr1 knockout mice [42–44] and thus may be one contributing factor for the gamma band alterations observed in the present study.

Our functional connectivity analyses revealed reduced long-range functional connectivity in the alpha and beta bands, but enhanced shorter-range connectivity in the gamma band in FXS. The decreased functional connectivity in the alpha and beta bands parallels previous findings in FXS [16]. We did not however observe the increased connectivity within the theta band that has been reported, though we did observe increased theta gamma coupling. For the first time, we report increased connectivity in gamma band activity in FXS patients. A previous fmr1 KO mouse study examined cross-frequency theta-gamma coupling, but during a cognitive task and when computed in the same hippocampal electrode [24]. While related to focus of the present study, the differences in species, in rest vs task performance situations, and within rather than across distant brain sites are differences that future work will need to resolve to integrate the observations. Further translational work bridging preclinical and clinical findings is needed to more directly link clinical neurophysiological findings to observations seen in fmr1 KO mice.

Our observation of increased spatial extent of coherent gamma band activity across more distant electrode pairs suggests an increased cortical spread of neural excitability paralleling effects observed in slice preparation data but on a far greater spatial scale [7]. It aligns with observations of increased neural synchrony observed in fmr1 knockout mice during sleep and quiet wakefulness [6]. The pattern of reduced long range connectivity in the alpha and beta bands suggests that reduced top-down inhibitory regulation of neocortical sensory systems may contribute to increased neural excitability of sensory cortex in FXS.

Given the alterations we observed in EEG power and functional connectivity in FXS, we investigated the coupling between low frequency band activity that was abnormal (alpha and theta activity) and high-frequency gamma band activity both within and across electrodes. We did this to determine whether the pattern of findings seen in gamma power and connectivity was related to a disruption in top-down modulation. Based on EEG data, it is not possible to determine whether a local circuit dysfunction is causing or resulting from the altered pattern of reduced long-distance functional connectivity in FXS. However, previous studies have shown that low frequency oscillations (e.g., alpha, theta) provide top-down inhibitory and modulatory influences in large, distributed neural networks, whereas fast oscillations (e.g., gamma) at rest are more related to neurophysiological tone in local networks [45]. Thus, the reduced alpha power, connectivity, and amplitude coupling in FXS may represent a failure of top-down modulation provided by alpha band input that could reduce gamma power in sensory systems. Previous studies have characterized the functional role of alpha band activity as actively inhibiting the processing of sensory information at rest and when environmental cues are not task relevant [22]. Posterior alpha has been reported to provide top-down control especially in visual attention studies, and thalamus has been identified as an important source of cortical alpha oscillations [46]. Both simulation and experimental studies have demonstrated that lower frequency oscillation rhythms (e.g., alpha, theta) can sustain long-range synchronization [45, 47], while synchronous activity in higher oscillation rhythms (e.g., gamma) declines more rapidly with increasing distances [48]. As a result, slower oscillations are better suited for top-down modulation by synchronizing and organizing activity across different brain regions [45]. This is consistent with findings from a nonhuman primate study of V1 and V4 showing that gamma rhythms propagate in a feedforward fashion from early to higher level visual processing regions, whereas alpha rhythms propagate in a feedback fashion to primary visual cortex [49].

In contrast to the reduced upper alpha-to-gamma coupling, FXS showed strong theta-to-gamma coupling with atypical theta connectivity being related to lower levels of gamma power (Fig. 3). Thus, while alpha power and coupling were reduced, theta power and coupling were increased in FXS, indicating a fundamental alteration in the pattern of cortico-cortical connectivity that supports top-down modulation in sensory systems. Further clinical and preclinical studies are needed to fully clarify the meaning of this novel observation, but one possibility is that in the context of reduced inhibitory modulation of alpha oscillations on gamma band activity, a second long-distance regulatory circuitry operating in the theta band may be relied upon to downregulate high-frequency neural activity in the gamma band, a compensation which is only partially and variably successful given the observation of clinically relevant increased gamma power in FXS. As theta power phasically synchronizes neural activity across brain regions to support different types of higher level cognition [50], a tonic activation to suppress sensory hyperexcitability reflected in increased theta power at rest might limit that phasic modulation and thereby contribute to the severe intellectual limitations often seen in FXS. Reduced alpha power might also contribute to the severe intellectual limitation since alpha activity has been reported to positively correlate with cognitive parameters [51].

The functional role of theta oscillation is related to its neural sources in the prefrontal and anterior cingulate cortex (ACC) [52], which play important roles in inhibitory control of behavior, behavioral flexibility, and error monitoring [53, 54]. During tasks requiring top-down inhibition of attention or behavior, microelectrode recordings in superficial cingulate layers exhibit strong task-related theta activity [55]. In addition, intermittent theta-burst stimulation has been shown to increase cortical inhibition in rat neocortex by reducing parvalbumin expression in fast-spiking interneurons [56], and stimulation in theta frequency bands increases expression of GABA precursors in inhibitory cortical systems [57]. Our gamma amplitude coupling associations may represent neural system factors that in vivo impact local circuit neurophysiology known to be altered in FXS, such as alterations in metabotropic glutamate receptor (mGluR) activation believed to be a cause of neuronal hyperexcitability in FXS. Inhibitory interneurons in mouse neocortex have been reported to fire in the theta frequency during mGluR activation [44, 58]. In addition, FMRP is highly expressed in the hippocampus [59], and long-term potentiation (LTP) elicited by theta burst stimulation has been reported to be impaired in the CA1 hippocampal subfield in *fmr1* KO mice [60].

Interest in systems biology alterations to complement understanding of local circuit pathology may be important not only for comprehensive models of pathology in FXS, but because individual variability in system-level modulatory factors may contribute to the wide range of clinical phenotypes seen even in patients with full mutation. This variability might explain the inconsistent treatment response to drugs targeting mGluR and other mechanisms aiming to reduce neuronal hyperexcitability, which have had more consistently positive effects in animal models. In this context, our findings not only provide new mechanistic understanding of FXS but also suggest that EEG studies of FXS may provide biomarkers for delineating disease heterogeneity and predicting and tracking response in human and mouse models to drugs targeting neuronal hyperactivity. Such approaches are urgently needed to advance drug development and personalized medicine for FXS patients. Our observation that quantitative EEG alterations were related to the severity of social communication and sensory reactivity problems supports the potential clinical utility of this approach.

This study has certain limitations, including the wide age range (12–57 years old) and the fact that younger children were not assessed. Although FXS and control groups were age-matched and no significant age effects were observed in the data, studies with younger populations remain an important target for future research. Other effects such as sex differences and medication effects were not statistically significant, but further research is needed to address those issues. Third, our study did not compare resting state abnormalities in FXS directly with other developmental disabilities to establish specificity of deficits to FXS relative to general effects of intellectual or developmental disability. While the parallel findings from our study and preclinical work in *fmr1* KO mice suggest a relevance to FXS, more research is needed to determine whether similar findings might be seen in the subset of ASD patients who demonstrate sensory hypersensitivities or other signs of cortical excitability, as well as in multiple other neurodevelopmental disorders.

Conclusions

In summary, we found an abnormal U-shaped alteration of spectral power with reduced long-range inhibitory and enhanced excitatory shorter-range connectivity in FXS. Furthermore, we found stronger theta-to-gamma amplitude coupling in FXS, possibly serving as a compensatory response to reduced top-down alpha-band inhibitory modulation and intrinsic pathology of local neural circuit excitability in sensory systems. Taken in combination, our findings provide direct in vivo evidence in FXS patients of heightened cortical arousal, reduced top-down regulatory input in the alpha band, and increased modulation in the theta band that together may determine the level of circuit hyper-excitability in sensory cortex in vivo.

Additional files

Additional file 1: Table S1. EEG measurements in the combined FXS group and in both the medicated FXS and non-medicated FXS group. (DOCX 14 kb)

Additional file 2: Figure S1. (A) Scalp topographies of "local coupling", showing correlations in each electrode between relative power of activity in the theta, and lower and upper alpha power bands and gamma power for FXS and healthy control participants, with significant group differences presented in the bottom row ($p < 0.05$, corrected), with dark blue reflecting no group difference. (B) Mean and standard error of correlations for all electrodes showing group differences as are plotted in A. * denotes correlations of spectral power in theta and upper alpha bands with gamma band power that are significantly different from zero based on the results of permutation analyses at $p < 0.05$. (TIF 3754 kb)

Additional file 3: Figure S2. Scatter plot of each participant's values of coupling with gamma in theta and alpha band within electrodes for FXS and healthy control participants. Circle denotes female participants, plus (+) denotes male participants. (TIF 321 kb)

Additional file 4: Cross-frequency amplitude coupling within individual electrodes. (DOCX 19 kb)

Additional file 5: Figure S3. Scalp topographies of relative power spectrum are presented for *male* FXS and *male* healthy control participants per frequency band, with significant group differences presented in the bottom row ($p < 0.05$, corrected). Relative power represents the percentage of power in each frequency band divided by total power across 1–80 Hz. (TIF 5063 kb)

Additional file 6: Figure S4. (A) Significant group differences in connectivity strength between *male* FXS and *male* healthy control participants based on permutation tests ($p < 0.05$) show increased connectivity in FXS in the gamma band but reduced connectivity in the alpha (lower and upper) and beta range. (B) Mean and standard error of between-electrode distances for electrode pairs showing group differences (plotted in A) in lower alpha, upper alpha, beta, and gamma bands. * denotes significant differences in connectivity distances with significant group differences between bands at $p < 0.05$. (C) Bivariate scatter plots depict the relationship between averaged connectivity strength (dbWPLI) and averaged between-electrode distance for FXS (red dots) and Healthy Control participants (black dots). (TIF 3314 kb)

Additional file 7: Figure S5. (A) Scalp topographies of "global coupling", showing correlations between activity in the region showing the maximum relative power of activity in the theta, and lower and upper alpha power bands defined as the average of the power in that region of electrodes clusters (marked with *) and gamma power in all other electrodes for *male* FXS and *male* healthy control participants. Significant group differences are presented in the bottom row ($p < 0.05$, corrected), with dark blue reflecting no group difference. (B) Mean and standard error of correlations for all electrodes showing group differences as are plotted in A. * denotes correlations of spectral power in theta and upper alpha bands with gamma band power that are significantly different from zero based on the results of permutation analyses at $p < 0.05$. (TIF 3306 kb)

Additional file 8: Figure S6 (A) Scalp topographies of "local coupling", showing correlations in each electrode between relative power of activity in the theta, and lower and upper alpha power bands and gamma power for *male* FXS and *male* healthy control participants, with significant group differences presented in the bottom row ($p < 0.05$, corrected), with dark blue reflecting no group difference. (B) Mean and standard error of correlations for all electrodes showing group differences as are plotted in A. * denotes correlations of spectral power in theta and upper alpha bands with gamma band power that are significantly different from zero based on the results of permutation analyses at $p < 0.05$. (TIF 4297 kb)

Additional file 9: Figure S7. Scatter plots of each participant's values of power and connectivity in delta, theta, lower alpha, upper alpha, beta bands for FXS and healthy control participants. Circle denotes female participants, plus denotes male participants. (TIF 475 kb)

Acknowledgements

The authors would like to thank Rachel Greene, Savanna Sablich, and Melanie Soilleux for aid in data collection.

Funding

This work was supported by the National Institute of Health (grant number: U54 HD082008-01).

Authors' contributions

JW and JAS were involved in designing, collecting, analyzing, and interpreting the data and drafting the manuscript. LEE, MWM, DKB, EVP, CAE, and MJB were involved in data collection and in revising the manuscript. SPW conducted patient diagnostic assessments, provided consultation for interpretation of clinical data, and was involved in revising the manuscripts. All authors read and approved the final manuscript.

Competing interests

Dr. Mosconi consults to and has research funding from Novartis. Dr. Pedapati has research grant support from StatKing. Dr. Erickson has research grant support from Confluence Pharmaceuticals, The Roche Group, SynapDx, Stemina Bioscience, and Riovant Pharmaceuticals; he is a consultant to Confluence Pharmaceuticals, Neurotrope, and Fulcrum Pharmaceuticals, and he holds equity interest in Confluence Pharmaceuticals. Dr. Byerly is a consultant and has a research grant from Otsuka. Dr. Sweeney consulted to Takeda Pharmaceuticals.

Author details
[1]Department of Psychology, Zhejiang Normal University, 688 Yingbin Road, Jinhua, Zhejiang, China 321004. [2]Department of Pediatrics, Section of Developmental and Behavioral Pediatrics, University of Oklahoma Health Sciences Center, Oklahoma City, OK, USA. [3]Department of Psychology, University of Oklahoma, Norman, OK, USA. [4]Clinical Child Psychology Program and Schiefelbusch Institute for Life Span Studies, University of Kansas, Lawrence, KS, USA. [5]Department of Psychiatry, Center for Autism and Developmental Disabilities, University of Texas Southwestern Medical Center, Dallas, TX, USA. [6]Center for Glial-Neuronal Interactions, Neuroscience Graduate Program, Division of Biomedical Sciences, School of Medicine, University of California, Riverside, CA, USA. [7]Department of Psychiatry and Behavioral Neuroscience and Division of Psychiatry, Cincinnati Children's Hospital Medical Center, Cincinnati, OH, USA. [8]Center for Mental Health Research and Recovery, Montana State University, Bozeman, MT, USA. [9]Department of Psychiatry and Behavioral Neuroscience, University of Cincinnati, Cincinnati, OH, USA.

References
1. Ashley CJ, Wilkinson K, Reines D, Warren S. FMR1 protein: conserved RNP family domains and selective RNA binding. Science. 1993;262:563–6.
2. Bear MF. Therapeutic implications of the mGluR theory of fragile X mental retardation. Genes Brain Behav. 2005;4(6):393–8.
3. Heulens I, D'Hulst C, Braat S, Rooms L, Kooy RF. Involvement and therapeutic potential of the GABAergic system in the fragile x syndrome. Sci World J. 2010;10:2198–206.
4. Cea-Del Rio CA, Huntsman MM. The contribution of inhibitory interneurons to circuit dysfunction in Fragile X Syndrome. Front Cell Neurosci. 2014;8:1–7.
5. Contractor A, Klyachko VA, Portera-Cailliau C. Altered neuronal and circuit excitability in fragile X syndrome. Neuron. 2015;87(4):699–715.
6. Gonçalves JT, Anstey JE, Golshani P, Portera-Cailliau C. Circuit level defects in the developing neocortex of Fragile X mice. Nat Neurosci. 2013;16:903–9.
7. Gibson JR, Bartley AF, Hays SA, Huber KM. Imbalance of neocortical excitation and inhibition and altered UP states reflect network hyperexcitability in the mouse model of fragile X syndrome. J Neurophysiol. 2008;100:2615–26.
8. Strumbos JG, Brown MR, Kronengold J, Polley DB, Kaczmarek LK. Fragile x mental retardation protein is required for rapid experience-dependent regulation of the potassium channel Kv3.1b. J Neurosci. 2010;30(31):10263–71.
9. Kim H, Gibboni R, Kirkhart C, Bao S. Impaired critical period plasticity in primary auditory cortex of fragile x model mice. J Neurosci. 2013;33(40):15686–92.
10. Rotschafer S, Razak K. Altered auditory processing in a mouse model of fragile X syndrome. Brain Res. 2013;1506:12–24.
11. Rojas DC, Benkers TL, Rogers SJ, Teale PD, Reite ML, Hagerman RJ. Auditory evoked magnetic fields in adults with fragile X syndrome. Neuroreport. 2001;12:2573–6.
12. Castrén M, Paakkonen A, Tarkka IM, Ryynanen M, Partanen J. Augmentation of auditory N1 in children with fragile X syndrome. Brain Topogr. 2003;15:165–71.
13. Van der Molen MJW, Van der Molen MW, Ridderinkhof KR, Hamel BCJ, Curfs LMG, Ramakers GJA. Auditory change detection in fragile X syndrome males: a brain potential study. Clin Neurophysiol. 2012;123:1309–18.
14. Ethridge L, White S, Mosconi M, Wang J, Byerly M, Sweeney J. Reduced habituation of auditory evoked potentials indicate cortical hyper-excitability in Fragile X Syndrome. Transl Psychiatry. 2016;6(4):e787.
15. Van der Molen MJW, Van der Molen MW. Reduced alpha and exaggerated theta power during the resting-state EEG in fragile X syndrome. Biol Psychol. 2013;92:216–9.
16. Van der Molen MJW, Stam CJ, van der Molen MW. Resting-state EEG oscillatory dynamics in fragile X syndrome: abnormal functional connectivity and brain network organization. PloS ONE. 2014. doi:10.1371/journal.pone.0088451.
17. Traub RD, Cunningham MO, Glovell T, LeBeau FEN, Bibbig A, Buhl EH, et al. GABA-enhanced collective behavior in neuronal axons underlies persistent gamma-frequency oscillations. Proc Natl Acad Sci U S A. 2003;100:11047–52.
18. Kim T, Thankachan S, McKenna JT, McNally JM, Yang C, Choi JH, et al. Cortically projecting basal forebrain parvalbumin neurons regulate cortical gamma band oscillations. Proc Natl Acad Sci U S A. 2015;112:3535–40.
19. Sohal VS, Zhang F, Yizhar O, Deisseroth K. Parvalbumin neurons and gamma rhythms enhance cortical circuit performance. Nature. 2009;459:698–702.
20. Berzhanskaya J, Phillips MA, Gorin A, Lai C, Shen J, Colonnese MT. Disrupted cortical state regulation in a rat model of fragile X syndrome. Cerebral Cortex. 2016:1–15. doi:10.1093/cercor/bhv331.
21. Canolty RT, Knight RT. The functional role of cross-frequency coupling. Trends Cogn Sci. 2010;14:506–15.
22. Jensen O, Mazaheri A. Shaping functional architecture by oscillatory alpha activity: gating by inhibition. Front Hum Neurosci. 2010;4:1–8.
23. Min B, Park H. Task-related modulation of anterior theta and posterior alpha EEG reflects top-down preparation. BMC Neurosci. 2010;11(79):1-8.
24. Radwan B, Dvorak D, Fenton AA. Impaired cognitive discrimination and discoordination of coupled theta-gamma oscillations in Fmr1 knockout mice. Neurobiol Dis. 2016;88:125–38.
25. Brown C, Dunn W. Adolescent-Adult Sensory Profile: user's manual. San Antonio: Therapy Skill Builders; 2002.
26. Rutter M, Bailey A, Lord C. SCQ: the Social Communication Questionnaire. Torrance: WPS; 2003.
27. Roid GH. Stanford-Binet Intelligence Scales, 5th edition (SB:V). Itasca: Riverside Publishing; 2003.
28. Wechsler D. Wechsler Abbreviated Scale of Intelligence (WASI). San Antonio: TX Harcourt Assessment; 1999.
29. Orekhova E, Elsabbagh M, Jones E, Dawson G, Charman T, Johnson M, et al. EEG hyper-connectivity in high-risk infants is associated with later autism. J Neurodev Disord. 2014;6:1–11.
30. Jasper HH. The ten twenty electrode system of the international federation. Electroencephalogr Clin Neurophysiol. 1958;10:371–5.
31. Delorme A, Makeig S. EEGLAB: an open source toolbox for analysis of single-trial EEG dynamics including independent component analysis. J Neurosci Methods. 2004;134(1):9–21.
32. Nolan H, Whelan R, Reilly R. FASTER: Fully automated statistical thresholding for EEG artifact rejection. J Neurosci Methods. 2010;192:152–62.
33. Cantero J, Atienza M, Salas R. Human alpha oscillations in wakefulness, drowsiness period, and REM sleep: different electroencephalographic phenomena within the alpha band. Clin Neurophysiol. 2002;32(1):54–71.
34. Groppe D, Urbach T, Kutas M. Mass univariate analysis of event-related brain potentials/fields I: a critical tutorial review. Psychophysiology. 2011;48(12):1711–25.
35. Vinck M, Oostenveld R, van Wingerden M, Battaglia F, Pennartz C. An improved index of phase-synchronization for electrophysiological data in the presence of volume-conduction, noise and sample-size bias. Neuroimage. 2011;55(4):1548–65.
36. Murias M, Webb S, Greenson J, Dawson G. Resting state cortical connectivity reflected in EEG coherence in individuals with autism. Biol Psychiatry. 2007;62(3):270–3.
37. Jensen O, Colgin L. Cross-frequency coupling between neuronal oscillations. Trends Cogn Sci. 2007;11(7):267–9.
38. Mazaheri A, Nieuwenhuis I, van Dijk H, Jensen O. Prestimulus alpha and mu activity predicts failure to inhibit motor responses. Hum Brain Mapp. 2009;30:1791–800.
39. Wang J, Barstein J, Ethridge LE, Mosconi M, Takarae Y, Sweeney J. Resting state EEG abnormalities in autism spectrum disorders. J Neurodev Disord. 2013;5:1–14.
40. Salkoff DB, Zagha E, Yüzgeç Ö, McCormick DA. Synaptic mechanisms of tight spike synchrony at gamma frequency in cerebral cortex. J Neurosci. 2015;35(28):10236–51.
41. Hiyoshi T, Kambe D, Karasawa J, Chaki S. Differential effects of NMDA receptor antagonists at lower and higher doses on basal gamma band oscillation power in rat cortical electroencephalograms. Neuropharmacology. 2014;85:384–96.
42. Yun S, Trommer B. Fragile X mice: reduced long-term potentiation and N-Methyl-D-Aspartate Receptor-Mediated neurotransmission in dentate gyrus. J Neurosci Res. 2011;89:176–82.
43. Eadie B, Cushman J, Kannangara T, Fanselow M, Christie B. NMDA receptor hypofunction in the dentate gyrus and impaired context discrimination in adult fmr1 knockout mice. Hippocampus. 2012;22:241–54.
44. Bostrom C, Majaess N, Morch K, White E, Christie B. Rescue of NMDAR-Dependent synaptic plasticity in Fmr1 knock-out mice. Cereb Cortex. 2015;25:271–9.
45. Von Stein A, Sarnthein J. Different frequencies for different scales of cortical integration: from local gamma to long range alpha/theta synchronization. Int J Psychophysiol. 2000;38(3):301–13.
46. Hughes SW, Crunelli V. Thalamic mechanisms of EEG alpha rhythms and their pathological implications. Neuroscientist. 2005;11(4):357–72.
47. Kopell N, Ermentrout G, Whittington M, Traub R. Gamma rhythms and beta rhythms have different synchronization properties. Proc Natl Acad Sci U S A. 2000;97(4):1867–72.
48. Bullock T. Temporal fluctuations in coherence of brain waves. Proc Natl Acad Sci U S A. 1995;92:11568–72.

49. Kerkoerle T, Self M, Dagnino B, Gariel-Mathis M, Poort J, van der Togt C, et al. Alpha and gamma oscillations characterize feedback and feedforward processing in monkey visual cortex. Proc Natl Acad Sci U S A. 2014;111:14332–41.

50. Başar E, Başar-Eroglu C, Karakaş S, Schürmann M. Gamma, alpha, delta, and theta oscillations govern cognitive processes. Int J Psychophysiol. 2001;39(2):241–8.

51. Jaušovec N, Jaušovec K. Correlations between ERP parameters and intelligence: a reconsideration. Biol Psychol. 2000;55(2):137–54.

52. Asada H, Fukuda Y, Tsunoda S, Yamaguchi M, Tonoike M. Frontal midline theta rhythms reflect alternative activation of prefrontal cortex and anterior cingulate cortex in humans. Neurosci Lett. 1999;274(1):29–32.

53. Hanslmayr S, Pastötter B, Bäuml K, Gruber S, Wimber M, Klimesch W. The electrophysiological dynamics of interference during the Stroop task. J Cogn Neurosci. 2008;20(2):215–25.

54. D'Cruz A-M, Ragozzino ME, Mosconi MW, Pavuluri MN, Sweeney JA. Human reversal learning under conditions of certain versus uncertain outcomes. Neuroimage. 2011;56(1):315–22.

55. Wang C, Ulbert I, Schomer D, Marinkovic K, Halgren E. Responses of human anterior cingulate cortex microdomains to error detection, conflict monitoring, stimulus-response mapping, familiarity, and orienting. J Neurosci. 2005;25(3):604–13.

56. Benali A, Trippe J, Weiler E, Mix A, Petrasch-Parwez E, Girzalsky W, et al. Theta-burst transcranial magnetic stimulation alters cortical inhibition. J Neurosci. 2011;31:1193–203.

57. Trippe J, Mix A, Aydin-Abidin S, Funke K, Benali A. Theta burst and conventional low-frequency rTMS differentially affect GABAergic neurotransmission in the rat cortex. Exp Brain Res. 2009;199:411–21.

58. Fanselow E, Richardson K, Connors B. Selective, state-dependent activation of somatostatin-expressing inhibitory interneurons in mouse neocortex. J Neurophysiol. 2008;100:2640–52.

59. Feng Y, Gutekunst C, Eberhart D, Yi H, Warren S, Hersch S. Fragile X mental retardation protein: nucleocytoplasmic shuttling and association with somatodendritic ribosomes. J Neurosci. 1997;17:1539–47.

60. Lauterborn J, Christopher S, Kramár E, Chen L, Pandyarajan V, Lynch G, et al. Brain-derived neurotrophic factor rescues synaptic plasticity in a mouse model of fragile X syndrome. J Neurosci. 2007;27(40):10685–94.

12

Load matters: neural correlates of verbal working memory in children with autism spectrum disorder

Vanessa M. Vogan[1,2†], Kaitlyn E. Francis[1†], Benjamin R. Morgan[1], Mary Lou Smith[3] and Margot J. Taylor[1,3*] (iD)

Abstract

Background: Autism spectrum disorder (ASD) is a pervasive neurodevelopmental disorder characterised by diminished social reciprocity and communication skills and the presence of stereotyped and restricted behaviours. Executive functioning deficits, such as working memory, are associated with core ASD symptoms. Working memory allows for temporary storage and manipulation of information and relies heavily on frontal-parietal networks of the brain. There are few reports on the neural correlates of working memory in youth with ASD. The current study identified the neural systems underlying verbal working memory capacity in youth with and without ASD using functional magnetic resonance imaging (fMRI).

Methods: Fifty-seven youth, 27 with ASD and 30 sex- and age-matched typically developing (TD) controls (9–16 years), completed a one-back letter matching task (LMT) with four levels of difficulty (i.e. cognitive load) while fMRI data were recorded. Linear trend analyses were conducted to examine brain regions that were recruited as a function of increasing cognitive load.

Results: We found similar behavioural performance on the LMT in terms of reaction times, but in the two higher load conditions, the ASD youth had lower accuracy than the TD group. Neural patterns of activations differed significantly between TD and ASD groups. In TD youth, areas classically used for working memory, including the lateral and medial frontal, as well as superior parietal brain regions, increased in activation with increasing task difficulty, while areas related to the default mode network (DMN) showed decreasing activation (i.e., deactivation). The youth with ASD did not appear to use this opposing cognitive processing system; they showed little recruitment of frontal and parietal regions across the load but did show similar modulation of the DMN.

Conclusions: In a working memory task, where the load was manipulated without changing executive demands, TD youth showed increasing recruitment with increasing load of the classic fronto-parietal brain areas and decreasing involvement in default mode regions. In contrast, although they modulated the default mode network, youth with ASD did not show the modulation of increasing brain activation with increasing load, suggesting that they may be unable to manage increasing verbal information. Impaired verbal working memory in ASD would interfere with the youths' success academically and socially. Thus, determining the nature of atypical neural processing could help establish or monitor working memory interventions for ASD.

Keywords: Autism spectrum disorder, Verbal working memory, Cognitive load, Executive functioning, fMRI

* Correspondence: margot.taylor@sickkids.ca
†V. M. Vogan and K. E. Francis contributed equally to this work.
[1]Diagnostic Imaging & Research Institute, Hospital for Sick Children, 555 University Avenue, Toronto, Ontario M5G 1X8, Canada
[3]Department of Psychology, University of Toronto, 100 St. George St., Toronto, Ontario M5S 3G3, Canada
Full list of author information is available at the end of the article

Background

Autism spectrum disorder (ASD) is a neurodevelopmental disorder characterised by diminished social reciprocity and communication skills, as well as the presence of stereotyped and restricted behaviours [1]. There is considerable evidence that individuals with ASD also have impaired executive and cognitive function [1–8]. The deficits in executive processing may contribute to the autistic symptomology, as proposed by the 'executive dysfunction theory' of ASD [5, 6]. Prior literature on the neural underpinnings of ASD, as well as the cognitive difficulties that follow, suggests that working memory (WM) impairments are associated with functional abnormalities in the frontal lobe, especially prefrontal cortical activity [3, 7, 9–12]. The protracted frontal lobe maturation means that the functions relying on the frontal lobes are particularly vulnerable to developmental disturbances [13, 14].

Working memory is the ability to temporarily store and manipulate information [15, 16]. WM is seen as an essential element of cognitive control [16–19], critical for learning and academic achievement [20], as well as social competency [21]. Previous literature suggests that individuals with ASD have greater difficulty with visuo-spatial than verbal WM, which is more often comparable to typically developing (TD) individuals [22–24]. Prior work also reports, however, that WM in ASD is intact for simple memory tasks [22–26] including simple verbal WM [27], but impaired on more complex tasks [22, 23, 25, 26, 28] including verbal WM [29], compared to typically developing (TD) individuals, or broadly compromised [30]. A number of studies found that when performing WM tasks of increasing complexity or cognitive load, children with ASD were impaired compared to TD children [8, 26, 29].

The neuroimaging literature has identified a system of lateral prefrontal, premotor and posterior parietal cortices underlying WM function [31, 32], with children showing more widespread activation patterns than adults [33]. During a verbal WM two-back task, Nagel et al. [34] found that children (ages 10–16 years) recruited the left frontal and temporal lobes. Similarly, Thomason et al. [35] used a verbal WM block design task and observed that children (ages 7–12 years) showed activation in the left frontal and parietal cortical regions, but activation in these regions was reduced compared to adults.

Few studies have used neuroimaging to investigate verbal WM in ASD, with most studies using visual-spatial tasks (e.g., [10, 12, 36, 37]); this, our understanding of the neural correlates underlying verbal WM deficits in ASD, particularly in children, remains modest. Koshino et al. [9] used a letter matching task and found that, despite comparable behavioural performance, adults with ASD showed right-lateralised activation in the dorsolateral prefrontal cortex (dlPFC) and parietal and inferior temporal areas, whereas TD adults showed bilateral dlPFC activation and less posterior activity. Following a multi-pronged analysis approach, the authors concluded that TD adults used verbal encoding strategies to complete the task, whereas adults with ASD used nonverbal and visually oriented strategies with their WM network shifted towards a right hemisphere dominance.

The 'n-back' protocol is commonly used to manipulate cognitive load while studying WM [9, 10, 27, 32, 38–45]. The typical n-back task involves viewing a series of stimuli, then indicating whether the current stimulus is the same as the one presented 'n' (1, 2, 3, etc.) trials before. The difficulty level is indexed by the total number of interfering items between repeating stimuli. By increasing load in this manner, different mental strategies required to complete the task are also employed, including executive functioning and procedural strategies. Manipulating both WM and other cognitive functions across load makes WM-specific changes difficult to quantify and link to specific brain regions. In the present study, we used a one-back letter matching task (LMT) [46–48] that avoids these confounds. LMT holds executive function constant across difficulty levels, while systematically manipulating memory load, which better isolates the effects of cognitive load on verbal WM. A developmental investigation of LMT in typically developing children and adults showed an opposing cognitive processing system, with increasing cognitive load and increasing recruitment of brain areas related to WM, while decreasing activation of areas in the default mode network (DMN); adults showed larger load-dependent changes than children in the bilateral superior parietal gyri, inferior/dorsolateral prefrontal and left middle frontal gyri [48].

Limited neuroimaging studies exist to examine the impact of WM load on brain activity in ASD. In a recent investigation by Rahko et al. [44], adolescents with ASD (ages 11–18 years) were observed to have reduced modulation of brain activity with increasing cognitive load in the insula, motor and auditory and somatosensory cortices compared to TD adolescents during a visuo-spatial n-back WM task. An earlier study by Vogan et al. [47] utilising a colour matching task (a visuo-spatial version of LMT) showed that children with ASD (ages 7–13 years) demonstrated reduced modulation in the dlPFC, medial premotor cortex and precuneus with increasing cognitive load.

The current study used functional magnetic resonance imaging (fMRI) with a verbal WM task to explore neural systems underlying WM, and the effects of cognitive load, in children and young adolescents with and without ASD. In this study, the cognitive load was manipulated by increasing task difficulty level (see the "Methods" section for full task description). We hypothesised that children with

ASD would perform with a lower accuracy than their matched TD controls on the LMT with increasing cognitive load. Moreover, we expected that children with ASD would under-recruit frontal and parietal cortical regions related to verbal WM, relative to TD children, and that the difference would increase with greater cognitive demand. We predicted that cortical activity would be linearly modulated (increasing in WM areas, decreasing in DMN areas) by task difficulty; however, we anticipated that the youth with ASD would have a less pronounced pattern of linear activation/deactivation.

Methods

Participants

Ninety one participants (47 ASD, 44 TD) were recruited through community support centres, parent support groups, email listservs, hospital ads and schools for this study. Six TD participants and 20 ASD participants were excluded from analyses due to inadequate task performance; see below (lines 197–202) for our threshold for task performance (ASD = 12, TD = 2), protocol completion (ASD = 5, TD = 2) and excessive movement (ASD = 3, TD = 0), and two TDs were excluded for age-matching. The age- and sex-matched sample was composed of 27 children with ASD (5 girls and 22 boys) and 30 TD children (8 girls and 22 boys) aged 9 to 16 years old. Although groups differed slightly on IQ as determined by the Wechsler Abbreviated Scale of Intelligence [49], $t_{(39)} = 2.16$, $p = 0.04$, both groups had IQs within the average range, see Table 1 for additional participant characteristics.

Participants were not included in the study with any significant psychiatric comorbidities [1], medical illnesses, neurological disorders, prematurity, colour blindness, uncorrected vision, IQ < 80 or any standard MRI contraindicators, such as ferromagnetic implants. TD participants were also not included if they had a history of learning disability, developmental delay, a sibling with ASD or attention deficit hyperactivity disorder (ADHD). These factors were not the current primary diagnosis for any of the ASD subjects.

Informed consent, MRI scanning, and the cognitive and clinical testing involved in this study were carried out at the Hospital for Sick Children in Toronto. All the experimental procedures used were approved by the hospital's Research Ethics Board. All participants gave informed verbal assent, and a parent or legal guardian of all participants gave informed written consent.

ASD clinical diagnosis was confirmed through expert clinical judgement and the Autism Diagnostic Observation Schedule (ADOS) [50] for all participants with ASD. The ADOS was conducted by a trained individual with established inter-rater research reliability.

Letter matching task

The LMT is a verbal WM task. LMT is presented visually to participants and has linguistic/phonological features. Participants attended to letters embedded in a global "A" figure. Participants were taught to focus only on the eight relevant letters (A, B, E, H, K, M, N, T) presented in uppercase and to ignore irrelevant letters "O" and "P" (Fig. 1). The task was designed with both relevant and irrelevant letters, as well as the irrelevant global letter, since tasks containing misleading or irrelevant features evoke interference and elicit cognitive control, which has been shown to provide more reliable measures of WM capacity [47, 51]. The number 'n' of relevant letters in the figure, referred to as capacity, increased by one item for each increasing difficulty level. Difficulty level was assigned $n + 2$ to account for these cognitive control and executive functions. LMT is a one-back task in which participants were instructed to identify relevant letter(s) and remember if the letter(s) in the current stimulus figure matched those from the previous figure, disregarding letter repetition and location. Repetition of both irrelevant and relevant letters within a stimulus was usual (see Fig. 1), and although the numbers and placement of the letters changed, the participants always ignored the same two letters, O and P. Stimuli were presented one at a time for 3 s, during which time children indicated their response using a dual-key MRI compatible keypad in their right hand; one button for the same relevant letters embedded in

Table 1 Demographic and neuropsychological test characteristics of the sample

Variables	ASD		TD		Significant test
	%	Mean (SD)	%	Mean (SD)	
Demographic data					
Sex (% male)	81		73		$\chi^2_{(1)} = 0.54$, $p = 0.46$
Age		12.56 (1.46)		12.96 (1.89)	$t_{(54)} = 0.91$, $p = 0.37$
Full-scale IQ		105.52 (14.41)		112.27 (7.91)	$t_{(39)} = 2.16$, $p = 0.04*$
ADOS total[a]		11.89 (4.30)		N/A	

*$p < 0.05$
[a]ADOS scores range from 3 to 20 with greater symptom severity reflected by higher scores

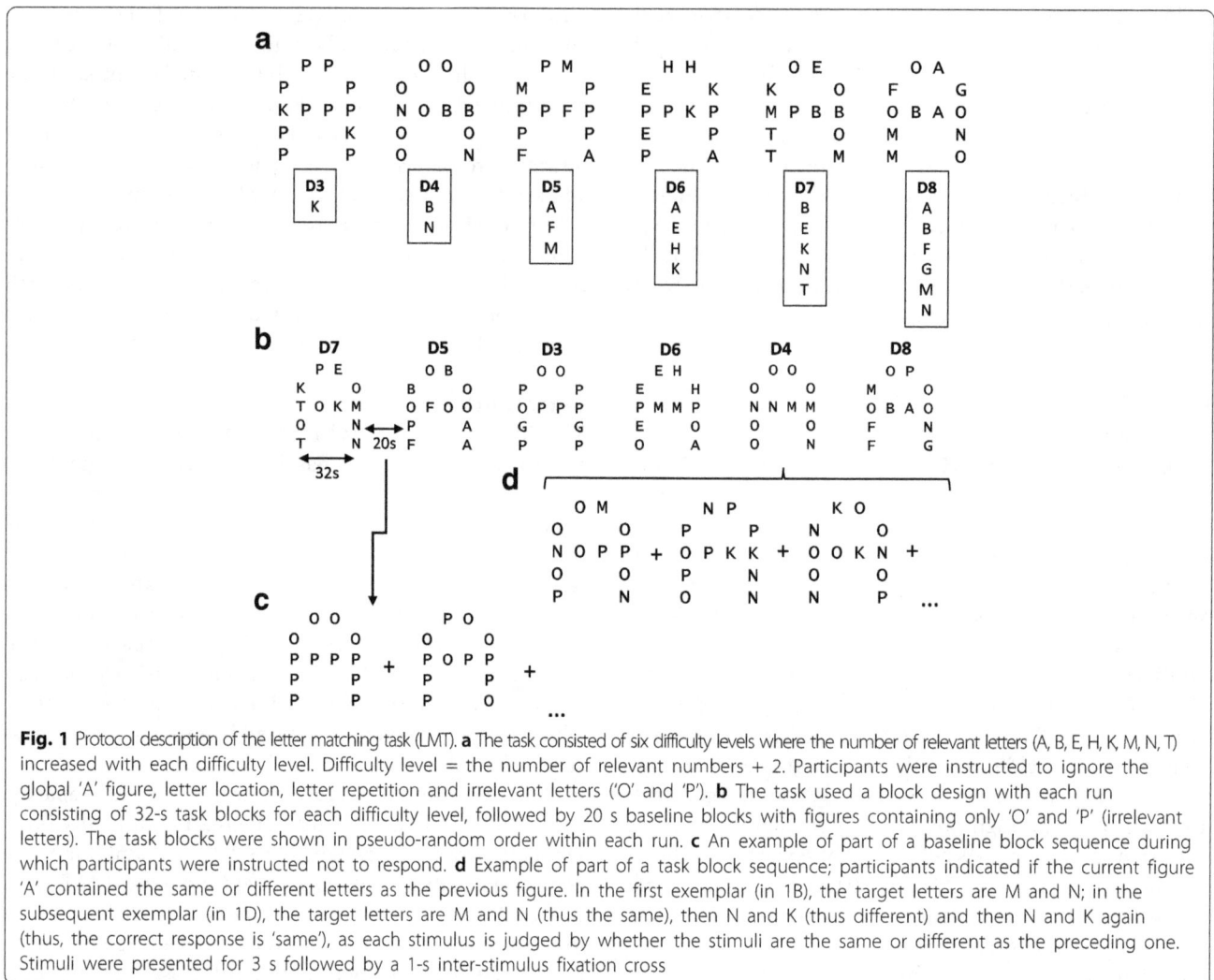

Fig. 1 Protocol description of the letter matching task (LMT). **a** The task consisted of six difficulty levels where the number of relevant letters (A, B, E, H, K, M, N, T) increased with each difficulty level. Difficulty level = the number of relevant numbers + 2. Participants were instructed to ignore the global 'A' figure, letter location, letter repetition and irrelevant letters ('O' and 'P'). **b** The task used a block design with each run consisting of 32-s task blocks for each difficulty level, followed by 20 s baseline blocks with figures containing only 'O' and 'P' (irrelevant letters). The task blocks were shown in pseudo-random order within each run. **c** An example of part of a baseline block sequence during which participants were instructed not to respond. **d** Example of part of a task block sequence; participants indicated if the current figure 'A' contained the same or different letters as the previous figure. In the first exemplar (in 1B), the target letters are M and N; in the subsequent exemplar (in 1D), the target letters are M and N (thus the same), then N and K (thus different) and then N and K again (thus, the correct response is 'same'), as each stimulus is judged by whether the stimuli are the same or different as the preceding one. Stimuli were presented for 3 s followed by a 1-s inter-stimulus fixation cross

the stimulus as the previous stimulus and one button for different. A 1-s inter-stimulus interval during which a fixation cross was presented followed the task stimuli. The baseline trials included presentations in the same configuration as the task stimuli, except that the stimuli only included the irrelevant letters (O and P) in varying configurations. They were presented with the same timing as the task, but for 20 s; thus, only five stimuli per block (see Fig. 1c). All children were trained and completed practice trials successfully with an accuracy of at least 80% prior to performing the task in the scanner.

Twenty-four task and 24 baseline blocks (168 total task trials) were displayed over four runs. Each run included a 32-s block for each of the six difficulty levels; each task block consisted of eight stimuli of the same difficulty level. The levels were randomised for each run, with the same order of runs presented to all participants. The task blocks alternated with the 20-s baseline blocks, where participants were taught to look but not respond to the figures. Items were only correct if subjects

responded correctly within 3 s of stimulus onset. The fMRI session took approximately 22 min, during which reaction time and accuracy were recorded as behavioural data.

Participants were excluded from the analyses if they did not complete at least three runs of the task, with an accuracy of at least 70% (averaged across their runs) on the two easiest levels (D3 and D4). Participants were also required to have at least two runs where at least 50% of the blocks were 70% accurate, to ensure that participants were performing better than chance (50%). Motion was considered acceptable if participants moved less than 1.5 mm from their average head position in a minimum of 60% of the volume within a task block.

Image acquisition

All images were acquired on a 3T Siemens Trio MRI system with a 12-channel head coil. Foam padding was used to provide head motion restriction and stabilisation. fMRI scans were a single-shot echo planar imaging sequence (axial; FOV = 192 × 192 × 150 mm; 3 × 3 × 5 mm voxels; TR/TE/FA = 2000/30/70). The visual stimuli for the task (LMT) were shown using MR-compatible goggles. Stimuli were displayed, and performance was documented using presentation software (Neurobehavioral Systems Inc., Berkeley, CA, USA). Structural scans were used as anatomical references, collected as a high-resolution T1-weighted 3D MP-RAGE image (sagittal; FOV = 2000/30/70 mm; 1 mm iso voxels; TR/TE/TI/FA = 2300/2.96/900/9). During the structural scan, participants used MR-compatible goggles and earphones to watch a movie of their choice.

Behavioural data analyses

Both TD and ASD groups performed poorly on difficulty levels 7 and 8 (D7 and D8), (TD: D7—M = 0.59, SD = 0.15; D8—M = 0.58, SD = 0.13; ASD: D7—M = 0.53, SD = 0.11; D8—M = 0.49, SD = 0.14). D7 and D8 were therefore excluded from the analyses, and the first four difficulty levels (D3 to D6) were analysed. Averages across runs for each group were generated for accuracy and response times at each difficulty level, which were analysed using two-way mixed ANOVAs with difficulty level (D3, D4, D5 and D6) as a within-subject factor and group (ASD and TD) as a between-subject factor.

fMRI data analyses

fMRI data were preprocessed using tools from FMRIB's Software Library: FSL [52] and AFNI [53]. The initial three volumes were discarded from each run to ensure scanner stabilisation. 3dvolreg was used for interleaved slice-timing and McFlirt motion correction; the data were smoothed in place using a 6-mm FWHM Gaussian kernel and temporally filtered (0.01–0.2 Hz) then converted to percent signal change from baseline volumes. Images were registered to the Montreal Neurological Institute (MNI) 152 brain template. The maximum Euclidean displacement (MD) travelled by any brain voxel was calculated for each volume from the six rigid body transformation parameters. This MD metric was used to identify volumes with motion surpassing the minimum motion threshold. Each subject's average MD was used to examine group motion differences (TD: M = 0.47, SD = 0.40; ASD: M = 0.50, SD = 0.47; $t_{(51)}$ = 0.25, ns.).

Data analyses were performed using FSL fMRI expert analysis tool (FEAT) [54]. The data were fit to a block-design general linear model combined with a gamma function used to model haemodynamic changes, with D3 to D6 task parameters. IQ and age were both assessed as confounding variables using FSL FEAT and were both found to have no significant impact on BOLD response during LMT. Linear trend analyses were performed using levels D3 to D6 with fixed-effects higher level modelling to examine areas that linearly modulated as a function of task difficulty. Linear trend analyses

were chosen as this was the approach used in prior studies with the same type of working memory protocols [48, 55, 56]. Individual subjects' results were averaged across runs, then between-group comparisons were conducted using FMRIB's Local Analysis of Mixed Effects-1 (FLAME-1) [52]. Using FLAME-1 allowed us to acquire between-subject variance estimation, thus increasing our capacity to identify real activation [54]. Cluster-based thresholding was determined by $Z > |2.3|$ as well as a corrected cluster significance threshold of $p_{corr} < 0.05$ to identify significant activations. Regions of interest (ROIs) were identified by examining local maxima of regions showing significant variation between TD and ASD groups in the linear trend analyses, for visualisation only. Spherical ROIs with 6-mm radii centred on the local maxima of cohort difference maps were created from which average percent signal change and standard error scores were derived. The average peak cluster signal change for both the TD and ASD groups was plotted as a function of difficulty to examine visually the verbal working memory activation patterns with increasing cognitive load.

Results
Behavioural data

There was a weak but significant effect of group on accuracy, $F(1,55)$ = 4.06, p = 0.049, in which TD children performed slightly better than children with ASD. There was a significant main effect of difficulty level on accuracy, with accuracy decreasing as a function of difficulty, $F(2.50, 165)$ = 80.26, $p < 0.001$ (Greenhouse-Geisser corrected degrees of freedom). There was also a significant group × level interaction, $F(2.50,165)$ = 2.98, p = 0.043 (Greenhouse-Geisser corrected), in which group differences in performance became larger with increasing task difficulty (see Fig. 2a). Post hoc t tests revealed that group performance did not differ on D3 ($t(55)$ = 0.12, p = 0.91) and D4 ($t(55)$ = 1.45, p = 0.15), whereas TD children performed somewhat better than children with ASD on D5 ($t(55)$ = 2.15, p = 0.04) and D6 ($t(55)$ = 2.14, p = 0.04).

There was no significant effect of group on response times, $F(1,55)$ = 0.29, p = 0.59, or on group × level interaction effect, $F(1.81, 165)$ =2.70, p = 0.077 (Greenhouse-Geisser corrected degrees of freedom). There was a significant effect of load on response times, $F(1.81, 165)$ = 83.82, $p < 0.001$ (Greenhouse-Geisser corrected), with response times increasing as a function of difficulty across groups (see Fig. 2b).

Within-group fMRI results

Typically developing children showed significantly increasing activation as a function of increasing cognitive load (i.e. positive linear trend between BOLD signal and

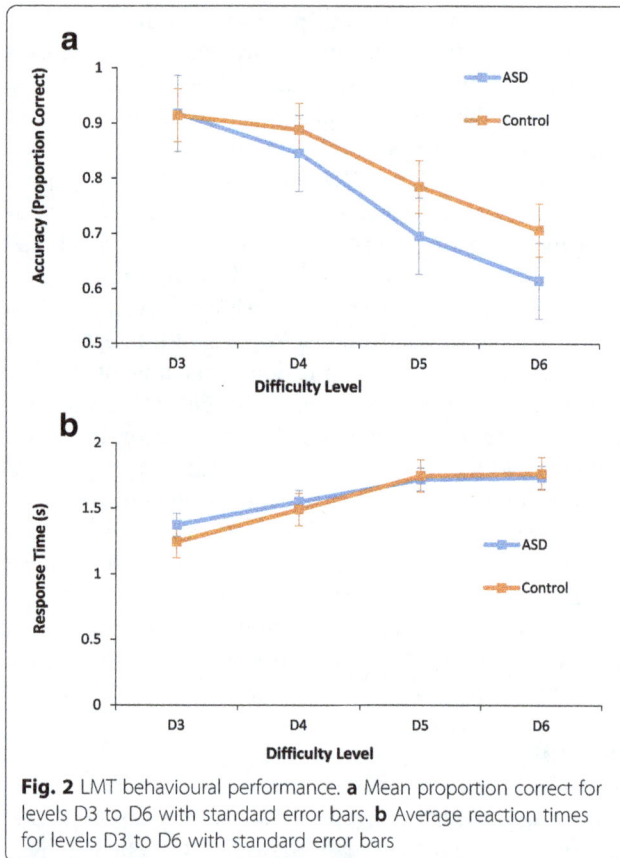

Fig. 2 LMT behavioural performance. **a** Mean proportion correct for levels D3 to D6 with standard error bars. **b** Average reaction times for levels D3 to D6 with standard error bars

difficulty level) in the occipital, parietal, fusiform, cingulate and frontal areas (Fig. 3; see Table 2 for a complete list). Regions that showed decreasing activation as a function of load (i.e. negative linear relations between BOLD signal and difficulty level) included the medial frontal, anterior cingulate, bilateral temporal and parietal gyri and precuneus and cingulate cortices (Table 2 and Fig. 3).

Children with ASD showed increasing activation with greater WM load in the occipital gyri, fusiform, precuneus and inferior frontal gyrus (Fig. 3; see Table 3 for a complete list). Areas that showed decreasing activation across task difficulty included the parietal lobule, middle temporal, cingulate, precuneus and frontal gyri (Fig. 3 and Table 3).

Between-group comparison

TD children had significantly stronger positive linear relations between activation and cognitive load compared to children with ASD in the bilateral prefrontal cortex, precuneus and inferior parietal lobule (Table 4; Fig. 4). In these regions, TD children showed increasing activation with increasing task difficulty, whereas the ASD group failed to show a positive linear trend (see Fig. 5 for graphs of the percent signal change of the ROIs of cortical areas that had significant between-group differences in linear patterns). There were no areas where the

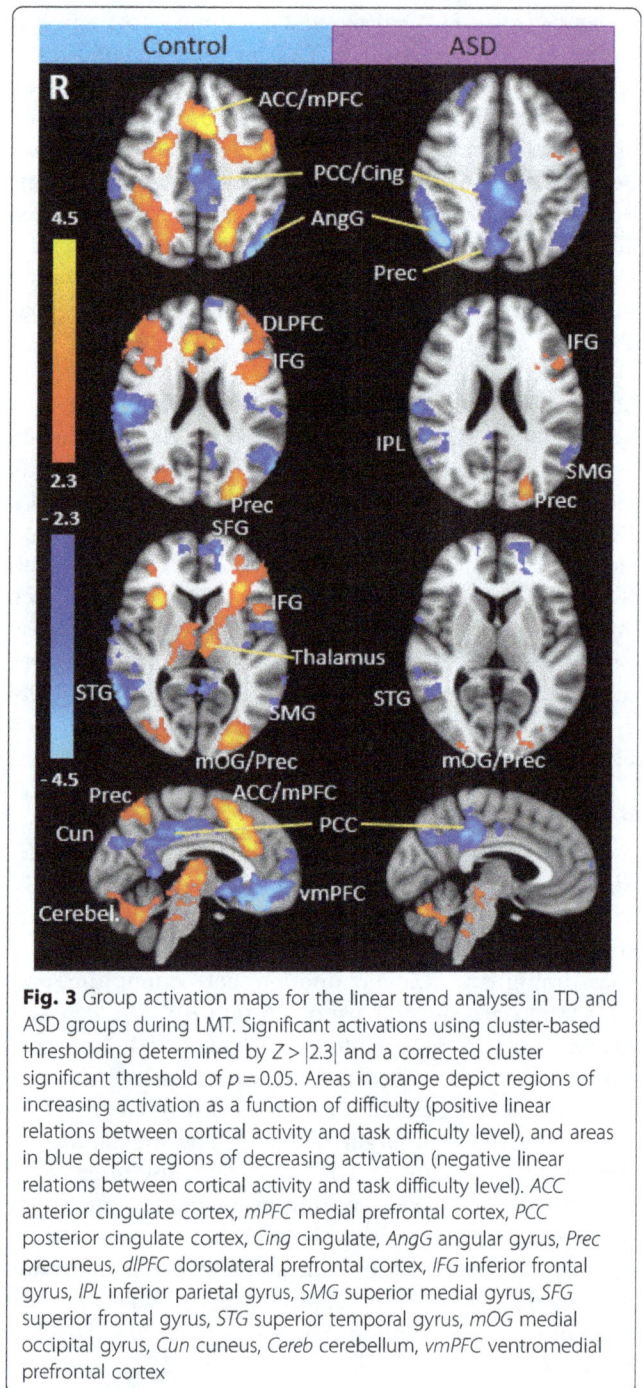

Fig. 3 Group activation maps for the linear trend analyses in TD and ASD groups during LMT. Significant activations using cluster-based thresholding determined by $Z > |2.3|$ and a corrected cluster significant threshold of $p = 0.05$. Areas in orange depict regions of increasing activation as a function of difficulty (positive linear relations between cortical activity and task difficulty level), and areas in blue depict regions of decreasing activation (negative linear relations between cortical activity and task difficulty level). *ACC* anterior cingulate cortex, *mPFC* medial prefrontal cortex, *PCC* posterior cingulate cortex, *Cing* cingulate, *AngG* angular gyrus, *Prec* precuneus, *dlPFC* dorsolateral prefrontal cortex, *IFG* inferior frontal gyrus, *IPL* inferior parietal gyrus, *SMG* superior medial gyrus, *SFG* superior frontal gyrus, *STG* superior temporal gyrus, *mOG* medial occipital gyrus, *Cun* cuneus, *Cereb* cerebellum, *vmPFC* ventromedial prefrontal cortex

ASD group showed greater linear activation across task difficulty than TD children. There were no significant differences between groups in the patterns of deactivation with increasing cognitive load.

Discussion

Protracted development of the frontal lobes in combination with vulnerability to neurodevelopmental disturbances emphasises the need for deeper understanding of

Table 2 Linear trend analyses across difficulty levels for TD children

	Voxels	MNI coordinates			Z value	p value	Hem.	Region
		x	y	z				
Regions where activation increases with difficulty (increasing BOLD signal)	14,922	− 28	− 76	− 4	4.81	6.31×10^{-25}	L	Middle occipital gyrus
	x	− 24	− 62	52	4.73		L	Superior parietal lobule
	x	− 26	− 72	− 10	4.51		L	Fusiform gyrus
	x	− 20	− 92	16	4.5		L	Cuneus
	x	28	− 58	58	4.44		R	Inferior parietal lobule
	14,033	− 8	18	42	5.41	6.92×10^{-24}	L	Cingulate gyrus
	x	− 40	2	30	4.96		L	Inferior frontal gyrus
	x	10	22	38	4.83		R	Cingulate gyrus
	x	− 4	28	28	4.76		L	Anterior cingulate cortex
	3447	50	32	32	4.57	9.29×10^{-9}	R	Middle frontal gyrus
	x	32	18	3	4.47		R	Insula
Regions where activation decreases with difficulty (decreasing BOLD signal)	5355	2	38	− 22	5.38	4.32×10^{-12}	R	Medial frontal gyrus
	x	− 6	40	− 12	4.74		L	Medial frontal gyrus
	x	− 14	34	− 16	4.51		L	Inferior frontal gyrus
	x	6	62	− 6	4.5		R	Superior frontal gyrus
	x	2	14	− 6	4.41		R	Anterior cingulate cortex
	5165	− 60	− 26	− 18	4.72	8.85×10^{-12}	L	Middle temporal gyrus
	x	− 40	− 78	40	4.54		L	Precuneus/angular gyrus
	x	− 56	− 62	30	4.46		L	Angular gyrus
	4472	60	− 22	20	4.84	1.31×10^{-10}	R	Supramarginal gyrus
	x	66	− 30	34	4.56		R	Inferior parietal lobule
	x	60	− 56	2	4.45		R	Middle temporal gyrus
	x	68	− 38	12	4.24		R	Superior temporal gyrus
	3615	− 16	− 48	36	4.25	4.5×10^{-9}	L	Cingulate gyrus
	x	2	− 44	34	4.04		R	Cingulate gyrus

the function of these regions with typical and atypical development. Previous research has been centred on WM in adolescents and adults with ASD, leaving a gap in our understanding of WM in children with ASD. This is the first study to investigate the neural correlates of verbal WM in children and young adolescents with ASD compared to TD youth and examine the impact of cognitive load.

The TD group showed increasing recruitment of the brain areas classically linked to WM as a function of increasing cognitive demand and decreasing activation in regions associated with the DMN. The group with ASD, however, did not show this opposing system of cognitive processing. Specifically, TD children recruited the prefrontal and parietal cortical regions, areas directly correlated with verbal WM [3, 32, 38, 41, 42, 57], as a function of cognitive load significantly more than children with ASD who only demonstrated load-dependent deactivation in DMN regions. In a qualitative examination of

activation patterns, we observed a larger spread of activation in children in this study compared to adults from Vogan et al.'s [48] study. This is consistent with the study by Geier et al. [33], who performed a visual spatial working memory oculomotor delayed-response task with adults, adolescents and children, and found that while all three age groups showed recruitment of a common network including the frontal, parietal and temporal regions, children and adolescents showed a wider distribution in addition to that network.

The behavioural data showed comparable performance on D3 and D4 between the TD and ASD groups; however, TD children performed with a higher accuracy on D5 and D6. These between-group differences emerging at higher cognitive loads are consistent with the literature suggesting that WM in children with ASD, when compared with TD children, is similar for simpler tasks but deficient for more complex tasks or those with greater cognitive demand [8, 22–25, 27, 29].

Table 3 Linear trend analyses across difficulty levels for children with ASD

	Voxels	MNI coordinates			Z value	p value	Hem.	Region
		x	y	z				
Regions where activation increases with difficulty (increasing BOLD signal)	2170	−28	−76	−6	4.25	3.64×10^{-6}	L	Middle occipital gyrus
	x	−24	−68	−6	4.09		L	Lingual gyrus/fusiform gyrus
	x	−28	−54	−6	3.91		L	Lingual gyrus
	x	−20	−86	12	3.85		L	Cuneus/middle occipital gyrus
	x	−22	−86	22	3.82		L	Precuneus
	1120	−2	−74	−26	4.19	1.31×10^{-3}	L	Cerebellar vermis
	x	28	−72	−10	3.62		R	Fusiform/lingual gyrus
	x	0	−58	−32	3.51		L	Culmen/cerebellar vermis
	x	−10	−64	−30	3.16		L	Cerebellum
	960	6	−28	−12	4.29	3.68×10^{-3}	R	Thalamus
	x	6	−34	−20	4.01		R	Culmen
	x	−8	−24	−12	3.43		L	Thalamus
	x	0	−34	−46	3.42		L	Brain-stem
	x	−2	−34	−30	3.41		L	Culmen
	610	−42	−4	26	4.04	4.4×10^{-2}	L	Inferior frontal gyrus
	x	−58	18	32	3.89		L	Middle frontal gyrus
	x	−38	22	18	3.05		L	Insula/inferior frontal gyrus
Regions where activation decreases with difficulty (decreasing BOLD signal)	3908	42	−68	42	4.92	1.31×10^{-9}	R	Inferior parietal/angular gyrus
	x	48	−58	40	4.52		R	Inferior parietal lobule
	x	48	−50	36	4.49		R	Angular gyrus
	x	48	−46	36	4.46		R	Supramarginal gyrus
	x	46	−44	0	4.1		R	Middle temporal gyrus
	3816	2	−32	44	4.38	1.92×10^{-9}	R	Cingulate gyrus
	x	−6	−38	38	4.19		L	Cingulate gyrus
	x	6	−68	36	4.02		R	Precuneus
	x	12	−46	30	3.79		R	Cingulate gyrus
	x	−16	−24	44	3.73		L	Cingulate gyrus
	1810	−64	−40	30	4.37	2.38×10^{-5}	L	Inferior parietal lobule
	x	−56	−56	34	3.97		L	Angular gyrus
	843	−12	62	12	4.07	8.14×10^{-3}	L	Medial frontal gyrus
	x	−22	66	14	3.77		L	Middle frontal gyrus
	x	−18	52	8	3.58		L	Superior frontal gyrus
	x	16	58	4	3.33		R	Superior frontal gyrus
	x	−20	42	4	3.32		L	anterior cingulate
	604	22	58	18	3.44	4.6×10^{-2}	R	superior frontal gyrus
	x	24	52	32	3.29		R	middle frontal gyrus

Results from linear trend analyses from D3 to D6 for children with ASD. Areas that increased as a function of difficulty level are associated largely with visual processing, whereas areas that decreased as a function of difficulty level are associated with the default mode network. MNI coordinates represent the peak Z value of the cluster, X peak local maximas within cluster

The ASD youth did not show comparable increasing activity in frontal-parietal regions with increased memory load, as the TD group. The frontal areas (BA 9) and inferior parietal lobe are classic areas for working memory [32], and activity in this WM task in the TD group was expected. The further activity that was greater in the TD group than the ASD group in the cingulate and precuneus could be due to increased recruitment of cognitive control mechanisms due to task difficulty, as both the anterior cingulate cortex (ACC) and precuneus are

Table 4 Regions of significant differences between TD and ASD groups

Voxels	MNI coordinates			Z value	p value	Hem.	Region
	x	y	z				
1341	− 10	40	26	3.38	3.37×10^{-4}	L	Medial frontal gyrus
x	− 14	8	50	3.32		L	Cingulate gyrus
x	− 16	6	62	3.26		L	Superior frontal gyrus
1175	38	− 36	44	3.58	9.25×10^{-4}	R	Inferior parietal lobule
1095	14	− 52	46	3.7	1.53×10^{-3}	R	Precuneus
x	− 6	− 62	52	3.32		L	Precuneus
833	54	36	22	3.73	8.73×10^{-3}	R	Middle frontal gyrus
x	28	42	38	3.16		R	Superior frontal gyrus

Results from between group comparisons of the linear trend analyses from D3 to D6. All regions reported are areas where TD children showed greater positive linear relations between cortical activity and difficulty level (increasing BOLD signal with increasing task difficulty) than children with ASD. There were no areas where children with ASD showed greater linear relations between cortical activity and difficulty level than TD children. MNI coordinates represent the peak Z values of the cluster; X peak local maximas within cluster

key hubs in cognitive networks. The differences between the groups were despite both completing the task successfully. Although the accuracy of the ASD group was lower than the TD group at the two higher load levels, they were performing the task similarly at D3 and D4 and were still at acceptable levels for D5 and D6. This suggests that the ASD group had unconventional utilisation of the brain areas for the WM task. This is concordant with the model that activation is more idiosyncratic in those with ASD, as reported elsewhere [58]. This leads to the usual regions not being seen in the ASD group analysis, and the more typical regions emerging as more active in the TD group in the group comparison. With a larger study, idiosyncratic patterns could be investigated specifically to determine if there are ASD subgroups with distinct alternative strategies.

Following on from this notion, future larger studies should also determine the role of other cognitive steps or strategies that may differ between TD and ASD groups that could influence WM performance. We included irrelevant aspects in the stimuli, to allow better determination of WM [51], but irrelevant details may also impact selective filtering and attention, which has been linked to working memory capacity [59]. As some researchers have found heightened visual processing in those with ASD [60, 61] particularly in relation to local features [62], this visual strategy may emerge more commonly in an ASD group and potentially impact strategy, and hence underlying neural recruitment. Future work could include assessments of visual processing skills (see [63]) and use that as a means of subgrouping participants by cognitive processing preferences.

A number of studies have reported atypical DMN activation in ASD [64–67], including an earlier investigation with the similar but visuo-spatial colour task (CMT) [55]. The DMN is a well-established network of the brain regions that are active during rest or non-task periods and show decreased BOLD signals during tasks [68], particularly tasks that are cognitively demanding. This modulation is believed to contribute to more efficient cognitive processing, and DMN regions are expected to deactivate with increasing task difficulty. The fact that here we saw no difference between the ASD and the TD groups in the decreasing activation of DMN regions with increasing task load could be due to a slightly older age range than previous studies, suggesting that DMN modulation may 'catch up' in children with ASD as they move into the teenage years. This is supported by a similar longitudinal protocol with somewhat older cohort [56], where the DMN modulation increased compared to 2 years earlier. These combined results indicate that the DMN modulation develops in ASD, albeit later than in the TD group, while the working memory processes remain distinct.

A limitation of the current study was the use of only linear models in the analyses. This was chosen as this is a subsequent study from our normative series [48], and a sister study to two other papers using a colour matching task [55, 56] all of which used the same analytic procedures, and we wanted to be able to relate the findings across the studies. Other approaches could be used in the future that investigate non-linear changes as a function of group (e.g. [69]) or with WM load, such as logarithmic changes that would be seen as rapidly increasing activation and then a plateau. Another limitation is that we had to exclude children who could not stay still in the scanner and who did not perform adequately on the task to ensure brain behaviour-related activation. By doing so, we were unable to include lower functioning children with ASD, and thus, our results are generalizable to higher functioning children only. There was also, on average, a lower IQ in the ASD youth and greater IQ variability. This is typical of this population, but even when IQ was covaried, the effects remained,

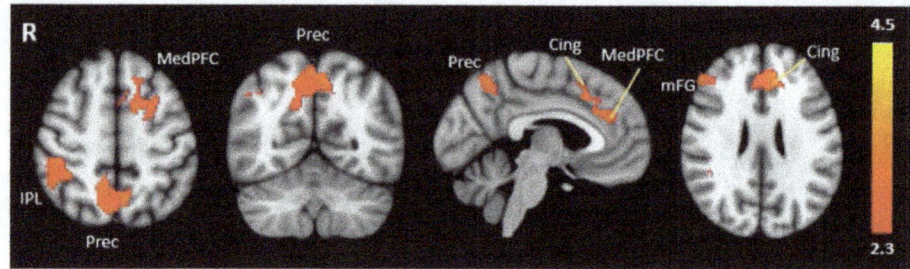

Fig. 4 Results from between-group comparisons. Significant activations using cluster-based thresholding determined by $Z > |2.3|$ and a corrected cluster significant threshold of $p = 0.05$. Areas in red/orange depict regions where the control children showed greater linear activation trends across difficulty level in the negative or positive direction than children with ASD. *medPFC* medial prefrontal cortex, *Cing* cingulate, *Prec* precuneus, *IPL* inferior parietal gyrus, *mFG* middle frontal gyrus

suggesting that the effects were robust within the higher IQ range, despite the group differences in IQ. Further fMRI investigations are required with less demanding protocols to understand verbal WM function in low functioning children with ASD, who may present unique neural profiles. Finally, we had a wide age range in the study. We matched groups on age and age did not contribute to group effects. Nevertheless, smaller age ranges are ideal, and with a larger sample, age-related effects could be explored.

Conclusions

The results from this study have several important implications. Our findings that children with ASD, relative to TD children, demonstrate inadequate modulation of neural capacity suggest that they could become overwhelmed with increasing verbal information. Impaired verbal working memory in ASD would have important academic and social implications. Specially, verbal WM difficulties could interfere with children's ability to recall verbal information from conversations and social interactions, as well as to learn verbal material from classroom lessons or follow instructions. Determining the neural deficits of WM in children with ASD will help us understand the origins of the behaviours associated with ASD. Brain functional abnormalities in ASD may drive behavioural symptoms and give rise to cognitive impairments. Thus, exploring the neural correlates of WM contributes to knowledge of the ASD behavioural phenotypes. Finally, our study helps determine the nature of atypical neurodevelopment, which could help establish or monitor interventions for WM function in ASD.

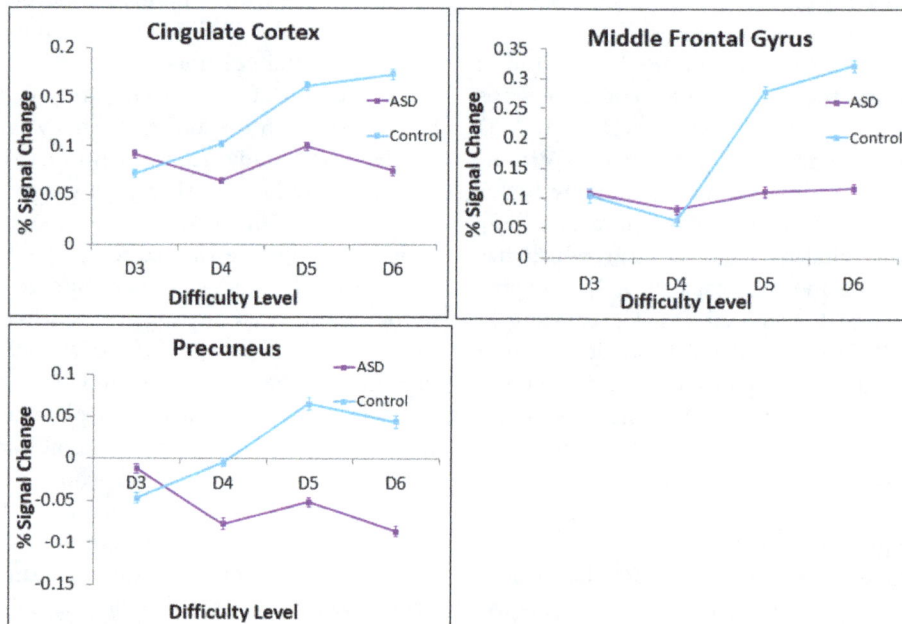

Fig. 5 Mean peak cluster percent signal changes and standard errors plotted as a function of difficulty level. Areas where children with ASD differed significantly from TD children in the linear trend analyses

Abbreviations
ADOS: Autism Diagnostic Observation Schedule; ASD: Autism spectrum disorder; BOLD: Brain-oxygen-level dependent; D3, D4 etc.: Difficulty level 3, difficulty level 4, etc.; dlPFC: Dorsolateral prefrontal cortex; DMN: Default mode network; fMRI: Functional magnetic resonance imaging; FWHM: Full width half maximum; LMT: Letter matching task; MD: Maximum Euclidean displacement; MNI: Montreal Neurological Institute; PFC: Prefrontal cortex; ROIs: Regions of interest; TD: Typically developing; WM: Working memory

Acknowledgements
We would like to thank first the families and children for their participation. Many thanks to Rachel Leung for administering the ADOS-R and ADOS-2 and Dr. Jessica Brian for reviewing the assessments. Warmest thanks to our MRI technologists, Tammy Rayner and Ruth Weiss, for all their incredible help in data acquisition. Lastly, thank you to Crescent School, Toronto, for their support and participation in this project.

Funding
This research was funded by the Canadian Institutes of Health Research (CIHR) grants MOP-106582 and MOP-142379.

Authors' contributions
VV is responsible for the recruitment, data acquisition, analysis and interpretation and writing and editing of the manuscript. KF also contributed significantly to the data analyses, interpretation and writing and editing of the manuscript. BM participated in the fMRI analysis and revising the manuscript. MS advised on patient testing, study design and revising the manuscript. MT initiated the study and participated in the design, analyses and writing and revising of the manuscript. All authors read and approved the final manuscript.

Competing interests
The authors declare that they have no competing interests.

Author details
[1]Diagnostic Imaging & Research Institute, Hospital for Sick Children, 555 University Avenue, Toronto, Ontario M5G 1X8, Canada. [2]Department of Applied Psychology and Human Development, Ontario Institute for Studies in Education, University of Toronto, 252 Bloor Street West, Toronto, Ontario M56 1V6, Canada. [3]Department of Psychology, University of Toronto, 100 St. George St., Toronto, Ontario M5S 3G3, Canada.

References
1. American Psychiatric Association. Diagnostic and statistical manual of mental disorders (5th ed.). Arlington: American Psychiatric Publishing; 2013.
2. Barnard L, Muldoon K, Hasan R, O'Brien G, Stewart M. Profiling executive dysfunction in adults with autism and comorbid learning disability. Autism. 2008;12:125–41.
3. Greene CM, Braet W, Johnson KA, Bellgrove MA. Imaging the genetics of executive function. Biol Psychol. 2008;79:30–42.
4. Happe F, Booth R, Charlton R, Hughes C. Executive function deficits in autism spectrum disorders and attention-deficit/hyperactivity disorder: examining profiles across domains and ages. Brain Cogn. 2006;61:25–39.
5. Hill EL. Executive dysfunction in autism. Trends Cogn Sci. 2004;8:26–32.
6. Joseph RM. Neuropsychological frameworks for understanding autism. Int Rev Psychiatry. 1999;11:309 24.
7. Luna B, Minshew NJ, Garver KE, Lazar NA, Thulborn KR, Eddy WF, Sweeney JA. Neocortical system abnormalities in autism: an fMRI study of spatial working memory. Neurology. 2002;59:834–40.
8. Russo N, Flanagan T, Iarocci G, Berringer D, Zelazo PD, Burack JA. Deconstructing executive deficits among persons with autism: implications for cognitive neuroscience. Brain Cogn. 2007;65:77–86.
9. Koshino H, Carpenter PA, Minshew NJ, Cherkassky VL, Keller TA, Just MA. Functional connectivity in an fMRI working memory task in high-functioning autism. Neuroimage. 2005;24:810–21.
10. Koshino H, Kana RK, Keller TA, Cherkassky VL, Minshew NJ, Just MA. fMRI investigation of working memory for faces in autism: visual coding and underconnectivity with frontal areas. Cereb Cortex. 2008;18:289–300.
11. O'Hearn KAM, Ordaz S, Luna B. Neurodevelopment and executive function in autism. Dev Psychopathol. 2008;20:1103–32.
12. Silk TJ, Rinehart N, Bradshaw JL, Tonge B, Egan G, O'Boyle MW, Cunnington R. Visuospatial processing and the function of prefrontal-parietal networks in autism spectrum disorders: a functional MRI study. Am J Psychiatry. 2006; 163:1440–3.
13. Powell KB, Voeller KK. Prefrontal executive function syndromes in children. J Child Neurol. 2004;19:785–97.
14. Sowell ER, Thompson PM, Leonard CM, Welcome SE, Kan E, Toga AW. Longitudinal mapping of cortical thickness and brain growth in normal children. J Neurosci. 2004;24:8223–31.
15. O'Hare ED, Lu LH, Houston SM, Bookheimer SY, Sowell ER. Neurodevelopmental changes in verbal working memory load-dependency: an fMRI investigation. Neuroimage. 2008;42:1678–85.
16. Baddeley A. Working memory. Science. 1992;255:556–9.
17. Case R. Exploring the Conceptual Underpinnings of Children's Thought and Knowledge. Hillsdale: Erlbaum; 1992.
18. Engle RW, Tuholski SW, Laughlin JE, Conway AR. Working memory, short-term memory, and general fluid intelligence: a latent-variable approach. J Exp Psychol Gen. 1999;128:309–31.
19. Graf P, Uttl B, Dixon R. Prospective and retrospective memory in adulthood. In: Graf P, Ohta N, editors. Lifespan development of human memory. Cambridge: MIT Press; 2002. p. 257-82.
20. TP A. Working memory, but not IQ, predicts subsequent learning in children with learning difficulties. Eur J Psychol Assess. 2009;25:92–8.
21. Dennis M, Agostino A, Roncadin C, Levin H. Theory of mind depends on domain-general executive functions of working memory and cognitive inhibition in children with traumatic brain injury. J Clin Exp Neuropsychol. 2009;31:835–47.
22. Ozonoff S, Strayer DL. Further evidence of intact working memory in autism. J Autism Dev Disord. 2001;31:257–63.
23. Russell J, Jarrold C, Henry L. Working memory in children with autism and with moderate learning difficulties. J Child Psychol Psychiatry. 1996; 37:673–86.
24. Steele SD, Minshew NJ, Luna B, Sweeney JA. Spatial working memory deficits in autism. J Autism Dev Disord. 2007;37:605–12.
25. Bennetto L, Pennington BF, Rogers SJ. Intact and impaired memory functions in autism. Child Dev. 1996;67:1816–35.
26. Minshew NJ, Goldstein G. The pattern of intact and impaired memory functions in autism. J Child Psychol Psychiatry. 2001;42:1095–101.
27. Williams DL, Goldstein G, Carpenter PA, Minshew NJ. Verbal and spatial working memory in autism. J Autism Dev Disord. 2005;35:747–56.
28. Williams DL, Goldstein G, Minshew NJ. The profile of memory function in children with autism. Neuropsychology. 2006;20:21–9.
29. Gabig CS. Verbal working memory and story retelling in school-age children with autism. Lang Speech Hear Serv Sch. 2008;39:498–511.
30. Southwick JS, Bigler ED, Froehlich A, Dubray MB, Alexander AL, Lange N, Lainhart JE. Memory functioning in children and adolescents with autism. Neuropsychology. 2011;25:702–10.
31. Fletcher PC, Henson RN. Frontal lobes and human memory: insights from functional neuroimaging. Brain. 2001;124:849–81.
32. Owen AM, McMillan KM, Laird AR, Bullmore E. N-back working memory paradigm: a meta-analysis of normative functional neuroimaging studies. Hum Brain Mapp. 2005;25:46–59.
33. Geier CF, Garver K, Terwilliger R, Luna B. Development of working memory maintenance. J Neurophysiol. 2009;101:84–99.

34. Nagel BJ, Herting MM, Maxwell EC, Bruno R, Fair D. Hemispheric lateralization of verbal and spatial working memory during adolescence. Brain Cogn. 2013;82:58–68.

35. Thomason ME, Race E, Burrows B, Whitfield-Gabrieli S, Glover GH, Gabrieli JD. Development of spatial and verbal working memory capacity in the human brain. J Cogn Neurosci. 2009;21:316–32.

36. Damarla SR, Keller TA, Kana RK, Cherkassky VL, Williams DL, Minshew NJ, Just MA. Cortical underconnectivity coupled with preserved visuospatial cognition in autism: evidence from an fMRI study of an embedded figures task. Autism Res. 2010;3:273–9.

37. Kana RK, Liu Y, Williams DL, Keller TA, Schipul SE, Minshew NJ, Just MA. The local, global, and neural aspects of visuospatial processing in autism spectrum disorders. Neuropsychologia. 2013;51:2995–3003.

38. Carlson S, Martinkauppi S, Rama P, Salli E, Korvenoja A, Aronen HJ. Distribution of cortical activation during visuospatial n-back tasks as revealed by functional magnetic resonance imaging. Cereb Cortex. 1998;8:743–52.

39. Cohen JD, Perlstein WM, Braver TS, Nystrom LE, Noll DC, Jonides J, Smith EE. Temporal dynamics of brain activation during a working memory task. Nature. 1997;386:604–8.

40. de Vries M, Geurts HM. Beyond individual differences: are working memory and inhibition informative specifiers within ASD? J Neural Transm (Vienna). 2014;121:1183–98.

41. Fuster JM. Prefrontal neurons in networks of executive memory. Brain Res Bull. 2000;52:331–6.

42. Kwon H, Reiss AL, Menon V. Neural basis of protracted developmental changes in visuo-spatial working memory. Proc Natl Acad Sci U S A. 2002; 99:13336–41.

43. Nelson CA, Monk CS, Lin J, Carver LJ, Thomas KM, Truwit CL. Functional neuroanatomy of spatial working memory in children. Dev Psychol. 2000;36: 109–16.

44. Rahko JS, Vuontela VA, Carlson S, Nikkinen J, Hurtig TM, Kuusikko-Gauffin S, Mattila ML, Jussila KK, Remes JJ, Jansson-Verkasalo EM, et al. Attention and working memory in adolescents with autism spectrum disorder: a functional MRI study. Child Psychiatry Hum Dev. 2016;47:503–17.

45. Urbain CM, Pang EW, Taylor MJ. Atypical spatiotemporal signatures of working memory brain processes in autism. Transl Psychiatry. 2015;5:e617.

46. Arsalidou M, Pascual-Leone J, Johnson J, Morris D, Taylor MJ. A balancing act of the brain: activations and deactivations driven by cognitive load. Brain Behav. 2013;3:273–85.

47. Powell TL, Vogan VM, Arsalidou M, Taylor MJ. Controlled interference and assessments of developmental working memory capacity: Evidence from the letter and colour matching tasks. Child Dev Res. 2014;6(1):19.

48. Vogan VM, Morgan BR, Powell TL, Smith ML, Taylor MJ. The neurodevelopmental differences of increasing verbal working memory demand in children and adults. Dev Cogn Neurosci. 2016;17:19–27.

49. Wechsler D. Wechsler intelligence scale for children. San Antonia: Psychological Corporation; 2003.

50. Lord C, Risi S, Lambrecht L, Cook EH Jr, Leventhal BL, DiLavore PC, Pickles A, Rutter M. The autism diagnostic observation schedule-generic: a standard measure of social and communication deficits associated with the spectrum of autism. J Autism Dev Disord. 2000;30:205–23.

51. P-LJ AM, Johnson J. Misleading cues improve developmental assessment of working memory capacity: the colour matching tasks. Cogn Dev. 2010;25:262–77.

52. Woolrich MW, Behrens TE, Beckmann CF, Jenkinson M, Smith SM. Multilevel linear modelling for FMRI group analysis using Bayesian inference. Neuroimage. 2004;21:1732–47.

53. Cox RW. AFNI: software for analysis and visualization of functional magnetic resonance neuroimages. Comput Biomed Res. 1996;29:162–73.

54. Woolrich MW, Jbabdi S, Patenaude B, Chappell M, Makni S, Behrens T, Beckmann C, Jenkinson M, Smith SM. Bayesian analysis of neuroimaging data in FSL. Neuroimage. 2009;45:S173–86.

55. Vogan VM, Morgan BR, Lee W, Powell TL, Smith ML, Taylor MJ. The neural correlates of visuo-spatial working memory in children with autism spectrum disorder: effects of cognitive load. J Neurodev Disord. 2014;6:19.

56. Vogan VM, Morgan BR, Smith ML, Taylor MJ. Functional changes during visuo-spatial working memory in autism spectrum disorder: 2-year longitudinal fMRI study: Autism; 2018. In Press

57. Baddeley A. Working memory: looking back and looking forward. Nat Rev Neurosci. 2003;4:829–39.

58. Byrge L, Dubois J, Tyszka JM, Adolphs R, Kennedy DP. Idiosyncratic brain activation patterns are associated with poor social comprehension in autism. J Neurosci. 2015;35:5837–50.

59. Vogel EK, McCollough AW, Machizawa MG. Neural measures reveal individual differences in controlling access to working memory. Nature. 2005;438:500–3.

60. Mottron L, Burack JA, Iarocci G, Belleville S, Enns JT. Locally oriented perception with intact global processing among adolescents with high-functioning autism: evidence from multiple paradigms. J Child Psychol Psychiatry. 2003;44:904–13.

61. Mottron L, Dawson M, Soulieres I, Hubert B, Burack J. Enhanced perceptual functioning in autism: an update, and eight principles of autistic perception. J Autism Dev Disord. 2006;36:27–43.

62. Plaisted K, Saksida L, Alcantara J, Weisblatt E. Towards an understanding of the mechanisms of weak central coherence effects: experiments in visual configural learning and auditory perception. Philos Trans R Soc Lond Ser B Biol Sci. 2003;358:375–86.

63. Dakin S, Frith U. Vagaries of visual perception in autism. Neuron. 2005; 48:497–507.

64. Chen CP, Keown CL, Jahedi A, Nair A, Pflieger ME, Bailey BA, Muller RA. Diagnostic classification of intrinsic functional connectivity highlights somatosensory, default mode, and visual regions in autism. Neuroimage Clin. 2015;8:238–45.

65. Kennedy DP, Redcay E, Courchesne E. Failing to deactivate: resting functional abnormalities in autism. Proc Natl Acad Sci U S A. 2006;103:8275–80.

66. Lynch CJ, Uddin LQ, Supekar K, Khouzam A, Phillips J, Menon V. Default mode network in childhood autism: posteromedial cortex heterogeneity and relationship with social deficits. Biol Psychiatry. 2013;74:212–9.

67. Washington SD, Gordon EM, Brar J, Warburton S, Sawyer AT, Wolfe A, Mease-Ference ER, Girton L, Hailu A, Mbwana J, et al. Dysmaturation of the default mode network in autism. Hum Brain Mapp. 2014;35:1284–96.

68. Raichle ME. The brain's default mode network. Annu Rev Neurosci. 2015;38:433–47.

69. Vakorin VA, Doesburg SM, Leung RC, Vogan VM, Anagnostou E, Taylor MJ. Developmental changes in neuromagnetic rhythms and network synchrony in autism. Ann Neurol. 2017;81:199–211.

13

Attention and motor deficits index non-specific background liabilities that predict autism recurrence in siblings

Sabine E. Mous[1,2], Allan Jiang[2], Arpana Agrawal[2] and John N. Constantino[2*]

Abstract

Background: Recent research has demonstrated that subclinical autistic traits of parents amplify the effects of deleterious mutations in the causation of autism spectrum disorder (ASD) in their offspring. Here, we examined the extent to which two neurodevelopmental traits that are non-specific to ASD—inattention/hyperactivity and motor coordination—might contribute to ASD recurrence in siblings of ASD probands.

Methods: Data from a quantitative trait study of 114 ASD probands and their brothers, 26% of whom also had ASD, were analyzed. Autistic trait severity was ascertained using the Social Responsiveness Scale-2, attention/hyperactivity problems using the Achenbach System of Empirically Based Assessment, and motor coordination (in a subset of participants) using the Developmental Coordination Disorder Questionnaire.

Results: Among siblings (affected and unaffected), both categorical recurrence of ASD (Nagelkerke $R^2 = 0.53$) and quantitative ASD trait burden ($R^2 = 0.55$) were predicted by sibling ADHD and motor coordination impairment scores, even though these traits, on average, were not elevated among the unaffected siblings.

Conclusions: These findings in a clinical family cohort confirm observations from general population studies that inattention/hyperactivity and motor impairment—axes of behavioral development that are non-specific to ASD, and often appreciable before ASD is typically diagnosed—jointly account for over 50% of the variation in autistic impairment of siblings, whether ascertained quantitatively or categorically. This finding within a sibling design suggests that background ASD susceptibilities that are inherited but non-specific ("BASINS") may contribute to additive genetic liability in the same manner that ASD-specific susceptibilities (such as parental subclinical ASD traits and deleterious mutations) engender ASD risk.

Keywords: Autism, ADHD, Motor coordination, Sibling recurrence, Family studies

Background

Autism spectrum disorder (ASD) is characterized by difficulties in social communication and restricted interests or repetitive behaviors. Recent epidemiologic research demonstrated that ASD traits are continuously distributed in the general population [1, 2] and are highly heritable; clinical autistic syndromes may arise from extreme aggregations of such continuously distributed traits or from the highly deleterious effects of genetic variants as occur in monogenic or oligogenic ASD syndromes [3]. Recently,

significant advances in scientific understanding of the nature of the influence of common variation were made on the basis of two strategic trans-generational family studies. The first demonstrated that in the setting of de novo mutations conferring ASD risk (patients with de novo 16p11.2 deletions and their first degree relatives), the level of impairment of the individual with the mutation was significantly amplified if the *genetic background* as indexed by the bi-parental mean for subclinical autistic traits was in the *upper range of normal* [4]. The second, in a large epidemiologic sample, demonstrated that when both parents exhibited autistic trait aggregation in the upper quintile of the *normal distribution*, the risk for clinical-level ASD affectation of offspring was doubled [5].

* Correspondence: constantino@wustl.edu
[2]Division of Child Psychiatry, Department of Psychiatry, Washington University School of Medicine, 660 South Euclid Avenue, Campus Box 8504, St Louis, MO 63110, USA
Full list of author information is available at the end of the article

Many previous studies have demonstrated the aggregation of *non-ASD-specific* neurodevelopmental impairments (e.g. motor or attentional impairment) in individuals affected by ASD, even though these inherited neurodevelopmental problems are not included in the DSM5 diagnostic criteria for autism spectrum disorder [6–8]. As yet, the nature and direction-of-effect of the genetic and developmental overlap between ASD and ADHD or between ASD and motor impairment remain incompletely specified. Although family and twin studies strongly suggest shared additive genetic liabilities between ASD and ADHD, findings from candidate gene, linkage, and genome-wide association studies are mixed [9]. Supporting causal overlap, molecular genetic studies have revealed highly pleiotropic effects of rare deleterious mutations—for example, those involving FMR1, TSC1/ TSC2, NF1, and the 22q11 deletion—which have been variously associated with ADHD or ASD across individual carriers [10–12]. Furthermore, a large population-based twin study indicated that a substantial proportion of the genetic susceptibility for ASD symptomatology is shared with that for ADHD symptomatology, with almost 60% of the genetic influences shared by both disorders [13]. Tempering the notion of causal overlap, however, a recent genome-wide association study, using large case–control ASD and ADHD samples, did *not* identify significant overlap in common variant liability [14]. Here, it is important to recognize that very few common variants in this study were *individually* associated with either disorder at a level reaching genome-wide significance. Shared familial transmission of ASD and ADHD has been suggested in a study showing that mothers with an ADHD diagnosis did not only have an increased risk of having a child with ADHD but also had a 2.5-fold increased risk of having a child with ASD [15]. Furthermore, studies suggest that siblings of children with ASD not only have a 20-fold relative risk of also developing ASD [16] but also have an increased risk of developing ADHD. In a recently published study of such co-aggregation, it was shown that 5.3% of the ASD-affected probands had at least one sibling with an ADHD diagnosis, versus 1.5% of the non-ASD-affected probands (adjusted risk ratio 3.7) [17]. Another study showed that the prevalence of an ADHD diagnosis was 15% among dizygotic co-twins of children with ASD [13], while the most recent US estimates place the general population prevalence of ADHD between 5 and 8%. Similarly, higher ASD symptom levels have been reported in siblings of children with ADHD [18].

Regarding motor coordination, a majority of children with ASD manifest some degree of impairment [19], the severity of which has been found to be strongly correlated with the degree of social communication impairment [8, 20, 21]. This is extremely important, because the measurement of motor impairment is far less likely to be confounded with measurement of social impairment than might be the case for other behavioral comorbidities. To this effect, shared additive genetic influences of ASD and developmental coordination disorder (DCD) have been demonstrated previously, showing that ASD and DCD shared about 40% of their respective genetic influences and that about 30% of children with an ASD diagnosis also met the criteria for a DCD diagnosis [13]. Similarly, a clear overlap between ADHD and DCD was found; among children with ADHD, the prevalence of DCD was about 10 times higher compared to the general population, and a similarly heightened prevalence of ADHD was reported in children with DCD [13]. Other genetically informative studies have demonstrated that both ADHD symptoms and motor problems are highly heritable [22].

Finally, a separate body of research has explored neurodevelopmental correlates of the co-occurrence of ADHD symptoms and motor impairments, beginning with specific groups of clinically ascertained patients for whom the term "DAMP syndrome" (deficits in attention, motor proficiency, and perception) was coined [23]. These patients were found to have substantially higher frequencies of clinical-level autistic symptomatology compared to children in the general population or children with ADHD symptoms only [23, 24]. When these associations were tested within an epidemiologic sample (in a study that actually excluded patients with ASD), Reiersen and colleagues similarly demonstrated that co-occurrence of attention problems and motor coordination impairments was associated with substantially elevated autistic trait burden [25].

In this study, we capitalized upon a sibling design to conduct a first ever analysis determining whether ADHD symptoms and impairments in motor coordination, which are non-specific to ASD, nevertheless represent a source of additive genetic background liability for ASD, when in the presence of inherited ASD-specific risk conferred by the status of being a later-born sibling of an ASD-affected proband. To our knowledge, no prior study has examined the extent to which quantitative variation in these traits among siblings in ASD-affected families contributes to ASD recurrence.

Methods

Sample

In total, there were 307 males in the original study sample. In families with multiple individuals diagnosed with ASD, proband status was assigned to the older affected brother. Monozygotic twins of probands, individuals with trisomy-21 and Fragile X syndrome, individuals without data, and individuals falling outside of age limits of instruments were excluded. For families with multiple male siblings of an affected proband, selection of the sibling was based on the amount of data available, the sibling closest-in-age to the proband, or using a random number generator. The final number of children included in the study was 228: 114 males with a clinical diagnosis of ASD and 114 of their male siblings (one per family). All were participants in a study of quantitative autistic traits over the life course [26]. The probands were recruited by their physicians (between 2003 and 2005) from either (a) the Washington University Child and Adolescent clinics or (b) from outpatient child psychiatry practices in the greater St. Louis metropolitan area. Any child with an ASD diagnosis documented by an expert clinician and who had at least one brother was eligible for inclusion. Diagnostic status of affected children was confirmed using the Autism Diagnostic Interview-Revised (ADI-R) [27]. The mean age at enrollment was 6.9 years (range 3–16 years) for the brothers and 7.1 years (range 3–18) for probands. The sample was 89% Caucasian, 4% Hispanic, 4% Asian, 2% African-American, and 1% other or bi-racial. Of the 114 siblings, 26% (n = 29) also had an ASD diagnosis and 94% (n = 107) were verbal.

Measures
Autistic traits
Autistic traits were assessed using the Social Responsiveness Scale-2 (SRS-2) [28] by parent and teacher report. The SRS-2 is a 65-item measure of quantitative autistic traits (QAT), using a 4-point Likert scale (not true, sometimes true, often true, almost always true) for each item. The SRS-2 items encompass both of the DSM-5 criterion domains for ASD (social communication/interaction and restricted/repetitive patterns of behavior, interests, or activities). Scores on the SRS-2 have been found to be highly heritable [29–31], extremely stable over time [26], continuously distributed in the general population [30], exhibit a unitary factor structure [32], and distinguish children with autism spectrum conditions from those with other child psychiatric conditions [33]. The SRS-2 yields a total problem score, which has been empirically validated by factor, cluster, and latent class analyses [32]. In this study, raw SRS-2 total scores were converted to standardized T scores (mean 50, SD 10), where higher scores indicate greater impairment. The total score is truncated at the low end of the scales, so that a T score of 30 is the minimum obtainable. A total T score of 76 or higher is consistent with severe clinical-level symptomatology, a T score of 60 through 75 subclinical, and a T score of 59 or less as normal.

The SRS-2 was completed by 113 parents of siblings, 107 parents of probands, 107 teachers of siblings, and 107 teachers of probands. Raw scores were converted to T scores (mean 50, SD 10). Higher scores indicate greater impairment.

Attention-deficit/hyperactivity symptoms
Attention-deficit/hyperactivity symptoms were assessed by parent and teacher report, using the Achenbach System of Empirically Based Assessment (ASEBA) [34, 35]. In the Child Behavior Checklist (CBCL) and Teacher Report Form (TRF), the primary caregiver and teacher are asked to report on the behavior of the child in the preceding months, using a 3-point Likert scale (not true, somewhat or sometimes true, and very true or often true) for each item. The CBCL and TRF 1.5–5 consist of 99 items, the CBCL 6–18 of 113 items, and the TRF 6–18 of 115 items. All versions yield a total problem score as well as scores on syndrome scales and DSM-oriented scales. In this study, the extensively validated DSM-oriented Attention-Deficit/Hyperactivity Problems (ADHP) Scale score was used. Raw scores were converted to standardized T scores (mean 50, SD 10). Higher T scores indicate greater impairment. The problem score is truncated at the low end of the scale, so that a T score of 50 is the minimum obtainable. A T score between 65 and 70 on the DSM-oriented scales is considered borderline clinical and a score above 70 as clinical.

In total, 114 parents completed the ASEBA CBCL in siblings and probands. The ASEBA TRF was completed by 106 teachers of siblings and 113 teachers of probands.

Motor proficiency
The Developmental Coordination Disorder Questionnaire (DCDQ'07; revised 2007 edition) was completed by parents on a subset of siblings (n = 39) and probands (n = 44). Data was only available in a subset of participants because the collection of DCDQ data was added to the study protocol after a first wave of patients had already completed their follow-up. The DCDQ is a 15-item questionnaire that ascertains gross and fine motor skill impairments that would contribute to a diagnosis of DCD [36]. Moderate correlations have been found between DCDQ scores and other measures of motor proficiency and visual motor integration (Movement Assessment Battery for Children; r = 0.55) [37] and the Beery Test of Visual-Motor Integration (r = .42) [38], supporting the construct (convergent) validity of the DCDQ. A previous study has also shown a strong correlation (r = 0.79) between total DCDQ and total Bruininks-Oseretsky Test of Motor Proficiency, Second Edition (BOT-2) scores in families with ASD, suggesting that the DCDQ can be used as a reliable proxy for the measurement of motor impairment in this population [8]. High internal consistency and predictive, construct, and concurrent validity and good sensitivity and specificity have been reported for the DCDQ [36, 39]. The DCDQ yields a raw total score (score range 15–75) which was

age-adjusted and incorporated into the analyses of this study; higher scores indicate better motor functioning.

Data analysis

All analyses were performed using the IBM SPSS Statistics, version 20 [40].

For descriptive purposes, independent samples t tests were performed to compare trait distributions between affected and unaffected children, as well as between siblings and probands. To study the extent to which trait variation was associated within families, intraclass correlation coefficients (ICC; two-way mixed, absolute agreement, average measure) between siblings and probands in each pair were calculated. Furthermore, to show the relation between the various measures, nonparametric bivariate correlations were calculated in the siblings. Finally, since DCDQ data was only available in a subset of participants, we performed an independent samples t test comparing the individuals with and without available DCDQ data on the SRS QAT and CBCL/TRF ADHP scores to rule out potential selection bias.

Next, we performed statistical prediction models. First, we examined the extent to which *ASD diagnostic status* of siblings could be predicted exclusively by the level of their attention and motor problems; hierarchical binary logistic regression analyses were performed. Finally, to assess whether *quantitative variation in autistic trait severity* among siblings could be predicted by attention and motor problems, hierarchical linear regression analyses were performed. To isolate the effect of non-ASD-specific additive genetic background liability for ASD, both the logistic and linear statistical prediction models were corrected for severity of affectation of the proband (acting as a proxy for inherited ASD-specific risk).

Results

Descriptives

Table 1 shows the descriptives of the sample and provides a comparison between probands and (unaffected + affected) siblings. In supplemental Additional file 1: Table S1 (online), the descriptives are presented according to ASD affectation status, comparing probands, affected siblings, and unaffected siblings. The results in Additional file 1: Table S1 show that as expected, mean QAT scores were significantly higher in ASD-affected than in unaffected individuals, with an about 3 SD difference in mean scores as reported by parents, and a 2 SD difference in mean scores as reported by teachers (SRS T score SD = 10). Among ASD-affected individuals, the mean ADHP scores were about 0.8 SD higher, reported by both parents and teachers (CBCL/TRF T score SD = 10). Also, ASD-affected and ASD-unaffected individuals differed significantly on the DCDQ. We emphasize here that the mean ADHP and DCDQ scores for unaffected siblings were well within the normal range and in keeping with means for the general population [34–36].

To study the extent to which variation in the respective traits was associated within families, intra-class correlation coefficients (ICC) were calculated (Table 1). We observed sibling correlations (ICC) on the order of 0.13–0.32 for QAT and ADHP, consistent with established heritability estimates for each of these parameters of child development and the expected attenuation of such correlations when both clinically affected and non-affected family members are included. In supplemental Additional file 1: Table S2 (online), ICC values are depicted for ASD concordant and discordant sibling pairs separately. As expected, ICC values are significantly larger in concordant sibling pairs.

Finally, an independent samples t test was performed, comparing the individuals with and without available DCDQ data on the SRS QAT and CBCL/TRF ADHP scores to rule out selection bias. We found no significant differences in autistic trait severity (t (218) = 0.25 and p = 0.800 and t (212) = −1.25 and p = 0.212 for parent and teacher report, respectively) or ADHD severity (t (226) = 0.17 and p = 0.867 and t (217) = −1.03 and p = 0.306 for parent and teacher report, respectively) between participants with or without DCDQ data.

Figure 1 displays the trait distributions of the three different measures. Scores were continuously distributed for both probands and siblings for all measures, with substantial floor effects for ADHP scores, as expected from rating systems in which T scores are truncated. Similarly, DCDQ motor proficiency scores exhibited a ceiling effect among unaffected siblings. Substantial pathological shifts in the distribution of ADHD and motor proficiency scores were appreciable for the probands, as well as for ASD-affected siblings, but not for unaffected siblings.

Bivariate (Spearman) correlations were calculated (Table 2). Correlations are presented here exclusively for the siblings as a group (affected and unaffected), because these variables are being explored to predict recurrence and to offer the widest and most representative distribution of scores in which to examine trait correlations.

A strong positive correlation was found between the teacher-reported SRS-2 autistic trait score and that of parent-reported SRS-2 autistic traits (r = 0.70), indicating high cross-informant validity of the scores in this sample of affected and unaffected children. A concomitantly low level of parent-teacher agreement on ADHD traits and the general superiority of teacher ratings for these symptoms motivated prioritization of teacher-report ADHD ratings in our prediction model. Differentiating the source of information for prediction (teachers) versus outcome (parents, clinicians) for the respective behavioral

Table 1 Descriptive statistics

	Siblings (unaffected + affected)		Probands		t (p)	Cohen's d^a	ICC (p)^b
	n	Mean (SD)	n	Mean (SD)			
SRS-2 score							
Parent	113	53.1 (15.1)	107	75.7 (12.3)	12.1 (<0.001)	1.64	0.15 (0.027)
Teacher	107	55.1 (15.0)	107	68.3 (10.8)	7.4 (<0.001)	1.01	0.32 (0.002)
CBCL/TRF ADHP score							
Parent	114	55.9 (8.0)	114	62.0 (9.4)	5.3 (<0.001)	0.70	0.20 (0.071)
Teacher	106	55.4 (7.6)	113	60.2 (7.7)	4.7 (<0.001)	0.63	0.13 (0.196)
DCDQ score							
Parent	39	60.2 (15.9)	44	44.2 (14.0)	−4.9 (<0.001)	1.07	0.01 (0.486)
	n (%)		n (%)		χ^2 (p)		Φ^a
Clinical diagnosis					137.8 (<0.001)		0.78
Autism	14 (12.3)		34 (29.8)				
ASD	15 (13.1)		80 (70.2)				
No ASD	85 (74.6)		0 (0.0)				
Expressive language					2.6 (0.104)		0.11
Nonverbal	3 (2.6)		8 (7.0)				
Verbal	107 (93.9)		97 (85.1)				
Missing	4 (3.5)		9 (7.9)				
ADOS-2 classification							
Autism	–		70 (61.4)				
ASD	–		17 (14.9)				
Non-spectrum	–		13 (11.4)				
Missing	–		14 (12.3)				

For SRS-2, CBCL, and TRF, a higher score indicates more severe impairment. For DCDQ, a higher score represents better functioning. For the SRS-2, a T score of 30 is the minimum obtainable. A total T score of 76 or higher is consistent with severe clinical-level symptomatology, a T score of 60 through 75 subclinical, and a T score of 59 or less as normal. For the CBCL and TRF, a T score of 50 is the minimum obtainable. A T score between 65 and 70 is considered borderline clinical and a score above 70 as clinical

SRS-2 Social Responsiveness Scale-2 (T score), *CBCL/TRF ADHP* DSM-oriented Attention-Deficit/Hyperactivity Problems Scale (T score), from Child Behavior Checklist and Teacher Report Form, *DCDQ* Developmental Disorder Coordination Questionnaire (adjusted total score), *ASD* autism spectrum disorder

^{a}Effect sizes reported as Cohen's d for t tests and phi (φ) for chi-square tests, with 0.1 considered a small effect, 0.3 a medium effect, and 0.5 or higher a large effect
^{b}Intraclass correlation coefficients (ICC; two-way mixed, absolute agreement, average measure) are provided, calculated between siblings and probands in each pair, depicting variation within families

indices of ADHP and QAT minimized effects of rater bias and optimized validity and interpretation of regression analysis results.

Attention-deficit/hyperactivity and motor traits predicting ASD diagnosis

Hierarchical binary logistic regression analyses were performed to examine the extent to which a categorical ASD diagnosis in a sibling could be predicted by teacher-reported ADHD symptom scores and parent-reported motor proficiency scores, controlling for proband ASD severity (Table 3).

Proband SRS-2 autistic trait score alone (model 1) did not predict sibling ASD diagnosis (χ^2 (1) = 0.556, p = 0.456, Nagelkerke R^2 = 0.022). The model improved dramatically when sibling ADHP score was added

(model 2a), resulting in significant overall fit of the model (χ^2 (2) = 8.013, p = 0.018, Nagelkerke R^2 = 0.283) and an overall correctly classified percentage of 80%. The TRF ADHP score was an important and highly significant predictor of ASD status (OR = 1.15, p = 0.033), showing that for each unit increase in TRF ADHP T score, the odds of an ASD diagnosis was increased by 15%. When sibling DCDQ motor proficiency score was added first to proband autistic trait score (model 2b), the model also improved, resulting in significant overall fit of the model (χ^2 (2) = 14.308, p = 0.001, Nagelkerke R^2 = 0.464) and an overall correctly classified percentage of 80%. The DCDQ score was an important and highly significant predictor of ASD status (OR = 0.91, p = 0.003), showing that for each unit increase in DCDQ motor proficiency score, the odds of an ASD diagnosis was decreased

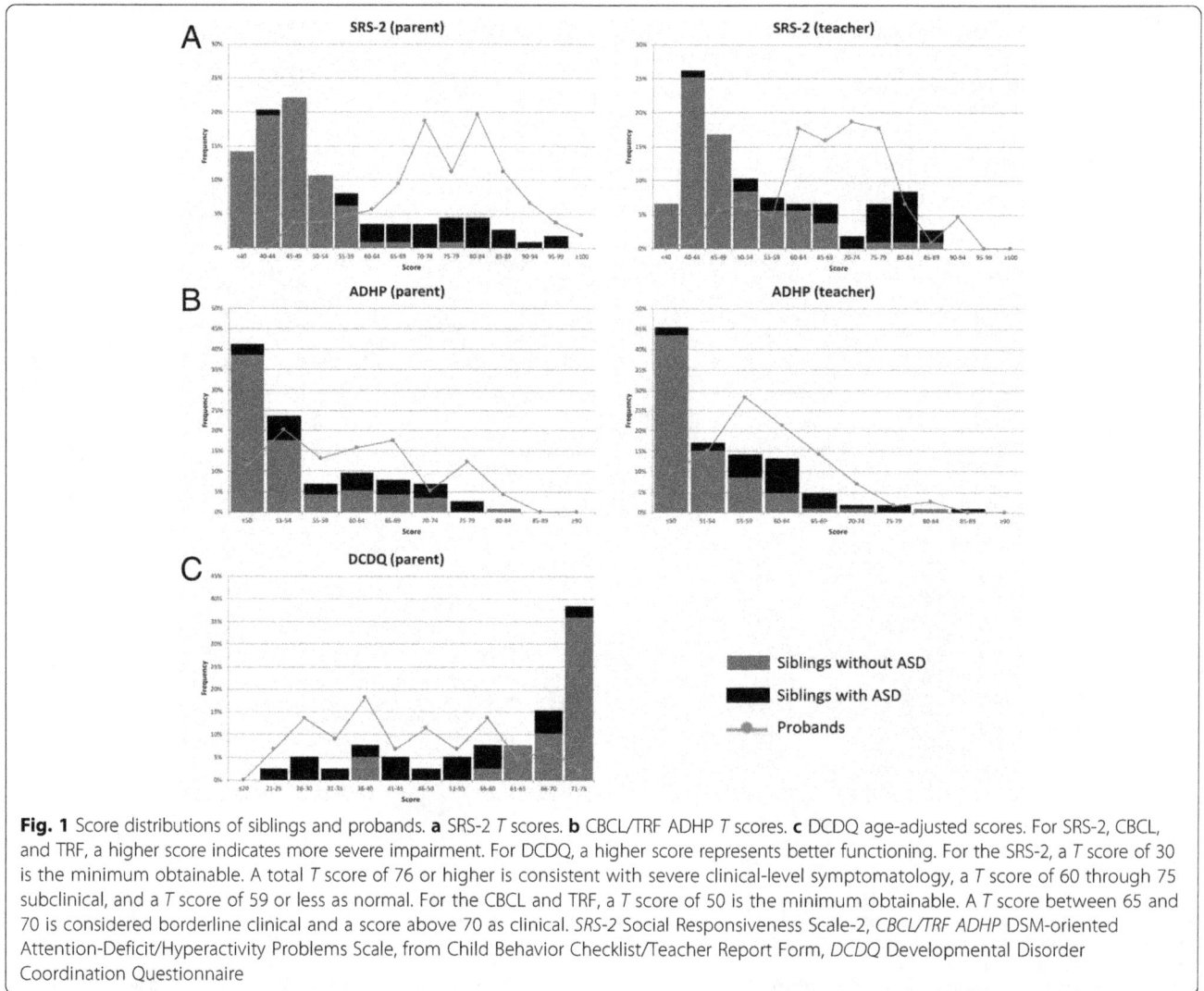

Fig. 1 Score distributions of siblings and probands. **a** SRS-2 *T* scores. **b** CBCL/TRF ADHP *T* scores. **c** DCDQ age-adjusted scores. For SRS-2, CBCL, and TRF, a higher score indicates more severe impairment. For DCDQ, a higher score represents better functioning. For the SRS-2, a *T* score of 30 is the minimum obtainable. A total *T* score of 76 or higher is consistent with severe clinical-level symptomatology, a *T* score of 60 through 75 subclinical, and a *T* score of 59 or less as normal. For the CBCL and TRF, a *T* score of 50 is the minimum obtainable. A *T* score between 65 and 70 is considered borderline clinical and a score above 70 as clinical. *SRS-2* Social Responsiveness Scale-2, *CBCL/TRF ADHP* DSM-oriented Attention-Deficit/Hyperactivity Problems Scale, from Child Behavior Checklist/Teacher Report Form, *DCDQ* Developmental Disorder Coordination Questionnaire

by 9%. When both sibling TRF ADHP and DCDQ motor proficiency scores were added (model 3), the model fit increased further (χ^2 (3) = 16.963, p = 0.001, Nagelkerke R^2 = 0.531) and an overall correctly classified percentage of 77% was achieved using these three variables. In this model, the DCDQ score (OR = 0.92, p = 0.010) was the most important predictor of ASD diagnostic status. To study potential interaction effects of the TRF ADHP score and the DCDQ score, analyses were repeated while adding an interaction term (model 4). Results show that the interaction term was insignificant and the model fit did not further improve (χ^2 (4) = 17.223, p = 0.002, Nagelkerke R^2 = 0.537). Finally, the analyses were repeated without the correction for proband ASD affectation severity

Table 2 Bivariate non-parametric (Spearman) correlations

	SRS-2 (parent)		SRS-2 (teacher)		CBCL ADHP (parent)		TRF ADHP (teacher)	
	r	*n*	*r*	*n*	*r*	*n*	*r*	*n*
SRS-2 (teacher)	0.70**	106						
CBCL ADHP (parent)	0.58**	113	0.42**	107				
TRF ADHP (teacher)	0.54**	105	0.70**	102	0.49**	106		
DCDQ (parent)	−0.65**	38	−0.56**	36	−0.33*	39	−0.54**	37

Note: siblings only. For SRS-2, CBCL, and TRF, a higher score indicates more severe impairment. For DCDQ, a higher score represents better functioning
SRS-2 Social Responsiveness Scale-2 (*T* score), *CBCL/TRF ADHP* DSM-oriented Attention-Deficit/Hyperactivity Problems Scale (*T* score), from Child Behavior Checklist and Teacher Report Form, *DCDQ* Developmental Disorder Coordination Questionnaire (adjusted total score)
*p < 0.05; **p < 0.01

Table 3 Logistic regression analyses predicting sibling diagnosis

	Model 1		Model 2a		Model 2b		Model 3		Model 4		Model 5	
	n = 35		n = 35		n = 35		n = 35		n = 35		n = 35	
	OR (95% CI)	p	OR (95% CI)	p	OR (95% CI)	p	OR (95% CI)	p	OR (95% CI)	p	OR (95% CI)	p
Proband SRS-2 score (teacher report)	1.02 (0.97–1.08)	0.461	1.02 (0.95–1.08)	0.609	1.01 (0.95–1.09)	0.729	1.02 (0.94–1.09)	0.678	1.02 (0.94–1.09)	0.678		
Sibling TRF ADHP score (teacher report)			1.15 (1.01–1.30)	0.033			1.09 (0.97–1.23)	0.144	1.09 (0.97–1.23)	0.159	1.09 (0.97–1.22)	0.155
Sibling DCDQ score (parent report)					0.91 (0.85–0.97)	0.003	0.92 (0.86–0.98)	0.010	0.92 (0.86–0.98)	0.013	0.92 (0.86–0.98)	0.009
TRF ADHP × DCDQ interaction									1.00 (0.98–1.01)	0.640		
Nagelkerke R^2	0.022		0.283		0.464		0.531		0.537		0.527	

Note: n = 35 for all models (only siblings with all data available were included). For SRS-2 and TRF, a higher score indicates more severe impairment. For DCDQ, a higher score represents better functioning

SRS-2 Social Responsiveness Scale-2 (T score), *TRF ADHP* DSM-oriented Attention-Deficit/Hyperactivity Problems Scale (T score), from Teacher Report Form, *DCDQ* Developmental Disorder Coordination Questionnaire (adjusted total score)

(model 5), showing the minimal contribution of this variable to the model as compared to model 3.

Supplemental analyses were performed including both teacher- and parent-reported ADHD measures. The fit of the complete model (including proband autistic trait severity, teacher- and parent-reported ADHD scores, and the motor proficiency score) was good (χ^2 (4) = 25.841, $p < 0.001$, Nagelkerke R^2 = 0.722), with an overall correctly classified percentage of 89% (Additional file 1: Table S3, online). Additional analyses with reversed reporters showed similar results to the original analyses (Additional file 1: Table S4, online). Also, similar results were found when analyses were repeated in the entire sample, thus not constrained to the set of participants with complete data (Additional file 1: Table S5, online). Finally, to study the specificity of our findings, analyses were repeated with the other available TRF DSM-oriented scales. The results showed that affective and oppositional defiant problems were also predictive of ASD diagnostic status, although less strong than ADHD problems (Additional file 1: Table S6, online).

Attention-deficit/hyperactivity and motor traits predicting autistic trait severity

Next, we examined the extent to which ADHP and DCDQ scores predicted quantitative autistic trait ratings among siblings of probands. We implemented hierarchical linear regression analyses in which sibling SRS-2 autistic trait severity (as reported by parents) was predicted by teacher-reported ADHP scores and parent-reported DCDQ motor proficiency score, controlling for teacher-reported proband SRS-2 autistic trait score (Table 4).

Again, proband SRS-2 autistic trait score alone (model 1) minimally accounted for sibling SRS-2 autistic trait severity (F (1.33) = 3.137, $p = 0.086$). When sibling TRF ADHP score was added to the model (model 2a), the model fit improved substantially (model 1 to 2a ΔR^2 = 0.204, $p = 0.005$). The overall model was significant (F (2.32) = 6575, $p = 0.004$) and explained 25% of the variance in SRS-2 autistic trait severity. In this model, the TRF ADHP score was a very strong predictor ($\beta = 0.45$, $p = 0.005$). When sibling DCDQ motor proficiency score was added first to proband SRS-2 autistic

Table 4 Linear regression analyses predicting parent-reported autistic trait severity in siblings

	Model 1		Model 2a		Model 2b		Model 3		Model 4		Model 5	
	n = 35		n = 35		n = 35		n = 35		n = 35		n = 35	
	β	p	β	p	β	p	β	p	β	p	β	p
Proband SRS-2 score (teacher report)	0.30	0.086	0.26	0.098	0.26	0.098	0.19	0.109	0.19	0.111		
Sibling TRF ADHP score (teacher report)			0.45	0.005			0.24	0.066	0.25	0.074	0.24	0.063
Sibling DCDQ score (parent report)					−0.68	<0.001	−0.60	<0.001	−0.60	<0.001	−0.62	<0.001
TRF ADHP × DCDQ interaction									0.03	0.793		
Adjusted R^2	0.059		0.247		0.517		0.554		0.540		0.530	

Note: n = 35 for all models (only siblings with all data available were included). For SRS-2 and TRF, a higher score indicates more severe impairment. For DCDQ, a higher score represents better functioning

SRS-2 Social Responsiveness Scale-2 (T score), *TRF ADHP* DSM-oriented Attention-Deficit/Hyperactivity Problems Scale (T score), from Teacher Report Form, *DCDQ* Developmental Disorder Coordination Questionnaire (adjusted total score)

trait score (model 2b), the model fit (F (2.32) = 19.200, $p < 0.001$) also improved significantly (models 1 to 2b ΔR^2 = 0.459, $p < 0.001$), explaining 52% of the variance in sibling SRS-2 autistic trait severity. When both sibling TRF ADHP score and DCDQ score were in the model (model 3), it appeared that adding the DCDQ score to the ADHP score significantly improved the model (models 2a to 3 ΔR^2 = 0.302, $p < 0.001$), while adding the ADHP score to the DCDQ score only marginally improved the model (models 2b to 3 ΔR^2 = 0.048, $p = 0.066$). The overall model fit including both sibling TRF ADHP score and DCDQ score was excellent (F (3.31) = 15.073, $p < 0.001$), and the proportion of explained variance showed that proband SRS-2 autistic trait score, sibling TRF ADHP score, and sibling DCDQ motor proficiency score jointly explained 55% of the variance in sibling SRS-2 autistic trait score. Again, the strongest predictor in this model was the DCDQ motor proficiency score (β = −0.60, $p < 0.001$). As in the logistic regression analyses, we also tested a model including the ADHP-by-DCDQ interaction term (model 4). Results show that the interaction term was insignificant and that the model fit decreased (F (4.30) = 10.983, $p < 0.001$, and models 3 to 4 ΔR^2 = 0.001, $p = 0.793$). A final analysis without correction for proband ASD affectation severity (model 5) again showed the minimal contribution of this variable to the model as compared to model 3.

Again, supplemental analyses were performed. First, analyses were repeated while both including teacher- and parent-reported ADHD measures, showing that up to 71% of the variance in autistic trait severity could be explained (Additional file 1: Table S7, online). Results remained similar to the original analyses when reversed reporters were used (Additional file 1: Table S8, online). When analyses were repeated in the entire sample, thus not constrained to the set of participants with complete data, all results remained identical (Additional file 1: Table S9, online). Also, the analyses were repeated exclusively predicting autistic trait severity in the unaffected siblings, and similar (but somewhat attenuated) results were found (Additional file 1: Table S10, online). Finally, specificity was studied, showing that affective and oppositional defiant problems were also predictive of autistic trait severity, although less strong than ADHD problems (Additional file 1: Table S11, online).

Discussion

In this contemporaneous analysis of symptom burden of non-ASD-specific neurodevelopmental traits and ASD recurrence in the siblings of affected probands, we observed that ADHD symptoms and motor coordination impairment jointly accounted for a large share of the variance (over 50%) in both categorical ASD recurrence

and quantitative trait severity. These findings in a clinical family cohort confirm observations from general population studies indicating that inattention/hyperactivity and motor coordination impairment—axes of behavioral development that exhibit trait-like stability, have been shown to be correlates of ASD symptomatology [41–45] and which were, *on average*, normal in the sibling group—account for approximately half of the variation in ASD recurrence, whether ascertained quantitatively or categorically, and controlling for the degree of ASD-specific background genetic liability indexed by the severity of affectation of the proband. Coupled with the observation of a lack of interaction effects between ADHD and motor coordination impairment, these findings suggest that ADHD and motor coordination impairments constitute contributors of additive risk for ASD, with motor coordination impairments adding the larger share.

This finding within a sibling design suggests that background ASD susceptibilities that are inherited but non-specific ("BASINS") may contribute additive genetic liability for autism in the same manner that ASD-specific susceptibilities (such as parental subclinical ASD traits and deleterious mutations) engender ASD risk. In this way, non-specific (genetic and environmental) influences may amplify the effect of ASD-specific susceptibility on autism severity (Fig. 2).

This particular role in contributing non-ASD-specific risk could potentially explain elements of "missing heritability" for autism and may help resolve *apparent* discrepancies between genetic epidemiologic (population-based) and molecular genetic (case–control) studies in estimating the extent of genetic overlap between autism and ADHD, since the latter depend upon disease-specific associations that reach a critical threshold of statistical significance and generally do not control for subclinical cross-trait aggregation among controls—the latter should be strongly considered for inclusion in future molecular genetic case–control studies.

It should be noted that BASINS are most likely not restricted to ADHD and motor impairments only; other non-ASD-specific phenotypes have also been associated with ASD diagnostic status and autistic trait severity. Furthermore, it should be noted that clinical scores on these non-ASD-specific measures may also arise from reciprocal influences of core ASD symptomatology on these traits over the course of early childhood development.

Beyond the issue of genetic overlap, these findings have important implications for the phenomenology of infant development and the clarification of early liabilities that might contribute to the development of autism. In recent studies of the early development of ASD among high-risk infant siblings of children with ASD, trajectories of delayed motor development have been shown to predict later ASD diagnosis [41–43]. Similarly,

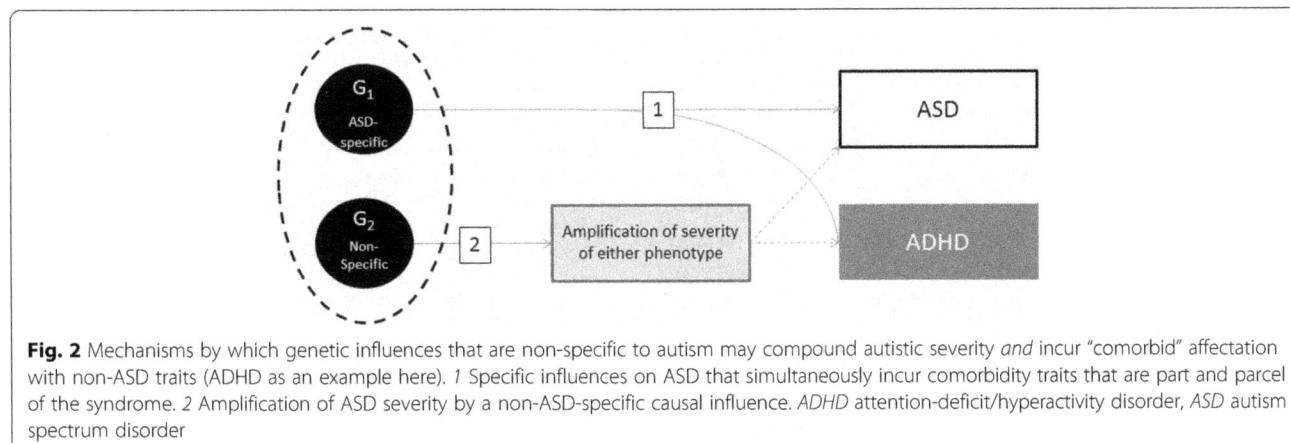

Fig. 2 Mechanisms by which genetic influences that are non-specific to autism may compound autistic severity *and* incur "comorbid" affectation with non-ASD traits (ADHD as an example here). *1* Specific influences on ASD that simultaneously incur comorbidity traits that are part and parcel of the syndrome. *2* Amplification of ASD severity by a non-ASD-specific causal influence. *ADHD* attention-deficit/hyperactivity disorder, *ASD* autism spectrum disorder

early abnormalities in visual social engagement predict ASD among high-risk infant siblings [44, 45]. Given the high prevalence of motor impairments and attention/hyperactivity problems in ASD, either or both might serve as important early targets for intervention, both with respect to reducing non-specific neurodevelopmental liabilities that may directly contribute to the syndrome (ASD) and to reducing so-called comorbidity in affected children. For example, studies have shown that developmental therapies targeted to the acquisition of motor skills may have broad-ranging positive effects on the development of executive functioning, reduce symptoms of inattention/hyperactivity, and improve social behavior [46, 47]. These and other findings strongly reinforce the clinical implication that children with any significant degree of ASD symptom burden or risk should be screened systematically for motor impairment and attention problems at the earliest juncture at which the respective conditions might be safely intervened and improved.

It remains unclear—and a potential clue to tracing the neural underpinnings of ASD—why the capacity for reciprocal social communication would track so closely with motor coordination and with variation in attention/hyperactivity. Although the timing of motor and attentional abnormalities makes it possible that they precede and contribute to the development of autistic symptomatology, the direction of effect between autism and these comorbidities cannot by any means be resolved by this study design, and this—along with the restriction of the available sample to males only—represents the most significant limitation of this study. Previous studies have construed motor impairment and ADHD symptomatology as "secondary comorbidities" to clinical ASD, but it is possible that ASD arises secondarily as a specific type of complication, decompensation, or epiphenomenon when a critical additive mass of neurodevelopmental liability compromises social maturation [48]. The fact that ADHD and motor coordination problems did not preferentially aggregate in the unaffected siblings of our ASD probands

(yet robustly predicted categorical and quantitative recurrence) raises the possibility that either (a) the direction of causation is actually from these secondary traits to ASD rather than the other way around or (b) a more fundamental developmental abnormality is responsible for the emergence of all three sets of correlated symptoms.

A further limitation of this study is that motor proficiency data were only available in a subset of participants, potentially attenuating the estimation of the true effect. Future, larger, prospective studies should examine these associations in a developmental context, which would allow for direction of causation to be more directly tested. Furthermore, our measures of ADHD symptoms and QAT were conducted by multi-informant questionnaire ratings rather than direct observation; we note however that the instruments used have been extensively validated and normed among many thousands of individuals in the general population [34, 35, 49, 50]. The use of independent informants minimized the effect of rater bias and optimized validity and interpretation of the results. Finally, although systematic measurements of IQ were not conducted in this study, only verbal, non-intellectually disabled siblings were eligible, and it has been well established that variation in QAT using the methods implemented in this study are unrelated to IQ within the normal range of variation in cognition in the general population [51].

Based on these and the previous findings, it will be important for the current generation of prospective studies of infant siblings of children with ASD to incorporate the evaluation of motor functioning and ADHD symptoms in longitudinal data collection. Relating early abnormalities in these functions to brain development, neurotransmitter systems, genetic variants, and other biomarkers may lend key insights into the biology of ASD.

Conclusions

To conclude, our findings in a clinical family cohort confirm observations from general population studies that inattention/hyperactivity and motor impairment—axes of behavioral development that are non-specific to ASD, and often appreciable before ASD is typically diagnosed—jointly account for over 50% of the variation in autistic impairment of siblings, whether ascertained quantitatively or categorically. This suggests that BASINS may contribute to additive genetic liability in the same manner that ASD-specific susceptibilities (such as parental subclinical ASD traits and deleterious mutations) engender ASD risk. Future biomarker and molecular genetic studies should strongly consider cross-trait ascertainment, particularly among controls, as a means of capturing "missing heritability" that might be tagged to genetic factors that are non-specific to ASD. Early interventions capable of improving or resolving early non-specific developmental liabilities that may contribute risk for ASD can be directly tested for their ability to ameliorate ASD severity, particularly among infants known to be at elevated risk.

Acknowledgements
The authors wish to thank the participating families for their generous investment of time and effort.

Funding
The research reported in this publication was supported by the Eunice Kennedy Shriver National Institute of Child Health & Human Development of the National Institutes of Health under award number U54 HD087011 to the Intellectual and Developmental Disabilities Research Center at Washington University. The content is solely the responsibility of the authors and does not necessarily represent the official views of the National Institutes of Health. Further financial support was provided by the Christopher Stephen and Johann Stephen Beimdiek Memorial Fund and the Sophia Children's Hospital Fund (Rotterdam, the Netherlands) under grant number SSWO B14-02 and through a Research Fellowship award.

Authors' contributions
SEM has contributed to the design of the study and the analysis and interpretation of the data and has written the manuscript. AJ has contributed to the design of the study and the analysis and interpretation of the data and has been involved in the drafting of the manuscript. AA has contributed to the design of the study and the interpretation of the data and has been involved in the revising of the manuscript. JNC has contributed to the conception and design of the study and the acquisition of the data and interpretation of the data and has been involved in drafting and revising of the manuscript. All authors have given final approval of the version to be published, have participated sufficiently in the work to take public responsibility for appropriate portions of the content, and have agreed to be accountable for all the aspects of the work in ensuring that questions related to the accuracy or integrity of any part of the work are appropriately investigated and resolved.

Competing interests
Dr. Constantino receives royalties from Western Psychological Services for commercial sales and distribution of the Social Responsiveness Scale-2. All other authors report no biomedical financial interests or potential conflicts of interest.

Author details
[1]Department of Child and Adolescent Psychiatry/Psychology, Sophia Children's Hospital, Erasmus Medical Center, Wytemaweg 80, 3015 CN Rotterdam, The Netherlands. [2]Division of Child Psychiatry, Department of Psychiatry, Washington University School of Medicine, 660 South Euclid Avenue, Campus Box 8504, St Louis, MO 63110, USA.

References
1. Constantino JN. The quantitative nature of autistic social impairment. Pediatr Res. 2011;69:55–62.
2. Robinson EB, Koenen KC, McCormick MC, Munir K, Hallett V, Happe F, et al. Evidence that autistic traits show the same etiology in the general population and at the quantitative extremes (5%, 2.5%, and 1%). Arch. Gen. Psychiatry. 2011;68:1113–21.
3. Constantino JN, Charman T. Diagnosis of autism spectrum disorder: reconciling the syndrome, its diverse origins, and variation in expression. Lancet Neurol. 2016;15:279–91.
4. Moreno-De-Luca A, Evans DW, Boomer KB, Hanson E, Bernier R, Goin-Kochel RP, et al. The role of parental cognitive, behavioral, and motor profiles in clinical variability in individuals with chromosome 16p11.2 deletions. JAMA Psychiat. 2015;72:119–26.
5. Lyall K, Constantino JN, Weisskopf MG, Roberts AL, Ascherio A, Santangelo SL. Parental social responsiveness and risk of autism spectrum disorder in offspring. JAMA Psychiat. 2014;71:936–42.
6. Antshel KM, Zhang-James Y, Faraone SV. The comorbidity of ADHD and autism spectrum disorder. Expert rev. Neurotherapeutics. 2013;13:1117–28.
7. Reiersen AM, Constantino JN, Volk HE, Todd RD. Autistic traits in a population-based ADHD twin sample. J Child Psychol Psychiatry. 2007;48:464–72.
8. Hilton CL, Zhang Y, Whilte MR, Klohr CL, Constantino J. Motor impairment in sibling pairs concordant and discordant for autism spectrum disorders. Autism. 2012;16:430–41.
9. Rommelse NNJ, Franke B, Geurts HM, Hartman CA, Buitelaar JK. Shared heritability of attention-deficit/hyperactivity disorder and autism spectrum disorder. Eur Child Adolesc Psychiatry. 2010;19:281–95.
10. Chung TK, Lynch ER, Fiser CJ, Nelson DA, Agricola K, Tudor C, et al. Psychiatric comorbidity and treatment response in patients with tuberous sclerosis complex. Ann Clin Psychiatry. 2011;23:263–9.
11. Garg S, Lehtonen A, Huson SM, Emsley R, Trump D, Evans DG, et al. Autism and other psychiatric comorbidity in neurofibromatosis type 1: evidence from a population-based study. Dev Med Child Neurol. 2013;55:139–45.
12. Niklasson L, Rasmussen P, Óskarsdóttir S, Gillberg C. Autism, ADHD, mental retardation and behavior problems in 100 individuals with 22q11 deletion syndrome. Res Dev Disabil. 2009;30:763–73.
13. Lichtenstein P, Carlström E, Råstam M, Gillberg C, Anckarsäter H. The genetics of autism spectrum disorders and related neuropsychiatric disorders in childhood. Am J Psychiatry. 2010;167:1357–63.
14. Cross-Disorder Group of the Psychiatric Genomics Consortium. Genetic relationship between five psychiatric disorders estimated from genome-wide SNPs. Nat Genet. 2013;45:984–94.
15. Musser ED, Hawkey E, Kachan-Liu SS, Lees P, Roullet JB, Goddard K, et al. Shared familial transmission of autism spectrum and attention-deficit/hyperactivity disorders. J Child Psychol Psychiatry. 2014;55:819–27.
16. Lauritsen MB, Pedersen CB, Mortensen PB. Effects of familial risk factors and place of birth on the risk of autism: a nationwide register-based study. J Child Psychol Psychiatry. 2005;46:963–71.
17. Jokiranta-Olkoniemi E, Cheslack-Postava K, Sucksdorff D, Suominen A, Gyllenberg D, Chudal R, et al. Risk of psychiatric and neurodevelopmental disorders among siblings of probands with autism spectrum disorders. JAMA Psychiat. 2016;73:622–9.
18. Nijmeijer JS, Hoekstra PJ, Minderaa RB, Buitelaar JK, Altink ME, Buschgens CJM, et al. PDD symptoms in ADHD, an independent familial trait? J Abnorm Child Psychol. 2009;37:443–53.
19. van Damme T, Simons J, Sabbe B, van West D. Motor abilities of children and adolescents with a psychiatric condition: a systematic literature review. World J Psychiatry. 2015;5:315–29.
20. Hilton C, Wente L, LaVesser P, Ito M, Reed C, Herzberg G. Relationship between motor skill impairment and severity in children with Asperger syndrome. Res Autism Spectr Disord. 2007;1:339–49.
21. Dziuk MA, Larson JCG, Apostu A, Mahone EM, Denckla MB, Mostofsky SH. Dyspraxia in autism: association with motor, social, and communicative deficits. Dev Med Child Neurol. 2007;49:734–9.
22. Fliers E, Vermeulen S, Rijsdijk F, Altink M, Buschgens C, Rommelse N, et al. ADHD and poor motor performance from a family genetic perspective. J Am Acad Child Adolesc Psychiatry. 2009;48:25–34.
23. Gillberg C. Deficits in attention, motor control, and perception: a brief review. Arch Dis Child. 2003;88:904–10.
24. Rasmussen P, Gillberg C. Natural outcome of ADHD with developmental coordination disorder at age 22 years: a controlled, longitudinal, community-based study. J Am Acad Child Adolesc Psychiatry. 2000;39:1424–31.

25. Reiersen AM, Constantino JN, Todd RD, Todd RD. Co-occurrence of motor problems and autistic symptoms in attention-deficit/hyperactivity disorder. J Am Acad Child Adolesc Psychiatry. 2008;47:662–72.

26. Constantino JN, Abbacchi AM, Lavesser PD, Reed H, Givens L, Chiang L, et al. Developmental course of autistic social impairment in males. Dev Psychopathol. 2009;21:127–38.

27. Lord C, Rutter M, Couteur AL. Autism diagnostic interview-revised: a revised version of a diagnostic interview for caregivers of individuals with possible pervasive developmental disorders. J Autism Dev Disord. 1994;24:659–85.

28. Constantino JN, Gruber CP. Social Responsiveness Scale, Second Edition (SRS-2). Torrance, CA: Western Psychological Services; 2012.

29. Constantino JN, Todd RD. Genetic structure of reciprocal social behavior. Am J Psychiatry. 2000;157:2043–5.

30. Constantino JN, Todd RD. Autistic traits in the general population: a twin study. Arch Gen Psychiatry. 2003;60:524–30.

31. Constantino JN, Todd RD. Intergenerational transmission of subthreshold autistic traits in the general population. Biol Psychiatry. 2005;57:655–60.

32. Constantino JN, Gruber CP, Davis S, Hayes S, Passanante N, Przybeck T. The factor structure of autistic traits. J Child Psychol Psychiatry. 2004;45:719–26.

33. Constantino JN, Przybeck T, Friesen D, Todd RD. Reciprocal social behavior in children with and without pervasive developmental disorders. J Dev Behav Pediatr. 2000;21:2–11.

34. Achenbach TM, Rescorla LA. Manual for the ASEBA School-Age Forms & Profiles. Burlington, VT: University of Vermont, Research Center for Children, Youth, & Families; 2001.

35. Achenbach TM, Rescorla LA. Manual for the ASEBA Preschool Forms & Profiles. Burlington, VT: University of Vermont, Research Center for Children, Youth, & Families; 2000.

36. Wilson BN, Crawford SG, Green D, Roberts G, Aylott A, Kaplan BJ. Psychometric properties of the revised Developmental Coordination Disorder Questionnaire. Phys Occup Ther Pediatr. 2009;29:182–202.

37. Henderson S, Sugden D. The movement assessment battery for children. London: The Psychological Corporation; 1992.

38. Beery K. The beery-Buktenica developmental test of visual-motor integration. 4th ed. Cleveland: Modern Curriculum Press; 1997.

39. Wilson B, Kaplan B, Crawford S, Campbell A, Dewey D. Reliability and validity of a parent questionnaire on childhood motor skills. Am J Occup Ther. 2000;54:484–93.

40. IBM Corp. IBM SPSS statistics for Macintosh, version 20.0. Armonk, NY: IBM Corp.; 2011.

41. Ozonoff S, Young GS, Belding A, Hill M, Hill A, Hutman T, et al. The broader autism phenotype in infancy: when does it emerge? J Am Acad Child Adolesc Psychiatry. 2014;53:398–407.

42. Landa RJ, Gross AL, Stuart EA, Bauman M. Latent class analysis of early developmental trajectory in baby siblings of children with autism. J Child Psychol Psychiatry. 2012;53:986–96.

43. Estes A, Zwaigenbaum L, Gu H, St John T, Paterson S, Elison JT, et al. Behavioral, cognitive, and adaptive development in infants with autism spectrum disorder in the first 2 years of life. J Neurodev Disord. 2015;7:24.

44. Jones W, Klin A. Attention to eyes is present but in decline in 2-6-month-old infants later diagnosed with autism. Nature. 2013;504:427–31.

45. Chawarska K, Macari S, Shic F. Decreased spontaneous attention to social scenes in 6-month-old infants later diagnosed with autism spectrum disorders. Biol Psychiatry. 2013;74:195–203.

46. Kamp CF, Sperlich B, Holmberg HC. Exercise reduces the symptoms of attention-deficit/hyperactivity disorder and improves social behaviour, motor skills, strength and neuropsychological parameters. Acta Paediatr. 2014;103:709–14.

47. Diamond A, Lee K. Interventions shown to aid executive function development in children 4 to 12 years old. Science. 2011;333:959–64.

48. Mahajan R, Dirlikov B, Crocetti D, Mostofsky SH. Motor circuit anatomy in children with autism spectrum disorder with or without attention deficit hyperactivity disorder. Autism Res. 2015;9:67–81.

49. Wigham S, McConachie H, Tandos J, Le Couteur AS. The reliability and validity of the social responsiveness scale in a UK general child population. Res Dev Disabil. 2012;33:944–50.

50. Bölte S, Poustka F, Constantino JN. Assessing autistic traits: cross-cultural validation of the social responsiveness scale (SRS). Autism Res. 2008;1:354–63.

51. Constantino JN, Lavesser PD, Zhang Y, Abbacchi AM, Gray T, Todd RD. Rapid quantitative assessment of autistic social impairment by classroom teachers. J Am Acad Child Adolesc Psychiatry. 2007;46:1668–76.

14

Reduced vagal tone in women with the *FMR1* premutation is associated with *FMR1* mRNA but not depression or anxiety

Jessica Klusek[1]* ⓘ, Giuseppe LaFauci[2], Tatyana Adayev[2], W. Ted Brown[3], Flora Tassone[4] and Jane E. Roberts[5]

Abstract

Background: Autonomic dysfunction is implicated in a range of psychological conditions, including depression and anxiety. The *fragile X mental retardation-1* (*FMR1*) premutation is a common genetic mutation that affects ~1:150 women and is associated with psychological vulnerability. This study examined cardiac indicators of autonomic function among women with the *FMR1* premutation and control women as potential biomarkers for psychological risk that may be linked to *FMR1*.

Methods: Baseline inter-beat interval and respiratory sinus arrhythmia (a measure of parasympathetic vagal tone) were measured in 35 women with the *FMR1* premutation and 28 controls. The women completed anxiety and depression questionnaires. *FMR1* genetic indices (i.e., CGG repeat, quantitative FMRP, *FMR1* mRNA, activation ratio) were obtained for the premutation group.

Results: Respiratory sinus arrhythmia was reduced in the *FMR1* premutation group relative to controls. While depression symptoms were associated with reduced respiratory sinus arrhythmia among control women, these variables were unrelated in the *FMR1* premutation. Elevated *FMR1* mRNA was associated with higher respiratory sinus arrhythmia.

Conclusions: Women with the *FMR1* premutation demonstrated autonomic dysregulation characterized by reduced vagal tone. Unlike patterns observed in the general population and in study controls, vagal activity and depression symptoms were decoupled in women with the *FMR1* premutation, suggesting independence between autonomic regulation and psychopathological symptoms that is atypical and potentially specific to the *FMR1* premutation. The association between vagal tone and mRNA suggests that molecular variation associated with *FMR1* plays a role in autonomic regulation.

Keywords: Fragile X carriers, Vagal tone, Heart rate, Physiological arousal, FMRP, *FMR1* mRNA

Background

The autonomic nervous system plays a fundamental role in health. Working in conjunction with other stress regulation systems, such as the hypothalamic-pituitary-adrenal axis and the immune system, the autonomic nervous system promotes adaptability to life stressors while helping the body maintain a well-controlled, functional physiological state [1]. Optimally, the sympathetic ("fight or flight") and parasympathetic ("rest and digest") branches of the autonomic nervous system work together in a coordinated and often antagonistic fashion to effectively respond to internal and external demands. When the dynamic interplay between the sympathetic and parasympathetic nervous systems is functioning well, the autonomic system serves a broad protective role, boosting the immune system, shielding against cardiovascular disease, and warding away psychopathology [2]. Conversely, dysfunction of the autonomic nervous system is associated with vulnerability to a host of physical and mental health disorders.

* Correspondence: klusek@mailbox.sc.edu
[1]Department of Communication Sciences and Disorders, University of South Carolina, Keenan Building, Suite 300, Columbia, SC 29208, USA
Full list of author information is available at the end of the article

The integrity of the autonomic system can be assessed objectively and non-invasively through peripheral measures of cardiac activity. The heart is innervated by the vagal nerve, which provides a pathway for brain-heart communication via connections in the brainstem and the sinoatrial node of the heart. The measurement of inter-beat interval (IBI; or the time between consecutive heart beats) provides an estimate of general arousal level influenced by both sympathetic and parasympathetic branches of the autonomic system [3]. A specific index of parasympathetic activity can be obtained by measuring heart rate variability patterns, which index parasympathetic influences on the heart via the vagal nerve [4]. Vagal tone can be estimated through descriptive measures of heart rate variability, as well as through the quantification of respiratory sinus arrhythmia (RSA), a measure of variability in the rise and fall of heart rate that occurs with respiration (see [5], for review).

Cardiac autonomic dysregulation in mood and anxiety disorders

Converging empirical and theoretical evidence supports cardiac autonomic indices as objective, non-invasive markers for mood and anxiety disorders (e.g., [6–9]). Dampened vagal tone is well documented in a major depressive disorder [10–13], and vagal level has also been shown to correlate with the continuous distribution of depression symptoms in non-clinical samples (e.g., [10, 14–16]). A number of reports demonstrate that depressed individuals with low vagal tone have greater symptom severity [17] and are less likely to recover or demonstrate symptomatic improvement [18, 19], and successful treatment for depression corresponds with vagal increases [20–22], albeit with some mixed findings (e.g., [23, 24]). Reduced cardiac vagal tone is also thought to represent a physiological pathway leading to anxiety. Low vagal tone relates to anxiety symptoms in non-clinical groups [25–27], and low vagal tone has been documented extensively among individuals with anxiety disorders, including populations affected by generalized anxiety disorder, panic disorder, and post-traumatic stress disorder (see [8, 9] for review).

Psychophysiological theories of vagal tone, such as the Polyvagal Theory [28, 29] and the Neurovisceral Integration Model [30, 31], support the integral role of the parasympathetic vagal system in emotional expression and regulation, accounting for reduced vagal level in mood and anxiety disorders—clinical conditions characterized by impaired emotional regulation [32]. A large body of literature suggests a mechanistic role of vagal tone in emotional regulation, coping, and social engagement [33, 34]. According to theory, vagal control is one component of a larger central autonomic network that serves to regulate defensive social behavior. The parasympathetic vagal system, in conjunction with other mechanisms, works to inhibit sympatho-excitatory threat circuits. When the vagal system is hypoactive, the body remains in a state of hypermobilization and defense, which increases "allostatic load," or wear and tear to the bodily system over time [35]. The ability to inhibit threat circuits via the vagus is compromised in disorders of impaired emotional regulation, such as anxiety and depression (see [36]).

Cardiac indices as biomarkers for psychological risk

The identification of biomarkers holds promise for furthering the prevention and treatment for complex mental health conditions such as anxiety and depression. Biomarkers, or measurable, endogenous traits that mark either the risk or manifestation of psychiatric illness [37], allow clinical groups to be deconstructed at the biological level, thus yielding information relevant to (1) the development of treatments targeted towards core mechanisms rather than symptoms, (2) the stratification of biological subgroups who are mostly likely to respond to targeted interventions, and (3) the identification of individuals who are most at risk, perhaps even before the onset of clinical symptoms [38]. A number of prior studies have put forth cardiac indicators of autonomic dysfunction as potentially useful biomarkers for anxiety and depression (e.g., [39, 40]) given that they co-occur with the clinical presentation of mood and anxiety disorders, are associated with symptoms in non-clinical samples, represent heritable and stable traits, are quantitative, and can be measured non-invasively and relatively quickly [41–44]. Thus, the study of cardiac activity in relation to depression and anxiety may prove useful in understanding the biological bases of these mental health conditions.

The *FMR1* premutation as a genetic model for psychological risk

Studying cardiac function within high-risk genetic groups can inform the intercorrelation between psychophysiological traits and unique genetic profiles. In this regard, the *fragile X mental retardation-1* (*FMR1*) premutation represents a particularly promising condition for study. This genetic condition is linked with significant psychological risk and may hold promise for uncovering genetic determinants for autonomic alterations. The *FMR1* premutation occurs when the trinucleotide (CGG) sequence on the *FMR1* gene of the X chromosome expands to 55–200 repeats [45]. This mutation is characterized by excess production of *FMR1* messenger RNA (mRNA), which causes neuronal toxicity [46–48]. The *FMR1* premutation expansion is highly prevalent, occurring in approximately 1 in 113–250 females and 1 in 250–810 males depending on ethnicity and world region [49–53]. Individuals with the *FMR1* premutation are at risk for passing the mutated gene to their children, which may undergo further expansions as it is transmitted through generations, increasing the severity of the disease. Risk for generational expansion is related to genetic factors such as CGG repeat size and the number of AGG anchors, as well as environmental factors such as maternal age [54, 55]. When the expansion extends beyond 200 CGG repeats, the gene becomes inactivated by methylation and fragile X syndrome results, a neurodevelopmental disorder affecting approximately 1 in 5000 individuals [56] that is associated with intellectual disability and autism spectrum disorder [57]. The present study focuses on women with the *FMR1* premutation, who show a well-documented psychological profile characterized by risk for depression and anxiety disorders. Research focused on women—and in particular mothers—with the *FMR1* premutation is important given that the *FMR1* premutation phenotype is associated with negative outcomes both for the affected individual as well as for their children with fragile X syndrome (e.g., [58, 59]).

Women with the *FMR1* premutation, referred to as "carriers" of fragile X, were once thought to be clinically unaffected; however, new evidence clearly supports clinical involvement in this group [60]. This includes risk for fragile X-specific conditions such as fragile X-associated primary ovarian insufficiency [61] and fragile X-associated tremor/ataxia syndrome (FXTAS), a late-onset neurodegenerative movement disorder characterized by tremors, gait ataxia, peripheral neuropathy, executive dysfunction, and cognitive decline that affects about 16% of women with the premutation [62]. A subset of women with the premutation may also present with certain cognitive deficits related to executive functioning, working memory [63], and symptoms of attention deficit-hyperactivity disorder [64], which may worsen with age [65, 66]. Social difficulties have also been documented in females with the *FMR1* premutation, such as social-language deficits [58, 67] and elevated rates of autism spectrum disorder [68]. Finally, a higher rate of immune-mediated disorders, sleep apnea, hypertension, migraines, and seizures has also been observed in individuals with the premutation (reviewed in [69]).

Psychological risk in the FMR1 premutation

Elevated rates of mood and anxiety disorders are one of the earliest and most consistently documented features of the *FMR1* premutation phenotype, with the risk for these conditions increasing significantly over time during adulthood [70]. Reported lifetime rates of major depressive disorder range from 12 to 54% in females with the premutation [70–75]. Lifetime rates of any anxiety disorder ranges from 25 to 47% [72, 74, 76]. This includes elevated lifetime rates of panic disorder [74, 75], social phobia [72, 74], and post-traumatic stress disorder [74]; although, findings vary somewhat depending on sample

characteristics and diagnostic instruments. Reported rates for current occurrence range from 5 to 13% for major depressive disorder [70, 75] and 13 to 50% for anxiety disorders [75–77].

Psychological risk in women with the *FMR1* premutation likely has a multifactorial basis, with both *FMR1* gene dysfunction and environmental factors, such as child-related challenges, mechanistically implicated in an additive or interactive manner. Chronic stressors associated with raising a child with a developmental disorder, such as elevated child problem behaviors, are linked to increased likelihood of anxiety disorders and major depression in women with the *FMR1* premutation [75, 78]. Yet, mental health problems in women with the *FMR1* premutation often proceed the birth of their child with fragile X syndrome [75] and women with the *FMR1* premutation who do not have a child affected by fragile X syndrome also show increased rates of psychological disorders [79], supporting genetic contributors to psychopathological risk that are independent of child-related stressors. Studies have begun to characterize specific *FMR1* genetic markers associated with psychiatric symptoms. A number of reports have documented that risk for depression in the *FMR1* premutation is highest among individuals with CGG repeat length within the midsize range [70, 75, 80, 81]. Seltzer et al. [81] also detected CGG-dependent sensitivity to the environmental context, where women with midsize CGG repeat length and above-average life stress showed greater vulnerability for depression and anxiety compared to women with higher or lower repeat lengths, whereas women with midsize CGG repeats and below-average life stress were the most resilient to depression and anxiety.

Psychological vulnerability may also be related to increased *FMR1* mRNA expression, which is present at up to eightfold normal levels and increases linearly with CGG repeat size in the premutation [82, 83]. Elevated mRNA levels were found to be associated with increased psychological symptoms and reduced amygdala activation in males with the premutation, and these associations were present even among male carriers without FXTAS, suggesting that the impact of mRNA toxicity is not exclusive to FXTAS [84, 85]. Levels of mRNA are also linked with the age of depression onset in individuals with the *FMR1* premutation, consistent with the hypothesis that mRNA toxicity builds over time, contributing to vulnerability [86]. Females may be more protected from mRNA toxicity, due to the presence of the second X chromosome. In females, a high activation ratio, or a high proportion of cells carrying the normal allele on the active X chromosome, can dilute the effects of the premutation allele [87] and has been associated with less severe clinical effects, such as lower parenting stress [88] and more typical patterns of cortisol stress responses [89]. Higher levels of mRNA are correlated with self-reported anxiety symptoms among women with the premutation, but only when the sample was restricted to women with an activation ratio of less than 0.5 [84].

Slightly reduced levels of fragile X mental retardation protein (FMRP) have also been reported among individuals with the *FMR1* premutation, particularly among individuals with high CGG repeats [90, 91]. FMRP is an mRNA-binding protein that regulates the translation of about one-third of the proteins in the pre- and post-synaptic proteomes, supporting its critical role in synaptic plasticity and the development and maintenance of neuronal circuits [92]. Its absence is thought to underlie the neurobehavioral impairments seen in the full mutation [93]. Yet, the phenotypic impact of reduced FMRP in the *FMR1* premutation is less clear. Until recently, FMRP level has been measured indirectly (e.g., by counting the percent of FMRP-positive lymphocytes, see [94]), limiting the ability to capture subtle variation in protein expression. No relationships have been detected between the percentage of lymphocytes staining positive for FMRP and psychological symptoms in males or females with the *FMR1* premutation [84]. However, new technological advances, such as the approach used in the present study, allow for quantitative measurement of actual FMRP levels in the blood and may lead to a new wave of discoveries into the role of FMRP in the clinical profile of the *FMR1* premutation. For instance, studies using quantitative FMRP have revealed relationships with neurobehavioral profiles, such as preliminary evidence of FMRP-mediated blunted amygdala responses that are associated with deficient social information processing in men [85].

Despite the documented links between *FMR1*-related variation and depression in the *FMR1* premutation, a number of studies have failed to detect molecular genetic correlates of anxiety in this group [70, 72, 77, 84, 86, 95, 96] and extant findings suggest a complex, multifactorial, epigenetic basis to anxiety symptom expression. Anxiety in women with the premutation has been linked with environmental factors such as child problem behaviors [75], with the impact of the stress of raising a child with fragile X syndrome moderated by variation on *CRHR1*, a gene involved in cortisol regulation [97]. Epigenetic changes associated with abnormal methylation have also been implicated, with one study showing that methylation of the CpG10-12 sites located at the *FMR1* intron 1 boundary predicted social anxiety with 92% sensitivity in women with the *FMR1* premutation [98]. Finally, anxiety in women with the premutation has been linked with neuroanatomical changes, specifically, with reduced hippocampal volume associated with elevated mRNA [99].

Autonomic function in the *FMR1* premutation

Given the elevated risk for depression and anxiety in the *FMR1* premutation and documented associations with

FMR1-associated genetic mechanisms, the *FMR1* premutation may represent a "portal" condition that can yield important information on the molecular genetic basis for autonomic alterations relevant to both individuals with and without *FMR1* mutations. This work may also inform prevention and treatment efforts specific to the *FMR1* premutation. The lack of useful biomarkers represents a critical barrier to targeted treatment for this group, given the incomplete penetrance of associated clinical effects. Should cardiac indicators account for inter-individual variability in psychological risk within this population, they may prove useful in identifying vulnerable subgroups who may benefit from targeted prevention efforts.

Although cardiac autonomic dysregulation is a robust, well-documented feature of fragile X syndrome (see [100], for review), no studies have examined cardiac autonomic integrity in the *FMR1* premutation. Yet, the clinical effects of the *FMR1* premutation are highly suggestive of autonomic impairment, such as increased rates of thyroid disorders, fibromyalgia, and hypertension—all conditions associated with autonomic dysfunction [101]. Moreover, symptoms consistent with autonomic dysfunction are common in FXTAS such as impotence, bowel and bladder incontinence, hypertension, and syncope [102]. Neuropathological involvement in the autonomic ganglion of the heart and autonomic neurons of the spinal cord has also been detected in postmortem studies of individuals with FXTAS [103, 104]. In the only study to date that employed direct measures of autonomic function in the premutation, Hessl and colleagues [105] detected dampened sympathetic reactivity to a social greeting task among a sample of 12 men with the premutation using measures of electrodermal response. No associations were detected between sympathetic activation and psychological symptoms or *FMR1* molecular measures (CGG repeat size and mRNA); although, conclusions were preliminary given the small sample.

The present study

Further investigation of autonomic nervous system activity among individuals with the *FMR1* premutation will help identify biophysiological pathways rooted in *FMR1* gene dysfunction, shedding light on biomarkers that may be linked with clinical impairment in this group. This work has implications for the identification of at-risk individuals based on specific biological markers and the potential to shift treatment efforts away from symptom-based approaches to target specific underlying mechanisms. In sum, investigations into cardiac indicators of autonomic function may provide insight into the intermediate functions of the *FMR1* gene that are coupled with psychological risk. The present study addressed the following questions:

1. Do cardiac markers of autonomic function (i.e., IBI and RSA) differ between women with the *FMR1* premutation and control women at baseline? *It was hypothesized that women with the FMR1 premutation would have elevated general arousal and reduced vagal tone when compared to controls, mirroring the physiological profile seen in the full mutation.*

2. Are cardiac markers of autonomic function related to symptoms of depression and anxiety among women with the *FMR1* premutation and control women? *It was hypothesized that low baseline vagal tone and high general arousal would relate to increased psychological symptoms in both groups.*

3. Are cardiac markers of autonomic function associated with *FMR1*-related genetic variation in women with the *FMR1* premutation? *Given the lack of prior research in this area, this aim was considered exploratory and specific hypotheses regarding gene-autonomic relationships were not made.*

Methods

Participants

Participants included 35 women with the *FMR1* premutation and 28 control women who were enrolled in a larger study of the social-language phenotype of women with the *FMR1* premutation. Inclusionary criteria for the broader study specified that all participants were native speakers of English, were mothers, and did not have an intellectual disability (i.e., IQ composite >80 on the Kaufman Brief Intelligence Test-II; [106]). Women who were pregnant were excluded from the study to control for pregnancy-related physiological changes (e.g., [107]). The women with the *FMR1* premutation were recruited through their children, who were participating in developmental studies of children with fragile X syndrome (PI's: Abbeduto, Roberts). Genetic status of the women with the *FMR1* premutation was confirmed through blood tests collected through this study ($n = 31$) or via medical records. The premutation was defined as an allele ranging from 55 to 200 CGG repeats on *FMR1*. Although it was beyond the scope of the present study to conduct genetic testing on control participants, 61% of controls completed genetic testing to rule out the *FMR1* premutation through dual enrollment in a related study. Control women had no known family history of fragile X-associated conditions and were mothers of typically developing children (i.e., children who had not been diagnosed or treated for any type of developmental delay or disorder, per participant report). Additionally, control women were excluded from the study if their child scored above the cut-off for autism spectrum disorder on the Social Communication Questionnaire [108]. Recruitment of controls was focused in the local community using flyers, social media, and word of mouth.

Descriptive and demographic information is presented in Table 1. The groups did not differ significantly on age, IQ, race, or household income. A higher proportion of women with the *FMR1* premutation were using psychotropic medications compared to the control women (48 vs 15%, $p = 0.008$). While the presence FXTAS was not an exclusionary criteria, none of the women reported a clinical diagnosis of FXTAS. The groups did not differ in self-reported functional symptoms of tremor measured

Table 1 Group characteristics

Variable	Group		
	Women with the *FMR1* Premutation ($n = 35$)	Control Women ($n = 28$)	Test of group differences (p value)
Age in years			
M (SD)	44.31(8.63)	41.70 (9.34)	0.251
Range	25.53–60.94	28.72–65.23	
IQ[a]			
M (SD)	104.26 (11.90)	104.57 (11.46)	0.928
Range	81.00–130.00	83.00–135.00	
Race			0.181
Caucasian	94%	85%	
African American	3%	15%	
American Indian	3%	–	
Household Income			
<20k	9%	12%	0.164
21–40k	12%	7%	
41–80k	33%	35%	
81–120k	12%	30%	
>121k	34%	11%	
Medication use			
Atypical antipsychotics	3%	–	0.008*
Classical antipsychotics	3%	–	
Antidepressants	48%	15%	
Mood stabilizers	7%	–	
Anti-anxiety	10%	–	
Stimulants	3%	4%	
Total stress percentile[b]			0.001*
M (SD)	62.12 (22.87)	34.64 (25.63)	
Range	4.00–96.00	1.00–88.00	
Tremor Disability Score[c]			0.508
M (SD)	4.30 (15.29)	2.06 (4.15)	
Range	0–77.42	0–12.90	

[a]Measured with the Kaufmann Brief Intelligence Test-II [106]
[b]Measured with the Parenting Stress Inventory-4 [112]
[c]Potential scores range from 0 to 100, with higher scores denoting greater functional disability associated with tremor
*$p < 0.05$

with the Tremor Disability Questionnaire [109], $p = 0.508$. Information on menopause status was also collected from the women with the *FMR1* premutation, as autonomic changes are observed among postmenopausal women (e.g., [110]) and the *FMR1* premutation is linked with early menopause [111]. Fifty-eight percent of the women in the *FMR1* premutation group had completed menopause, defined here as the cessation of menses for >1 year. Finally, the Parenting Stress Inventory-4 [112] was administered, given the reported relationships between parenting stress and maternal psychological health in other disability groups (e.g., [113]). Parenting stress was significantly elevated in the *FMR1* premutation group ($p = 0.001$).

Procedures

Assessments took place in a university laboratory setting. Baseline cardiac activity was the first assessment activity completed after consent was obtained. To control for the potential influences of circadian rhythm, assessments were conducted in the morning (generally starting at 9:00 a.m.). Participants were asked to refrain from drinking coffee for at least 1 h prior to the assessment. Procedures were approved by the Institutional Review Board of the University of South Carolina.

Measures
Cardiac autonomic activity

Cardiac activity was sampled during a 5-min baseline context where participants viewed a video of ocean waves that was designed for meditation and relaxation. Participants were instructed to "sit back and try to relax." Data were analyzed from the final 3 min of viewing, which allowed additional time for participants to "settle into" the task. Cardiac data were collected with an Actiwave Cardio monitor (CamNtech Ltd., Cambridge, UK), which samples activity via two electrodes placed on the participant's chest and internally records the ECG signal. Data were sampled at a rate of 1024 Hz. The IBI series was extracted from the ECG signal using QRSTool [114] with a threshold detection method. CardioEdit software (Brain-Body Center, University of Illinois at Chicago) was then used to edit artifacts and arrhythmias (<5%). Mean values for RSA and IBI were then extracted using CardioBatch software (Brain-Body Center, University of Illinois at Chicago). Briefly, CardioBatch samples sequential heart periods in 250 ms epochs and uses a 21-point moving polynomial algorithm to de-trend the data [115, 116]. The data are then bandpass filtered to extract variance associated with spontaneous breathing parameters (0.12–0.40 Hz), and RSA is estimated by transforming the variance to its natural logarithm. RSA and IBI were measured from 30 s epochs and then averaged for a total mean across the 3-min baseline period.

Depression symptom severity

Participants completed the Beck Depression Inventory-II [117], which is a 21-item questionnaire measuring self-reported symptoms of depression occurring over the last 2 weeks. Items are designed to reflect the defining symptoms of major depressive disorder as outlined in the Diagnostic and Statistical Manual for Mental Health Disorders [118] and are tallied to create a continuous index of depression symptom severity. The Beck depression inventory-II (BDI-II) demonstrates high test-retest reliability, internal consistency, and validity estimates (e.g., [119–121]). Nine women with the *FMR1* premutation obtained a score of 14 or higher on the BDI-II, which is considered indicative of clinical depression; no control women scored within this range.

Anxiety symptom severity

The Beck Anxiety Inventory [122] measured self-reported generalized anxiety symptoms occurring over the past week. This 21-item questionnaire provides a total score reflecting anxiety symptom severity, aligning with the criteria outlined in the Diagnostic and Statistical Manual for Mental Health Disorders [118]. The Beck anxiety inventory (BAI) has high internal consistency, adequate test-retest reliability, and evidence supporting convergent and discriminant validity [123, 124]. Scores above 9 are considered indicative of clinically significant anxiety; 12 women with the *FMR1* premutation and 3 control women scored above this cut-off.

FMR1 molecular measures

Genomic DNA was isolated from peripheral blood lymphocytes using standard methods (Qiagen, Valencia, CA). CGG repeat length was determined using polymerase chain reaction (PCR) and Southern Blot, as previously described [125, 126]. Activation ratio, or the percent of cells carrying the normal allele on the active X chromosome, was measured using an Alpha Innotech FluorChem 8800 Image Detection System [87]. Total RNA was isolated from 3 mL of blood collected in PAXgene® tubes. To determine the relative expression levels of the *FMR1* gene, qRT-PCR amplification was carried out on total RNA using custom-designed Taqman gene expression assays, for both the validated target *FMR1* gene and the reference genes (β-glucoronidase) in a 7900 Sequence detector (Applied Biosystems, Foster City, CA) as detailed in [87]. A quantitative index of FMRP was obtained by using a capture Luminex-based immunoassay to determine the amount of FMRP in peripheral blood lymphocytes (expressed in pg/ug of total lysate). This assay has been shown to have high accuracy with dried blood spots, peripheral lymphocytes, brain, and other human tissues [127, 128].

Data analysis

Analyses were conducted in SAS 9.4 [129]. The data were first examined for normality. Skewedness was detected for several variables; the Box-Cox transformation [130] was applied to find the optimal normalizing transformation for IBI ($\lambda = -0.50$), depression symptoms on the BDI-II ($\lambda = 0$), anxiety symptoms on the BAI ($\lambda = -0.25$), CGG repeat length ($\lambda = 0$), activation ratio ($\lambda = 1.50$), and mRNA ($\lambda = -1.50$); the data were transformed accordingly. The remaining variables were normally distributed and did not require transformation. Transformed values were used in all analyses. Descriptive statistics were computed and are presented in Tables 2 and 3. To explore potential confounds related to menopause status, t tests examined differences in the cardiac indices between the subgroups of pre- and postmenopausal women. Mean RSA and IBI did not differ by menopause status in the women with the FMR1 premutation (p's >0.172). Information on menopause status was not available for the control participants.

To test the first research question, general linear regression models tested group as a predictor of IBI and RSA. Covariates in the models included age, medication use (captured as the total number of psychotropic medications used), and parenting stress level (indexed by the total stress percentile on the Parenting Stress Inventory-4 [112]); these variables have been shown to influence cardiac functioning in prior work [27, 131–133]. Cohen's d effect sizes were computed for group differences [134]. In general, effect sizes of 0.32 or less are interpreted as "small," 0.33–0.55 "medium," and 0.56–1.20 "large" [135]. Then, a series of general linear models tested each of the cardiac variables, group, and their interaction as predictors of depression and anxiety symptoms, after controlling for age, medication use, and parenting stress level. False discovery was controlled by adjusting at the level of the

Table 2 Descriptive statistics

Variable	Group	
	FMR1 premutation	Control
IBI (untransformed) M (SD), range	816.20 (131.11), 540.27–1135.33	791.58 (137.04), 577.93–1193.69
IBI (transformed) M (SD), range	1.93 (0.01), 1.91–1.94	1.93 (0.01), 1.91–1.94
RSA M (SD), range	4.82 (1.44), 1.78–7.64	5.56 (0.97), 3.24–7.26
BDI-II (untransformed) M (SD), range	10.97 (7.84), 0–33.00	4.07 (3.66), 0–13.00
BDI-II (transformed) M (SD), range	2.56 (0.58), 1.39–3.61	1.99 (0.44), 1.38–2.83
BAI (untransformed) M (SD), range	7.96 (6.79), 0–24.00	3.72 (5.29), 0–23.00
BAI (transformed) M (SD), range	1.73 (0.35), 1.17–2.26	1.49 (0.29), 1.17–2.25

IBI inter-beat interval, RSA respiratory sinus arrhythmia, BDI-II Beck Depression Inventory, BAI Beck Anxiety Inventory

Table 3 Descriptive statistics: FMR1 molecular measures in the FMR1 premutation group

Variable	M (SD), range
CGG repeat length (untransformed)	95.81 (17.42), 64–147
CGG repeat length (transformed)	4.54 (0.18), 4.16–4.99
Quantitative FMRP	9.16 (3.99), 2.81–18.44
Activation ratio (untransformed)	0.60 (0.18), 0.10–0.90
Activation ratio (transformed)	−0.35 (0.13), −0.65 to −1.00
Messenger RNA (untransformed)	0.77 (0.19), 0.49–1.24
Messenger RNA (transformed)	0.68 (0.01), 0.68–0.70

model F test using the Benjamini-Hochberg correction procedure [136]. Interaction contrasts were estimated to determine the effect of the cardiac predictor on psychological symptoms at each level of group. Partial eta squared (η_p^2) effect sizes were computed. In general, values of η_p^2 at 0.01, 0.06, and 0.14 are considered "small," "medium," and "large," respectively [134].

Finally, exploratory Pearson correlations were conducted between the cardiac variables and the FMR1 molecular variables within the FMR1 premutation group. Significant correlations were followed with more sophisticated general linear models testing the molecular genetic variable as a predictor of the cardiac outcome, controlling for age, medication use, and parenting stress level. Because of the exploratory nature of this aim, we did not attempt to adjust for multiple comparisons in these analyses. Regression models including quadratic and cubic terms were also conducted to test for non-linear associations with CGG expansion size, considering recent reports of curvilinear associations with CGG repeat length (e.g., [75, 80]).

Results

Descriptive statistics

Means, standard deviations, and ranges for the cardiac indices and psychological symptoms are presented in Table 2. t tests indicated significant group differences for these variables, with the women with the FMR1 premutation presenting with higher levels of both depression symptoms (t [58.40] = 4.22, $p < 0.001$) and anxiety symptoms (t [53.83] = 2.74, $p = 0.007$). Table 3 presents the descriptive statistics of the FMR1 genetic data within the FMR1 premutation group.

Group comparisons on cardiac indicators

The combined effects of group, age, medication use, and parenting stress level accounted for significant variability in RSA, F (1, 51) = 2.84, $p = 0.033$, $R^2 = 0.18$. Group accounted for significant variability in RSA, with the women with the FMR1 premutation exhibiting lower RSA than controls, F (1, 51) = 4.17, $p = 0.046$. Cohen's d effect size was 0.54, consistent with a medium effect. The combined effects group, age, medication use, and parenting stress level did not account for significant variability in IBI, $F (1, 51) = 2.54$, $p = 0.051$, and $R^2 = 0.17$. Cohen's d for the group differences in IBI was 0.05, which is consistent with a small effect size. Regression coefficients are presented in Table 4, and group comparisons are presented in Fig. 1.

Relationship between cardiac activity and symptoms of anxiety and depression

A significant effect was detected for the overall model testing RSA as a predictor of depression symptoms ($F [6, 48] = 9.82$, $p = 0.004$, $R^2 = 0.55$). After controlling for age, medication use, and parenting stress level, the main effect for group was statistically significant, $F [1, 48] = 21.39$, $p < 0.001$, $\eta_p^2 = 0.31$. A significant group-by-RSA interaction term was also detected ($F [1, 48] = 7.83$, $p = 0.007$, with a η_p^2 effect size of 0.14 consistent with a large effect. Regression coefficients are presented in Table 5. Interaction contrasts confirmed that the effect of RSA on depression symptom severity differed by group; among the control women, decreased RSA was significantly associated with elevated depression symptoms with a medium-to-large effect ($F [1, 48] = 6.40$, $p = 0.015$, $\eta_p^2 = 0.12$), whereas the association between RSA and depression symptoms was not statistically significant in the women with the FMR1 premutation with a small effect size ($F [1, 48] = 1.83$, $p = 0.182$, $\eta_p^2 = 0.04$), see Fig. 2. The remaining models testing the cardiac variables as predictors of depression and anxiety symptoms did not indicate a significant effect of RSA, IBI, or their interactions with group on the psychological outcomes (see Tables 5 and 6).

Table 4 Regression coefficients depicting group membership as a predictor of cardiac autonomic indices

Effect	B	SE	t	p	R^2
Coefficients: RSA model					
Intercept	5.87	0.88	6.70	<0.001*	0.18
Group[a]	−0.75	0.37	−2.04	0.046*	
Age	−0.01	0.02	−0.44	0.659	
Medication use	−0.33	0.23	−1.48	0.144	
Parenting stress	<0.01	0.01	0.27	0.785	
Coefficients: IBI model					
Intercept	1.92	<0.01	466.47	<0.001*	0.17
Group[a]	<0.01	<0.01	0.16	0.876	
Age	<0.01	<0.01	2.92	0.005*	
Medication use	<0.01	<0.01	−1.11	0.272	
Parenting stress	<0.01	<0.01	0.47	0.641	

[a]The control group was set as the reference category
*$p < 0.05$

Relationship between cardiac autonomic activity and FMR1 molecular variation

Exploratory Pearson correlations between the genetic and cardiac variables within the FMR1 premutation group are presented in Table 7. Elevated mRNA was correlated with higher RSA ($r = 0.51$, $p = 0.009$). CGG repeat length was also positively correlated with RSA ($r = 0.57$, $p < 0.001$). Significant correlations were followed with general linear models including age, medication use, and parenting stress level as covariates. After including for these covariates, mRNA remained a significant predictor of RSA, $F (1, 18) = 4.88$, $p = 0.040$, with a η_p^2 of 0.21 which is consistent with a large effect, see Fig. 3. The general linear model testing CGG repeat length as a predictor of RSA did not show a significant effect of CGG repeat size after controlling for age, medication use, and parenting stress level; $F (1, 22) = 2.51$, $p = 0.128$, and $\eta_p^2 = 0.10$. Regression coefficients are presented in Table 8. Finally, general linear regression models including quadratic and cubic terms were run to test for non-linear CGG effects, with no significant non-linear CGG effects detected.

Discussion

Women with the FMR1 premutation are at substantially increased risk for depression and anxiety disorders, which are conditions associated with autonomic dysregulation in the general population. Given its single-gene basis, the FMR1 premutation may serve as a foothold to inform the genetic background for autonomic aberrations. This is the first study to examine cardiac autonomic function in women with the FMR1 premutation and its psychological and genetic correlates. Vagal tone was significantly depressed among the women with the FMR1 premutation, supporting impaired parasympathetic function in this group. Unlike the patterns observed in study controls and the general population, vagal tone and depression symptoms were unrelated in women with the FMR1 premutation, suggesting that the parasympathetic system is not serving its normal emotional regulatory functions in this group. Elevated FMR1 mRNA, which is typically associated with neuronal toxicity, was correlated with higher (i.e., "better") vagal tone among women with the FMR1 premutation. Results underscore the need for additional research to delineate the clinical correlates and predictive utility of autonomic markers in this high-risk group and their relationship with FMR1-related mechanisms.

Group comparisons on cardiac indices of autonomic function

This study provides the first evidence of reduced vagal tone in women with the FMR1 premutation, which could not be accounted for by elevated parenting stress or increased use of psychotropic medications. Dampened vagal tone is thought to indicate inflexibility of psychophysiological

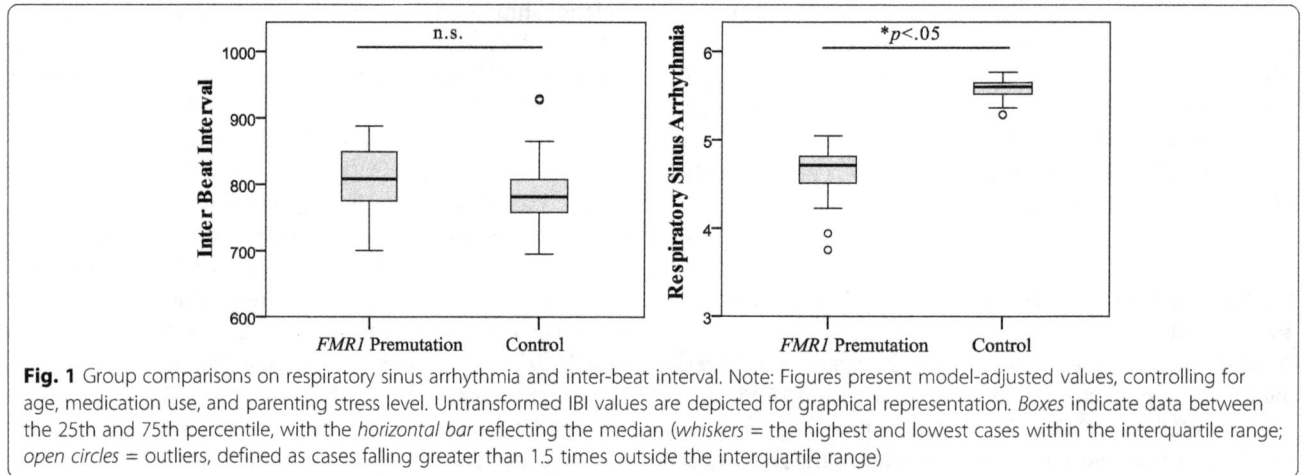

Fig. 1 Group comparisons on respiratory sinus arrhythmia and inter-beat interval. Note: Figures present model-adjusted values, controlling for age, medication use, and parenting stress level. Untransformed IBI values are depicted for graphical representation. *Boxes* indicate data between the 25th and 75th percentile, with the *horizontal bar* reflecting the median (*whiskers* = the highest and lowest cases within the interquartile range; *open circles* = outliers, defined as cases falling greater than 1.5 times outside the interquartile range)

resources that regulate affective information processing [137]. A large body of literature documents a supporting role of the vagus in emotional regulation and pro-social behavior. Adults with high vagal tone show greater self-regulatory capacity [138], better regulation of negative facial expressions [139, 140], increased perceived social support [141], and increased feelings of social integration and acceptance [142]. Vagal tone has also been shown to moderate the impact of negative life experiences, acting as a buffer to shield at risk individuals from negative emotional and physical consequences [143–145]. Moreover, an "upwards spiral" reciprocal causality effect has been suggested, where high vagal tone supports psychological well-being, which in turn promotes further vagal increases

Table 5 Regression coefficients testing RSA as a predictor of depression and anxiety symptom severity

Effect	β	SE	t	p	R^2
Coefficients: Depression Symptom Severity Model					
Intercept	3.64	0.60	6.10	<0.001*	0.55
RSA	−0.24	0.09	−2.53	0.015*	
Group[a]	−1.34	0.62	−2.16	0.036*	
Group × RSA	0.32	0.11	2.85	0.007*	
Age	−0.12	0.01	−2.27	0.028*	
Medication Use	0.06	0.09	0.72	0.477	
Parenting Stress	0.01	<0.01	3.85	<0.001*	
Coefficients: Anxiety Symptom Severity Model					
Intercept	2.04	0.42	4.87	<0.001*	0.41
RSA	−0.05	0.07	−0.78	0.437	
Group[a]	−0.23	0.43	−0.52	0.604	
Group × RSA	0.07	0.08	0.88	0.384	
Age	−0.01	<0.01	−2.21	0.032*	
Medication use	0.04	0.06	0.58	0.564	
Parenting stress	<0.01	<0.01	3.06	0.004*	

[a]The control group was set as the reference category
*$p < 0.05$

[146]. The finding of dampened vagal activity among women with the *FMR1* premutation suggests that these individuals may lack the physiological resources that are needed to support optimal social-adaptive outcomes. Blunted vagal tone may be a factor in the elevated risk for emotional and physical health conditions seen in this group. Additional research is needed to determine the utility of vagal tone in predicting individual differences in clinical risk. Penetrance is not complete in the *FMR1* premutation and the identification of a biomarker that can account for phenotypic variability would contribute significantly to prevention and treatment efforts.

Differential relationships between cardiac activity and psychological symptoms across groups

Vagal activity was not associated with depression symptoms in the women with the premutation, although, this relationship was observed in study controls and has been documented in the general population [14] and among individuals with clinically diagnosed mood disorders [10]. A similar decoupling between vagal tone and anxiety symptoms was observed in the *FMR1* premutation, which is contrary to a wealth of evidence supporting a link between vagal regulation and anxiety symptoms in other groups [8]. Together, these findings suggest that parasympathetic control of the heart via the vagal nerve is not only suboptimal (i.e., reduced in level) but also dysfunctional (i.e., not serving its normal functions) in women with the *FMR1* premutation. In other populations, the vagus is thought to play a mechanistic role in psychological vulnerability; when vagal tone is reduced, the body is unable to maintain an adaptive physiological state that promotes social engagement, leading to increased risk for emotional regulatory disorders [29]. Here, we found that vagal activity and psychological risk were not correlated in the *FMR1* premutation, despite the fact that vagal tone was reduced and psychological symptoms were increased. This may suggest different

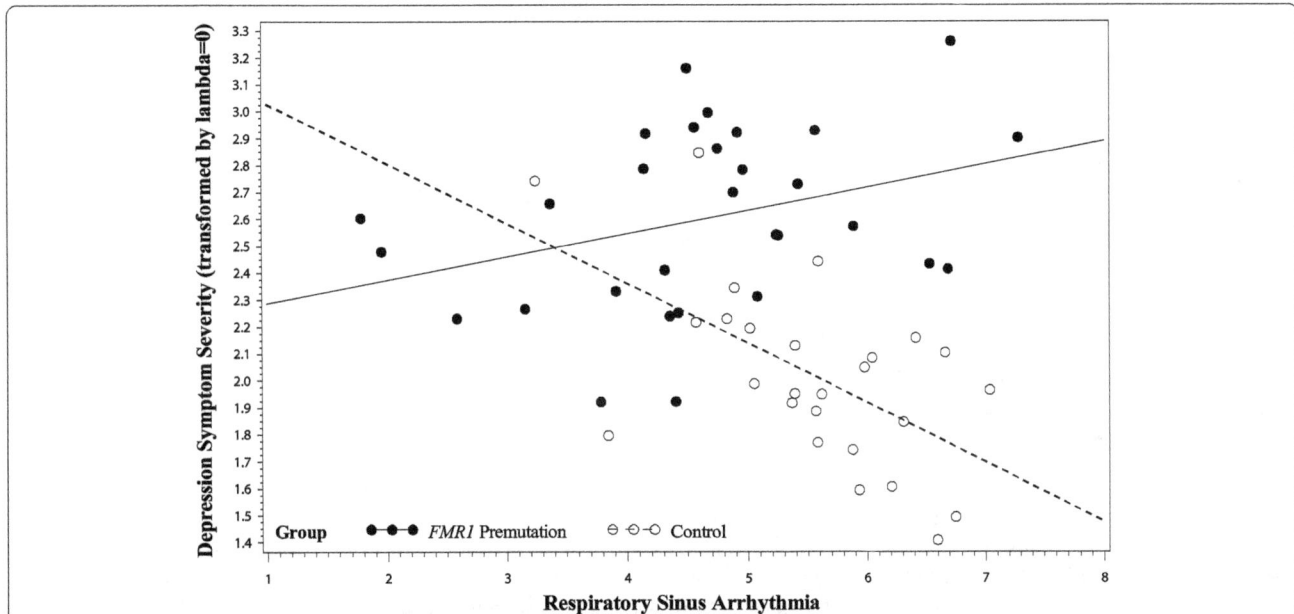

Fig. 2 Differential associations between respiratory sinus arrhythmia and depression symptom severity across groups. Note: Model-adjusted values are depicted, controlling for age, medication use, and parenting stress level

mechanistic underpinnings in the *FMR1* premutation and is consistent with distinct symptom profiles seen in this group (e.g., women with the premutation have a lower likelihood of recurrent major depressive episodes than women in the general population; Roberts et al., [75]). Future work incorporating measures of vagal reactivity may clarify relationships. The present study only

Table 6 Regression coefficients testing IBI as a predictor of depression and anxiety symptom severity

Effect	β	SE	t	p	R^2
Coefficients: Depression Symptom Severity Model					
Intercept	17.76	35.52	0.50	0.619	0.48
IBI	−7.96	18.49	−0.42	0.669	
Group[a]	−31.06	43.19	−0.72	0.476	
Group × IBI	16.30	22.39	0.73	0.470	
Age	−0.02	0.01	−2.11	0.040*	
Medication use	0.04	0.09	0.40	0.691	
Parenting stress	0.01	<0.01	3.46	0.001*	
Coefficients: Anxiety Symptom Severity Model					
Intercept	15.92	22.38	0.71	0.481	0.43
IBI	−7.33	11.65	−0.63	0.532	
Group[a]	−34.14	27.09	−1.26	0.214	
Group × IBI	17.77	14.04	1.27	0.212	
Age	−0.01	0.01	−2.13	0.039*	
Medication use	0.04	0.06	0.61	0.542	
Parenting stress	0.01	<0.01	3.10	0.003*	

[a]The control group was set as the reference category
*p < 0.05

included measures of tonic vagal activity, and some work suggests that task-related vagal modulation may be a more robust marker for depression than are baseline levels [39]. Future research may also investigate relationships among individuals who meet clinical thresholds for depression and anxiety, as opposed to investigating continuous symptom presentation across affected and unaffected individuals, as was done here, or among individuals with lifetime histories of depression and anxiety as opposed to current symptomatology.

Relationship between *FMR1* molecular variation and cardiac activity

It is unexpected that elevated *FMR1* mRNA was associated with higher (i.e., "better") vagal levels within the *FMR1* premutation group because mRNA is thought to be toxic to the neural system. So, why was elevated mRNA linked with superior vagal functioning in this sample? Undetected non-linear effects might explain this association, which would be consistent with evidence of CGG-dependent curvilinear risk patterns (i.e., [70, 75, 80, 81]) and the suggestion that maximal mRNA toxicity

Table 7 Genetic correlations with the cardiac activity in women with the FMR1 premutation

	CGG repeat length	Quantitative FMRP	Messenger RNA	Activation ratio
IBI	0.14	0.26	0.17	−0.01
RSA	0.57**	−0.17	0.51**	.07

IBI inter-beat interval, *RSA* respiratory sinus arrhythmia
**p < 0.01

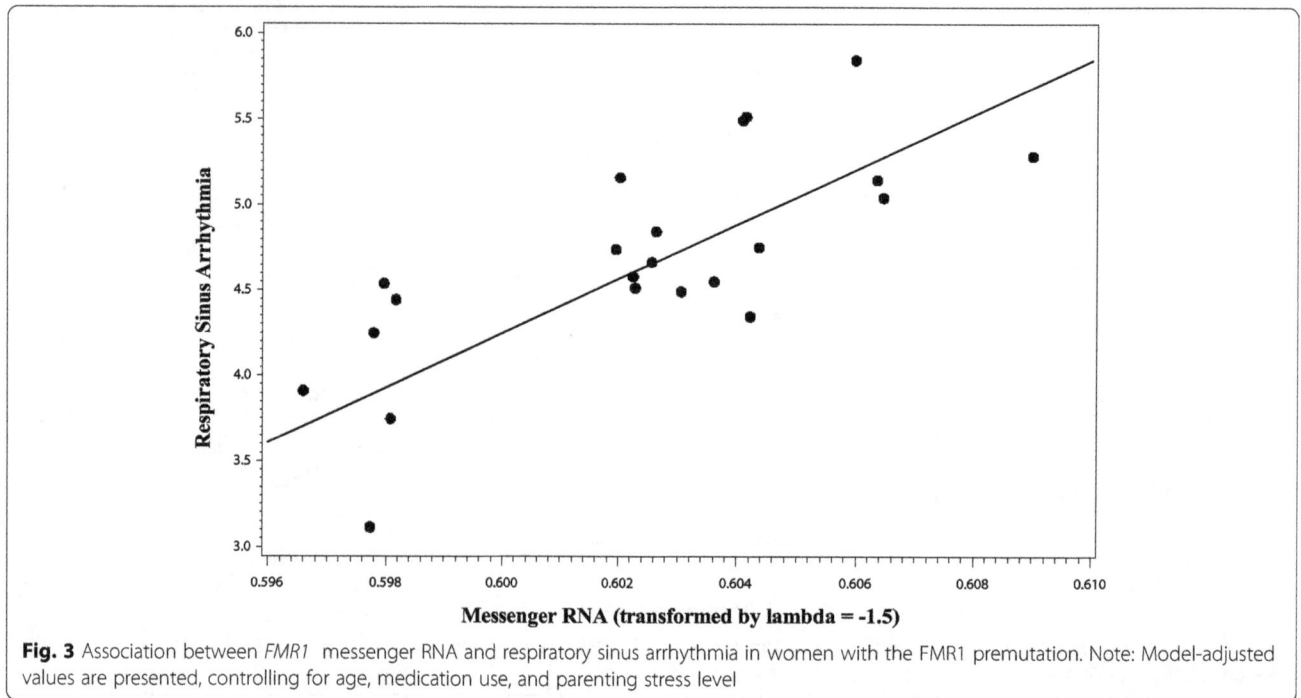

Fig. 3 Association between *FMR1* messenger RNA and respiratory sinus arrhythmia in women with the FMR1 premutation. Note: Model-adjusted values are presented, controlling for age, medication use, and parenting stress level

may occur within the mid-premutation range [80, 147]. However, an undetected curvilinear relationship seems unlikely, as the statistical tests and scatterplot distribution both suggest a linear association. The unexpected mRNA association underscores the complexity in untangling gene-brain-behavior relationships. *FMR1* mRNA toxicity is thought to involve the sequestration of other RNA binding proteins, which prevents the proteins of other genes from carrying out their normal functions [69]. Thus, *FMR1* does not function in isolation and the mechanisms by which *FMR1* variation leads to autonomic dysfunction are not straightforward. It is possible that the relationship

Table 8 Regression coefficients testing FMR1 mRNA and CGG repeat length as predictors of RSA

Effect	β	SE	t	p	R^2
Coefficients: *FMR1* mRNA predicting RSA					0.29
Intercept	−112.07	53.06	−2.11	0.049*	
mRNA	191.70	86.79	2.21	0.040*	
Age	0.04	0.06	0.78	0.444	
Medication use	−0.01	0.01	−0.69	0.497	
Parenting stress	−0.35	0.30	−1.17	0.256	
Coefficients: CGG repeat length predicting RSA					
Intercept	−5.74	7.76	−0.74	0.458	0.20
CGG repeat	2.52	1.59	1.58	0.128	
Age	−0.02	0.04	−0.42	0.679	
Medication use	<0.01	0.01	0.14	0.891	
Parenting stress	−0.59	0.30	−1.98	0.060	

*$p < 0.05$

between mRNA and vagal tone is driven by background gene dysfunction caused by protein sequestration associated with elevated mRNA. More research is needed to understand the inter-correlations between *FMR1* mRNA and other *FMR1* and non-*FMR1* mechanisms and their collective role in autonomic regulation.

Potential sex effects should also be considered, as much of our understanding of the functions of *FMR1* mRNA comes from work involving males with the premutation (e.g., [103, 148, 149]). The functions of mRNA and its neurodegenerative consequences may differ across males and females, which is consistent with evidence that FXTAS is less prevalent among females and characterized by less white matter disease, reduced brain atrophy, fewer astrocytic inclusions, and lower likelihood for dementia when compared to males [150–152]. Sex differences may be partially accounted for by random X inactivation in females, but the influence of sex-specific hormonal patterns must also be considered and has not yet been characterized. Longitudinal work will also be an informative next step, particularly given that *FMR1* mRNA gain-of-function is hypothesized to represent a degenerative, rather than developmental, mechanism, with toxicity building over time [153]. It should also be noted that mRNA levels were measured from peripheral blood lymphocytes and therefore might not necessarily reflect expression levels in relevant brain regions.

Findings did not support a relationship between cardiac activity and quantitatively measured FMRP levels in women with the premutation. No other studies have examined FMRP-autonomic relationships in the premutation, but these results are consistent with prior reports failing to detect a relationship between cardiac activity and the percent of lymphocytes staining positive for FMRP in males with the full mutation [154, 155]. One study did document a relationship between FMRP and vagal activity in females with the full mutation [155]; although, the significance of these findings are unclear as the association was only present when vagal tone was indexed using descriptive measures of heart rate variability but not when respiratory sinus arrhythmia was used, which is considered to be a more accurate measure of vagal tone [156, 157]. Overall, more research including larger samples is needed to determine whether FMRP is implicated in autonomic dysregulation in fragile X conditions.

Summary and directions

There are a number of future directions of this work. First, follow-up studies including more diverse samples and testing gender effects are needed. This study was limited by a relatively small sample, which may have reduced statistical power. Considering that the a priori power calculations for the larger study were based on by a different set of questions and assumptions, we reported effect sizes when possible to provide insight into the strength of the detected relationships. Given the novelty of the research question addressing the relationships between cardiac function and FMR1 molecular variation, this aim was considered exploratory and we did not attempt to correct for multiple comparisons. The exploratory associations detected here may be used to generate follow-up studies including more focused hypotheses. Follow-up work may also include more comprehensive investigation of associations with menopause, given that ~20% of women with the FMR1 premutation experience fragile X-associated primary ovarian insufficiency, and some research suggests changes in autonomic function following menopause (e.g., [110]). Finally, genotyping was not conducted on all controls and we cannot definitively rule out the presence of atypical CGG repeat numbers in this group, which could attenuate group differences.

It should also be noted that the premutation group consisted of mothers who had a child affected by fragile X syndrome, and results may not generalize to premutation carriers who do not have an affected child. While we covaried for parenting stress levels in our models, future work may more comprehensively examine the potential moderating role of parenting stress on the patterns observed here. Interactions with environmental factors such as social support should also be considered in future work, in light of evidence suggesting an "upwards spiral" reciprocal causality effect, where vagal tone and feelings of social connectedness reciprocally and prospectively predict one another [146]. Women with the FMR1 premutation report increased aloof personality traits [67] and heightened interpersonal sensitivity [95], which may interact with

the vagal system. Vagal tone may also be important for understanding the family environment, as women with the premutation are particularly susceptible to parenting stress [158], and low vagal tone is thought to magnify sensitivity to psychosocial stressors [159]. Furthermore, vagal tone has been shown to moderate the parenting behaviors of shy-anxious mothers, influencing child outcomes [160]. Recent work shows that disruption of other allostatic systems, such as the neuroendocrine system, directly impacts maternal responsivity in mothers who carry the FMR1 premutation [161]. Adopting a biobehavioral approach may be invaluable in parsing out the complex, multi-dimensional influences on individual and family risk factors in this population.

It should also be acknowledged that the autonomic system is one of the many bodily stress regulatory systems, and a multisystem approach is needed to account for how interactions and coordination across systems may influence findings. For instance, hypothalamic-pituitary-adrenal (HPA) axis function of the neuroendocrine system is blunted in women with the FMR1 premutation and is related to FMR1 variation [81, 89]. Some evidence suggests that the vagus plays an inhibitory role in the regulation of other allostatic systems, including the neuroendocrine system, with individuals with low vagal tone showing poor post-stress recovery of cardiovascular, neuroendocrine, and immune markers [162]. Better understanding of how these interacting systems function together will be important for developing targeted treatments.

Conclusions

In summary, the present study provides evidence that autonomic dysfunction extends to the premutation, highlighting autonomic dysregulation as a hallmark feature associated with defects on FMR1. Associations between FMR1-related variation and cardiac activity were detected, which sheds light on genetic determinants of autonomic alterations relevant to FMR1-associated conditions and the general population as well. Despite the elevated depression and anxiety symptoms, we observed independence between psychological symptoms and the autonomic system dysfunction in women with the FMR1 premutation group. This suggests that cardiac indices may have limited utility as biomarkers for anxiety and depression in this group. Yet, there is little understanding of the clinical consequences of autonomic dysregulation in this group and future studies may identify cardiac indices as useful markers for other clinical phenotypes associated with FMR1 gene dysfunction, such as FXTAS. The identification of biomarkers for clinical risk in the FMR1 premutation may improve early identification, tailored treatment, prevention, and the ability to predict which individuals are most at risk for late-onset symptom presentation. This study represents a first step in that direction.

Abbreviations

BAI: Beck anxiety inventory; BDI-II: Beck depression inventory-II; *FMR1*: *Fragile X mental retardation-1*; FMRP: Fragile X mental retardation protein; FXTAS: Fragile X-associated tremor/ataxia syndrome; IBI: Inter-beat interval; mRNA: Messenger RNA; RSA: Respiratory sinus arrhythmia

Acknowledgements

We would like to thank the women who participated in this study.

Funding

This research was supported by the National Institutes of Health (F32DC013934, PI: Klusek; R01MH090194, PI: Roberts; R01HD024356, PI: Abbeduto; R01HD02274, PI: Tassone), the Research Participant Registry Core of the Carolina Institute for Developmental Disabilities (P30HD03110), and the IDDRC Administrative Core (U54HD079125).

Authors' contributions

JK conceived the study and lead the data collection, analysis, and interpretation. JER provided guidance on study design, data collection, and interpretation. GL, TA, WTB, and FT contributed to the collection and interpretation of the genetic data. JK drafted the manuscript. All authors contributed to the interpretation of the results and critical revising of the manuscript. All authors read and approved the final manuscript.

Competing interests

The authors declare that they have no competing interests.

Author details

[1]Department of Communication Sciences and Disorders, University of South Carolina, Keenan Building, Suite 300, Columbia, SC 29208, USA. [2]Department of Developmental Biochemistry, New York State Institute for Basic Research in Developmental Disabilities, 1050 Forest Hill Road, Staten Island, NY 10314, USA. [3]Department of Human Genetics, New York State Institute for Basic Research in Developmental Disabilities, 1050 Forest Hill Road, Staten Island, NY 10314, USA. [4]UC Davis MIND Institute, University of California Davis, 2825 50th Street, Sacramento, CA 95817, USA. [5]Department of Psychology, University of South Carolina, 1512 Pendleton Street, Columbia, SC 29208, USA.

References

1. McEwen BS. Stress, adaptation, and disease: allostasis and allostatic load. Ann N Y Acad Sci. 1998;840:33–44.
2. Lovallo WR. Stress and health: Biological and psychological interactions. 3rd ed. Tousand Oaks: Sage Publications; 2015.
3. Jänig W, McLachlan EM. Neurobiology of the autonomic nervous system. In: Autonomic Failure: A Textbook of Clinical Disorders of the Autonomic Nervous System Oxford. 2013. p. 21–34.
4. Shaffer F, McCraty R, Zerr CL. A healthy heart is not a metronome: an integrative review of the heart's anatomy and heart rate variability. Front Psychol. 2014;5:1040.
5. Grossman P, Taylor EW. Toward understanding respiratory sinus arrhythmia: relations to cardiac vagal tone, evolution and biobehavioral functions. Biol Psychol. 2007;74:263–85.
6. Appelhans BM, Luecken LJ. Heart rate variability as an index of regulated emotional responding. Rev Gen Psychol. 2006;10:229.
7. Nardelli M, Valenza G, Cristea IA, Gentili C, Cotet C, David D, Lanata A, Scilingo EP. Characterizing psychological dimensions in non-pathological subjects through autonomic nervous system dynamics. Front Comput Neurosci. 2015;9:37.
8. Friedman BH. An autonomic flexibility-neurovisceral integration model of anxiety and cardiac vagal tone. Biol Psychol. 2007;74:185–99.
9. Gorman JM, Sloan RP. Heart rate variability in depressive and anxiety disorders. Am Heart J. 2000;140:S77–83.
10. Carney RM, Blumenthal JA, Stein PK, Watkins L, Catellier D, Berkman LF, Czajkowski SM, O'Connor C, Stone PH, Freedland KE. Depression, heart rate variability, and acute myocardial infarction. Circulation. 2001;104:2024–8.
11. Kemp AH, Quintana DS, Felmingham KL, Matthews S, Jelinek HF. Depression, comorbid anxiety disorders, and heart rate variability in physically healthy, unmedicated patients: implications for cardiovascular risk. PLoS One. 2012;7:e30777.
12. Stapelberg NJ, Hamilton-Craig I, Neumann DL, Shum DHK, McConnell H. Mind and heart: heart rate variability in major depressive disorder and coronary heart disease—a review and recommendations. Aust N Z J Psychiatry. 2012;46:946–57.
13. Koenig J, Kemp AH, Beauchaine TP, Thayer JF, Kaess M. Depression and resting state heart rate variability in children and adolescents—a systematic review and meta-analysis. Clin Psychol Rev. 2016;46:136–50.
14. Hughes JW, Stoney CM. Depressed mood is related to high-frequency heart rate variability during stressors. Psychosom Med. 2000;62:796–803.
15. Vazquez L, Blood JD, Wu J, Chaplin TM, Hommer RE, Rutherford HJV, Potenza MN, Mayes LC, Crowley MJ. High frequency heart-rate variability predicts adolescent depressive symptoms, particularly anhedonia, across one year. J Affect Disord. 2016;196:243–7.
16. Koval P, Ogrinz B, Kuppens P, Van den Bergh O, Tuerlinckx F, Sütterlin S. Affective instability in daily life is predicted by resting heart rate variability. PLoS One. 2013;8:e81536.
17. Agelink MW, Boz C, Ullrich H, Andrich J. Relationship between major depression and heart rate variability: clinical consequences and implications for antidepressive treatment. Psychiatry Res. 2002;113:139–49.
18. Agelink MW, Klimke A, Cordes J, Sanner D, Kavuk I, Malessa R, Klieser E, Baumann B. A functional-structural model to understand cardiac autonomic nervous system (ANS) dysregulation in affective illness and to elucidate the ANS effects of antidepressive treatment. Eur J Med Res. 2004;9:37–50.
19. Chambers AS, Allen JJ. Vagal tone as an indicator of treatment response in major depression. Psychophysiology. 2002;39:861–4.
20. Balogh S, Fitzpatrick DF, Hendricks SE, Paige SR. Increases in heart rate variability with successful treatment in patients with major depressive disorder. Psychopharmacol Bull. 1993;29:201–6.
21. Carney RM, Freedland KE, Stein PK, Skala JA, Hoffman P, Jaffe AS. Change in heart rate and heart rate variability during treatment for depression in patients with coronary heart disease. Psychosom Med. 2000;62:639–47.
22. de Guevara MS, Schauffele SI, Nicola-Siri LC, Fahrer RD, Ortiz-Fragola E, Martinez-Martinez JA, Cardinali DP, Guinjoan SM. Worsening of depressive symptoms 6 months after an acute coronary event in older adults is associated with impairment of cardiac autonomic function. J Affect Disord. 2004;80:257–62.
23. Royster EB, Trimble LM, Cotsonis G, Schmotzer B, Manatunga A, Rushing NN, Pagnoni G, Auyeung SF, Brown AR, Schoenbeck J, et al. Changes in heart rate variability of depressed patients after electroconvulsive therapy. Cardiovasc Psychiatry Neurol. 2012;2012:794043.
24. Karpyak VM, Rasmussen KG, Hammill SC, Mrazek DA. Changes in heart rate variability in response to treatment with electroconvulsive therapy. J ECT. 2004;20:81–8.
25. Miu AC, Heilman RM, Miclea M. Reduced heart rate variability and vagal tone in anxiety: trait versus state, and the effects of autogenic training. Auton Neurosci. 2009;145:99–103.
26. Watkins LL, Grossman P, Krishnan R, Sherwood A. Anxiety and vagal control of heart rate. Psychosom Med. 1998;60:498–502.
27. Brosschot JF, Van Dijk E, Thayer JF. Daily worry is related to low heart rate variability during waking and the subsequent nocturnal sleep period. Int J Psychophysiol. 2007;63:39–47.
28. Porges SW. The polyvagal theory: phylogenetic contributions to social behavior. Physiol Behav. 2003;79:503–13.
29. Porges SW. The polyvagal perspective. Biol Psychol. 2007;74:116–43.

30. Thayer JF, Lane RD. A model of neurovisceral integration in emotion regulation and dysregulation. J Affect Disord. 2000;61:201–16.

31. Thayer JF, Lane RD. Claude Bernard and the heart–brain connection: further elaboration of a model of neurovisceral integration. Neurosci Biobehav Rev. 2009;33:81–8.

32. Campbell-Sills L, Barlow DH. Incorporating emotion regulation into conceptualizations and treatments of anxiety and mood disorders. In: Gross JJ, editor. Handbook of Emotion Regulation. New York: Guilford Press; 2007. p. 542–59.

33. Thayer JF, Hansen AL, Saus-Rose E, Johnsen BH. Heart rate variability, prefrontal neural function, and cognitive performance: the neurovisceral integration perspective on self-regulation, adaptation, and health. Ann Behav Med. 2009;37:141–53.

34. Porges SW, Furman SA. The early development of the autonomic nervous system provides a neural platform for social behavior: a polyvagal perspective. Infant Child Dev. 2011;20:106–18.

35. McEwen BS, Wingfield JC. The concept of allostasis in biology and biomedicine. Horm Behav. 2003;43:2–15.

36. Thayer JF, Brosschot JF. Psychosomatics and psychopathology: looking up and down from the brain. Psychoneuroendocrinology. 2005;30:1050–8.

37. Beauchaine TP. The role of biomarkers and endophenotypes in prevention and treatment of psychopathological disorders. Biomark Med. 2009;3:1–3.

38. Beauchaine TP, Neuhaus E, Brenner SL, Gatzke-Kopp L. Ten good reasons to consider biological processes in prevention and intervention research. Dev Psychopathol. 2008;20:745.

39. Yaroslavsky I, Rottenberg J, Kovacs M. Atypical patterns of respiratory sinus arrhythmia index an endophenotype for depression. Dev Psychopathol. 2014;26:1337–52.

40. Beauchaine TP. Respiratory sinus arrhythmia: a transdiagnostic biomarker of emotion dysregulation and psychopathology. Curr Opin Psychol. 2015;3:43–7.

41. Boomsma DI, Plomin R. Heart rate and behavior of twins. Merrill-Palmer Q (1986). 1986;32:141–51.

42. Doussard-Roosevelt JA, Montgomery LA, Porges SW. Short-term stability of physiological measures in kindergarten children: respiratory sinus arrhythmia, heart period, and cortisol. Dev Psychobiol. 2003;43:230–42.

43. Fracasso MP, Porges SW, Lamb ME, Rosenberg AA. Cardiac activity in infancy: reliability and stability of individual differences. Infant Behav Dev. 1994;17:277–84.

44. Kupper NH, Willemsen G, van den Berg M, de Boer D, Posthuma D, Boomsma DI, de Geus EJ. Heritability of ambulatory heart rate variability. Circulation. 2004;110:2792–6.

45. Maddalena A, Richards CS, McGinniss MJ, Brothman A, Desnick RJ, Grier RE, Hirsch B, Jacky P, McDowell GA, Popovich B. Technical standards and guidelines for fragile X: the first of a series of disease-specific supplements to the Standards and Guidelines for Clinical Genetics Laboratories of the American College of Medical Genetics. Genet Med. 2001;3:200–5.

46. Hagerman PJ, Hagerman RJ. Fragile X-associated tremor/ataxia syndrome. Ann N Y Acad Sci. 2015;1338:58–70.

47. Oh SY, He F, Krans A, Frazer M, Taylor JP, Paulson HL, Todd PK. RAN translation at CGG repeats induces ubiquitin proteasome system impairment in models of fragile X-associated tremor ataxia syndrome. Hum Mol Genet. 2015;24:4317–26.

48. Todd PK, Oh SY, Krans A, He F, Sellier C, Frazer M, Renoux AJ, Chen K-c, Scaglione KM, Basrur V. CGG repeat-associated translation mediates neurodegeneration in fragile X tremor ataxia syndrome. Neuron. 2013; 78:440–55.

49. Fernandez-Carvajal I, Walichiewicz P, Xiaosen X, Pan R, Hagerman PJ, Tassone F. Screening for expanded alleles of the FMR1 gene in blood spots from newborn males in a Spanish population. J Mol Diagn. 2009;11:324–9.

50. Hantash FM, Goos DM, Crossley B, Anderson B, Zhang K, Sun W, Strom CM. FMR1 premutation carrier frequency in patients undergoing routine population-based carrier screening: Insights into the prevalence of fragile X syndrome, fragile X-associated tremor/ataxia syndrome, and fragile X-associated primary ovarian insufficiency in the United States. Genet Med. 2011;13:39–45.

51. Seltzer MM, Baker MW, Hong J, Maenner M, Greenberg J, Mandel D. Prevalence of CGG expansions of the FMR1 gene in a US population-based sample. Am J Med Genet B Neuropsychiatr Genet. 2012;159B:589–97.

52. Tassone F, long KP, Tong T-H, Lo J, Gane LW, Berry-Kravis E, Nguyen D, Mu LY, Laffin J, Bailey DB. FMR1 CGG allele size and prevalence ascertained through newborn screening in the United States. Genome Med. 2012;4:100.

53. Toledano-Alhadef H, Basel-Vanagaite L, Magal N, Davidov B, Ehrlich S, Drasinover V, Taub E, Halpern GJ, Ginott N, Shohat M. Fragile-X carrier screening and the prevalence of the premutation and full-mutation carriers in Israel. Am J Hum Genet. 2001;69:351–60.

54. Yrigollen CM, Martorell L, Durbin-Johnson B, Naudo M, Genoves J, Murgia A, Polli R, Zhou L, Barbouth D, Rupchock A, et al. AGG interruptions and maternal age affect FMR1 CGG repeat allele stability during transmission. J Neurodev Disord. 2014;6:1–12.

55. Nolin SL, Glicksman A, Ersalesi N, Dobkin C, Brown WT, Cao R, Blatt E, Sah S, Latham GJ, Hadd AG. Fragile X full mutation expansions are inhibited by one or more AGG interruptions in premutation carriers. Genet Med. 2014;17:358–64.

56. Coffee B, Keith K, Albizua I, Malone T, Mowrey J, Sherman SL, Warren ST. Incidence of fragile X syndrome by newborn screening for methylated FMR1 DNA. Am J Hum Genet. 2009;85:503–14.

57. Hagerman RJ, Hagerman PJ. Fragile X syndrome: Diagnosis, treatment, and research. Taylor & Francis US; 2002.

58. Klusek J, McGrath SE, Abbeduto L, Roberts JE. Pragmatic language features of mothers with the FMR1 premutation are associated with the language outcomes of adolescents and young adults with fragile X syndrome. J Speech Lang Hear Res. 2016;59:49–61.

59. Wheeler A, Hatton D, Reichardt A, Bailey D. Correlates of maternal behaviours in mothers of children with fragile X syndrome. J Intellect Disabil Res. 2007;51:447–62.

60. Tassone F, Hagerman PJ, Hagerman RJ. Fragile X premutation. J Neurodev Disord. 2014;6:1–4.

61. Allingham-Hawkins DJ, Babul-Hirji R, Chitayat D, Holden JJA, Yang KT, Lee C, Hudson R, Gorwill H, Nolin SL, Glicksman A, et al. Fragile X premutation is a significant risk factor for premature ovarian failure: the international collaborative POF in fragile X study—preliminary data. Am J Med Genet. 1999;83:322–5.

62. Rodriguez-Revenga L, Madrigal I, Pagonabarraga J, Xuncla M, Badenas C, Kulisevsky J, Gomez B, Mila M. Penetrance of FMR1 premutation associated pathologies in fragile X syndrome families. Eur J Hum Genet. 2009;17:1359–62.

63. Shelton AL, Cornish K, Kraan C, Georgiou-Karistianis N, Metcalfe SA, Bradshaw JL, Hocking DR, Archibald AD, Cohen J, Trollor JN. Exploring inhibitory deficits in female premutation carriers of fragile X syndrome: through eye movements. Brain Cogn. 2014;85:201–8.

64. Kraan CM, Hocking DR, Georgiou-Karistianis N, Metcalfe SA, Archibald AD, Fielding J, Trollor J, Bradshaw JL, Cohen J, Cornish KM. Impaired response inhibition is associated with self-reported symptoms of depression, anxiety, and ADHD in female FMR1 premutation carriers. Am J Med Genet B Neuropsychiatr Genet. 2014;165:41–51.

65. Goodrich-Hunsaker NJ, Wong LM, McLennan Y, Srivastava S, Tassone F, Harvey D, Rivera SM, Simon TJ. Young adult female fragile X premutation carriers show age- and genetically-modulated cognitiveimpairments. Brain Cogn. 2011;75:255–60.

66. Goodrich-Hunsaker NJ, Wong LM, McLennan Y, Tassone F, Harvey D, Rivera SM, Simon TJ. Adult female fragile X premutation carriers exhibit age- and CGG repeat length-related impairments on an attentionally-based enumeration task. Front Hum Neurosci. 2011;5:63.

67. Losh M, Klusek J, Martin GE, Sideris J, Parlier M, Piven J. Defining genetically meaningful language and personality traits in relatives of individuals with fragile X syndrome and relatives of individuals with autism. Am J Med Genet B Neuropsychiatr Genet. 2012;159B:660–8.

68. Clifford S, Dissanayake C, Bui QM, Huggins R, Taylor AK, Loesch DZ. Autism spectrum phenotype in males and females with fragile X full mutation and premutation. J Autism Dev Disord. 2007;37:738–47.

69. Hagerman R, Hagerman P. Advances in clinical and molecular understanding of the FMR1 premutation and fragile X-associated tremor/ataxia syndrome. Lancet Neurol. 2013;12:786–98.

70. Roberts JE, Tonnsen BL, McCary LM, Ford AL, Golden RN, Bailey DB. Trajectory and Predictors of Depression and Anxiety Disorders in Mothers with the FMR1 Premutation. Biol Psychiatry. 2016;79:85.

71. Thompson NM, Rogeness GA, McClure E, Clayton R, Johnson C. Influence of depression on cognitive functioning in fragile X females. Psychiatric Res. 1996;64:97–104.

72. Franke P, Leboyer M, Gansicke M, Weiffenbacj O. Genotype-phenotype relationship in female carriers of the premutation and full mutation of FMR-1. Psychiatry Res. 1998;90:113–27.

73. Reiss A, Freund L, Abrams MT, Boehm C, Kazazian H. Neurobehavioral effects of the fragile X premutation in adult women: a controlled study. Am J Hum Genet. 1993;52:884–94.

74. Bourgeois JA, Seritan AL, Casillas EM, Hessl D, Schneider A, Yang Y, Kaur I, Cogswell JB, Nguyen DV, Hagerman RJ. Lifetime prevalence of mood and anxiety disorders in fragile X premutation carriers. J Clin Psychiatry. 2011;72:175–82.

75. Roberts JE, Bailey DB, Mankowski J, Ford A, Weisenfeld LA, Heath TM, Golden RN. Mood and anxiety disorders in females with the FMR1 premutation. Am J Med Genet B Neuropsychiatr Genet. 2009;150B:130–9.

76. Hunter JE, Rohr JK, Sherman SL. Co-occurring diagnoses among FMR1 premutation allele carriers. Clin Genet. 2010;77:374–81.

77. Cordeiro L, Abucayan F, Hagerman R, Tassone F, Hessl D. Anxiety disorders in fragile X premutation carriers: preliminary characterization of probands and non-probands. Intractable Rare Dis Res. 2015;4:123–30.

78. Roberts JE, Tonnsen BL, McCary LM, Ford AL, Golden RN, Bailey DB. Trajectory and predictors of depression and anxiety disorders in mothers with the FMR1 premutation. Biol Psychiatry. 2016;79:850–7.

79. Franke P, Maier W, Hautzinger M, Weiffenbach O, Gänsicke M, Iwers B, Poustka F, Schwab SG, Froster U. Fragile-X carrier females: evidence for a distinct psychopathological phenotype? Am J Med Genet A. 1996;64:334–9.

80. Loesch D, Bui M, Hammersley E, Schneider A, Storey E, Stimpson P, Burgess T, Francis D, Slater H, Tassone F. Psychological status in female carriers of premutation FMR1 allele showing a complex relationship with the size of CGG expansion. Clin Genet. 2015;87:173–8.

81. Seltzer MM, Barker ET, Greenberg JS, Hong J, Coe C, Almeida D. Differential sensitivity to life stress in FMR1 premutation carrier mothers of children with fragile X syndrome. Health Psychol. 2012;31:612–22.

82. Allen EG, He W, Yadav-Shah M, Sherman SL. A study of the distributional characteristics of FMR1 transcript levels in 238 individuals. Hum Genet. 2004;114:439–47.

83. Tassone F, Beilina A, Carosi C, Albertosi S, Bagni C, Li L, Glover K, Bentley D, Hagerman PJ. Elevated FMR1 mRNA in premutation carriers is due to increased transcription. RNA. 2007;13:555–62.

84. Hessl D, Tassone F, Loesch DZ, Berry-Kravis E, Leehey MA, Gane LW, Barbato I, Rice C, Gould E, Hall DA, et al. Abnormal elevation of FMR1 mRNA is associated with psychological symptoms in individuals with the fragile X premutation. Am J Med Genet B Neuropsychiatr Genet. 2005;139:115–21.

85. Hessl D, Wang JM, Schneider A, Koldewyn K, Le L, Iwahashi C, Cheung K, Tassone F, Hagerman PJ, Rivera SM. Decreased FMRP expression underlies amygdala dysfunction in carriers of the fragile X premutation. Biol Psychiatry. 2011;70:859–65.

86. Seritan AL, Bourgeois JA, Schneider A, Mu Y, Hagerman RJ, Nguyen DV. Ages of onset of mood and anxiety disorders in fragile X premutation carriers. Curr Psychiatr Rev. 2013;9:65–71.

87. Tassone F, Hagerman RJ, Taylor AK, Gane LW, Godfrey TE, Hagerman PJ. Elevated levels of FMR1 messenger RNA in carrier males: a new mechanism of involvement in the fragile X syndrome. Am J Hum Genet. 2000;66:6–15.

88. Tonnsen BL, Cornish KM, Wheeler AC, Roberts JE. Maternal predictors of anxiety risk in young males with fragile X. Am J Med Genet B: Neuropsychiatr Genet. 2014;165B:299–409.

89. Hartley SL, Seltzer MM, Hong J, Greenberg JS, Smith L, Almeida D, Coe C, Abbeduto L. Cortisol response to behavior problems in FMR1 premutation mothers of adolescents and adults with fragile X syndrome: a diathesis-stress model. Int J Behav Dev. 2012;36:53–61.

90. Kenneson A, Zhang F, Hagedorn CH, Warren ST. Reduced FMRP and increased FMR1 transcription is proportionally associated with CGG repeat number in intermediate-length and premutation carriers. Hum Mol Genet. 2001;10:1449–54.

91. Primerano B, Tassone F, Hagerman RJ, Hagerman P, Amaldi F, Bagni C. Reduced FMR1 mRNA translation efficiency in fragile X patients with premutations. RNA. 2002;8:1482–8.

92. Darnell JC, Van Driesche SJ, Zhang C, Hung KY, Mele A, Fraser CE, Stone EF, Chen C, Fak JJ, Chi SW, et al. FMRP stalls ribosomal translocation on mRNAs linked to synaptic function and autism. Cell. 2011;146:247–61.

93. Penagarikano O, Mulle JG, Warren ST. The pathophysiology of fragile x syndrome. Annu Rev Genomics Hum Genet. 2007;8:109–29.

94. Schutzius G, Bleckmann D, Kapps-Fouthier S, di Giorgio F, Gerhartz B, Weiss A. A quantitative homogeneous assay for fragile X mental retardation 1 protein. J Neurodev Disord. 2013;5:8.

95. Johnston C, Eliez S, Dyer-Friedman J, Hessl D, Glaser B, Blasey C, Taylor A, Reiss A. Neurobehavioral phenotype in carriers of the fragile X premutation. Am J Med Genet. 2001;103:314–9.

96. Hunter JE, Allen EG, Abramowitz A, Rusin M, Leslie M, Novak G, Hamilton D, Shubeck L, Charen K, Sherman SL. Investigation of phenotypes associated with mood and anxiety among male and female fragile X premutation carriers. Behav Genet. 2008;38:493–502.

97. Hunter JE, Leslie M, Novak G, Hamilton D, Shubeck L, Charen K, Abramowitz A, Epstein MP, Lori A, Binder E, et al. Depression and anxiety symptoms among women who carry the FMR1 premutation: impact of raising a child with fragile X syndrome is moderated by CRHR1 polymorphisms. Am J Med Genet B Neuropsychiatr Genet. 2012;0:549–59.

98. Cornish KM, Kraan CM, Bui QM, Bellgrove MA, Metcalfe SA, Trollor JN, Hocking DR, Slater HR, Inaba Y, Li X. Novel methylation markers of the dysexecutive-psychiatric phenotype in FMR1 premutation women. Neurology. 2015;84:1631–8.

99. Adams PE, Adams JS, Nguyen DV, Hessl S, Brunberg JA, Tassone S, et al. Psychological symptoms correlate with reduced hippocampal volume in fragile X premutation carriers. Am J Med Genet. 2010;153B:775–85.

100. Klusek J, Roberts JE, Losh M. Cardiac autonomic regulation in autism and fragile X syndrome: a review. Psychol Bull. 2015;141:141–75.

101. Coffey SM, Cook K, Tartaglia N, Tassone F, Nguyen DV, Pan R, Bronsky HE, Yuhas J, Borodyanskaya M, Grigsby J, et al. Expanded clinical phenotype of women with the FMR1 premutation. Am J Med Genet A. 2008;146:1009–16.

102. Jacquemont S, Hagerman RJ, Leehey M, Grigsby J, Zhang L, Brunberg JA, Greco C, Des Portes V, Jardini T, Levine R, et al. Fragile X premutation tremor/ataxia syndrome: molecular, clinical, and neuroimaging correlates. Am J Hum Genet. 2003;72:869–78.

103. Greco CM, Berman RF, Martin RM, Tassone F, Schwartz PH, Chang A, Trapp BD, Iwahashi C, Brunberg J, Grigsby J, et al. Neuropathology of fragile X-associated tremor/ataxia syndrome (FXTAS). Brain. 2005;129:243–55.

104. Gokden M, Al-Hinti JT, Harik SI. Peripheral nervous system pathology in fragile X tremor/ataxia syndrome (FXTAS). Neuropathology. 2009;29:280–4.

105. Hessl D, Rivera S, Koldewyn K, Cordeiro L, Adams J, Tassone F, Hagerman PJ, Hagerman RJ. Amygdala dysfunction in men with the fragile X premutation. Brain. 2007;130:404–16.

106. Kaufman AS, Kaufman NL. Kaufman Brief Intelligence Test. 2nd ed. Los Angeles: Pearson Assessments; 2004.

107. DiPietro JA, Costigan KA, Gurewitsch ED. Maternal psychophysiological change during the second half of gestation. Biol Psychol. 2005;69:23–38.

108. Rutter M, Bailey A, Lord C. SCQ: The Social Communication Questionnaire. Los Angeles: Western Psychological Services; 2003.

109. Louis ED, Barnes LF, Wendt KJ, Albert SM, Pullman SL, Yu Q, Schneier FR. Validity and test-retest reliability of a disability questionnaire for essential tremor. Mov Disord. 2000;15:516–23.

110. Moodithaya SS, Avadhany ST. Comparison of cardiac autonomic activity between pre and post menopausal women using heart rate variability. Indian J Physiol Pharmacol. 2009;53:227–34.

111. Sullivan AK, Marcus M, Epstein MP, Allen EG, Anido AE, Paquin JJ, Yadav-Shah M, Sherman SL. Association of FMR1 repeat size with ovarian dysfunction. Hum Reprod. 2005;20:402–12.

112. Abidin RR. Parenting Stress Index, Fourth Edition Short Form (PSI-4-SF). Lutz: PAR, Inc; 2013.

113. Tomeny TS. Parenting stress as an indirect pathway to mental health concerns among mothers of children with autism spectrum disorder. Autism. 2016. doi:10.1177/1362361316655322.

114. Allen JJ, Chambers AS, Towers DN. The many metrics of cardiac chronotropy: a pragmatic primer and a brief comparison of metrics. Biol Psychol. 2007;74:243–62.

115. Porges SW, Bohrer RE. Analyses of periodic processes in psychophysiological research. In: Cacioppo JT, Tassinary LG, editors. Principles of Psychophysiology: Physical, Social, and Inferential Elements. New York: Cambridge University Press; 1990. p. 708–53.

116. Porges SW. Method and apparatus for evaluating rhythmic oscillations in aperiodic physiological response systems. (States U ed., vol. 4520944; 1985.

117. Beck AT, Steer RA, Brown GK. Beck Depression Inventory-II. San Antonio: Psychological Corporation; 1996. p. b9.

118. American Psychological Association. Diagnostic and Statistical Manual of Mental Disorders (DSM-IV). 4th ed. Washington: American Psychological Association; 1994.

119. Storch EA, Roberti JW, Roth DA. Factor structure, concurrent validity, and internal consistency of the beck depression inventory—second edition in a sample of college students. Depress Anxiety. 2004;19:187–9.

120. Sprinkle SD, Lurie D, Insko SL, Atkinson G, Jones GL, Logan AR, Bissada NN. Criterion validity, severity cut scores, and test-retest reliability of the Beck

Reduced vagal tone in women with the FMR1 premutation is associated with FMR1 mRNA...

175

Depression Inventory-II in a university counseling center sample. J Couns Psychol. 2002;49:381.

121. Osman A, Kopper BA, Barrios F, Gutierrez PM, Bagge CL. Reliability and validity of the Beck Depression Inventory-II with adolescent psychiatric inpatients. Psychol Assess. 2004;16:120.

122. Beck AT, Steer RA. Manual for the Beck Anxiety Scale. San Antonio: Pyschological Corportation; 1990.

123. Fydrich T, Dowdall D, Chambless DL. Reliability and validity of the Beck Anxiety Inventory. J Anxiety Disord. 1992;6:55–61.

124. de Beurs E, Wilson KA, Chambless DL, Goldstein AJ, Feske U. Convergent and divergent validity of the Beck Anxiety Inventory for patients with panic disorder and agoraphobia. Depress Anxiety. 1997;6:140–6.

125. Tassone F, Pan R, Amiri K, Taylor AK, Hagerman PJ. A rapid polymerase chain reaction-based screening method for identification of all expanded alleles of the fragile X (FMR1) gene in newborn and high-risk populations. J Mol Diagn. 2008;10:43–9.

126. Filipovic-Sadic S, Sah S, Chen L, Krosting J, Sekinger E, Zhang W, Hagerman PJ, Stenzel TT, Hadd AG, Latham GJ, Tassone F. A novel FMR1 PCR method for the routine detection of low abundance expanded alleles and full mutations in fragile X syndrome. Clin Chem. 2010;56:399–408.

127. LaFauci G, Adayev T, Kascsak R, Kascsak R, Nolin S, Mehta P, Brown WT, Dobkin C. Fragile X screening by quantification of FMRP in dried blood spots by a Luminex immunoassay. J Mol Diagn. 2013;15:508–17.

128. Adayev T, LaFauci G, Dobkin C, Caggana M, Wiley V, Field M, Wotton T, Kascsak R, Nolin SL, Glicksman A. Fragile X protein in newborn dried blood spots. BMC Med Genet. 2014;15:119.

129. SAS Institute: SAS Institute version 9.4. Cary NC; 2013.

130. Box GE, Cox DR. An analysis of transformations. J R Stat Soc Ser B (Methodological). 1964;26:211–52.

131. O'Brien P, Oyebode F. Psychotropic medication and the heart. Adv Psychiatr Treat. 2003;9:414–23.

132. Das S, O'Keefe JH. Behavioral cardiology: recognizing and addressing the profound impact of psychosocial stress on cardiovascular health. Curr Atheroscler Rep. 2006;8:111–8.

133. De Meersman RE, Stein PK. Vagal modulation and aging. Biol Psychol. 2007;74:165–73.

134. Cohen J. Statistical power analysis for the behavioral sciences. Hillsdale: L. Erlbaum Associates; 1988.

135. Lipsey MW. Design sensitivity: Statistical power for experimental research. Newbury Park: Sage; 1990.

136. Benjamini Y, Hochberg Y. Controlling the false discovery rate: a practical and powerful approach to multiple testing. J R Stat Soc Ser B Methodol. 1995;57:289–300.

137. Thayer JF, Ahs F, Fredrikson M, Sollers JJ, Wager TD. A meta-analysis of heart rate variability and neuroimaging studies: implications for heart rate variability as a marker of stress and health. Neurosci Biobehav Rev. 2012;36:747–56.

138. Segerstrom SC, Nes LS. Heart rate variability reflects self-regulatory strength, effort, and fatigue. Psychol Sci. 2007;18:275–81.

139. Demaree HA, Robinson JL, Everhart E, Schmeichel BJ. Resting RSA is associated with natural and self-regulated responses to negative emotional stimuli. Brain Cogn. 2004;56:14–24.

140. Kettunen J, Ravaja N, Naatanen P, Keltikangas-Jarvinen L. The relationship of respiratory sinus arrhythmia to the co-activation of autonomic and facial responses during the Rorschach test. Psychophysiology. 2000;37:242–50.

141. Schwerdtfeger AR, Schlagert H. The conjoined effect of naturalistic perceived available support and enacted support on cardiovascular reactivity during a laboratory stressor. Ann Behav Med. 2011;42:64–78.

142. Geisler FCM, Kubiak T, Siewert K, Weber H. Cardiac vagal tone is associated with social engagement and self-regulation. Biol Psychol. 2013;93:279–86.

143. El-Sheikh M, Harger J, Whitson SM. Exposure to interparental conflict and children's adjustment and physical health: the moderating role of vagal tone. Child Dev. 2001;72:1617–36.

144. Leary A, Katz LF. Coparenting, family-level processes, and peer outcomes: the moderating role of vagal tone. Dev Psychopathol. 2004;16:593–608.

145. El-Sheikh M. Parental drinking problems and children's adjustment: vagal regulation and emotional reactivity as pathways and moderators of risk. J Abnorm Psychol. 2001;110:499–515.

146. Kok BE, Fredrickson BL. Upward spirals of the heart: autonomic flexibility, as indexed by vagal tone, reciprocally and prospectively predicts positive emotions and social connectedness. Biol Psychol. 2010;85:432–6.

147. Ennis S, Ward D, Murray A. Nonlinear association between CGG repeat number and age of menopause in FMR1 premutation carriers. Eur J Hum Genet. 2006;14:253–5.

148. Tassone F, Iwahashi C, Hagerman PJ. FMR1 RNA within the intranuclear inclusions of fragile X-associated tremor/ataxia syndrome (FXTAS). RNA Biol. 2004;1:103–5.

149. Koldewyn K, Hessl D, Adams J, Tassone F, Hagerman PJ, Hagerman RJ, Rivera S. Reduced hippocampal activation during recall is associated with elevated FMR1 mRNA and psychiatric symptoms in men with the fragile X premutation. Brain Imaging Behav. 2008;2:105–16.

150. Tassone F, Greco CM, Hunsaker MR, Seritan AL, Berman RF, Gane LW, Jacquemont S, Basuta K, Jin LW, Hagerman PJ. Neuropathological, clinical and molecular pathology in female fragile X premutation carriers with and without FXTAS. Genes Brain Behav. 2012;11:577–85.

151. Seritan AL, Nguyen DV, Farias ST, Hinton L, Grigsby J, Bourgeois JA, Hagerman RJ. Dementia in fragile X-associated tremor/ataxia syndrome (FXTAS): comparison with Alzheimer's disease. Am J Med Genet B Neuropsychiatr Genet. 2008;147:1138–44.

152. Adams J, Adams P, Nguyen D, Brunberg J, Tassone F, Zhang W, Koldewyn K, Rivera S, Grigsby J, Zhang L. Volumetric brain changes in females with fragile X-associated tremor/ataxia syndrome (FXTAS). Neurology. 2007;69:851–9.

153. Kraan CM, Hocking DR, Bradshaw JL, Fielding J, Cohen J, Georgiou-Karistianis N, Cornish KM. Neurobehavioural evidence for the involvement of the FMR1 gene in female carriers of fragile X syndrome. Neurosci Biobehav Rev. 2013;37:522–47.

154. Roberts JE, Boccia ML, Bailey DB, Hatton DD, Skinner M. Cardiovascular indices of physiological arousal in boys with fragile X syndrome. Dev Psychobiol. 2001;39:107–23.

155. Hall SS, Lightbody AA, Huffman LC, Lazzeroni LC, Reiss AL. Physiological correlates of social avoidance behavior in children and adolescents with fragile X syndrome. J Am Acad Child Adolesc Psychiatry. 2009;48:320–9.

156. Grossman P, van Beek J, Wientjes C. A comparison of three quantification methods for the estimation of respiratory sinus arrhythmia. Psychophysiology. 1990;27:702–14.

157. Billman GE. Heart rate variability—a historical perspective. Front Physiol. 2011;2:1–13.

158. Lewis P, Abbeduto L, Murphy M, Richmond E, Giles N, Bruno L, Schroeder S, Anderson J, Orsmond G. Psychological well-being of mothers of youth with fragile X syndrome: syndrome specificity and within-syndrome variability. J Intellect Disabil Res. 2006;50:894–904.

159. McLaughlin KA, Rith-Najarian L, Dirks MA, Sheridan MA. Low vagal tone magnifies the association between psychosocial stress exposure and internalizing psychopathology in adolescents. J Clin Child Adolesc Psychol. 2015;44:314–28.

160. Root AE, Hastings PD, Rubin KH. The parenting behaviors of shy–anxious mothers: The moderating role of vagal tone. J Child Fam Stud. 2015;4:1–9.

161. Robinson AR, Roberts JE, McQuillin SD, Brady N, Warren S. Physiological correlates of maternal responsivity in mothers of preschoolers with fragile X syndrome. Am J Intellect Dev Disabil. 2016;121:111–20.

162. Weber CS, Thayer JF, Rudat M, Wirtz PH, Zimmermann-Viehoff F, Thomas A, Perschel FH, Arck PC, Deter HC. Low vagal tone is associated with impaired post stress recovery of cardiovascular, endocrine, and immune markers. Eur J Appl Physiol. 2010;109:201–11.

15

The effects of intranasal oxytocin on reward circuitry responses in children with autism spectrum disorder

R. K. Greene[1], M. Spanos[2,3,4,6,7], C. Alderman[2,4,6], E. Walsh[4], J. Bizzell[5,6], M. G. Mosner[1], J. L. Kinard[6], G. D. Stuber[4,8,9], T. Chandrasekhar[3,4], L. C. Politte[4,6], L. Sikich[2,3,4,7] and G. S. Dichter[1,4,6,10*]

Abstract

Background: Intranasal oxytocin (OT) has been shown to improve social communication functioning of individuals with autism spectrum disorder (ASD) and, thus, has received considerable interest as a potential ASD therapeutic agent. Although preclinical research indicates that OT modulates the functional output of the mesocorticolimbic dopamine system that processes rewards, no clinical brain imaging study to date has examined the effects of OT on this system using a reward processing paradigm. To address this, we used an incentive delay task to examine the effects of a single dose of intranasal OT, versus placebo (PLC), on neural responses to social and nonsocial rewards in children with ASD.

Methods: In this placebo-controlled double-blind study, 28 children and adolescents with ASD (age: $M = 13.43$ years, $SD = 2.36$) completed two fMRI scans, one after intranasal OT administration and one after PLC administration. During both scanning sessions, participants completed social and nonsocial incentive delay tasks. Task-based neural activation and connectivity were examined to assess the impact of OT relative to PLC on mesocorticolimbic brain responses to social and nonsocial reward anticipation and outcomes.

Results: Central analyses compared the OT and PLC conditions. During nonsocial reward anticipation, there was greater activation in the right nucleus accumbens (NAcc), left anterior cingulate cortex (ACC), bilateral orbital frontal cortex (OFC), left superior frontal cortex, and right frontal pole (FP) during the OT condition relative to PLC. Alternatively, during social reward anticipation and outcomes, there were no significant increases in brain activation during the OT condition relative to PLC. A Treatment Group × Reward Condition interaction revealed relatively greater activation in the right NAcc, right caudate nucleus, left ACC, and right OFC during nonsocial relative to social reward anticipation during the OT condition relative to PLC. Additionally, these analyses revealed greater activation during nonsocial reward outcomes during the OT condition relative to PLC in the right OFC and left FP. Finally, functional connectivity analyses generally revealed changes in frontostriatal connections during the OT condition relative to PLC in response to nonsocial, but not social, rewards.

Conclusions: The effects of intranasal OT administration on mesocorticolimbic brain systems that process rewards in ASD were observable primarily during the processing of nonsocial incentive salience stimuli. These findings have implications for understanding the effects of OT on neural systems that process rewards, as well as for experimental trials of novel ASD treatments developed to ameliorate social communication impairments in ASD.

Keywords: Autism spectrum disorder, Oxytocin, Reward, fMRI

* Correspondence: dichter@med.unc.edu
[1]Department of Psychology and Neuroscience, University of North Carolina at Chapel Hill, Chapel Hill, NC 27514, USA
[4]Department of Psychiatry, University of North Carolina at Chapel Hill School of Medicine, Chapel Hill, NC 27514, USA
Full list of author information is available at the end of the article

Background

Autism spectrum disorder (ASD) is a neurodevelopmental disorder characterized by impairments in social communication and interaction, as well as restricted and repetitive behaviors (APA [1]). Although various pharmacological treatments are commonly prescribed to treat associated symptoms of ASD (e.g., irritability, inattention, and aggression), there are currently no pharmacological treatments approved to treat the core features of the disorder [2–4].

The neuropeptide oxytocin (OT) has been shown to increase pro-social behaviors in human studies and in preclinical model organisms. Studies in typically developing individuals have shown that intranasal OT administration increases in-group trust [5] and interoceptive awareness [6] while also reducing fear [7]. Preclinical studies, on the other hand, have established the vital role of OT in sociality. For example, in mammalian nonhuman models, OT moderates or initiates paternal and reproductive behaviors, as well as other pro-social behaviors such as grooming and social recognition [8, 9].

Because of the need for effective treatments for core ASD symptoms, there has been increasing interest in the potential for OT to ameliorate social communication impairments in ASD. Some, but not all, studies of the effects of OT in ASD have reported benefits in social functioning, including enhanced emotion recognition [10], increased eye gaze [11], and enhanced feelings of trust in others [12]. Other studies, however, have failed to find clinical benefits of OT on primary social outcome measures [13, 14], and a recent trial found that the beneficial effects of OT on social functioning in ASD were moderated by pre-treatment endogenous OT levels, suggesting that OT may be beneficial for some, but not all, individuals with ASD [15].

Although there is emerging evidence that OT may be clinically beneficial for at least a significant subset of individuals with ASD, the mechanisms of action of OT are not well understood. One potential mechanism of action may be the capacity of OT to modulate sensitivity to, and the perceived salience of, external rewards that influence behavior and facilitate reward-based learning. Preclinical studies implicate the mesocorticolimbic dopamine system as a mechanism by which OT exerts its pro-social effects [16, 17]. This neural network is comprised of midbrain structures (the ventral tegmental area (VTA) and substantia nigra), the striatum, and cortical regions including the orbital frontal, anterior cingulate, and prefrontal cortices [18]. OT and mesocorticolimbic dopamine interact in such a manner that the activation of OT-responsive neurons in the VTA increases dopaminergic activity in the broader mesocorticolimbic system [19–21]. Furthermore, when administered an OT receptor agonist, mice demonstrate a subsequent decrease in dopaminergic release within the nucleus accumbens, reflecting the influence of OT on mesocorticolimbic dopamine transmission [19].

To date, no functional neuroimaging study has examined the effects of OT on the mesocorticolimbic system in response to rewards in ASD. However, two functional neuroimaging studies indicate the relevance of mesocorticolimbic brain regions to the potential mechanisms of action of OT in ASD. Gordon et al. [22] found increased activation in the ventral striatum, left posterior superior temporal sulcus, and left premotor cortex in ASD in response to acute intranasal OT administration during a socio-emotional recognition task and that these same brain regions showed decreased activation to nonsocial (i.e., object) judgements. Other research from this group found that intranasal OT administration increased functional connectivity between the ventral striatum and ventromedial prefrontal cortex in ASD in response to a biological motion task, underscoring the potential centrality of mesocorticolimbic brain regions to the mechanism of action of OT [23].

Although both of these studies highlight the potential relevance of reward-responsive mesocorticolimbic brain regions to the mechanism of action of OT in ASD, neither used a reward task to directly test this hypothesis. Thus, the goal of the present study was to extend these findings by assessing the impact of acute intranasal OT administration on response to rewards in ASD using social and nonsocial incentive delay tasks. Social and nonsocial incentive delay tasks have been used in multiple studies to investigate reward processing in ASD (for a review see [24]). These studies have consistently revealed reduced ventral striatal activation during social and nonsocial reward anticipation in ASD [25–28]. Although the pattern of mesocorticolimbic responses to rewards in ASD is complex (i.e., different studies with different sample characteristics have reported decreased ventral striatal responses to social, but not nonsocial, reward anticipation in ASD [27, 29] whereas others have reported decreased ventral striatal responses to nonsocial, but not social, reward anticipation in ASD [26]), it is clear that mesocorticolimbic responses to rewards in ASD are impaired and that incentive tasks are suitable to study the functional integrity of this system.

Participants in the current study completed functional neuroimaging scans after double-blind administration of OT or PLC, and responses to nonsocial and social rewards were examined. We hypothesized that intranasal OT administration, relative to PLC, would result in greater activation and connectivity within mesocorticolimbic brain regions (frontal lobes, amygdala, nucleus accumbens (NAcc), insula, thalamus, caudate nucleus, anterior cingulate cortex (ACC), and putamen) that have previously been found to be functionally impaired during reward processing in ASD [30]. We also hypothesized that the effects of OT would be more pronounced in the social, relative to nonsocial, reward context because of the putative pro-social effects of OT described earlier [22, 23]. Finally, we explored relations between neural response to OT, symptom severity, and salivary OT concentrations.

Methods
Participants
This protocol was approved by the Institutional Review Boards at the University of North Carolina at Chapel Hill and Duke University Medical Center, and informed consent was obtained from the parent or guardian of each participant before testing. Participants older than 11 also provided verbal and written assent. Participants were recruited through the Autism Research Registry maintained through the Carolina Institute for Developmental Disabilities. Exclusion criteria included a history of medical conditions associated with ASD, including Fragile X syndrome, tuberous sclerosis, neuro-fibromatosis, phenylketonuria, epilepsy and traumatic brain injury, full-scale intelligence < 70, and MRI contraindications.

The study enrolled 33 children and adolescents with ASD ages 10 to 17 years old. Diagnoses were based on a history of clinical diagnosis confirmed by proband assessment by a research reliable assessor via Module 3 or 4 of the Autism Diagnostic Observation Schedule, Second Edition (ADOS-2; [31]) using standard clinical algorithm cutoffs. Of the 33 individuals enrolled, data from 28 were analyzable (see Table 1): one participant elected to discontinue testing during the first visit, another was unable to complete the scan due to claustrophobia, and three participants were excluded due to excessive motion (see "Motion Correction" for details).

After providing informed consent, participants completed two fMRI sessions (one after OT administration and one after PLC administration, with the order of scans counter-balanced across participants). The two scan sessions were scheduled at least 72 h apart to minimize the possibility of carry-over effects of OT administration (mean time between scans = 15 days; range = 3–46 days). Participants were offered the opportunity to participate in an optional mock scan prior to the neuroimaging sessions. Families were compensated $50 for each visit attended.

Table 1 Participant characteristics

Characteristic	Mean	Standard deviation	Range
Age	13.43	2.36	10–17
Full-scale IQ	103.55	15.19	75–128
ADOS-2 calibrated severity score	8.46	1.29	7–10
SRS total *T* score	76.19	10.66	49–90
Sex	26 males, 2 females		

ADOS-2 calibrated severity scores were calculated for modules 3 and 4 using guidelines established by Gotham et al. [83] and Hus and Lord [84]
ADOS-2 Autism Diagnostic Observation Schedule, Second Edition

Drug protocol
Oxytocin (Syntocinon®, Novartis, Switzerland) and a matched solution containing no medication (PLC) were repackaged into identically appearing bottles. The administration sequence was counter-balanced by UNC Investigational Drug Service and Triangle Compounding Pharmacy, and OT and PLC were administered to participants by a blinded research assistant. A 24 international unit (IU)/mL dose of each solution was administered in alternating nostril insufflations (six total puffs) over the course of several minutes. This dose was the same as those used in multiple previous studies examining the effect of OT in adults, adolescents, and children with ASD [10, 11, 14, 22, 23]. Recent clinical and preclinical findings have demonstrated intranasal OT's ability to increase peripheral (i.e., cerebrospinal fluid, plasma) OT concentrations [32], while preclinical research has reported augmented brain OT levels following intranasal OT administration [33–35].

fMRI task
As described in Richey et al., participants completed two versions of an incentive delay tasks [36] such that nonsocial rewards (i.e., money) and social rewards (i.e., pictures of smiling faces) were presented as rewards on alternating runs. Participants were presented with two runs of the nonsocial reward condition and two runs of the social reward condition. On all runs, rewards could be won or not won (i.e., there was no "loss" condition). Face stimuli were smiling images from the NimStim set of facial expressions [37]. Each run began with a 10-s instructional screen indicating the forthcoming reward type (i.e., nonsocial or social), and the two task types were segregated by run to minimize the number of cues to be memorized.

Each trial consisted of (1) a 2000-ms cue indicating whether adequately quick responses to the bull's-eye would result in a "win" (a triangle) or not (a circle); (2) a 2000–2500-ms crosshair fixation; (3) a target bull's-eye presented for up to 500 ms that requires a speeded button press; (4) 3000 ms of feedback that indicated whether that trial was a "win" or not, with wins accompanied by either an image of money or a face; and (5) a variable length ITI crosshair resulting in a total trial duration of 12 s. Potential win and non-win trials were aperiodic and pseudorandomly ordered. Each 8-min run contained 40 trails, half of which were potential win trials. The task was adaptive such that participants were successful on two thirds of trials, regardless of individual differences in RTs (confirmed via inspection of behavioral data collected during scanning). Mean reaction times were calculated during practice trials prior to the scan and then entered into the fMRI paradigm to ensure that participants succeeded on 66% of their responses as described in [36].

During nonsocial runs, participants won $1 per trial if bull's-eye responses were adequately quick. During social runs, participants viewed a face image if bull's-eye responses were adequately quick. Coincident with feedback, cumulative win totals were presented. Participants were instructed to respond to all target bull's-eyes as quickly as possible to win on as many trials as possible and win or non-win outcomes were contingent on reaction times (RTs). Standard administration of incentive delay tasks involves showing participants' rewards that may be won prior to scanning [36]. Consistent with this procedure, participants were shown the money they could win based on scanner task performance and were informed that they would receive the total amount of money won during the scan. Prior to scanning, participants rated face stimuli on the dimensions of valence and arousal. Stimuli were presented using E-Prime presentation software version 2.0 (Psychology Software Tools Inc., Pittsburgh, PA, USA).

Prior to and immediately following each scan, participants were asked to rate face stimuli on the dimensions of valence, arousal, and trust using Qualtrics software (Qualtrics, Provo, UT) on a computer outside of the scanner (pre-scan ratings were completed prior to the nasal spray administration).

Imaging methods and preprocessing

Functional imaging data were acquired at the Duke-UNC Brain Imaging and Analysis Center (BIAC) on a 3.0-T General Electric (Waukesha, WI, USA) MR750 scanner system equipped with 50 mT/m gradients and an eight-channel head coil. High-resolution T1-weighted anatomical images were acquired with 256 axial slices using an FSPGR pulse sequence (TR = 8.16 ms, TE = 3.18 ms; flip angle = 12°; FOV = 256; image matrix = 256 mm^2; voxel size = 1 × 1 × 1 mm) for normalization and co-registration. Whole brain functional images were acquired with 64 axial slices oriented parallel to the AC-PC plane using a spiral-in SENSE sequence (TR = 1500 ms, TE = 30 ms; flip angle = 60°; FOV = 240; image matrix = 64 mm^2; voxel size = 3.75 × 3.75 × 4 mm). The first four volumes of each functional task were discarded to allow for steady state equilibrium.

Functional data were preprocessed using FSL version 5.0.1 (Oxford Centre for Functional Magnetic Resonance Imaging of the Brain (FMRIB), Oxford University, UK). Preprocessing was applied as follows: (1) brain extraction for non-brain removal [38], (2) motion correction using MCFLIRT [39], (3) spatial smoothing using a Gaussian kernel of FWHM 5 mm, (4) mean-based intensity normalization of all volumes by the same factor, and (5) high-pass filtering [40]. Functional images were co-registered to structural images in native space, and structural images were normalized into a standard stereotaxic space (Montreal Neurological Institute). Registrations used an intermodal registration tool [38, 40]. Voxel-wise temporal autocorrelation was estimated and corrected using FMRIB's Improved Linear Model [41].

Motion correction

Consistent with motion thresholds used in Gordon et al. [22], runs with maximum motion > 3 mm along any of six axes (i.e., x, y, z, pitch, yaw, and roll) were excluded from analyses. Due to excessive motion (> 3 mm), some participants only had one social and/or nonsocial reward condition run per scan. Participants were only included in the final analyses if they had at least one nonsocial and one social run that met motion criteria for both their OT and PLC scans. Either due to motion or the participant's ability to stay in the scanner for the entire length of the scan, 17 of the 56 scans had less than four total runs. Sixty-six percent of runs included in analyses had < 1.0 mm of motion in any axis (pitch, roll, yaw, x, y, z), 26% had 1.0–1.99 mm of motion, and 8% had motion between 2.0 and 2.9 mm. In addition to conducting motion correction using MCFLIRT [39], time points with large motion, as defined by FSL, were entered into the general linear model (GLM) model as additional confound variables within first-level analyses using FSL's motion outlier detection program (http://fsl.fmrib.ox.ac.uk/fsl/fslwiki/FSLMotionOutliers). Following motion correction, paired t tests were used to compare differences in motion between OT and PLC groups: there was equivalent motion for mean and maximum values along all six axes (i.e., x, y, z, pitch, yaw, and roll), all p values > .05.

fMRI analysis

Planned analyses included (1) treatment group (OT vs. PLC) differences in frontostriatal functional activation and connectivity in response to social reward anticipation and outcomes; (2) treatment group differences in frontostriatal functional activation and connectivity in response to nonsocial reward anticipation and outcomes; (3) treatment group differences in frontostriatal functional activation in response to nonsocial relative to social reward anticipation and outcomes, conducted also with a small volume correction for the striatum alone given the centrality of this region for reward processing; and (4) correlations between frontostriatal functional activation and connectivity with ASD symptoms and salivary OT analyses.

Supplemental analyses included (1) main effects of OT and PLC separately on whole brain functional activation in response to nonsocial and social reward anticipation and outcomes, (2) treatment group (OT vs. PLC) differences in frontostriatal structural activation in response to social and nonsocial reward anticipation and outcomes,

(3) correlations between structural activation with ASD symptoms, and (4) treatment group differences in frontostriatal functional connectivity of structurally defined clusters in response to social and nonsocial reward anticipation and outcomes.

Small volume corrections

For all analyses, anticipation and outcome phases were analyzed separately. Key anatomical regions within the reward system (superior frontal gyrus, medial frontal gyrus, orbitofrontal gyrus, paracingulate gyrus, amygdala, nucleus accumbens (NAcc), insula, thalamus, caudate nucleus, anterior cingulate cortex (ACC), and putamen) were defined a priori for small volume correction. These regions were generated separately for the right and left hemispheres in FSL using the Harvard–Oxford cortical and subcortical structural probabilistic atlases. Masks were thresholded at 25%, binarized, and then combined into a single mask using fslmaths. For planned main effect analyses (i.e., nonsocial and social reward conditions analyzed independently) and planned interaction analyses (i.e., nonsocial > social, social > nonsocial), voxels were considered significant if they passed a threshold of $p < .005$ and were part of a 39-voxel cluster of contiguous significant voxels, resulting in a cluster-corrected $p < .05$. This cluster size was determined by performing 1000 Monte Carlo simulations using 3dClustSim [42]. Interaction analyses (e.g., nonsocial > social) also included an analysis using a small volume correction that included only the striatum given our a priori interest in the striatum. Due to this small volume correction, interaction clusters within the striatum were considered significant if they passed a statistical threshold of $p < .005$ and were part of a 17-voxel cluster of contiguous significant voxels, resulting in a cluster-corrected threshold of $p < .05$ (again determined by performing 1000 Monte Carlo simulations using 3dClustSim [42]). Localizations were based on Harvard–Oxford cortical and subcortical structural probabilistic atlases as implemented in FSLView version 5.0.1, and all activations were visualized with MRIcron (https://www.nitrc.org/projects/mricron/).

Activation analyses

Whole brain general linear model (GLM) activation analyses were conducted using the FSL expert analysis tool (FEAT). For ROI analyses, each participant's condition-specific mean percent signal change was calculated for both the social and nonsocial conditions. Within-participant activation differences were analyzed for treatment effects using paired t tests and using a 2 (Treatment Group: OT, PLC) × 2 (Reward Condition: nonsocial, social) ANOVA (see Additional file 1: Supplementary Materials). Structural ROI activation results are also provided in Additional file 1: Supplementary Materials.

Connectivity analyses

Task-based functional connectivity was analyzed using a generalized psychophysiological interaction (gPPI) approach due to its improved power, sensitivity, and specificity in detecting context-dependent functional connectivity [43, 44]. Functional seeds were derived from activation clusters showing significant OT > PLC effects. These seeds were supplemented with structural left and right NAcc seeds because of the centrality of the NAcc to the mesocorticolimbic reward processing system [36], once again defined using the Harvard–Oxford subcortical structural probabilistic atlas. Voxel-wise models evaluated whole-brain connectivity with these seeds. For each participant, mean fMRI time courses (i.e., physiological regressors) were extracted from seed regions for each task run using *fslmeants* in FSL, then multiplied by each psychological regressor of interest (i.e., Trial Type: reward, non-reward) to form the PPI interaction terms. The gPPI model included physiological and psychological regressors, as well as their interaction terms to describe the unique effect of these interactions above and beyond the main effect of seed time courses and reward conditions. Our contrasts of interest evaluated the reward condition alone. No additional preprocessing procedures were completed beyond what has been described above. Supplemental analyses examined functional connectivity with anatomically defined right and left NAcc using the same procedures described for the functional connectivity analyses (see Additional file 1: Supplementary Materials).

Symptom analyses

Symptom analyses examined interactions between ASD symptom severity, measured by the Social Responsiveness Scale (SRS) [45], and functional activation and connectivity in the OT relative to PLC condition, conducted by including demeaned SRS values as a covariate within frontostriatal general linear models within the ASD group. Supplementary analyses examined interactions between ASD symptoms and structural activation, as well as functional activation of structurally defined clusters (see Additional file 1: Supplementary Materials).

Salivary analyses

Saliva samples were collected using pediatric oral swabs (Salimetrics) prior to each nasal drug administration (i.e., OT and PLC) and immediately following the fMRI scan (time between samples in minutes $M = 85$; $SD = 9$). During each sample, participants were asked to place the swab under their tongue for approximately 1 min or until it was saturated with saliva. Samples were stored on ice for up to 2 h to liquid extraction and were permanently stored at -70 °C (see Additional file 1:

Supplementary Materials for a more detailed description of the salivary analyses).

Results

Face image ratings

Participants rated the faces seen in the social reward condition on the dimensions of valence, arousal, and trust prior to and immediately following each scan. Results from a 2 (Treatment Group: OT, PLC) × 2 (Time point: pre- or post-scan) ANOVA revealed a main effect of time point for the dimension of trust, such that participants were more likely to rate the faces as more trustworthy at the post-scan rating ($M = 5.07$; SD = 1.59) compared to the pre-scan rating ($M = 4.86$; SD = 1.63), regardless of treatment condition, $F(1,54) = 8.37$, $p = .006$ (see Fig. 1). Additionally, a main effect of time point for the dimension of arousal was observed, reflecting that participants perceived the faces at the post-scan rating ($M = 5.04$; SD = 1.75) to be more arousing than those at the pre-scan rating ($M = 4.91$; SD = 1.80) across treatment groups, $F(1,54) = 4.42$, $p = .040$. No other main effects or interactions between treatment group and time point for the perceived valence, arousal, or trust of the faces were significant, all p values > .05.

Task reaction times

Reaction times (RTs) to task bull's-eyes are depicted in Fig. 2 and were evaluated via a 2 (Treatment Group: OT, PLC) × 2 (Reward Condition: nonsocial, social) × 2 (Trial Type: reward, non-reward) mixed ANOVA. There was a main effect for trial type, $F(1,54) = 18.67$, $p < .0001$, such that individuals responded more quickly to trials during which they could receive a reward ($M = 226.49$; SD = 59.73) compared to trials in which they could not receive a reward ($M = 242.03$; SD = 60.91). No other main effects or interactions between treatment group, reward condition, and trial type were significant, all p values > .05.

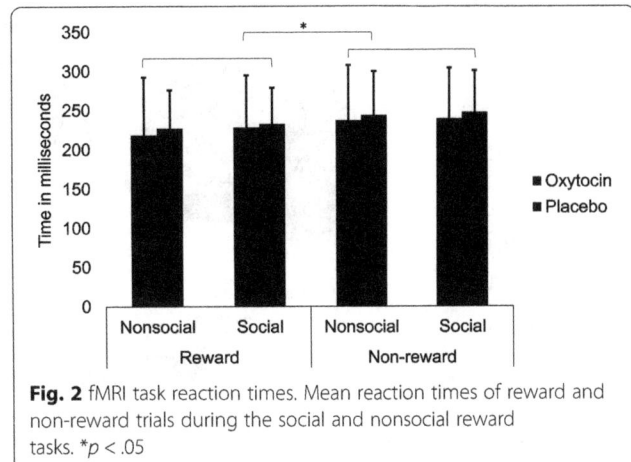

Fig. 2 fMRI task reaction times. Mean reaction times of reward and non-reward trials during the social and nonsocial reward tasks. *$p < .05$

Functional activation analyses

Nonsocial reward

During nonsocial reward anticipation, there were no regions with relatively decreased activation in the OT relative to the PLC condition. However, there were several clusters with greater activation during nonsocial reward anticipation in the OT condition relative to PLC, including the right NAcc, right frontal pole (FP), left ACC, left superior frontal cortex, and bilateral orbital frontal cortex (OFC) (see Fig. 3 and Table 2).[1] Significant increases in activation were observed during nonsocial reward outcomes after OT relative to PLC administration in the right OFC and left FP (see Fig. 4).

Supplementary analyses for OT and PLC conditions separately are presented in Additional file 1: Supplementary Materials and visualized within Additional file 2: Figure S1 and Additional file 3: Figure S2. These simple effects analyses revealed that both groups showed activation in mesocorticolimbic reward processing regions in response to the social and nonsocial incentive delay tasks.

Social reward

During social reward outcomes, there was significantly decreased activation in the right frontal pole in the OT condition relative to the PLC condition. There were no other clusters with significant changes in activation during social anticipation or social outcomes in the OT condition relative to the PLC condition (see Additional file 1: Supplementary Materials and Additional file 4: Figure S3 for structural activation results for social and nonsocial reward anticipatory and outcomes).

Treatment Group × Reward Condition Interaction

We next evaluated the impact of OT, relative to PLC, on nonsocial versus social reward processing by evaluating a Treatment Group × Reward Condition interaction general linear model. OT increased activation in the

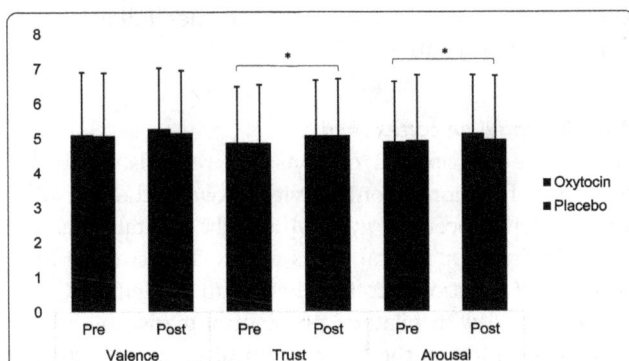

Fig. 1 Subjective ratings of faces. Average ratings of valence, arousal, and trust of faces. Valence = 0 (extremely unpleasant) to 8 (extremely pleasant); arousal = 0 (not at all aroused) to 8 (extremely aroused); trust = 0 (not at all trustworthy) to 8 (extremely trustworthy). *$p < .05$

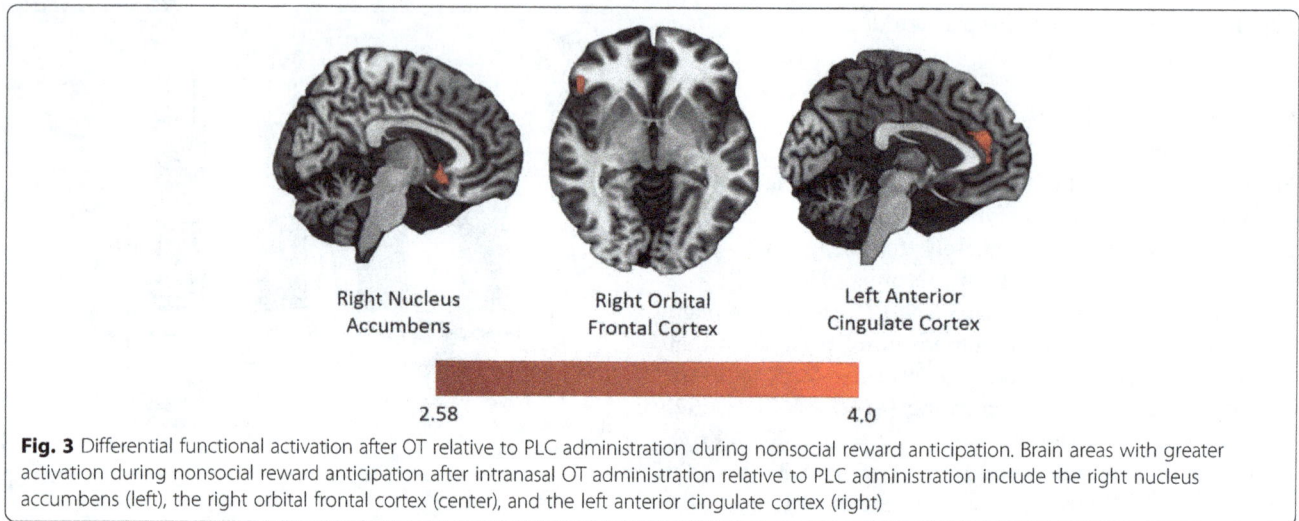

Fig. 3 Differential functional activation after OT relative to PLC administration during nonsocial reward anticipation. Brain areas with greater activation during nonsocial reward anticipation after intranasal OT administration relative to PLC administration include the right nucleus accumbens (left), the right orbital frontal cortex (center), and the left anterior cingulate cortex (right)

right caudate nucleus, left ACC, bilateral FP, right insular cortex, and right OFC in response to nonsocial compared to social reward outcomes (see Table 2). Planned analyses within the striatal small volume revealed greater activation during nonsocial relative to social reward anticipation after intranasal OT relative to PLC in the right NAcc. There were no regions with greater activation during social relative to nonsocial reward anticipation or outcomes after intranasal OT relative to PLC.

Correlations between functional activation and ASD symptoms

Increased ASD symptom severity, as measured by SRS total scores, was associated with greater activation in the right FP and the right ACC during nonsocial reward anticipation and greater activation in the right precentral gyrus and left caudate nucleus during nonsocial reward outcome following the administration of OT relative to PLC (see Fig. 5 and Table 3). This finding within the left caudate nucleus was corroborated by structural activation analyses (see Additional file 1: Supplementary Materials). There were no relations between symptom severity and brain activation in the anticipation or outcome phases of the social reward condition.

Functional connectivity analyses

Given the prominent roles of the NAcc and ACC in reward processing [46, 47], functional connectivity analyses were seeded by the right NAcc and left ACC functional clusters that showed increased activation to OT relative to PLC during nonsocial reward anticipation in the functional activation analyses. Because there were no clusters that differentiated conditions in the social reward condition, functional connectivity results are only reported for connectivity in the nonsocial reward condition (functional connectivity of structurally defined

clusters is presented in Additional file 1: Supplementary Materials).

Right nucleus accumbens seed

During nonsocial reward anticipation, OT relative to PLC administration resulted in increased functional connectivity between the right NAcc seed and the right frontal pole (see Fig. 6), whereas OT-induced decreases in functional connectivity were observed between the right NAcc seed and the left precentral gyrus and the right superior frontal gyrus (see Table 4). These findings were further corroborated by functional connectivity analyses of structurally defined clusters using a structural right NAcc seed (see Additional file 1: Supplementary Materials and Additional file 5: Figure S4). During nonsocial reward outcomes, increased functional connectivity was observed between the right NAcc and the right OFC and left FP in response to OT relative to PLC. Finally, decreased functional connectivity was exhibited between the right NAcc and right postcentral gyrus during nonsocial reward outcomes following OT administration relative to PLC.

Anterior cingulate cortex seed

During the anticipation of nonsocial rewards, there was decreased functional connectivity between the left ACC and the left precentral gyrus, the right frontal pole, and the right superior frontal gyrus after OT relative to PLC. Attenuated functional connectivity with the left ACC was also observed with bilateral postcentral gyrus, the left inferior frontal gyrus, the left precentral gyrus, and the left medial frontal gyrus during nonsocial reward outcomes following OT relative to PLC (Table 5). No increases in connectivity were exhibited with the left ACC for nonsocial reward anticipation or outcomes, all p values > .05.

Table 2 Effects of oxytocin on functional activation

Phase	Reward condition	Region	Hem	k	BA	x	y	z	Z max
OT > PLC									
Anticipation	Nonsocial	Frontal pole	R	316	10	41	95	38	3.99
		Anterior cingulate cortex	L	182	32	46	83	46	3.97
		Superior frontal cortex	L	83	–	49	74	65	3.31
		Orbital frontal cortex	R	76	–	23	79	30	3.26
		Orbital frontal cortex	L	52	–	58	72	27	3.16
		Nucleus accumbens	R	56	–	43	72	30	3.42
	Nonsocial > social	Anterior cingulate cortex	L	441	–	46	84	46	3.91
		Frontal pole	L	69	–	54	91	29	3.12
		Frontal pole	R	40	–	38	87	56	3.17
		Insular cortex	R	65	47	25	72	31	3.24
		Caudate nucleus	R	64	–	42	67	36	3.11
		Orbital frontal cortex	R	47	–	29	76	29	3.34
		Nucleus accumbens	R	21	–	42	71	30	3.09
Outcome	Nonsocial	Frontal pole	L	42	–	55	91	52	3.28
		Orbital frontal cortex	R	39	–	21	75	30	3.35
OT < PLC									
Outcome	Social	Frontal pole	R	50	–	24	91	37	3.29

Hem hemisphere, *k* cluster size in voxels, *BA* Brodmann area; *Z max* maximum *z*-value

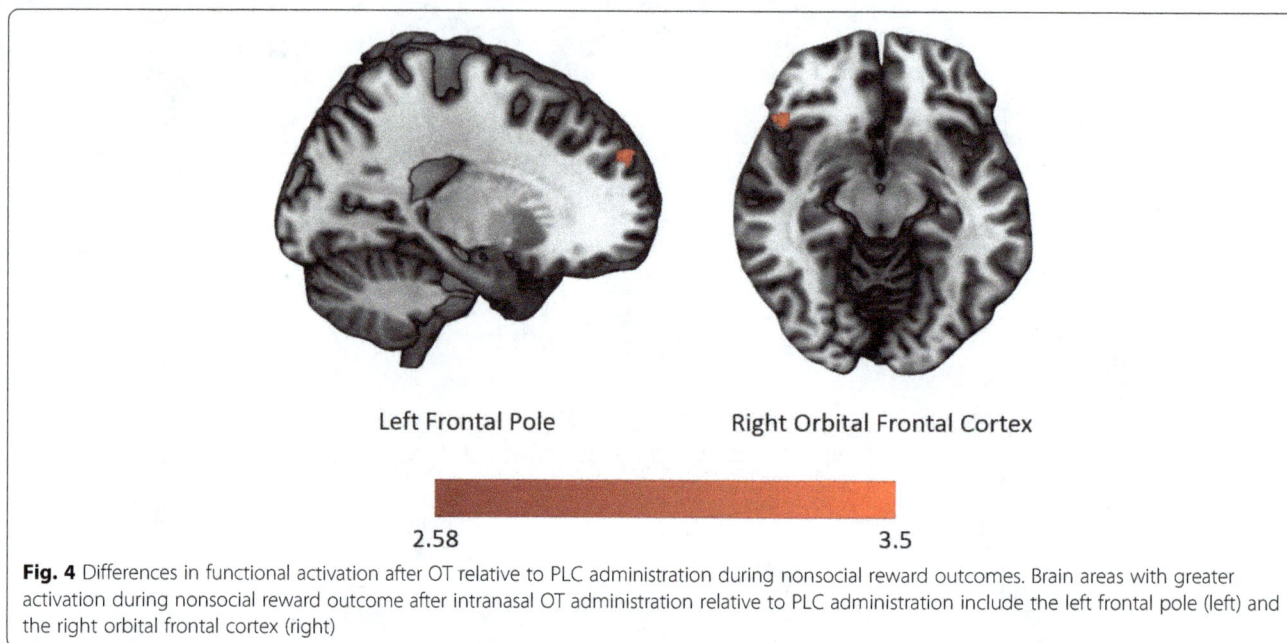

Left Frontal Pole   **Right Orbital Frontal Cortex**

2.58   3.5

Fig. 4 Differences in functional activation after OT relative to PLC administration during nonsocial reward outcomes. Brain areas with greater activation during nonsocial reward outcome after intranasal OT administration relative to PLC administration include the left frontal pole (left) and the right orbital frontal cortex (right)

Correlations between functional connectivity and ASD symptoms

For the right NAcc and left ACC seeds, greater ASD symptom severity, measured by SRS total scores, was associated with increased connectivity with the right postcentral gyrus during nonsocial reward outcomes following OT relative to PLC (see Table 6). During nonsocial reward anticipation, there were no significant correlations between SRS scores and connectivity with the right NAcc or left ACC following OT relative to PLC.

Salivary OT

To examine changes in OT concentration levels, salivary samples were collected prior to OT administration and immediately following the fMRI scan. There were considerable individual differences in the magnitude of salivary OT change from baseline to post-scan following OT administration, and, thus, one outlier was removed from salivary analyses due to significantly elevated OT concentration levels (754.17 pg/ml) in the PLC condition. After the removal of this outlier, as expected, there was a significant increase in mean peripheral OT levels following OT administration relative to PLC, $t = 3.57$; $p = 0.0016$ (see Fig. 7).

Because of the primary role of the NAcc in reward processing [46], correlation analyses examined relations between changes in peripheral OT and neural activation within the right NAcc functional activation cluster identified in the nonsocial anticipation activation analysis. This revealed a significant positive correlation indicating

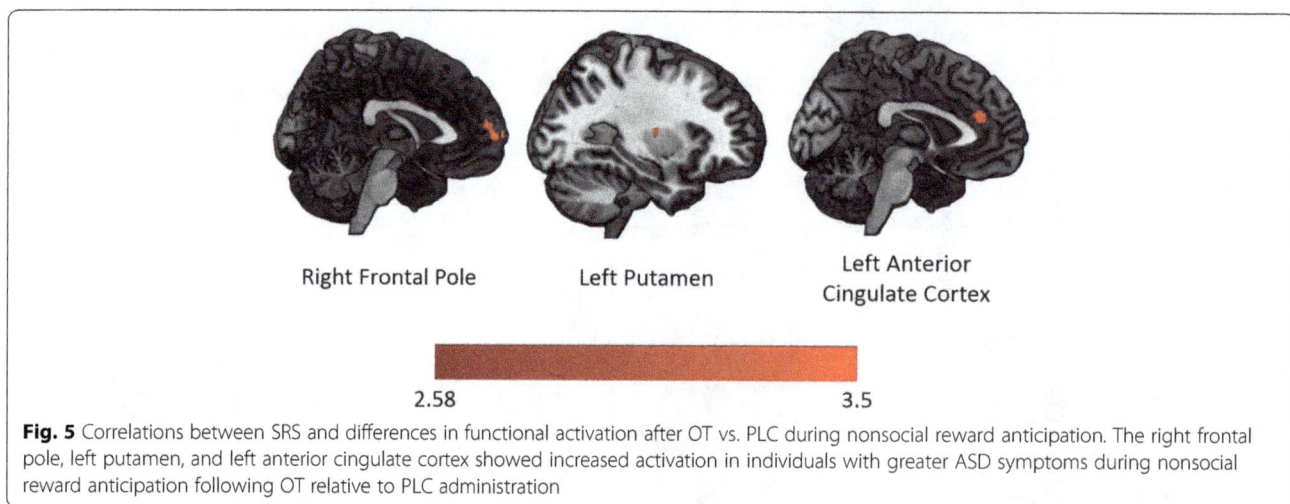

Right Frontal Pole   **Left Putamen**   **Left Anterior Cingulate Cortex**

2.58   3.5

Fig. 5 Correlations between SRS and differences in functional activation after OT vs. PLC during nonsocial reward anticipation. The right frontal pole, left putamen, and left anterior cingulate cortex showed increased activation in individuals with greater ASD symptoms during nonsocial reward anticipation following OT relative to PLC administration

Table 3 Correlations between ASD symptoms and functional activation to oxytocin relative to placebo

Phase	Reward condition	Region	Hem	k	BA	x	y	z	Z max
Anticipation	Nonsocial	Frontal pole	R	95	10	41	95	38	3.53
		Anterior cingulate cortex	L	82	32	46	83	46	3.41
Outcome	Nonsocial	Precentral gyrus	R	48	–	18	59	51	3.29
		Caudate nucleus	L	51	–	58	63	47	3.27

Hem hemisphere, *k* cluster size in voxels, *BA* Brodmann area, *Z max* maximum z-value

that individuals with greater changes in peripheral OT concentrations following OT administration showed greater increased activation within the right NAcc functional activation cluster during nonsocial reward anticipation, $r = 0.56$; $p = 0.005$ (see Fig. 8). However, when a significant outlier (2 SD's > the salivary group mean; 3 SD's > the activation group mean) was removed, the relation was no longer significant, $r = 0.26$; $p = 0.23$.[2]

Discussion

The purpose of this investigation was to examine the effects of acute intranasal OT administration on functional activation and connectivity within mesocorticolimbic brain regions during the anticipation and receipt of social and nonsocial rewards in ASD. OT administration, relative to PLC administration, was associated with increased activity in the right NAcc, the right FP, the left ACC, the left superior frontal cortex, and bilateral OFC during anticipation of nonsocial rewards. These findings combined with prior

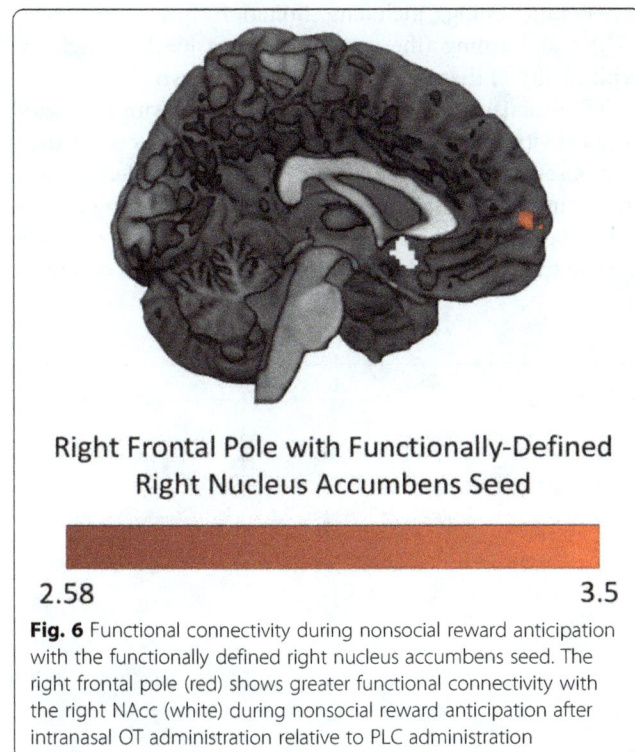

Right Frontal Pole with Functionally-Defined Right Nucleus Accumbens Seed

2.58   3.5

Fig. 6 Functional connectivity during nonsocial reward anticipation with the functionally defined right nucleus accumbens seed. The right frontal pole (red) shows greater functional connectivity with the right NAcc (white) during nonsocial reward anticipation after intranasal OT administration relative to PLC administration

ASD research demonstrating increased activation in the NAcc following OT administration during a social judgment task [22] suggest that whether OT impacts social or nonsocial processing is contingent on task context. In addition, the correlation between salivary OT concentrations and changes in right NAcc activation indicates that this region may be particularly sensitive to the acute effects of OT (though this correlation was not significant following removal of an outlier). This is consistent with preclinical findings, which indicate that the NAcc is among several neural regions with the highest OT receptor density [48].

Although we found increased left ACC activation after OT administration during nonsocial reward anticipation, Watanabe and colleagues [49] reported increased ACC activation after OT administration during a social judgment task, reflecting the task-dependent nature of the effects of OT on neural responses to social or nonsocial processing. Our finding of increased activation of OFC, a region with an established role in reward processes documented in preclinical and clinical studies [50, 51], during the anticipation and receipt of nonsocial rewards after OT administration is consistent with prior findings that ASD is characterized by attenuated OFC activation during nonsocial reward anticipation [26] and suggests a remediation of this pattern in ASD after OT.

In contrast to previous studies examining the neural impact of OT in response to social stimuli in individuals with ASD [22, 23], we did not find evidence of increased activity in mesocorticolimbic regions during social reward processing following OT administration. Further, interaction analyses showed increased activity in the right nucleus accumbens and right caudate nucleus during nonsocial reward anticipation relative to social reward anticipation. The lack of effects of OT in the social reward conditions are surprising and stand in contrast to preclinical findings that OT enhances neural responses to a range of social stimuli, including conditioned social preference [52–54] and reproductive behaviors [55, 56] as well of the prosocial effects of OT in ASD [57]. These unexpected findings highlight that OT may serve to increase neural activations in response to nonsocial rewards. These effects are consistent with preclinical findings that the impact of OT is apparent in the context of a certain nonsocial rewards, including food cues [58, 59] and place preferences [60, 61], and it may be the

Table 4 Functional connectivity with the right NAcc seed

Phase	Reward condition	Region	Hem	k	BA	x	y	z	Z max
OT > PLC									
Anticipation	Nonsocial	Frontal pole	R	45	–	39	95	39	3.39
Outcome		Orbital frontal cortex	R	82	–	22	75	31	3.96
		Frontal pole	L	41	9	54	92	52	3.19
OT < PLC									
Anticipation	Nonsocial	Precentral gyrus	L	266	–	54	62	63	3.64
		Superior frontal gyrus	R	53	–	37	63	69	3.6
Outcome		Postcentral gyrus	R	42	–	19	58	51	3.4

Hem hemisphere, *k* cluster size in voxels, *BA* Brodmann area, *Z max* maximum z-value

case that the clinical benefits of OT on social functioning in ASD (e.g., enhanced emotion recognition and increased eye gaze) reflect the influence of OT on mesocorticolimbic reward processing systems that mediate nonsocial incentive salience processing, reward valuation, and reward-based learning [62] rather than responses specifically to social rewards. Alternatively, it may be the case that the static social rewards used in this study impeded our capacity to detect OT-related neural changes given that dynamic stimuli have been shown to be more potent elicitors of social impairments in ASD than static stimuli [63]. Future studies that evaluate the impact of OT on neural responses to dynamic social rewards will be needed to evaluate this possibility.

We observed significant correlations between ASD symptom severity and increased activity within the right frontal pole and the left ACC during nonsocial reward anticipation in response to OT relative to PLC. Additionally, during nonsocial reward outcomes, increases in the left caudate nucleus and right precentral gyrus activity after OT relative to PLC were significantly correlated with symptom severity. The postcentral gyrus also showed greater connectivity with both the right NAcc and left ACC functional seeds as ASD symptom severity increased. These regions may be most responsive to neural effects of OT administration in individuals with more severe ASD presentations. Alternatively,

these associations suggest that the impact of OT on responses to nonsocial rewards may be conditional on ASD symptom severity. These associations may also reflect mechanisms described by Parker and colleagues [15] which revealed that individuals with ASD with lower endogenous levels of OT benefited the most from OT. Thus, it may be the case that individuals with greater ASD symptoms demonstrated greater regional activation changes during reward anticipation in response to OT. It is noteworthy that symptom correlations with neural responses to nonsocial reward anticipation were apparent in brain regions (FP and ACC) implicated in higher-order executive processing [64] and known to show functional impairments in ASD in the context of cognitive control tasks [65, 66]. Conversely, regions showing symptom correlations with neural responses to social reward anticipation involved regions implicated in other functioning, including imitation (precentral gyrus [67]) and learning (the caudate nucleus [68]), though the replicability of these patterns is not yet known.

OT administration was associated broadly with decreased connectivity with functional seeds. Decreased connectivity was observed between the right NAcc and the left precentral gyrus and the right superior frontal gyrus during the anticipation of nonsocial rewards as well as with the postcentral gyrus during nonsocial reward outcomes

Table 5 Functional connectivity with the left ACC seed

Phase	Reward condition	Region	Hem	k	BA	x	y	z	Z max
OT < PLC									
Anticipation	Nonsocial	Precentral gyrus	L	206	–	58	58	63	3.86
		Frontal pole	R	197	–	30	83	48	3.34
		Superior frontal gyrus	R	39	–	37	63	69	3.66
Outcome		Postcentral gyrus	R	179	–	21	57	51	3.72
			L	90	3	75	57	50	3.13
		Inferior frontal gyrus	L	55	–	70	78	42	3.64
		Precentral gyrus	L	49	–	73	64	54	3.13
		Medial frontal gyrus	L	42	6	57	66	59	3.09

Hem hemisphere, *k* cluster size in voxels, *BA* Brodmann area, *Z max* maximum z-value

Table 6 Correlations between ASD symptoms and functional connectivity for oxytocin relative to placebo

Phase	Reward condition	Region	Hem	k	BA	x	y	z	Z max
Right NAcc seed									
Outcome	Nonsocial	Postcentral gyrus	R	74	–	18	58	51	3.37
Left ACC seed									
Outcome	Nonsocial	Postcentral gyrus	R	131	–	18	58	51	3.5

Hem hemisphere, *k* cluster size in voxels, *BA* Brodmann area, *Z max* maximum z-value

following OT administration relative to PLC. Further, OT-induced attenuation in functional connectivity was observed between the left ACC functional seed and the left precentral gyrus, the right frontal pole, and the right superior frontal gyrus during nonsocial reward anticipation. During nonsocial reward outcomes, decreased functional connectivity was observed between the left ACC and bilateral postcentral gyrus, left inferior frontal gyrus, left precentral gyrus, and left medial frontal gyrus following OT relative to PLC. Resting state functional connectivity findings suggest that ASD is largely characterized by increased frontostriatal connectivity relative to typically developing controls [69–72], and the results of the present study suggest that OT

may normalize these increased frontostriatal functional connections.

There were additional findings of increased functional connectivity after OT administration, including increased connectivity between the right NAcc and the right FP during nonsocial reward anticipation. OT-induced increased connectivity between the right NAcc and right FP was also reported by Gordon et al. [23] using a biological motion task. This finding across two different task contexts highlights a neural pathway by which OT may exert a therapeutic effect by potentiating neural connectivity. The FP plays a critical role in the cognitive processing of future events [73], a process that may

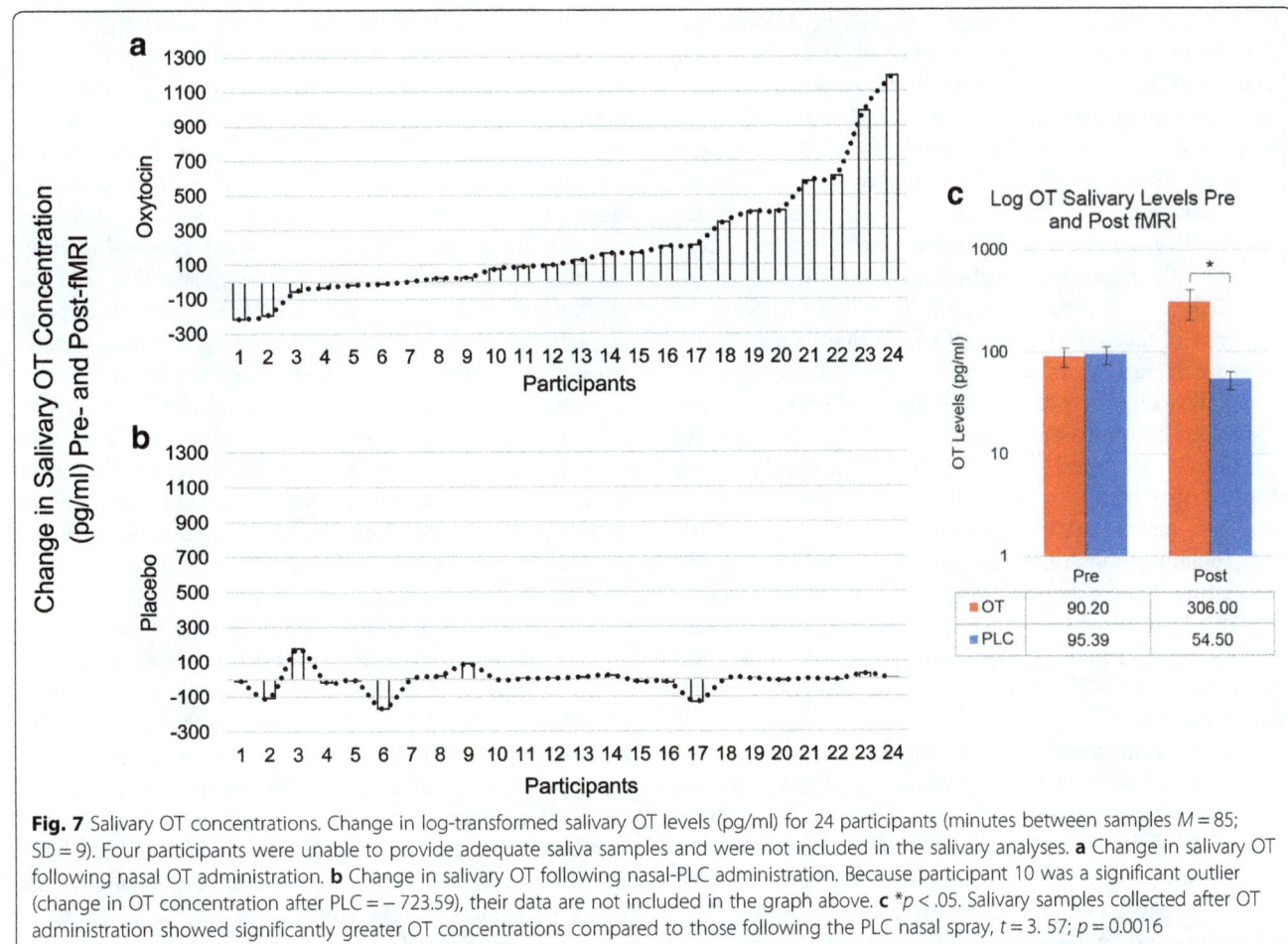

Fig. 7 Salivary OT concentrations. Change in log-transformed salivary OT levels (pg/ml) for 24 participants (minutes between samples $M = 85$; SD = 9). Four participants were unable to provide adequate saliva samples and were not included in the salivary analyses. **a** Change in salivary OT following nasal OT administration. **b** Change in salivary OT following nasal-PLC administration. Because participant 10 was a significant outlier (change in OT concentration after PLC = − 723.59), their data are not included in the graph above. **c** *$p < .05$. Salivary samples collected after OT administration showed significantly greater OT concentrations compared to those following the PLC nasal spray, $t = 3.57$; $p = 0.0016$

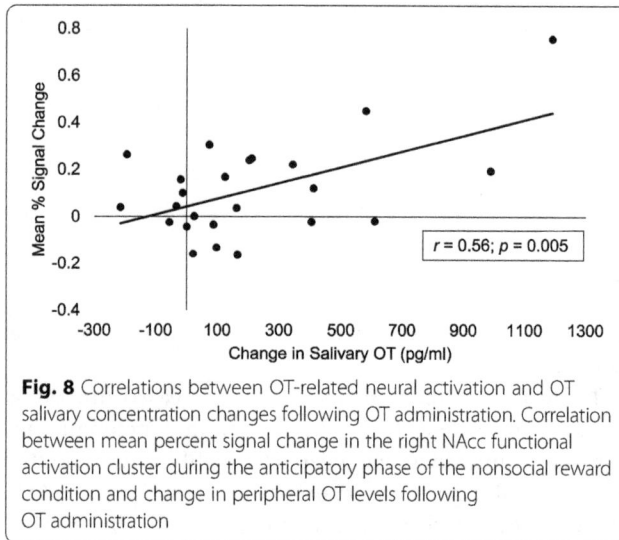

Fig. 8 Correlations between OT-related neural activation and OT salivary concentration changes following OT administration. Correlation between mean percent signal change in the right NAcc functional activation cluster during the anticipatory phase of the nonsocial reward condition and change in peripheral OT levels following OT administration

be particularly relevant to reward contexts. Additionally, the right NAcc demonstrated relatively greater connectivity with the right FP and right OFC during nonsocial reward outcomes following OT administration relative to PLC, though the directionality of this effect was unexpected given that increased functional connectivity between the striatum and the OFC has been reported in ASD during resting-state functional connectivity [69]. It is also noteworthy that the effects of OT on the NAcc and ACC exhibited right-lateralized effects given evidence of right lateralization of functional neural responses to social and nonsocial stimuli in ASD [74, 75], though it should be noted that incentive delay tasks do not reliably evoke greater activation in one hemisphere or the other but rather tend to evoke bilateral reward-related frontostriatal activations [76].

Ratings of faces in the social task revealed a significant increase in ratings of trustworthiness and arousal for faces following the scan. These main effects were not moderated by treatment group (i.e., OT, PLC), indicating that individuals rated faces they had seen previously as more trustworthy across both treatment groups. Previous studies have reported that individuals with ASD reliably understand the concept of trustworthiness and distinguish trustworthy versus non-trustworthy faces [77, 78]. Our results suggest that familiarity with faces may increase ratings of trustworthiness and arousal for individuals with ASD. No effects were observed for ratings of valence.

Task reaction times showed increased speed of responses to reward relative to non-reward trials, with no significant interactions of treatment group (OT, PLC) or Reward Type (nonsocial, social). These findings are consistent with reports of decreased reaction times for reward compared to non-reward trial in ASD [79]. Delmonte and colleagues [79] reported no relation

between reward condition (e.g., nonsocial vs. social) and reaction times. However, this stands in contrast with other ASD reward studies that have reported faster reaction times in response to nonsocial rewards compared to social rewards [26, 80]. This discrepancy may reflect different ages of participants across studies: the current study and others showing no differences in reaction times based on reward condition were conducted in child and adolescent populations, whereas those showing faster responses for nonsocial versus social rewards were completed using adult participants. This may suggest that during development, nonsocial rewards may begin to have increased salience relative to social rewards in individuals with ASD. This might be related to increased awareness of the relationship between money and acquiring objects of interest and/or to increased demands in financial responsibility for adults living independently. This developmental interaction should be noted in future studies examining differential responses to nonsocial versus social rewards in ASD. It may also be useful to explore the salience of other nonsocial rewards in ASD.

In addition to the substantive findings reported here, these results have implications for future experimental therapeutic trials that seek to evaluate novel ASD therapeutics. The National Institute of Health has emphasized the use of translational research to speed the discovery of treatments through pipelines that evaluate the potential for novel compounds to engage brain targets relevant to disease etiology [81]. In addition to providing substantive results about the neural impact of acute intranasal OT administration on reward processing brain systems, the present study also suggests that optimal approaches to evaluate novel ASD treatments with putative effects on brain systems that support social reward processing may not be constrained to evaluating responses to only social stimuli. Rather, novel pro-social ASD therapeutics may exert their influence on relevant brain targets in a range of social and/or nonsocial contexts. In this regard, these results provide preliminary data to guide the development of optimal targets for use in future experimental therapeutics trials that evaluate novel ASD social communication treatments.

The present study had some limitations. Developmental stage plays a particularly important moderating role in the strength of functional connectivity patterns in individuals with ASD, with younger individuals showing increased connectivity compared to adolescents and adults with ASD [82]. Future studies with large sample sizes will be needed to examine the moderating effect of developmental stage on the effects of OT on brain activation and connectivity in ASD. Additionally, the effects of prolonged OT administration are likely to be distinct from the effects of a single dose, and future research should examine the effect of chronic OT administration on neural functioning in ASD. Additionally, the order of social and nonsocial runs was not randomized across participants in this study. Because the current study found no behavioral changes due to a single OT administration, interpretations regarding associations between behavioral and neural effects of OT must be cautious. Finally, because all participants in the present study met a minimum IQ cutoff of 70, findings from this study may be restricted to individuals with ASD with higher cognitive ability.

Conclusions

Despite these limitations, these findings indicate a mechanistic role for the mesocorticolimbic system in the potentially therapeutic effect of oxytocin in individuals with ASD. These findings align with prior studies that highlight the important role of enhanced functioning of striatal regions as a potential mechanism of action of OT [22, 23] and extend this area of research into the domain of striatal functioning in response to reward-based tasks. When the present findings are considered along with these prior fMRI studies, it appears that the role of the mesocorticolimbic system in the effects of OT on neural functioning is not confined to social rewards but may extend to nonsocial responses more broadly, depending on task contexts.

Endnotes

[1]Similar analyses during the anticipation of nonsocial rewards were conducted after removing both female participants, as well as a participant with outlying salivary OT concentrations (see Figure 7a). Results from these analyses remained statistically significant within all regions reported in Table 2. Therefore, all activation results include both females and the participant with outlying salivary OT levels.

[2]We thank an anonymous reviewer for highlighting this. This outlier was not the same outlier as the one mentioned in the previous salivary analyses examining treatment group (OT vs. PLC) differences in OT concentrations.

Additional files

Additional file 1: Supplementary Analyses & Results.

Additional file 2: Figure S1. Functional activation during the anticipatory phase of the nonsocial and social tasks for OT and PLC.

Additional file 3: Figure S2. Functional activation during the outcome phase of the nonsocial and social tasks for OT and PLC.

Additional file 4: Figure S3. Structural activation in striatal regions during the anticipation and outcome of nonsocial and social rewards. Frontostriatal structural activation during nonsocial (left) and social (right) reward anticipation and outcome after intranasal OT relative to PLC

administration. In the nonsocial reward condition, the right NAcc showed relatively increased activation during reward anticipation following OT relative to PLC administration. No significant differences in activation were observed during nonsocial outcomes following OT relative to PLC administration. In the social reward conditions, none of the regions queried showed differential activation during either the anticipation or outcome phases after intranasal OT relative to PLC administration. NAcc = nucleus accumbens. *$p < .05$.

Additional file 5: Figure S4. Functional connectivity with structurally defined right NAcc during nonsocial reward anticipation. The right frontal pole (red) shows greater structural connectivity with the right NAcc (white) during nonsocial reward anticipation after intranasal OT administration relative to PLC administration.

Abbreviations

ACC: Anterior cingulate cortex; ADOS: Autism Diagnostic Observation Schedule; ASD: Autism spectrum disorder; FEAT: FSL expert analysis tool; fMRI: Functional magnetic resonance imaging; FP: Frontal pole; GLM: General linear model; gPPI: Generalized psychophysiological interaction; NAcc: Nucleus accumbens; OFC: Orbital frontal cortex; OT: Oxytocin; PLC: Placebo; ROI: Region of interest; SRS: Social Responsiveness Scale; WASI: Wechsler Abbreviated Scales of Intelligence

Acknowledgements

We thank the many dedicated families and staff who have graciously offered their valuable time to the benefit of this study. We thank the MRI technologists Susan Music, Natalie Goutkin, and Luke Poole for the assistance with the data acquisition and BIAC Director Allen Song for the assistance with the various aspects of this project. We also thank Dr. Lucina Uddin, Dr. Jason Nomi, Dr. Shruti Vij, Catherine Burrows, Taylor Bolt, and Willa Voorhies for their assistance with conducting the functional connectivity analyses.

Funding

Support for this project was provided by the Clinical Translational Core of U54 HD079124. GSD was supported by U54 HD079124 and MH110933. Functional neuroimaging analytic training was supported by an accelerator grant from the Autism Science Foundation (RKG). EW was supported by T32AT003378. JB was supported by HD079124. JKL was supported by T32-HD40127. GDS was supported by DA032750 and HD079124. The funding bodies did not have any role in the design, collection, analyses, and interpretation of data or in writing the manuscript.

Authors' contributions

GSD, LS, and GDS contributed to the study conception and study design. RKG collected all the fMRI data, acquired the behavioral data, and assisted with regulatory responsibilities. RKG and GSD were responsible for the analysis and interpretation of the data, as well as drafting the manuscript. LS made substantial contributions to the interpretation of data. MS and LS were responsible for overseeing the collection of behavioral data and critically revised the manuscript for important intellectual content. CA was responsible for the acquisition of behavioral data and managed regulatory responsibilities. LCP and TC were responsible for the collection of behavioral and diagnostic data and critically revised the manuscript for important intellectual content. EW and JB contributed to the fMRI analysis and interpretation. MGM and JLK were involved in the interpretation of fMRI data and critically revised the manuscript for important intellectual content. All authors read and approved the final manuscript.

Competing interests

The authors declare that they have no competing interests.

Author details

[1]Department of Psychology and Neuroscience, University of North Carolina at Chapel Hill, Chapel Hill, NC 27514, USA. [2]Duke Clinical Research Institute, Duke University, Durham, NC 27705, USA. [3]Duke Center for Autism and Brain Development, Duke University, Durham, NC 27705, USA. [4]Department of Psychiatry, University of North Carolina at Chapel Hill School of Medicine, Chapel Hill, NC 27514, USA. [5]Duke-UNC Brain Imaging and Analysis Center, Duke University Medical Center, Durham, NC 27705, USA. [6]Carolina Institute for Developmental Disabilities, University of North Carolina at Chapel Hill School of Medicine, Chapel Hill, NC 27514, USA. [7]Department of Psychiatry and Behavioral Sciences, Duke University Medical Center, Durham, NC 27705, USA. [8]Department of Cell Biology and Physiology, University of North Carolina at Chapel Hill School of Medicine, Chapel Hill, NC 27514, USA. [9]Neuroscience Center, University of North Carolina at Chapel Hill School of Medicine, Chapel Hill, NC 27514, USA. [10]Department of Psychiatry, University of North Carolina at Chapel Hill School of Medicine, CB 7155, Chapel Hill, NC 27599-7155, USA.

References

1. American Psychiatric Association. Diagnostic and statistical manual of mental disorders. 5th ed. Washington: American Psychiatric Association; 2013.
2. Jesner OS, Aref-Adib M, Coren E. Risperidone for autism spectrum disorder. Cochrane Libr. 2007;1:CD005040.
3. Farmer C, Thurm A, Grant P. Pharmacotherapy for the core symptoms in autistic disorder: current status of the research. Drugs. 2013;73:303–14.
4. Dove D, Warren Z, McPheeters ML, Taylor JL, Sathe NA, Veenstra-VanderWeele J. Medications for adolescents and young adults with autism spectrum disorders: a systematic review. Pediatrics. 2012;130:717–26.
5. Kosfeld M, Heinrichs M, Zak PJ, Fischbacher U, Fehr E. Oxytocin increases trust in humans. Nature. 2005;435:673–6.
6. Quattrocki E, Friston K. Autism, oxytocin and interoception. Neurosci Biobehav Rev. 2014;47:410–30.
7. Kirsch P, Esslinger C, Chen Q, Mier D, Lis S, Siddhanti S, Gruppe H, Mattay VS, Gallhofer B, Meyer-Lindenberg A. Oxytocin modulates neural circuitry for social cognition and fear in humans. J Neurosci. 2005;25:11489.
8. Carter CS, Grippo AJ, Pournajafi-Nazarloo H, Ruscio MG, Porges SW. Oxytocin, vasopressin and sociality. Progress Brain Res. 2008;170:331–6.
9. Insel TR, Fernald RD. How the brain processes social information: searching for the social brain. Annu Rev Neurosci. 2004;27:697–722.
10. Guastella AJ, Einfeld SL, Gray KM, Rinehart NJ, Tonge BJ, Lambert TJ, Hickie IB. Intranasal oxytocin improves emotion recognition for youth with autism spectrum disorders. Biol Psychiatry. 2010;67:692–4.
11. Guastella AJ, Mitchell PB, Dadds MR. Oxytocin increases gaze to the eye region of human faces. Biol Psychiatry. 2008;63:3–5.
12. Andari E, Duhamel J-R, Zalla T, Herbrecht E, Leboyer M, Sirigu A. Promoting social behavior with oxytocin in high-functioning autism spectrum disorders. Proc Natl Acad Sci U S A. 2010;107:4389–94.
13. Anagnostou E, Soorya L, Chaplin W, Bartz J, Halpern D, Wasserman S, Wang AT, Pepa L, Tanel N, Kushki A. Intranasal oxytocin versus placebo in the treatment of adults with autism spectrum disorders: a randomized controlled trial. Molecular autism. 2012;3:16.
14. Dadds MR, MacDonald E, Cauchi A, Williams K, Levy F, Brennan J. Nasal oxytocin for social deficits in childhood autism: a randomized controlled trial. J Autism Dev Disord. 2014;44:521–31.
15. Parker KJ, Oztan O, Libove RA, Sumiyoshi RD, Jackson LP, Karhson DS, Summers JE, Hinman KE, Motonaga KS, Phillips JM, et al. Intranasal oxytocin treatment for social deficits and biomarkers of response in children with autism. Proc Natl Acad Sci. 2017;114:8119.
16. Love TM. Oxytocin, motivation and the role of dopamine. Pharmacol Biochem Behav. 2014;119:49–60.
17. Hung LW, Neuner S, Polepalli JS, Beier KT, Wright M, Walsh JJ, Lewis EM, Luo L, Deisseroth K, Dölen G, Malenka RC. Gating of social reward by

18. oxytocin in the ventral tegmental area. Science. 2017;357:1406.
18. Haber SN, Knutson B. The reward circuit: linking primate anatomy and human imaging. Neuropsychopharmacology. 2010;35:4–26.
19. Melis MR, Melis T, Cocco C, Succu S, Sanna F, Pillolla G, Boi A, Ferri GL, Argiolas A. Oxytocin injected into the ventral tegmental area induces penile erection and increases extracellular dopamine in the nucleus accumbens and paraventricular nucleus of the hypothalamus of male rats. Eur J Neurosci. 2007;26:1026–35.
20. Melis MR, Succu S, Sanna F, Boi A, Argiolas A. Oxytocin injected into the ventral subiculum or the posteromedial cortical nucleus of the amygdala induces penile erection and increases extracellular dopamine levels in the nucleus accumbens of male rats. Eur J Neurosci. 2009;30:1349–57.
21. Xiao L, Priest MF, Nasenbeny J, Lu T, Kozorovitskiy Y. Biased oxytocinergic modulation of midbrain dopamine systems. Neuron. 2017;95:368–84. e365
22. Gordon I, Vander Wyk BC, Bennett RH, Cordeaux C, Lucas MV, Eilbott JA, Zagoory-Sharon O, Leckman JF, Feldman R, Pelphrey KA. Oxytocin enhances brain function in children with autism. Proc Natl Acad Sci. 2013;110:20953–8.
23. Gordon I, Jack A, Pretzsch CM, Vander Wyk B, Leckman JF, Feldman R, Pelphrey KA. Intranasal oxytocin enhances connectivity in the neural circuitry supporting social motivation and social perception in children with autism. Sci Rep. 2016;6.
24. Kohls G, Schulte-Rüther M, Nehrkorn B, Müller K, Fink GR, Kamp-Becker I, Herpertz-Dahlmann B, Schultz RT, Konrad K. Reward system dysfunction in autism spectrum disorders. Soc Cogn Affect Neurosci. 2012;8:565–72.
25. Dichter GS, Felder JN, Green SR, Rittenberg AM, Sasson NJ, Bodfish JW. Reward circuitry function in autism spectrum disorders. Soc Cogn Affect Neurosci. 2012;7:160–72.
26. Dichter GS, Richey JA, Rittenberg AM, Sabatino A, Bodfish JW. Reward circuitry function in autism during face anticipation and outcomes. J Autism Dev Disord. 2012;42:147–60.
27. Scott-Van Zeeland AA, Dapretto M, Ghahremani DG, Poldrack RA, Bookheimer SY. Reward processing in autism. Autism Res. 2010;3(2):53–67.
28. Richey JA, Rittenberg A, Hughes L, Damiano CR, Sabatino A, Miller S, Hanna E, Bodfish JW, Dichter GS. Common and distinct neural features of social and non-social reward processing in autism and social anxiety disorder. Soc Cogn Affect Neurosci. 2013;9:367–77.
29. Stavropoulos KKM, Carver LJ. Reward anticipation and processing of social versus nonsocial stimuli in children with and without autism spectrum disorders. J Child Psychol Psychiatry. 2014;55:1398–408.
30. Schmitz N, Rubia K, van Amelsvoort T, Daly E, Smith A, Murphy DGM. Neural correlates of reward in autism. Br J Psychiatry. 2008;192:19–24.
31. Lord C, Rutter M, PC DL, Risi S, Gotham K, Bishop S. Autism diagnostic observation schedule, second edition (ADOS-2) manual (part I): modules 1-4. Torrance: Western Psychological Services; 2012.
32. Striepens N, Kendrick KM, Hanking V, Landgraf R, Wüllner U, Maier W, Hurlemann R. Elevated cerebrospinal fluid and blood concentrations of oxytocin following its intranasal administration in humans. Sci Rep. 2013;3:3440.
33. Tanaka A, Furubayashi T, Arai M, Inoue D, Kimura S, Kiriyama A, Kusamori K, Katsumi H, Yutani R, Sakane T. Delivery of oxytocin to the brain for the treatment of autism spectrum disorder by nasal application. Mol Pharm. 2018;15(3):1105–11.
34. Neumann ID, Maloumby R, Beiderbeck DI, Lukas M, Landgraf R. Increased brain and plasma oxytocin after nasal and peripheral administration in rats and mice. Psychoneuroendocrinology. 2013;38:1985–93.
35. Dal Monte O, Noble PL, Turchi J, Cummins A, Averbeck BB. CSF and blood oxytocin concentration changes following intranasal delivery in macaque. PLoS One. 2014;9:e103677.
36. Knutson B, Fong GW, Adams CM, Varner JL, Hommer D. Dissociation of reward anticipation and outcome with event-related fMRI. Neuroreport. 2001;12:3683–7.
37. Tottenham N, Tanaka JW, Leon AC, McCarry T, Nurse M, Hare TA, Marcus DJ, Westerlund A, Casey B, Nelson C. The NimStim set of facial expressions: judgments from untrained research participants. Psychiatry Res. 2009;168:242–9.
38. Smith SM, Jenkinson M, Woolrich MW, Beckmann CF, Behrens TE, Johansen-Berg H, Bannister PR, De Luca M, Drobnjak I, Flitney DE. Advances in functional and structural MR image analysis and implementation as FSL. NeuroImage. 2004;23:S208–19.

39. Smith SM. Fast robust automated brain extraction. Hum Brain Mapp. 2002; 17:143–55.

40. Jenkinson M, Bannister P, Brady M, Smith S. Improved optimization for the robust and accurate linear registration and motion correction of brain images. NeuroImage. 2002;17:825–41.

41. Jenkinson M, Smith S. A global optimisation method for robust affine registration of brain images. Med Image Anal. 2001;5:143–56.

42. Ward BD. Simultaneous inference for fMRI data. AFNI 3dDeconvolve Documentation, Medical College of Wisconsin. 2000.

43. Cisler JM, Bush K, Steele JS. A comparison of statistical methods for detecting context-modulated functional connectivity in fMRI. NeuroImage. 2014;84:1042–52.

44. McLaren DG, Ries ML, Xu G, Johnson SC. A generalized form of context-dependent psychophysiological interactions (gPPI): a comparison to standard approaches. NeuroImage. 2012;61:1277–86.

45. Constantino JN, Gruber CP. Social responsiveness scale, (SRS-2). Los Angeles: Western Psychological Services Google Scholar; 2012.

46. Knutson B, Adams CM, Fong GW, Hommer D. Anticipation of increasing monetary reward selectively recruits nucleus accumbens. J Neurosci. 2001; 21:RC159.

47. Bush G, Vogt BA, Holmes J, Dale AM, Greve D, Jenike MA, Rosen BR. Dorsal anterior cingulate cortex: a role in reward-based decision making. Proc Natl Acad Sci. 2002;99:523.

48. Insel TR, Shapiro LE. Oxytocin receptor distribution reflects social organization in monogamous and polygamous voles. Proc Natl Acad Sci. 1992;89:5981.

49. Watanabe T, Abe O, Kuwabara H, Yahata N, Takano Y, Iwashiro N, Natsubori T, Aoki Y, Takao H, Kawakubo Y. Mitigation of sociocommunicational deficits of autism through oxytocin-induced recovery of medial prefrontal activity: a randomized trial. JAMA psychiatry. 2014;71:166–75.

50. Tremblay L, Schultz W. Relative reward preference in primate orbitofrontal cortex. Nature. 1999;398:704–8.

51. Rolls ET. The orbitofrontal cortex and reward. Cereb Cortex. 2000;10:284–94.

52. Choe HK, Reed MD, Benavidez N, Montgomery D, Soares N, Yim YS, Choi GB. Oxytocin mediates entrainment of sensory stimuli to social cues of opposing valence. Neuron. 2015;87:152–63.

53. Kent K, Arientyl V, Khachatryan MM, Wood RI. Oxytocin induces a conditioned social preference in female mice. J Neuroendocrinol. 2013;25:803–10.

54. Kosaki Y, Watanabe S. Conditioned social preference, but not place preference, produced by intranasal oxytocin in female mice. Behav Neurosci. 2016;130:182.

55. Borrow AP, Cameron NM. The role of oxytocin in mating and pregnancy. Horm Behav. 2012;61:266–76.

56. Nakajima M, Görlich A, Heintz N. Oxytocin modulates female sociosexual behavior through a specific class of prefrontal cortical interneurons. Cell. 2014;159:295–305.

57. Yamasue H, Domes G. Oxytocin and Autism Spectrum Disorders. Current Topics in Behavioral Neurosciences. Berlin, Heidelberg: Springer; 2017.

58. Herisson FM, Waas JR, Fredriksson R, Schiöth HB, Levine AS, Olszewski PK. Oxytocin Acting in the Nucleus Accumbens Core Decreases Food Intake. J Neuroendocrinol. 2016;28.

59. Klockars A, Brunton C, Li L, Levine AS, Olszewski PK. Intravenous administration of oxytocin in rats acutely decreases deprivation-induced chow intake, but it fails to affect consumption of palatable solutions. Peptides. 2017;93:13–9.

60. Moaddab M, Hyland BI, Brown CH. Oxytocin enhances the expression of morphine-induced conditioned place preference in rats. Psychoneuroendocrinology. 2015;53:159–69.

61. Subiah CO, Mabandla MV, Phulukdaree A, Chuturgoon AA, Daniels WM. The effects of vasopressin and oxytocin on methamphetamine-induced place preference behaviour in rats. Metab Brain Dis. 2012;27:341–50.

62. Daniel R, Pollmann S. A universal role of the ventral striatum in reward-based learning: evidence from human studies. Neurobiol Learn Mem. 2014;114:90–100.

63. Chevallier C, Parish-Morris J, McVey A, Rump KM, Sasson NJ, Herrington JD, Schultz RT. Measuring social attention and motivation in autism spectrum disorder using eye-tracking: stimulus type matters. Autism Res. 2015;8:620–8.

64. Mansouri FA, Buckley MJ, Mahboubi M, Tanaka K. Behavioral consequences of selective damage to frontal pole and posterior cingulate cortices. Proc Natl Acad Sci U S A. 2015;112:E3940–9.

65. Agam Y, Joseph RM, Barton JJ, Manoach DS. Reduced cognitive control of response inhibition by the anterior cingulate cortex in autism spectrum disorders. NeuroImage. 2010;52:336–47.

66. Dichter GS. Functional magnetic resonance imaging of autism spectrum disorders. Dialogues Clin Neurosci. 2012;14:319–51.

67. Wu H, Tang H, Ge Y, Yang S, Mai X, Luo YJ, Liu C. Object words modulate the activity of the mirror neuron system during action imitation. Brain Behav. 2017;7:e00840.

68. Chiu YC, Jiang J, Egner T. The caudate nucleus mediates learning of stimulus-control state associations. J Neurosci. 2017;37:1028–38.

69. Delmonte S, Gallagher L, O'Hanlon E, Mc Grath J, Balsters JH. Functional and structural connectivity of frontostriatal circuitry in autism spectrum disorder. Front Hum Neurosci. 2013;7:430.

70. Di Martino A, Kelly C, Grzadzinski R, Zuo X-N, Mennes M, Mairena MA, Lord C, Castellanos FX, Milham MP. Aberrant striatal functional connectivity in children with autism. Biol Psychiatry. 2011;69:847–56.

71. Turner KC, Frost L, Linsenbardt D, McIlroy JR, Müller R-A. Atypically diffuse functional connectivity between caudate nuclei and cerebral cortex in autism. Behav Brain Funct. 2006;2:34.

72. Dajani DR, Uddin LQ. Local brain connectivity across development in autism spectrum disorder: a cross-sectional investigation. Autism Res. 2016;9:43–54.

73. Okuda J, Fujii T, Ohtake H, Tsukiura T, Tanji K, Suzuki K, Kawashima R, Fukuda H, Itoh M, Yamadori A. Thinking of the future and past: the roles of the frontal pole and the medial temporal lobes. NeuroImage. 2003;19:1369–80.

74. Di Martino A, Ross K, Uddin LQ, Sklar AB, Castellanos FX, Milham MP. Functional brain correlates of social and nonsocial processes in autism spectrum disorders: an activation likelihood estimation meta-analysis. Biol Psychiatry. 2009;65:63–74.

75. Pantelis PC, Byrge L, Tyszka JM, Adolphs R, Kennedy DP. A specific hypoactivation of right temporo-parietal junction/posterior superior temporal sulcus in response to socially awkward situations in autism. Soc Cogn Affect Neurosci. 2015;10:1348–56.

76. Liu X, Hairston J, Schrier M, Fan J. Common and distinct networks underlying reward valence and processing stages: a meta-analysis of functional neuroimaging studies. Neurosci Biobehav Rev. 2011;35:1219–36.

77. Caulfield F, Ewing L, Burton N, Avard E, Rhodes G. Facial trustworthiness judgments in children with ASD are modulated by happy and angry emotional cues. PLoS One. 2014;9:e97644.

78. Ewing L, Caulfield F, Read A, Rhodes G. Appearance-based trust behaviour is reduced in children with autism spectrum disorder. Autism. 2015;19:1002–9.

79. Delmonte S, Balsters JH, McGrath J, Fitzgerald J, Brennan S, Fagan AJ, Gallagher L. Social and monetary reward processing in autism spectrum disorders. Molecular Autism. 2012;3:7.

80. Rademacher L, Krach S, Kohls G, Irmak A, Gründer G, Spreckelmeyer KN. Dissociation of neural networks for anticipation and consumption of monetary and social rewards. NeuroImage. 2010;49:3276–85.

81. Insel TR, Gogtay N. National Institute of Mental Health clinical trials: new opportunities, new expectations. JAMA Psychiatry. 2014;71(7):745–6.

82. Uddin LQ, Supekar K, Menon V. Reconceptualizing functional brain connectivity in autism from a developmental perspective. Front Hum Neurosci. 2013;7:458.

83. Gotham K, Pickles A, Lord C. Standardizing ADOS scores for a measure of severity in autism spectrum disorders. J Autism Dev Disord. 2009;39:693–705.

84. Hus V, Lord C. The autism diagnostic observation schedule, module 4: revised algorithm and standardized severity scores. J Autism Dev Disord. 2014;44:1996–2012.

Motor problems in children with neurofibromatosis type 1

André B. Rietman[1,6*], Rianne Oostenbrink[2], Sanne Bongers[1], Eddy Gaukema[5], Sandra van Abeelen[5], Jos G. Hendriksen[5], Caspar W. N. Looman[4], Pieter F. A. de Nijs[1] and Marie-Claire de Wit[3]

Abstract

Background: Children with the neurogenetic disorder neurofibromatosis type 1 (NF1) often have problems with learning and behaviour. In both parent reports and neuropsychological assessment, motor problems are reported in approximately one third to one half of the children with NF1. Studies using broad motor performance test batteries with relatively large groups of children with NF1 are limited. The aim of this cross-sectional observational study was to describe the severity of motor problems in children with NF1 and to explore the predictive value of demographics, intelligence, and behavioural problems.

Methods: From 2002 to 2014, 69 children with NF1, aged 4 to 16 years (age = 9.5 ± 2.8 years; 29 girls) had a motor, psychological, and neurological evaluation in an NF1 expertise centre. Data were collected about (1) motor performance (M-ABC: Movement Assessment Battery for Children), (2) intelligence, and (3) emotional and behavioural problems as rated by parents.

Results: Sixty-one percent of these children scored within the clinical range of the M-ABC. In ordinal logistic regression analyses, motor problems were associated with symptoms of attention-deficit/hyperactivity disorder (ADHD), symptoms of autism spectrum disorder (ASD), and externalising behavioural problems. Motor outcome was not predicted by age, intelligence, scoliosis, hypotonia, nor hypermobility.

Conclusions: Motor problems are among the most common comorbid developmental problems in children with NF1, and these problems do not diminish with age. Because of their impact on daily functioning, motor problems need to be specifically addressed in diagnosis, follow-up, and treatment of NF1.

Keywords: Neurofibromatosis type 1, Motor problems, DCD, Emotional and behavioural problems, Intelligence

Background

Neurofibromatosis type 1 (NF1) is an autosomal dominant neurogenetic disorder with an incidence of at least 1:2700 [1]. Although NF1 is defined by cutaneous and neurological symptoms such as café-au-lait spots and neurofibromas, the most common complications in childhood are deficits of cognition and of social and emotional development [2]. The prevalence of neuropsychiatric problems such as attention-deficit/hyperactivity disorder (ADHD) and autism spectrum disorder (ASD) is much larger than in the general population [3]. In both parent reports and neuropsychological assessments, motor problems are reported in approximately one third to one half of the children with NF1 [4, 5]. Almost 30% of children with NF1 had received occupational therapy [6], and over 40% receive remedial teaching for motor problems at school [7]. NF1-related skeletal and muscular abnormalities, such as scoliosis, pseudo-arthrosis, decreased bone strength, and reduced muscle strength may be associated with motor problems in NF1 [5]. Motor problems can hinder a child's participation at school and in play, sports, and peer-group activities, but they may also affect social and emotional

* Correspondence: a.rietman@erasmusmc.nl
[1]Department of Child and Adolescent Psychiatry/Psychology, ENCORE NF1 Expertise Centre for Neurodevelopmental Disorders, Erasmus Medical Centre–Sophia Children's Hospital, Rotterdam, The Netherlands
[6]Department of Child and Adolescent Psychiatry/Psychology, Sophia Children's Hospital, Room Sp 2478, P.O. Box 20603000 CB Rotterdam, The Netherlands
Full list of author information is available at the end of the article

development [8]. In our expertise centres for NF1, motor problems are among the most common complaints, which is the reason for the structural assessment of motor skills presented in this study.

Previous studies on motor skills in NF1 have often used selective tests, targeting only parts of the motor domain [2, 9]. Studies using a small selection of motor or constructional tests do not show the full range of motor problems in children with NF1. Broader test batteries for both fine and gross motor skills have been used in a limited number of smaller studies [5, 10] or when focusing on young children [4, 11]. Recently, [9] a broad test battery (the BOT-2) was used with 46 children, from 7 to 17 years old, to establish correlations between problems in motor and cognitive domains. In this study, cognition was associated with balance, gait, running speed, and agility in children with NF1. A shared abnormal neurodevelopmental process underlying cognitive and motor abilities in NF1 was hypothesised [9].

A study on a large group of children and adolescents with NF1, using a broad test battery for motor performance, could inform health care professionals not only about the association between motor problems and cognitive development but also about the association with the emotional and behavioural problems often present in NF1. Our cross-sectional study aims to describe the presence and severity of motor problems in children and adolescents with NF1 and to explore the associations between these motor problems and background variables, intelligence, and emotional and behavioural problems.

Methods
Procedure and patients
The Kempenhaeghe Centre for Neurological Learning Disabilities (CNL) is an expertise centre for children with neurological learning disabilities such as NF1. At school age, a paediatric neurologist evaluates all patients at least once. Patients are offered additional evaluations by a neuropsychologist and a physiotherapist. Patients without any complaints about motor performance were not included in this study. Next to this, we did not re-evaluate the motor performance of patients who already had serious motor problems according to a recent evaluation by a physiotherapist using the Movement-ABC in a different institute. The selection process is depicted in Fig. 1. We used medical and psychological patient files from 2002 to 2014 of 4- to 16-year-old patients who met the National Institutes of Health (NIH) diagnostic criteria for NF1 [12] and who were evaluated by a physiotherapist using the Movement Assessment Battery for Children version 1 [13] or 2 [14] (M-ABC-1 or 2). Exclusion criteria were segmental NF1, symptomatic pathology of the CNS, deafness or severely impaired vision, pseudarthrosis, insufficient command of the Dutch language, or an IQ below the range covered by the Wechsler Intelligence Scale for Children, third edition, Dutch version (WISC-III-NL [15]; total IQ below 48).

Clinical data were registered by a paediatrician of Erasmus Medical Centre, Sophia Children's Hospital during annual follow-up, by a paediatric neurologist from CNL and by psychologists from both centres. All children were evaluated according to a standardised protocol, routinely applied to all children with NF1 visiting the expertise centre. Familial or sporadic NF1 was determined from family history. In clinical assessments by the paediatric neurologist and the psychologist, the presence of neurologic, orthopaedic, or neuropsychiatric problems such as hypotonia, hypermobility, and scoliosis were recorded. Classifications of ADHD and ASD were based on neuropsychological assessment and on information from parents and teachers, using DSM-IV [16] criteria. Writing problems were reported by parents. Socio-

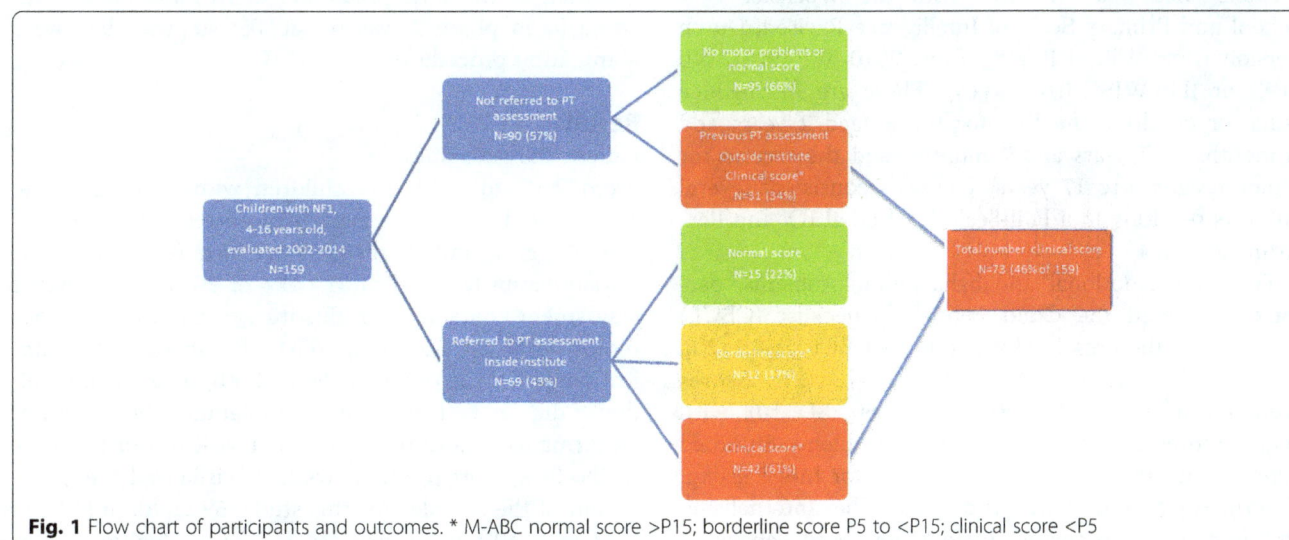

Fig. 1 Flow chart of participants and outcomes. * M-ABC normal score >P15; borderline score P5 to <P15; clinical score <P5

economic status (SES) was derived from the zip code of the child's home address using a standard Dutch classification system [17]. For the participating patients, a formal review and waiver was given by the medical ethical human research ethics committees of both the Erasmus Medical Centre and the CNL.

Instruments

The Movement ABC, [13, 14] an instrument measuring the presence and severity of motor problems, is one of the most frequently and widely used standardised assessments of motor skills, also used in diagnosing developmental coordination disorder (DCD). To assess motor performance, the physiotherapist administered the M-ABC-1 [13] (2002-2010) or 2 [14] (2010-2014). The M-ABC assesses three components: manual dexterity, ball skills (catching and throwing), and balance (static and dynamic). The M-ABC is designed to identify and describe impairments in the motor performance of children and adolescents aged 4 to 12 (M-ABC-1) or 3 to 16 (M-ABC-2). The M-ABC-2 is an updated version of the M-ABC-1, not only the age range but also the sample size, have been expanded and more information on psychometric qualities has been acquired. Results on both tests are expressed in a score, with any child scoring below the 6th percentile of the normative sample being recorded as falling within the clinical range indicating serious movement difficulties. Scores from the 6th to the 15th percentile (approximately between 1.5 and 2.0 SD below average) are labelled as borderline, indicating that the child is at risk of motor problems. Above the 15th percentile, the child is unlikely to have movement difficulties. Additionally, the M-ABC-2 also provides norm-referenced standardised scores for the component and the total scores. The M-ABC-2 has good reliability (ICC = .95 to .98).

Intelligence was measured with the Wechsler Preschool and Primary Scale of Intelligence-Revised, Dutch version (first WPPSI-R [18], from 2010 WPPSI-III-NL [19]) or the WISC-III-NL [15]. These are intelligence tests for children, the first for those aged 2 years and 6 months to 7 years and 7 months, and the second for children aged 6 to 17 years. The tests consist of several subtests resulting in a Full-Scale IQ, Verbal IQ, and Performance IQ.

To assess emotional and behavioural problems, parents completed the Child Behavior Checklist (CBCL) using either the preschool version, the CBCL/1½-5 [20], or the school-aged version, CBCL/6-18 [21]. Scores were converted to T scores (mean 50, SD 10), with higher scores corresponding to more problems. Summed scores result in three broadband scales for Internalising, Externalising, and Total Problems. The Internalising Problems scale comprises anxious/depressed behaviour,

withdrawn/depressed behaviour, and somatic complaints. The Externalising Problems scale comprises rule-breaking behaviour and aggressive behaviour. The Total Problems scale is a combination of both the Internalising and Externalising Problems scales, together with scales for Social Problems, Thought Problems, and Attention Problems. T scores between 59 and 62 fall within a borderline clinical range, whilst T scores of 63 and higher fall within the clinical range. All tests were administered in their Dutch versions, using Dutch normative samples.

Statistical analysis

All data were analysed using SPSS, version 21 [22], and R [23]. Proportions of groups were compared using chi-square (χ^2) tests. Effect sizes were calculated using Cohen's d, [24] when comparing the NF1 sample with the test manual normative sample, with .20 interpreted as a small effect size, .50 as medium, and .80 as large.

Since the common outcome for both versions of the M-ABC was the classification into three consecutive categories (normal, borderline, or clinical), ordinal logistic regression analysis was performed to find predictors of these three categories of motor outcome. For this, a two-phase strategy was followed. In phase 1, all separate variables from Table 1 were tested in univariable ordinal regression analyses with M-ABC classification as the dependent variable. Since this phase served as an initial, broad selection of potential predictors, α in phase 1 was set at .20 [25]. In phase 2, multivariable ordinal regression models were constructed for every block of variables from Tables 1 and 2, containing all significant variables from phase 1. Blocks were defined as demographics, neuropsychiatric problems, emotional and behavioural problems, and cognition. Variables shown to be significant contributors in the final models were regarded as the final predictors of M-ABC motor outcome (α in phase 2 was set at .05; stepwise backward elimination procedure).

Results
Patient characteristics
From 2002 to 2014, 159 children with NF1 aged 4 to 16 years old visited the expertise centre. Ninety (57% of 159; 46 girls and 44 boys) were not referred to the physiotherapist, of which 31 (34% of 90) had a previous assessment outside our institute, indicating serious motor problems, according to M-ABC scores in the clinical range. Of the other 59 (66% of 90), parents and children did not have any complaints about motor performance before or during their visit to our institute. In the flow chart of Fig. 1, we have visualised the distribution of the sample. For this study, 69 children (43% of 159) with NF1 were included for PT evaluation in our

Table 1 Characteristics of children with NF1

Variable	
Demographic characteristics	n = 69 Frequency (%)
Age	8.7 (4.1)[a]
Gender	
Male	40 (58)
Female	29 (42)
Type of education	
Regular education	48 (70)
Special education	21 (30)
Social economic status [b]	0.34 (1.29)[a]
Mode of inheritance NF1	
De novo mutation	39 (57)
Familial mutation	29 (42)
Unknown	1 (1)
Neuropsychiatric problems	
Attention-deficit/hyperactivity disorder (ADHD)	
ADHD combined type	25 (36)
ADHD inattentive type	11 (16)
ADHD hyperactive/impulsive type	2 (3)
Total	38 (55)
Using stimulant medication	18 (26)
Autism spectrum disorder (PDD-NOS)	7 (10)
Neurologic and orthopaedic problems	
Hypotonia	14 (20)
Hypermobility (Beighton criteria)	13 (19)
Scoliosis	7 (10)

[a]Median (interquartile range)
[b]Average SES in 2010 = 0.17; higher scores indicate higher SES

institute, 29 girls, and 40 boys. This group is indicated in the box 'Referred to PT assessment' in Fig. 1. Ages ranged from 4 years to 15 years and 11 months, with a median age of 8 years and 8 months (IQR = 4 years and 1 month) (Table 1). Sixty-seven children were right handed. Eighteen out of 38 of the children with a DSM-IV-TR classification of ADHD (47%) used stimulant medication. Seven children had an ASD classification, all of them with a comorbid ADHD classification. Intelligence, emotional and behavioural problems, and standard scores of the M-ABC-2 are presented in Table 2.

Twenty-four children (41%) had emotional and behavioural problem scores within the clinical range, with large effect sizes for internalising problems and medium effect sizes for externalising problems. Parents of 11 children (16%) did not return CBCLs. These children were left out of analyses using CBCL scores as predictors. Compared to the normative sample, the distribution of intelligence scores was shifted approximately one

SD to the left, and total IQ scores ranged from 58 to 123. Effect sizes were large for performance IQ and medium for verbal IQ compared to the normative population. Effect sizes for all motor scales were large.

Motor problems

Thirty-five of 69 children (51%) were assessed with the M-ABC version 1, 34 (49%) with version 2. The comparison between children tested with these two versions showed no significant differences in the distribution of scores between the percentile classification categories for the total scores (χ^2 (2) = 3.08, p = .21), nor for distributions of Hand, Ball, or Balance scale scores. For the purpose of ordinal regression analyses, both groups were combined. Figure 2 presents the distribution of the classifications in all motor scales. Overall, 42 (61%) children with NF1 scored within the clinical range (below 6th percentile) of the M-ABC.

In ordinal regression analysis, age was found not to be a significant predictor of motor outcome. The proportion of children scoring in the 'borderline' or 'clinical' range of the M-ABC was 67% of children from 4 to 6 years old, 82% of children from 7 to 11 years old, and 79% of adolescents from 12 to 16 years old.

In univariable ordinal regression analysis (Table 3; phase 1 with α set at .20), a higher probability of borderline or clinical motor problems was predicted by type of education, classifications of ADHD or ASD, hypermobility, Performance IQ, Total IQ, and CBCL Internalising, Externalising, and Total Problems. In all univariable models, the test of parallel lines failed to reach significance, meaning that effects of all separate variables were the same for normal versus borderline and borderline versus clinical scores.

In multivariable ordinal regression analyses (Table 4; phase 2 with α set at .05), single variables within one block (type of education and hypermobility) had p values above α = .05 and so could not be used in multivariable models. In three blocks, final models yielded a limited amount of significant predictors. Since all seven children with an ASD classification scored within the clinical range, the odds ratio of having borderline or clinical M-ABC scores could not be calculated and so ASD was left out of multivariable analyses. Also, the multivariable ordinal regression of ADHD and ASD could not be performed because all seven children with ASD classifications also had an ADHD classification. We compared the distribution of the M-ABC classification between the groups without ADHD or ASD versus the group with only ADHD versus the group with both ADHD and ASD using a chi-squared test. This distribution did not differ significantly (χ^2 (4, N = 69) = 7.53, p = .11), indicating that all three groups contributed independently to the distribution of motor problems.

Table 2 Scores and frequencies for emotional and behavioural problems, intelligence and motor performance

Domain	Number	Mean	SD[a]	BCR[b] (%)	CR[b] (%)	ES[c]
Parent-rated emotional and behavioural problems[d]						
Internalising problems	58	59	10	19	37	0.9***
Externalising problems	58	55	12	8	27	0.5**
Total problems	58	61	11	10	41	1.0***
Intelligence[e]						
Verbal IQ	68	92	15			0.5***
Performance IQ	68	88	14			0.8***
Total IQ	69	89	13			0.8***
Movement ABC-1 and 2 ($n = 69$)						
Classification normal[f]	15 (22%)					
Classification borderline[f]	12 (17%)					
Classification clinical[f]	42 (61%)					
Movement ABC-2[g] ($n = 34$)						
Manual dexterity	34	5.8	3.3			1.3***
Ball skills	34	6.7	3.6			1.0***
Balance	33	5.7	3.0			1.4***
Total	34	4.8	3.2			1.7***

[a]*SD* Standard deviation
[b]*BCR/CR* Percentage of scores in borderline clinical range/clinical range
[c]*ES* effect size (Cohen's *d*); Significance compared to normative sample **$p < .01$; ***$p < .001$
[d]*T* scores (population mean = 50; SD = 10; higher scores reflect more problems)
[e]IQ scores (population mean = 100; SD = 15; higher scores reflect better performance)
[f]M-ABC normal score >P15; borderline score P5 to <P15; clinical score <P5
[g]Standard-scores (population mean = 10; SD = 3; higher scores reflect better performance)

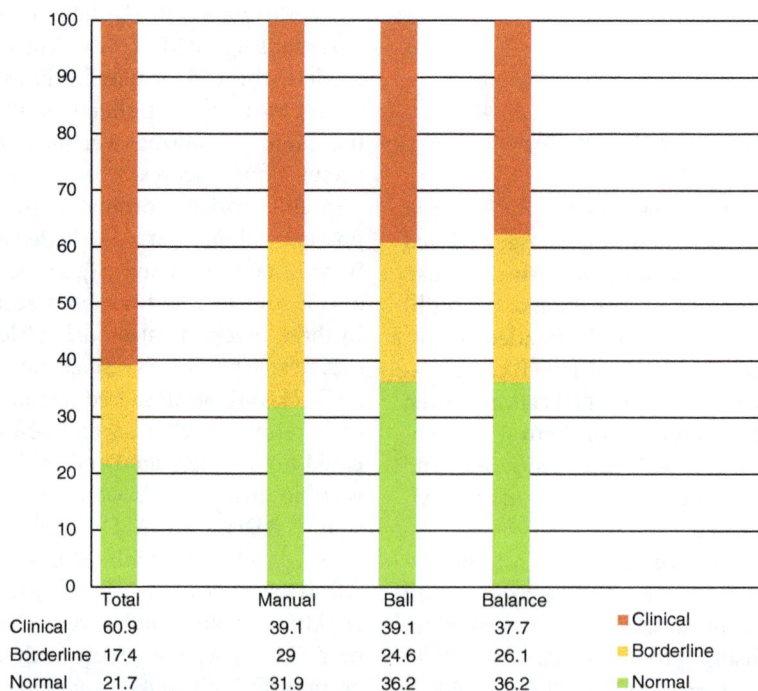

	Total	Manual	Ball	Balance
Clinical	60.9	39.1	39.1	37.7
Borderline	17.4	29	24.6	26.1
Normal	21.7	31.9	36.2	36.2

Fig. 2 Classification of motor problems based on Movement ABC percentile scores ($n = 69$). *Clinical*: percentage of children with movement difficulty- scores below 6th percentile. *Borderline*: percentage of children with scores from 6th to 15th percentile. *Normal*: percentage of children with no movement difficulty scores above 15th percentile

Table 3 Univariable ordinal logistic regression with separate variables predicting motor outcome (Movement ABC total scores; $n = 69$)

Variable	Number	B (SE)	95% CI of odds ratio			Wald	R^2	p
			Lower	OR	Upper			
Age	69	0.08 (0.09)	0.77	0.93	1.12	4.31	.01	.429
Gender	69	0.56 (0.49)	0.22	0.57	1.49	1.31	.02	.253
Type of education	69	0.84 (0.58)	0.14	0.43	1.35	2.08	.04	.135[#]
Social economic status	69	−0.10 (0.19)	0.77	1.10	1.59	0.29	.01	.595
Mode of inheritance	69	−0.42 (0.49)	0.59	1.53	3.95	0.76	.01	.383
ADHD	69	1.01 (0.49)	0.14	0.36	0.96	4.22	.07	.038[*]
Using stimulant medication	69	−0.35 (0.54)	0.49	1.41	4.05	0.41	.01	.523
Autism spectrum disorder[a]	69	–	–	NA	–	–	.12	.035[**]
Hypotonia	69	0.28 (0.60)	0.23	0.76	2.47	0.21	<.01	.644
Hypermobility	69	0.98 (0.70)	0.10	0.38	1.49	1.94	.04	.140[#]
Scoliosis	69	0.25 (0.79)	0.28	1.28	5.97	0.10	<.01	.755
Writing problems at school	69	−0.20 (0.50)	0.46	1.22	3.25	0.16	<.01	.694
CBCL Internalising problems	58	−0.04 (0.03)	0.99	1.04	1.09	2.23	.04	.134[#]
CBCL Externalising problems	58	−0.04 (0.02)	0.10	1.04	1.09	3.30	.07	.063[#]
CBCL Total problems	58	−0.05 (0.03)	1.00	1.05	1.10	3.65	.08	.051[#]
Verbal IQ	68	0.01 (0.02)	0.96	0.99	1.02	0.41	.01	.519
Performance IQ	68	0.03 (0.02)	0.94	0.97	1.01	2.43	.04	.115[#]
Total IQ	69	0.03 (0.02)	0.94	0.97	1.01	2.10	.04	.141[#]

R^2 Nagelkerke pseudo R^2
p values of likelihood ratio chi-square; [#]$p < .20$; [*]$p < .05$; [**]$p < .01$
[a]As there were no cases in cells with normal M-ABC-scores for children with an ASD classification, the estimate was minus infinity

Table 4 Multivariable backward ordinal logistic regression with variables from separate blocks predicting motor outcome (Movement ABC total classification; $n = 69$)

Variables	Number	B (SE)	95% CI of OR			Wald	R^2	p value
			Lower	OR	Upper			
Neuropsychiatric problems								
ADHD	69	1.01 (0.49)	0.14	0.36	0.96	4.22	.07	.038[*]
Autism spectrum disorder[a]	69	–	–	NA	–	–	.12	.035[*]
Emotional and behavioural problems								
Model 1	58						.07	.168
Internalising problems		−0.01 (0.03)	0.95	1.01	1.08	0.10		.757
Externalising problems		−0.04 (0.03)	0.98	1.04	1.10	1.44		.235
Model 2	58							
Externalising problems		−0.04 (0.02)	0.10	1.04	1.09	3.30	.07	.063
Intelligence								
Model 1	68						.04	.289
Performance IQ		0.03 (0.03)	0.91	0.97	1.04	0.71		.401
Total IQ		0.001 (0.03)	0.94	1.00	1.07	0.001		.973
Model 2	68							
Performance IQ		0.03 (0.02)	0.94	0.97	1.01	2.43	.04	.115

OR odds ratio, NA not applicable, R^2 Nagelkerke pseudo R^2
p values of likelihood ratio chi-square; [*]$p < .05$
[a]As there were nog cases in cells with normal M-ABC-scores for children with an ASD classification, the estimate was minus infinity

The Externalising Problems scale was approaching significance as a predictor of motor outcome ($p = .063$). With low scores for Externalising Problems, the probability of a clinical score on the M-ABC was low. Children without externalising problems on the CBCL only had a 23% chance of a clinical score on the M-ABC, whilst children with externalising problems scores in the clinical range had an 81% chance, as is shown in Fig. 3. Finally, intelligence (i.e. Performance IQ) was not found to be significantly associated with total motor problems.

Exploratory univariable linear regression analyses, with motor outcome on the M-ABC-2 as a continuous dependent variable ($n = 34$), found significant associations with independent variables: Internalising Problems scale (F (1,26) = 5.21; $p = .031$; $R^2 = .17$; $\beta = -.13$); Externalising Problems scale (F (1,26) = 6.99; $p = .014$; $R^2 = .21$; $\beta = -.12$); and Total Problems scale (F (1,26) = 6.15; $p = .020$; $R^2 = .19$; $\beta = -.13$), again indicating that an increase in emotional and behavioural problems is associated with a decrease in motor proficiency. Residuals for these regressions were normally distributed.

Discussion

Our study shows that motor problems frequently occur in our group of children with NF1: 61% of these 69 children have serious motor problems and another 17% score within the borderline range. In the part of our cohort not evaluated in the expertise centre ($n = 90$), 31 were already identified as having motor problems, resulting in an overall 46% (73/159) with serious motor problems. The distribution of these groups and outcomes is visualised in Fig. 1 in the box with 'Total number clinical

score'. Previous studies using broad motor test batteries found smaller or comparable proportions. One study in a comparable age range found 54% (14 out of 26 children) scoring between one and two standard deviations below average and another 27% (7/26) scored below 2 SD [6]. When comparing studies, one should realise that the cut-offs of the P5 and the P15 correspond to z scores of 1.65 and 1.04 below average in the standard normal distribution.

Next to ADHD [26] and ASD symptoms [27], motor problems seem to be among the most common comorbid developmental problems of children with NF1. We found motor problems in a broad range of domains, comparable to the problems found in DCD [8].

In our attempt to find predictors of motor outcome, we did not find a significant contribution of demographic characteristics such as age, gender, or SES. A previous comparable study in a smaller sample did not find effects for age or gender either [6]. We also did not find associations with neurological and orthopaedic problems such as hypotonia, hypermobility, or scoliosis. Given the broad variability in these characteristics within our population (Table 1), we think our study population had sufficient power to detect potential associations if they existed. There was a limited association between (performance) intelligence and motor performance. Previous research [4] found that motor coordination and motor speed contributed to the performance on some subtests of the WISC. However, in our study, we used a broader motor test battery such as the M-ABC and children were found to have serious motor problems in general, regardless of their overall intelligence. Since a previous study [9] found that poorer balance skills were associated with a reduced perceptual reasoning index, we performed an additional univariable ordinal logistic regression to specifically find out whether balance skills on the M-ABC were associated with performance IQ. Only a weak association was found with an odds ratio of 0.97 (95% CI, 0.93 to 1.00), Wald χ^2 (1) = 3.774, $p = .052$). Whether this finding is a reflection of an abnormal neurodevelopmental process, underlying these abilities in children with NF1, may be a subject for future research.

Recent studies do provide evidence for a relation between motor experience and cognitive development in the first 3 years of life when at the same time this relation becomes less clear in older children [28]. The fact that we did not find a significant effect of age on motor performance may presumably be caused by the fact we included children from 4 to 16 years old.

Externalising behavioural problems might be associated with motor outcome. This association was found to be significant in additional explorative analyses with standard scores of the children tested with the M-ABC-2. Also, ADHD was a significant predictor of motor

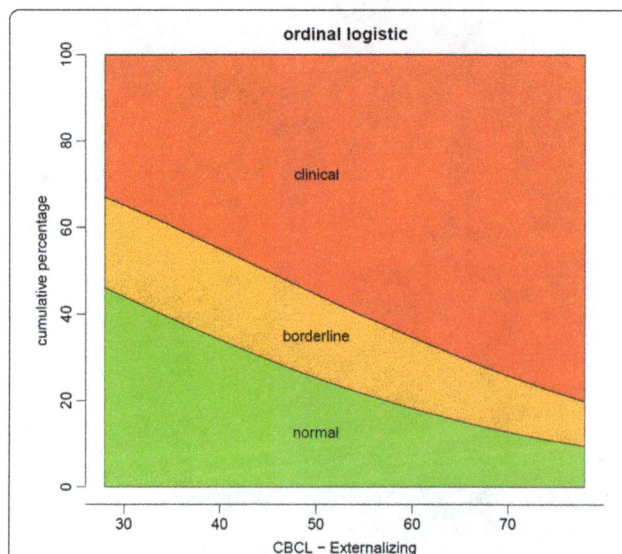

Fig. 3 Relationship between cumulative percentages of classification of total motor scores and scores on CBCL Externalising problems scale

outcome, and all children with an ASD classification had severe motor problems. Previous studies also found that motor problems often occur in children with emotional, behavioural, and pervasive developmental disorders [29, 30]. The co-occurrence of motor and behavioural problems could be an indicator of a more severe neurologic phenotype [31]. It is, however, unclear what the direction of the association between behavioural and motor problems is. Longitudinal and treatment studies could elucidate this issue. Neuropsychiatric and motor problems have a large impact on participation in daily life, even more so when these problems occur simultaneously.

Limitations

Although NF1 is relatively rare, we succeeded in gathering data on the motor performance of 69 children over a 12-year period. However, our sample size is still small considering the number of variables incorporated into the regression analyses of this study. For this reason, there is a risk of overfitting, and care should be taken when drawing conclusions regarding the predictive value of variables. To avoid unnecessary assessments, we did not evaluate the motor performance of children who recently had such an assessment. In addition, since the assessment of motor performance was on a voluntary basis, children without any motor complaints were not required to visit our physiotherapist. For these reasons, we cannot exclude selection bias. We tried to correct for this bias by calculating the total amount of children scoring in the clinical range (Fig. 1).

The cross-sectional design limits interpretations regarding the effect of age on motor performance. Probably, longitudinal research will be able to express this relationship in a more decisive way.

During the time period of this study, there was a move by physiotherapists in the Netherlands from using the first version of the Movement-ABC to the second version. For this reason, we were dependent on the categorical classification of motor problems as a primary outcome measure. This is a consequence of continuous sampling over a long period of time. One should be careful when combining data from both tests since the M-ABC-2 is an elaboration of the M-ABC-1, resulting in differences between both instruments [32]. Because the age range of the M-ABC was the starting point of this study, we used the two age-appropriate versions of the Wechsler scales and of the CBCL. Although the correlation between both versions is high, [19, 20] future research in larger groups could benefit from the selection of smaller age ranges.

For this study, we collected data from medical records. This resulted in missing information (as is shown in Table 2), particularly regarding emotional and behavioural problems, most likely because some parents failed to return questionnaires. Since all children were assessed using a standardised protocol, other data are relatively complete.

The proportion of children with ADHD symptoms is comparable to that in other studies, [26] but the percentage of children with ASD symptomatology in our study (10%) is somewhat lower than former prevalence estimates (21–40%) [33]. In the group with ASD, all children appeared to have severe motor problems. Although this may suggest clinical relevance, we interpret this observation with care, due to the small sample size.

Clinical implications and recommendations

Developmental motor problems are frequently overlooked in clinical practice, yet they can have a considerable impact on children's lives [34]. Using a broad motor assessment in a large cohort of children with NF1, we showed a high prevalence of serious motor problems. These problems seem to be independent of age or intelligence. When children with NF1 show serious motor problems, the diagnosis of DCD might be considered as a comorbid problem. This is especially important in helping to recognise the impact of motor problems on daily life and in allocating the correct treatment. Although the DSM-IV-TR [16] states that in DCD, 'the disorder is not due to a general medical condition', to our opinion NF1 does not have to be regarded as such. DCD could be used in practice as a descriptive diagnosis stressing the impact of motor problems on daily life.

Concerning participation in daily life, children with NF1 often experience problems with writing [4, 35]. It is important to find out whether people with NF1 experience further such difficulties in daily functioning such as in activities of daily living, play, sports, or with driving. This is of great importance since a decrease in participation could not only affect the practice of motor skills but also the development of social skills and quality of life in general.

Assessment and treatment of motor problems in NF1, especially in children with behavioural and social problems, should be considered at a young age, using a broad motor assessment battery. Early motor intervention can have a beneficial effect on behavioural problems, as is indicated by a study showing that in ADHD, [36] motor-affected children receiving physiotherapy presented less frequently with comorbid emotional and behavioural problems. The impact of physiotherapy and psychological therapy on motor functioning, motor participation, and emotional and behavioural problems in children with both NF1 and motor problems is unknown. However, considering the larger potential for plasticity at a young age, referral to both a physiotherapist and a psychologist could be considered at a young age in children with NF1.

Conclusions

More than half of the children with NF1 in this sample had severe motor problems. These problems seem to be independent of age or intelligence. Next to ADHD and ASD, motor problems are among the most frequent co-morbid developmental problems in children with NF1. In this study, ADHD and ASD symptomatology, and externalising behavioural problems are associated with motor problems. The combination of both motor and behavioural problems might result in a more severe phenotype of NF1. Because of their impact on participation in daily life, motor problems need to be specifically addressed in diagnosis, follow-up, and treatment of children with NF1.

Abbreviations

ADHD: Attention-deficit/hyperactivity disorder; ASD: Autism spectrum disorder; CBCL: Child Behavior Checklist; CNL: Kempenhaeghe Centre for Neurological Learning Disabilities; DCD: Developmental coordination disorder; DSM-IV: Diagnostic and statistical manual of mental disorders; IQ: Intelligence quotient; M-ABC-1 or 2: Movement Assessment Battery for Children version 1 or 2; NF1: Neurofibromatosis type 1; SES: Socio-economic status; WISC-III-NL: Wechsler Intelligence Scale for Children, third version for the Netherlands; WPPSI-III-R: Wechsler Preschool and Primary Scale of Intelligence—Third version for the Netherlands

Acknowledgements

We would like to thank all the children and families for participating in this study. A special thank you to Bethany Nicholson for her assistance and expertise, and Alma Weber and Annick Laridon for including many patients and for the assistance during study conduct. We also thank clinicians throughout the Netherlands for referring patients.

Funding

This study was not supported by any grant.

Authors' contributions

ABR planned and conceptualised the study, drafted the initial manuscript, performed all of the statistical analyses, created all of the tables, and edited the final manuscript as submitted. SB participated in the planning of the study, participated in drafting the initial manuscript, and assisted with statistical analyses. EG, SvA, JGH, and PFAdN participated in the interpretation of the results and edited the final manuscript as submitted. CWNL assisted with statistical analyses and edited the final manuscript as submitted. RO and M-CdW supervised the study design and the analysis, participated in the interpretation of the results, and edited the final manuscript as submitted. All authors approved the final manuscript as submitted.

Competing interests

The authors declare that they have no competing interests.

Author details

[1]Department of Child and Adolescent Psychiatry/Psychology, ENCORE NF1 Expertise Centre for Neurodevelopmental Disorders, Erasmus Medical Centre–Sophia Children's Hospital, Rotterdam, The Netherlands. [2]Department of General Paediatrics, ENCORE NF1, Erasmus Medical Centre–Sophia Children's Hospital, Rotterdam, The Netherlands. [3]Department of Paediatric Neurology, ENCORE NF1, Erasmus Medical Centre–Sophia Children's Hospital, Rotterdam, The Netherlands. [4]Department of Public Health, Erasmus Medical Centre, Rotterdam, The Netherlands. [5]Kempenhaeghe Centre for neurological learning disabilities, Heeze, The Netherlands. [6]Department of Child and Adolescent Psychiatry/Psychology, Sophia Children's Hospital, Room Sp 2478, P.O. Box 20603000 CB Rotterdam, The Netherlands.

References

1. Evans DG, Howard E, Giblin C, Clancy T, Spencer H, Huson SM, et al. Birth incidence and prevalence of tumor-prone syndromes: estimates from a UK family genetic register service. Am J Med Genet A. 2010;152A(2):327–32. doi: 10.1002/ajmg.a.33139.
2. Lehtonen A, Howie E, Trump D, Huson SM. Behaviour in children with neurofibromatosis type 1: cognition, executive function, attention, emotion, and social competence. Dev Med Child Neurol. 2013;55(2):111–25. doi:10. 1111/j.1469-8749.2012.04399.x.
3. Garg S, Lehtonen A, Huson SM, Emsley R, Trump D, Evans DG, et al. Autism and other psychiatric comorbidity in neurofibromatosis type 1: evidence from a population-based study. Dev Med Child Neurol. 2013;55(2):139–45. doi:10.1111/dmcn.12043.
4. Soucy EA, Gao F, Gutmann DH, Dunn CM. Developmental delays in children with neurofibromatosis type 1. J Child Neurol. 2012;27(5):641–4. doi:10.1177/ 0883073811423974.
5. Johnson BA, MacWilliams BA, Carey JC, Viskochil DH, D'Astous JL, Stevenson DA. Motor proficiency in children with neurofibromatosis type 1. Pediatr Phys Ther. 2010;22(4):344–8. doi:10.1097/PEP.0b013e3181f9dbc8.
6. Hyman SL, Shores A, North KN. The nature and frequency of cognitive deficits in children with neurofibromatosis type 1. Neurology. 2005;65(7): 1037–44. doi:10.1212/01.wnl.0000179303.72345.ce.
7. Krab LC, Aarsen FK, de Goede-Bolder A, Catsman-Berrevoets CE, Arts WF, Moll HA, et al. Impact of neurofibromatosis type 1 on school performance. J Child Neurol. 2008;23(9):1002–10. doi:10.1177/0883073808316366.
8. Skinner RA, Piek JP. Psychosocial implications of poor motor coordination in children and adolescents. Hum Mov Sci. 2001;20(1-2):73–94.
9. Champion JA, Rose KJ, Payne JM, Burns J, North KN. Relationship between cognitive dysfunction, gait, and motor impairment in children and adolescents with neurofibromatosis type 1. Dev Med Child Neurol. 2014; 56(5):468–74. doi:10.1111/dmcn.12361.
10. Hofman KJ, Harris EL, Bryan RN, Denckla MB. Neurofibromatosis type 1: the cognitive phenotype. J Pediatr. 1994;124(4):S1–8.
11. Lorenzo J, Barton B, Acosta MT, North K. Mental, motor, and language development of toddlers with neurofibromatosis type 1. J Pediatr. 2011; 158(4):660–5. doi:10.1016/j.jpeds.2010.10.001.
12. NIH nioh. Neurofibromatosis. NIH Consens Statement 1987 Jul 13-15. 1987; 6(12):1-19.
13. Henderson SE, Sugden DA. Movement assessment battery for children manual. London: The Psychological Corporation Ltd.; 1992.
14. Henderson S, Sugden D, Barnett A. Movement assessment battery for children-2 second edition [Movement ABC-2]. London: The Psychological Corporation; 2007.
15. Kort W, Schittekatte M, Dekker PH, Verhaeghe P, Compaan EL, Bosmans M et al. WISC-III NL; Wechsler intelligence scale for children, derde Editie NL. Handleiding en verantwoording Londen: Harcourt Assessment; 2005.
16. Association AP. Diagnostic and statistical manual of mental disorders: DSM-IV-TR. Washington, DC: American Psychiatric Association; 2000.
17. Knol FA. Statusontwikkeling van wijken in Nederland 1998-2010 (Dutch; 'Status development in districts in the Netherlands 1998-2010'). The Hague, the Netherlands: Social and Cultural Planbureau, 2012.
18. G. van der Steene AB. Wechsler Preschool and Primary Scale of Intelligence- Revised, Dutch version (WPPSI-R), manual. Lisse: Swets and Zeitlinger BV; 1997.
19. Weschler D, Hendriksen J, Hurks P. WPPSI-III-NL, Wechsler preschool and primary scale of intelligence. Nederlandse bewerking. London: Pearson Assessment and Information BV; 2009.
20. Achenbach T, Rescorla LA. Multicultural Supplement to the Manual for the ASEBA Preschool Forms & Profiles. Burlington: University of Vermont, Research Center for Children, Youth and Families; 2010.
21. Verhulst F, Van der Ende, J. Handleiding ASEBA: Vragenlijsten voor Leeftijden 6 t/m 18 jaar. Rotterdam: ASEBA Nederland; 2013.
22. IBMCorp. IBM SPSS Statistics for Windows, Version 20.0. Armonk, NY: IBM Corp.; 2011.
23. Team RDC. R: A language and environment for statistical computing. Vienna, Austria: R Foundation for Statistical Computing; 2008.

24. Cohen J. Statistical power analysis for the behavioral sciences. New York: Academic Press, New York; 1988.

25. Steyerberg E. Clinical prediction models: a practical approach to development, validation, and updating. New York: Springer; 2009.

26. Mautner VF, Kluwe L, Thakker SD, Leark RA. Treatment of ADHD in neurofibromatosis type 1. Dev Med Child Neurol. 2002;44(3):164–70.

27. Garg S, Plasschaert E, Descheemaeker MJ, Huson S, Borghgraef M, Vogels A, et al. Autism spectrum disorder profile in neurofibromatosis type I. J Autism Dev Disord. 2015;45(6):1649–57. doi:10.1007/s10803-014-2321-5.

28. Libertus K, Hauf P. Editorial: motor skills and their foundational role for perceptual, social, and cognitive development. Front Psychol. 2017;8:301. doi:10.3389/fpsyg.2017.00301.

29. Emck C, Bosscher R, Beek P, Doreleijers T. Gross motor performance and self-perceived motor competence in children with emotional, behavioural, and pervasive developmental disorders: a review. Dev Med Child Neurol. 2009;51(7):501–17. doi:10.1111/j.1469-8749.2009.03337.x.

30. Fliers E, Rommelse N, Vermeulen SH, Altink M, Buschgens CJ, Faraone SV, et al. Motor coordination problems in children and adolescents with ADHD rated by parents and teachers: effects of age and gender. J Neural Transm (Vienna). 2008;115(2):211–20. doi:10.1007/s00702-007-0827-0.

31. Peters LH, Maathuis CG, Hadders-Algra M. Children with behavioral problems and motor problems have a worse neurological condition than children with behavioral problems only. Early Hum Dev. 2014;90(12):803–7. doi:10.1016/j.earlhumdev.2014.09.001.

32. Brown T, Lalor A. The movement assessment battery for children—second edition (MABC-2): a review and critique. Phys Occup Ther Pediatr. 2009; 29(1):86–103. doi:10.1080/01942630802574908.

33. Garg S, Plasschaert E, Descheemaeker MJ, Huson S, Borghgraef M, Vogels A et al. Autism spectrum disorder profile in neurofibromatosis type I. J Autism Dev Disord. 2014. doi:10.1007/s10803-014-2321-5.

34. Baird G, Santosh PJ. Interface between neurology and psychiatry in childhood. J Neurol Neurosurg Psychiatry. 2003;74 Suppl 1:i17–22.

35. Gilboa Y, Josman N, Fattal-Valevski A, Toledano-Alhadef H, Rosenblum S. The handwriting performance of children with NF1. Res Dev Disabil. 2010; 31(4):929–35. doi:10.1016/j.ridd.2010.03.005.

36. Fliers EA, Franke B, Lambregts-Rommelse NN, Altink ME, Buschgens CJ, der Nijhuis-van Sanden MW, et al. Undertreatment of motor problems in children with ADHD. Child Adolesc Ment Health. 2009;15(2):85–90. doi:10. 1111/j.1475-3588.2009.00538.x.

Neurophysiological correlates of holistic face processing in adolescents with and without autism spectrum disorder

Sandra Naumann[1]* ⓘ, Ulrike Senftleben[2], Megha Santhosh[3], James McPartland[4] and Sara Jane Webb[5]

Abstract

Background: Face processing has been found to be impaired in autism spectrum disorders (ASD). One hypothesis is that individuals with ASD engage in piecemeal compared to holistic face processing strategies. To investigate the role of possible impairments in holistic face processing in individuals with autism, the current study investigated behavioral and electroencephalography (EEG) correlates of face processing (P1/N170 and gamma-band activity) in adolescents with ASD and sex-, age-, and IQ-matched neurotypical controls.

Methods: Participants were presented with upright and inverted Mooney stimuli; black and white low information faces that are only perceived as faces when processed holistically. Participants indicated behaviorally the detection of a face. EEG was collected time-locked to the presentation of the stimuli.

Results: Adolescents with ASD perceived Mooney stimuli as faces suggesting ability to use holistic processing but displayed a lower face detection rate and slower response times. ERP components suggest slowed temporal processing of Mooney stimuli in the ASD compared to control group for P1 latency but no differences between groups for P1 amplitude and at the N170. Increases in gamma-band activity was similar during the perception of the Mooney images by group, but the ASD group showed prolonged temporal elevation in activity.

Conclusion: Overall, our results suggest that adolescents with ASD were able to utilize holistic processing to perceive a face within the Mooney stimuli. Delays in early processing, marked by the P1, and elongated elevation in gamma activity indicate that the neural systems supporting holistic processing are slightly altered suggesting a less automatic and less efficient facial processing system.

Keywords: ASD, Gamma-band activity, Holistic face processing, P1, N170

Background

The processing of social information in faces is crucial to communicate effectively with others [1, 2]. Faces possess two types of configural information: first-order information (repeated in every face; e.g., two eyes, above a nose, above a mouth) to enable early face detection [3, 4], and emerging second-order properties (variations in spacing between the features) to extract inter-face variance and to discriminate between faces [3, 5–7]. In configural processing, a face is therefore perceived from lower features to emergent features. In contrast, holistic processing assumes that faces are perceived immediately as undifferentiated wholes without going from first-to second-order features [7]. Configural and holistic processing have been assumed to play parallel roles within face processing [8].

Further interest in face processing is fueled by neurodevelopmental conditions such as autism spectrum disorders (ASDs), which are characterized by early and pervasive social communication and interaction impairments [9]. Individuals with ASD show an enhanced reliance on, or a greater scanning of, unusual face parts (i.e., mouth instead of eyes) [10–12]. The integration of visual information into a meaningful whole may be

* Correspondence: sandra.naumann@hu-berlin.de
[1]Berlin School of Mind and Brain, Humboldt-Universität zu Berlin, Berlin, Germany
Full list of author information is available at the end of the article

impeded by processing predominantly first- rather than second-order features leading to a part-based processing style [13–15].

Face inversion paradigms have been used to examine holistic and configural processing in ASD (e.g., [15]). The inversion of a human face may disrupt configural processing [16, 17]. The extraction of first-order information remains intact regardless of stimulus' orientation [3]. In face inversion tasks, accuracy rates for upright faces compared to inverted faces were higher for neurotypical controls [5]. For upright stimuli, holistic and configural strategies may work together, which contributes to higher accuracy rates, whereas a stronger reliance on first-order features is necessary for inverted faces, which contributes to lower accuracy levels. In contrast, individuals with ASD displayed similar detection rates for upright and inverted faces [18]. This pattern of results supports the idea of a part-based processing strategy in which individuals with ASD predominantly rely on first-order information for upright and inverted face stimuli. Reaction time analyses of face inversion paradigms complement these findings as controls are faster in making their decisions compared to individuals with ASD (e.g., [19]). There have been, however, contrasting results which demonstrate similar face detecting rates in both groups [15, 20, 21] or even better performance in the ASD group compared to controls [20]. In fact, a recent systematic review suggested an intact face inversion effect for the ASD group in most studies [22].

Individuals with ASD may engage in similar face processing strategies as controls [12], but due to a lack of attention to faces from an early age [2], individuals with ASD may develop less expertise in face identification and discrimination [23]. Similar face detection rates for controls and the ASD group were also observed when cueing to relevant parts of the face [10]. Researchers have therefore suggested a quantitative instead of a qualitative difference of face perception in ASD [22, 24].

The disentanglement of holistic and configural processes is another challenge of face inversion tasks [7]. To address this, studies employ the Mooney face task to specifically trigger holistic processes [16, 19, 25, 26]. Mooney stimuli give rise to faces by the two-tone composition of black and white parts [16]. Extensive binding and holistic processes are required to perceive them as faces because they contain few explicit local features [25, 27, 28]. Upright presented Mooney stimuli are thought to recruit more efficient holistic processes, whereas inverted Mooney stimuli severely hinder face abstraction [8, 29]. As before, some studies reported a face inversion effect with Mooney stimuli for the ASD group (e.g., [20]), while others failed to find it (e.g., [19]).

Part of the discrepancy in these result patterns may be related to the inclusion of individuals spanning broad age bands. Holistic face processing was suggested to be impaired in children with ASD (aged 8 to 13 years) who displayed lower accuracy for inverted compared to upright face stimuli [21] and showed less sensitivity to configuration of the faces potentially due to holistic processing deficit or a lack of expertise with faces [30]. McPartland et al. (2004) demonstrated ERP differences in basic face vs. house comparisons in adolescents and adults 15 to 42 years; however, Webb et al. (2012) in adults 18-to-44-year-olds with ASD did not find altered face vs. house ERP activity but did find differences between groups in face inversion processing [23]. In a sample of 9-to 45-year-olds with ASD, O'Connor et al. (2005) found that the younger group with ASD (9 to 15 years) displayed no difference in task performance (compared to the controls), whereas adults with ASD (18 to 45 years) showed deficits across all emotion categories, which the authors suggested reflected indicating a general facial configuration deficit for adults with ASD [17]. One possible source of confound in these papers is the inclusion of the transitional stage of adolescence within either the child or adult groups. It may be of importance to examine manifestations and trajectories of face processing differences separately for adolescents, particularly as orientation processing and some aspects of holistic processing may become mature in childhood (e.g., [31]), but other neural markers of face sensitivity do not become mature until late-adolescence [32].

General face processing differences in adolescents with and without ASD may be represented by altered patterns at the neural level, specifically in the ERP components P1 and N170 which reflect attentional and perceptual aspects of the neural circuitry of face perception [1, 12, 33, 34]. Of importance, based on the latency of these components, this neural activity often precedes behavioral responses about face stimuli. The P1 event-related potential (ERP) component is a positive deflection around 100 ms associated with visual attention [35, 36]. In children and young adolescents with ASD compared to controls, Hileman et al. (2011) found smaller P1 amplitudes (but not latency) for inverted compared to upright faces while Neuhaus et al. (2016) found an inversion effect in the control group for latency (but not amplitude) which was not apparent in children and adolescents with ASD [37]. Within an adult sample, differences in P1 amplitude (but not latency) for inversion across groups were reported [38].

The N170 component reflects face categorical processing (relative to other objects), as well as eye featural sensitivity [39, 40]. In 3- to 4- and 3- to 6-year-old children with ASD, N170 latencies were longer and amplitudes smaller compared to controls in face vs. object perception tasks [2, 41]. Studies of early and late adolescence in ASD displayed a similar pattern of delayed N170 latencies without differences in N70 amplitudes to faces compared to controls [42], but this was not found in another report [37]. It is possible, that the inconsistent finding of a face inversion effect in behavior and ERPs is also associated with the underlying developmental trajectory of holistic processing and with different stimulus types and comparisons altering the extent to which the sources contributing to the P1 or N170 are implicated.

Additional EEG signal properties may inform our understanding of the mechanisms of holistic processing. The rhythmic synchronization of neural discharges in the gamma-band (> 25 Hz) relates to the 'binding problem' that is, the question of how various visual features are integrated to a coherent object representation [26, 43, 44]. It is associated with the pyramidal network's synchronization of excitatory and inhibitory interneurons [43]. Gamma-band activity (GBA) has also been connected to working memory and visual attention processes [43, 45]. The match-and-utilization model (MUM) predicts that meaningful objects such as upright faces lead to stronger GBA compared to inverted faces [46]. GBA in the lower range (25–45 Hz, 150–250 ms) has been shown to be sensitive to inversion of faces with lower activity for inverted compared to upright faces [39] and greater for faces compared to scrambled faces in neurotypical controls around 200 ms [4, 47]. Adults with ASD displayed lower levels of GBA in the lower gamma-band over occipital areas within a passive face viewing task with peak differences between 250 and 450 ms [45] or during a Mooney face inversion task between 100 and 300 ms [19]. GBA of adults with ASD was not sensitive to inversion of face in the lower gamma-band range at frontal sites, whereas controls showed a larger burst for upright faces [48]. These abnormalities in GBA may underlie disruptions in face processing in ASD at a very basic level [45].

Taken together, there are documented differences in face processing in behavioral and neural activity in children and adults with ASD but less is known about holistic face processing during adolescence as most studies have included adolescents either with younger or adult participants rather than as a targeted group. This may be an age period of particular importance as the P1 and N170 (amplitude, latency, and response characteristics) as a marker of early stage face processing becomes adult-like in the quality of the response pattern but still quantitatively differs in amplitude and latency [32]. Therefore, we aimed at investigating behavioral (detection rate/response times) and neurophysiological correlates (P1/N170 component/gamma-band activity) of holistic face processing in a narrow range sample of adolescents with ASD and sex-, age-, and IQ-matched neurotypical controls. EEG was collected while adolescents completed an inversion task with Mooney stimuli.

If adolescents with neurotypical development show effective holistic processes, and in contrast, holistic processing is impaired in the ASD group, then we predict that (1) slower response times as well as reduced face detection rates would occur in the ASD group compared to controls, suggestive of reduced holistic face perception and stronger focus on first-order features. (2) P1 latency would not be modulated by Mooney stimuli detected as faces, whereas P1/N170 amplitudes and N170 latencies to Mooney stimuli detected as faces would be slower and of less amplitude in ASD compared to controls. (3) Controls but not the ASD group would display greater P1/N170 amplitude and faster N170 latency to stimuli perceived as face compared to non-face responses. (4) Gamma power in the lower gamma-band range (25–45 Hz; associated with perceptual binding) would be smaller in the ASD compared to the control group in early and late time windows for anterior and posterior clusters.

Methods
Participants
The local Institutional Review Board approved the protocol, all adolescents provided written assent, and a parent provided written consent for participation. Adolescents with ASD met research diagnostic criteria based on the Autism Diagnostic Observation Schedule (ADOS) [49], criteria on the social and communication domains of the Autism Diagnostic Interview-Revised (ADI-R) [50], and DSM-IV criteria based on expert clinical diagnostic judgment [51]. Adolescents with typical development had no history of developmental delay or concerns about autism-related behaviors. Exclusionary criteria for adolescents with ASD and controls included performance IQ scores < 80 (Wechsler Intelligence Scale III; WISC), known genetic disorders, seizures, significant sensory or motor impairment, major physical abnormalities, serious head injury, and use of anticonvulsant or barbiturate medications. Performance IQ was employed as criteria because the tasks across the full protocol focused on non-verbal visual processing. Additional exclusionary criteria for controls included birth or developmental abnormalities, psychotropic medication usage, and a first-degree relative with ASD. Sixty-eight adolescents were enrolled in the study. Participants were matched based on their age and sex followed by bin-matching with regard to their performance IQ during the screening session. Thirty participants were excluded from the final analysis: 8 participants were disqualified after enrollment (non-compliance or too low IQ), 8 datasets had EEG file errors that resulted in unusable data, 6 had significant EEG artifacts (e.g., excessive movement), and 8 did not show visible ERP components after averaging. The final sample consisted

of 19 controls and 19 participants with ASD. No group differences for age, gender, or performance IQ were detected. There were no significant differences in characteristics between those that were included in the analysis and those that were not (ps > .05). Demographic characteristics are provided in Table 1.

Apparatus and stimuli

The current study used a set of 50 Mooney face stimuli (5.9° by 7.9°), which are degraded, 2-tone pictures of human faces [52] (see Fig. 1, Mooney face stimulus examples). They were presented upright and inverted to manipulate holistic face perception.

Procedure

Adolescents completed a training block, consisting of four trials in which Mooney stimuli were either presented upright (n = 2) or inverted (n = 2). They were asked to indicate whether they perceived a face or not. During the training trials, the goal was to practice mapping the right/left button press to the decision of face/ no face. After the mapping was understood, adolescents started with the actual task in which they saw a random sequence of upright and inverted Mooney stimuli. Participants were asked to answer as spontaneously and quickly as possible. Face and no face button position was balanced across participants.

The experiment consisted of 200 trials, presented in four 50 image blocks. A break of participant-determined length separated each block. In each trial, a gray background was presented for 500 ms (baseline) followed by a Mooney stimulus for 500 ms displayed on a gray background. The inter-trial interval (ITI) varied between 2000 and 2500 ms. Adolescents could indicate their decision across the entire stimulus presentation and ITI.

Electrophysiological recordings

EEG was recorded with a 128-channel Geodesic Sensor NetAmps 200 in Net Station 2.0 (Electric Geodesic, Inc. Eugene OR), with a sampling rate of 500 Hz, and experimental control through E-Prime 1.0 software. In a dimly-lit, sound-attenuated room, adolescents sat approximately 24 inches from the stimulus monitor and

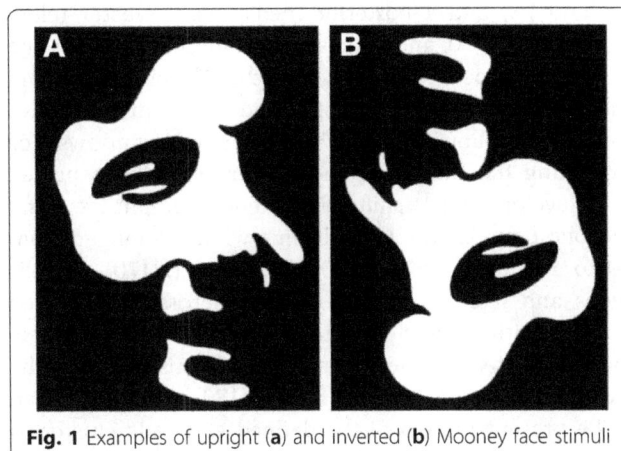

Fig. 1 Examples of upright (**a**) and inverted (**b**) Mooney face stimuli

used buttons 1 (left most button, left index finger) and 5 (right most button, right index finger) on a 5-button box for experimental response.

Processing

All procedures were conducted with MATLAB's Toolbox EEGLAB (The MathWorks, Natick, MA). Re-sampling of the data to 250 Hz and filtering (0.1 Hz highpass; 100 Hz lowpass; 60 Hz notch) preceded the exclusion of bad channels (impedances over 200 KOhm, drifting channels). Data was re-referenced to average reference, segmented into epochs (– 500 to 1000 ms) for each condition and baseline-corrected to 500 ms pre-stimulus interval. Hand editing was done as a first artifact rejection step to address "non-stereotyped" noise (e.g., pulling the cap) prior to conducting an independent component analysis (ICA). With the help of the EEGLAB plugin SASICA [53], components such as those containing electrical noise, ocular, or head movements were identified. Visual inspection served as final judgment on rejecting bad components. Lastly, excluded channels were interpolated using spherical interpolation.

ERP data

Based on a study of Webb et al. (2012), amplitudes for the P1 and N170 component in adolescents were chosen from a posterior medial left cluster (electrodes 65, 70,

Table 1 Means and standard deviations for gender, age, and IQ scores of controls and the ASD group

	Controls (N = 19)		ASD group (n = 19)		χ^2/t value	p value
	Mean	SD	Mean	SD		
Gender (M:F)	16:3		16:3		$\chi^2(1) = 0.000$	1.000
Age (years)	13.950	1.268	14.000	1.667	$t(36) = 0.110$	.913
P IQ	112.790	16.755	115.737	14.681	$t(36) = 0.577$	.568
FS IQ	113.630	17.150	109.370	13.039	$t(36) = -0.863$	.394

Note. *ASD* = autism spectrum disorder, *P IQ* = Wechsler Intelligence Scale III Performance IQ, *FS IQ* = Wechsler Intelligence Scale III Full Performance, *SD* = standard deviation

71, and 75) and a posterior medial right cluster (electrodes 83, 84, 90, and 91; also see Additional file 1). The first positive peak was defined as the P1 component and the N170 component was specified as the first negative deflection following the P1. Temporal windows for extracting the ERP components were visually inspected for developmental shifts in latency, amplitude, and morphology [32, 42]. Overall time windows ranged from 70 to 170 ms (P1) and 120 to 220 ms (N170). Amplitudes and latencies were extracted across the selected clusters within the designated time windows separately for the clusters of the left and right hemisphere for the P1 and N170 component. P1 and N170 components had to be present in 50% of the defined electrode cluster to be further included. Data was separately inspected for upright presented stimuli (trials face response: $M = 65.210$, SD = 11.928; trials no face response: $M = 17.820$, SD = 9.320) and inverted presented stimuli (trials face response: $M = 44.000$, SD = 20.254; trials no faces response: $M = 37.530$, SD = 15.446). At least 20 trials in a condition were necessary to be included in further analyses. Instead of peak amplitude, mean P1 amplitude was calculated to account for the noise level of the waveform [54]. To account for influences of the preceding P1, adjusted N170 amplitudes and latencies were calculated by subtracting the P1 peak amplitude from the N170 peak amplitude, and the P1 peak latency from the N170 peak latency [55]. Lastly, grand average waveforms were calculated for both groups.

Time-frequency-analysis

Gamma-band power (25–45 Hz) was calculated in 50 linear steps using complex Morlet wavelets (c.f. [56]). The wavelets were defined as $(\sigma_t \sqrt{\pi})^{-\frac{1}{2}} \exp(-\frac{t^2}{2\sigma_f^2}) \exp(2i\pi f_0 t)$, with $\sigma_f = 1/2\pi\sigma_t$, where t is time, f_0 is frequency, and where σ_f and σ_t denote the length of the wavelet in the frequency and time domain. The ratio f_0/σ_f was set to 5. We focused on induced gamma (i.e., non phase-locked gamma power) by obtaining time-frequency transforms of single epochs first and then averaging them across trials for each condition (c.f. [57, 58]). The time-frequency data was normalized to baseline (– 350 to – 50 ms) by applying a Z-transform, where the difference between signal and baseline was divided by the standard deviation of the baseline according to formula (1):

$$Z_{tf} = \frac{\text{activity}_{tf} - \overline{\text{baseline}}_{tf}}{\sqrt{n^{-1} \sum_{i=1}^{n} \left(\text{baseline}_{tf} - \overline{\text{baseline}}_{tf}\right)^2}}$$

in which Z denotes Z value, t denotes time, f frequency, and n denotes the number of time points in the baseline. Z values from the electrode clusters of interest included the P1/N170 posterior inferior left and right clusters.

Based on visual inspection of the scalp map distribution, an anterior left and anterior right cluster was added (left cluster electrodes 19, 23, 24, and 27; right cluster electrodes 2, 3, 9, and 10). Further, based on the time-frequency plots, two time windows were identified for analysis (50–200 ms; 200–350). Signal was averaged separately for clusters across the 25–45 Hz band and for each time window. These values were then averaged across participants for each group.

Statistical analysis

After processing, too few participants had data available for upright Mooney faces not detected as faces. This condition was therefore not included. Thus, we examined the contrasts of face responses to upright and inverted stimuli and face "no face" responses for inverted stimuli within the ERP and gamma analyses.

For face detection rates and reaction times, trials were averaged based on stimulus' orientation (upright/inverted) for stimuli detected as faces. They were submitted to repeated-measures analyses of variances (ANOVA) with orientation (upright/inverted) as within-factor and group (ASD group/controls) as between-factor.

To contrast ERP responses for face responses to upright and inverted stimuli, mean P1 amplitudes and latencies and adjusted N170 amplitudes and latencies were entered into separate repeated-measures ANOVA including the factors orientation (upright/inverted) and hemisphere (left/right) as within-factors and group (ASD group/controls) as between-factor.

To compare face to no face responses, mean P1 amplitudes and latencies and adjusted N170 amplitudes and latencies were averaged for these categories within the inverted condition. Afterwards, values were submitted to separate repeated-measures ANOVA with percept (face/no face) and hemisphere (left/right) as within-factors and group (ASD group/controls) as between-factor.

To compare GBA responses, a repeated-measures ANOVA with the within factors percept (face/no face), time window (50–200 ms/ 200–350 ms), cluster (anterior/posterior), and hemisphere (left/right) as well as the between factor group (ASD group/controls) was calculated.

All statistical analyses were performed with the IBM (Armank, NY) SPSS Statistics 14.0 software package and MATLAB (The MathWorks, Natick, MA). All analyses were followed up with inclusion of FS IQ or age as a covariate; these covariates did not change the results and findings are reported without the covariates. Significant main effects and interactions were followed by subsequent 1-way ANOVAs for the groups or by post hoc Bonferroni-corrected contrasts. For all analyses, the significance level was set at $\alpha < 0.05$.

Results

Behavioral performance

Detection rate

As hypothesized, Controls detected significantly more Mooney stimuli as faces compared to participants with ASD ($F(1, 36) = 6.272$, $p < .05$, $\eta_p^2 = .148$). Both groups identified more Mooney stimuli as faces in the upright compared to the inverted presentation ($F(1, 36) = 37.316$, $p < .001$, $\eta_p^2 = .982$). There was no orientation × group interaction ($F(1, 36) = 0.089$, $p = .768$, $\eta_p^2 = .148$) (Fig. 2).

Response time

In line with our hypothesis, the control group was faster than the ASD group to detect a face for upright and inverted Mooney stimuli ($F(1, 36) = 6.106$, $p < .05$, $\eta_p^2 = .145$). Both groups were faster to detect an upright Mooney stimulus as opposed to an inverted Mooney stimulus as a face ($F(1, 36) = 92.506$, $p < .001$, $\eta_p^2 = .720$).

There was no group x orientation interaction ($F(1, 36) = 0.159$, $p = .692$, $\eta_p^2 = .004$) (Table 2).

ERP analysis for face decisions in upright vs. inverted stimuli

P1 latency

In contrast to our hypothesis, a between-group comparison revealed a significant effect for group ($F(1, 36) = 5.692$, $p < .05$, $\eta_p^2 = .137$) with controls compared to the ASD group displaying faster P1 latencies for trials with a face decision. There was no effect of orientation ($F(1, 36) = 0.907$, $p = .347$, $\eta_p^2 = .025$) or interaction of group × orientation ($F(1, 36) = 0.004$, $p = .950$, $\eta_p^2 = .000$). When averaged across group and orientation, no hemisphere differences were detected ($F(1, 36) = 2.899$, $p = .097$, $\eta_p^2 = .075$), nor interactions with group ($F(1, 36) = 0.450$, $p = .507$, $\eta_p^2 = .012$) or orientation ($F(1, 36) = 0.529$, $p = .472$, $\eta_p^2 = .014$). The significant 3-way interaction of group × orientation × hemisphere ($F(1, 36) = 9.339$, $p < .05$, $\eta_p^2 = .206$) led to subsequent 1-way ANOVAs separated for group. None of the contrasts (separated by group) displayed significant outcomes.

P1 amplitude

Contrary to expectations, the ASD group showed similar P1 amplitudes compared to controls when Mooney stimuli were detected as faces ($F(1, 36) = 1.068$, $p = .308$, $\eta_p^2 = .029$). There was no main effect of orientation ($F(1, 36) = 1.013$, $p = .321$, $\eta_p^2 = .027$), nor interaction with group ($F(1, 36) = 3.014$, $p = .091$, $\eta_p^2 = .077$). P1 amplitudes did not differ across hemisphere ($F(1, 36) = 0.944$, $p = .338$, $\eta_p^2 = .026$). No significant interactions of hemisphere × group ($F(1, 36) = 0.243$, $p = .625$, $\eta_p^2 = .007$), hemisphere × orientation ($F(1, 36) = 0.000$, $p = .998$, $\eta_p^2 = .000$), nor hemisphere × group × orientation ($F(1, 36) = 1.337$, $p = .255$, $\eta_p^2 = .036$) were observed.

N170 latency

Faster latencies were expected for controls compared to the ASD group when detecting a face. In contrast to our hypothesis, the ASD group showed similar N170 latencies compared to controls ($F(1, 36) = 0.796$, $p = .378$,

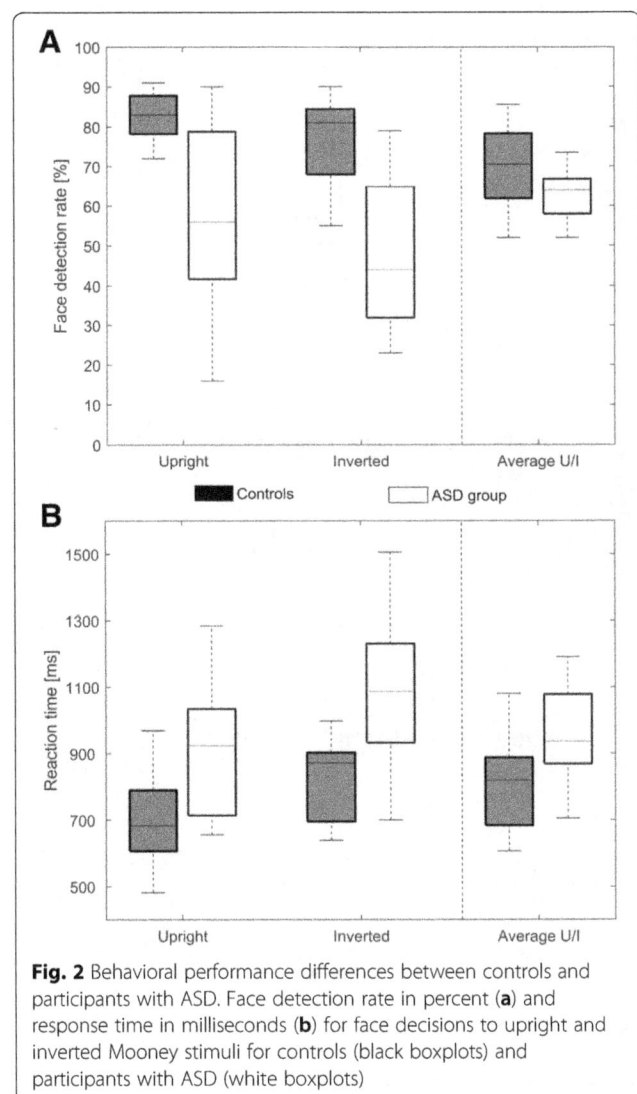

Fig. 2 Behavioral performance differences between controls and participants with ASD. Face detection rate in percent (**a**) and response time in milliseconds (**b**) for face decisions to upright and inverted Mooney stimuli for controls (black boxplots) and participants with ASD (white boxplots)

Table 2 Means and standard deviations for face detection rate and reaction times for controls and the participants with ASD

	Controls ($n = 19$)		ASD group ($n = 19$)	
	Mean	SD	Mean	SD
Hits upright stimuli (hus) (%)	81.250	8.097	75.474	12.607
Hits inverted inverted (his) (%)	56.200	21.279	47.737	18.624
Reaction time hus (ms)	829.979	196.972	952.684	221.415
Reaction time his (ms)	1049.970	226.513	1188.531	221.813

Note. *ASD* = autism spectrum disorder, *SD* = standard deviation

$\eta_p^2 = .022$), not influenced by orientation ($F(1, 36) = 2.191$, $p = .147$, $\eta_p^2 = .057$). No group × orientation interaction ($F(1, 36) = 0.280$, $p = .600$, $\eta_p^2 = .008$) or differences between hemispheres ($F(1, 36) = 2.338$, $p = .245$, $\eta_p^2 = .037$) were detected. Hemisphere did not interact with group ($F(1, 36) = 1.396$, $p = .245$, $\eta_p^2 = .037$) or orientation ($F(1, 36) = 0.121$, $p = .730$, $\eta_p^2 = .335$). The 3-way interaction of group × orientation × hemisphere was not significant ($F(1, 36) = 3.673$, $p = .063$, $\eta_p^2 = .093$).

N170 amplitude

Contrary to expectations, controls and participants with ASD showed similar N170 amplitudes when detecting faces within the Mooney stimuli ($F(1, 36) = 0.492$, $p = .488$, $\eta_p^2 = .013$). Orientation did not influence N170 amplitudes ($F(1, 36) = 0.393$, $p = .535$, $\eta_p^2 = .011$) or interact with group ($F(1, 36) = 0.780$, $p = .383$, $\eta_p^2 = .021$). A significant difference between hemispheres ($F(1, 36) = 18.135$, $p < .001$, $\eta_p^2 = .335$) indicated larger N170 amplitudes in the right compared to the left cluster ($p < .001$). There was no interaction of hemisphere × group ($F(1, 36) = 2.031$, $p = .163$, $\eta_p^2 = .053$), hemisphere × orientation ($F(1, 36) = 0.001$, $p = .979$, $\eta_p^2 = .000$), nor hemisphere × orientation × group ($F(1, 36) = 0.155$, $p = .696$, $\eta_p^2 = .004$).

ERP analysis for face vs. no face decisions in inverted Mooney stimuli
P1 latency

Contrary to expectations, a main effect of group ($F(1, 36) = 5.349$, $p < .05$, $\eta_p^2 = .129$) indicated longer latencies for the ASD group compared to controls across conditions. Latencies were not modulated by percept ($F(1, 36) = 0.704$, $p = 407$, $\eta_p^2 = .019$) or a percept × group interaction ($F(1, 36) = 0.028$, $p = .868$, $\eta_p^2 = .001$), indicating that the latency difference was not due to face detection differences. The effect of hemisphere was not significant ($F(1, 36) = 3.249$, $p = .080$, $\eta_p^2 = .083$), nor did hemisphere interact with percept ($F(1, 36) = 0.088$, $p = .769$, $\eta_p^2 = .002$), group ($F(1, 36) = 0.767$, $p = .387$, $\eta_p^2 = .021$) or display 3-way interaction ($F(1, 36) = 2.818$, $p = .102$, $\eta_p^2 = .073$) (Fig. 3).

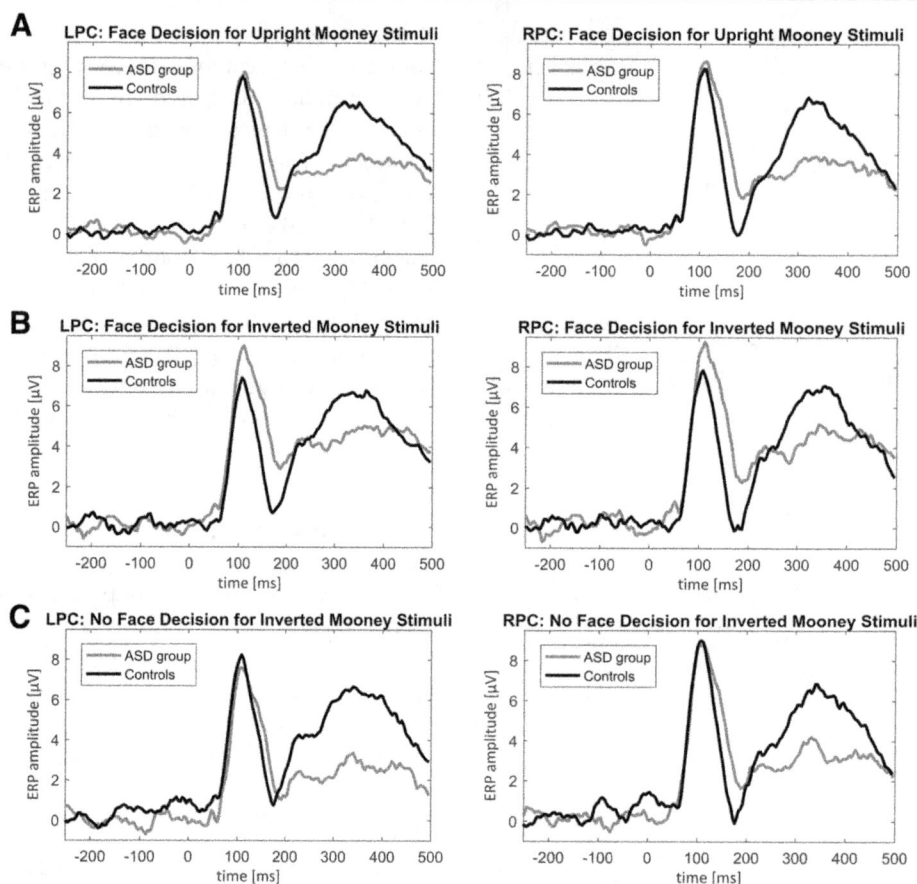

Fig. 3 ERP differences for face and no face decisions between groups. ERP plots are represented for face decisions in upright Mooney stimuli (**a**), face decisions in inverted Mooney stimuli (**b**), and no face decisions in inverted Mooney stimuli (**c**) separately for the left posterior cluster (LPC) and right posterior cluster (RPC) for controls (gray line) and the ASD group (black line)

P1 amplitude

In contrast to our hypothesis, there was no significant main effect of group suggesting that P1 amplitudes for face vs. no face decision did not differ between controls and the ASD group ($F(1, 36) = 0.558$, $p = .460$, $\eta_p^2 = .015$). Percept did not yield a significant effect ($F(1, 36) = 0.105$, $p = .748$, $\eta_p^2 = .003$). A significant percept × group interaction was observed ($F(1, 36) = 5.699$, $p < .05$, $\eta_p^2 = .137$); however, post hoc analyses showed no difference of percept for controls ($p = .153$) or the ASD group ($p = .063$). The effect of hemisphere was significant ($F(1, 36) = 7.953$, $p < .05$, $\eta_p^2 = .181$). Amplitudes in the right cluster were larger compared to the left cluster ($p > .05$). Hemisphere did not interact with group ($F(1, 36) = 0.026$, $p = .872$, $\eta_p^2 = .001$), nor percept ($F(1, 36) = 0.977$, $p = .330$, $\eta_p^2 = .026$), nor a 3-way interaction ($F(1, 36) = 1.346$, $p = .254$, $\eta_p^2 = .036$).

N170 latency

We expected similar N170 latencies for face and no face decisions for the ASD group which were hypothesized to be delayed compared to controls. In contrast to our hypothesis, controls and participants with ASD displayed similar N170 latencies ($F(1, 36) = 0.155$, $p = .696$, $\eta_p^2 = .004$). N170 latencies were not modulated by percept ($F(1, 36) = 1.670$, $p = .204$, $\eta_p^2 = .044$) or percept × group interaction ($F(1, 36) = 1.670$, $p = .204$, $\eta_p^2 = .044$). None of the factors (hemisphere: $F(1, 36) = 1.604$, $p = .213$, $\eta_p^2 = .043$; hemisphere × group: $F(1, 36) = 1.313$, $p = .259$, $\eta_p^2 = .035$; hemisphere × percept: $F(1, 36) = 0.018$, $p = .893$, $\eta_p^2 = .001$, hemisphere × percept × group: $F(1, 36) = 1.495$, $p = .229$, $\eta_p^2 = .040$) reached significance.

N170 amplitude

Contrary to expectations, controls showed similar N170 amplitudes compared to the ASD group ($F(1, 36) = 0.922$, $p = .343$, $\eta_p^2 = .025$). There was no effect of percept ($F(1, 36) = 0.019$, $p = .892$, $\eta_p^2 = .001$), nor did percept interact with group ($F(1, 36) = 1.049$, $p = .313$, $\eta_p^2 = .028$). A significant effect for hemisphere ($F(1, 36) = 20.744$, $p < .001$, $\eta_p^2 = .366$) was observed, indicating that larger N170 values were found within the right cluster ($p < .001$). There was no interaction of hemisphere × group ($F(1, 36) = 0.250$, $p = .620$, $\eta_p^2 = .007$), hemisphere × percept ($F(1, 36) = 0.386$, $p = .539$, $\eta_p^2 = .011$) or hemisphere × percept × group ($F(1, 36) = 0.566$, $p = .121$, $\eta_p^2 = .065$).

Summary ERP analysis

To summarize our ERP results, controls and individuals with ASD showed similar P1 and N170 morphologies. They only differed with regard to their P1 latencies. Controls displayed faster latencies than the ASD group

for face decisions across inverted and upright Mooney stimuli and for face vs. no face decision for inverted Mooney stimuli. Across groups, N170 amplitudes were larger in the right hemisphere for face decisions. For the face vs. no face contrast in inverted Mooney stimuli, P1 amplitudes were larger in the right compared to the left cluster.

Time frequency analyses face vs. no face decisions in inverted Mooney stimuli

We hypothesized larger GBA for controls compared to the ASD group. Contrary to expectations, groups did not differ in their general GBA ($F(1, 36) = 0.407$, $p = .528$, $\eta_p^2 = .011$). Whether they detected a face or not did not influence GBA levels ($F(1, 36) = 0.049$, $p = .826$, $\eta_p^2 = .001$), nor was there a percept × group interaction ($F(1, 36) = 0.056$, $p = .814$, $\eta_p^2 = .002$). GBA levels significantly differed across time ($F(1, 36) = 7.888$, $p < .01$, $\eta_p^2 = .158$) with larger activity in the early (50–200 ms) compared to the later time window (200–350 ms). The significant time × group interaction ($F(1, 36) = 5.392$, $p < .05$, $\eta_p^2 = .110$) indicates that controls showed larger GBA levels within the first time window ($p < .001$), whereas GBA levels for the ASD group were equal across time ($p = .742$). None of the effects of hemisphere reached significance (hemisphere: $F(1, 36) = 0.393$, $p = .535$, $\eta_p^2 = .011$; hemisphere × group: $F(1, 36) = 0.003$, $p = .986$, $\eta_p^2 = .000$; hemisphere × percept: $F(1, 36) = 0.081$, $p = .778$, $\eta_p^2 = .002$; hemisphere × time: $F(1, 36) = 0.079$, $p = .781$, $\eta_p^2 = .002$). GBA levels were larger for anterior compared to the posterior cluster ($F(1, 36) = 8.799$, $p < .01$, $\eta_p^2 = .189$). There was no significant cluster × group interaction ($F(1, 36) = 1.690$, $p = .202$, $\eta_p^2 = .036$), nor cluster × percept interaction ($F(1, 36) = 0.084$, $p = .774$, $\eta_p^2 = .002$). GBA levels of clusters did, however, differ between time windows ($F(1, 36) = 10.389$, $p < .001$, $\eta_p^2 = .223$). A larger reduction of activity from the early to the later time window in posterior ($p < .001$), but not within the anterior cluster ($p = .368$), was detected. Cluster did not interact with hemisphere ($F(1, 36) = 0.005$, $p = .983$, $\eta_p^2 = .000$). No significant 3- or 4-way interactions were observed.

Summary time frequency analysis

Groups did not differ in their general GBA to Mooney stimuli, regardless of orientation or percept. Controls displayed significant decreases in GBA levels in frontal clusters across time. This decrease in GBA did not occur in participants with ASD. For both groups, GBA was larger for the anterior cluster and activity showed larger decreases at the posterior compared to the anterior cluster across time (Fig. 4).

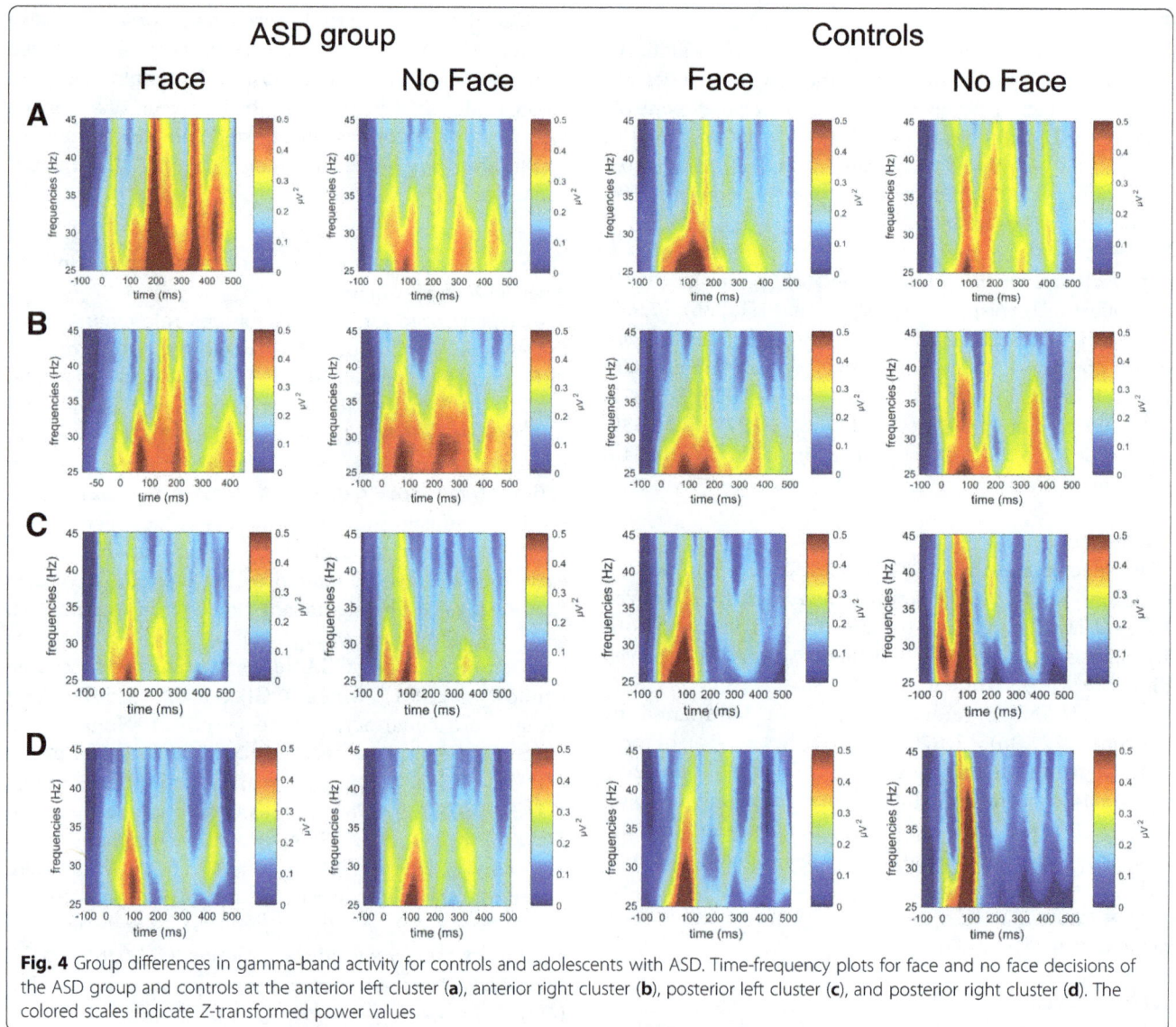

Fig. 4 Group differences in gamma-band activity for controls and adolescents with ASD. Time-frequency plots for face and no face decisions of the ASD group and controls at the anterior left cluster (**a**), anterior right cluster (**b**), posterior left cluster (**c**), and posterior right cluster (**d**). The colored scales indicate Z-transformed power values

Discussion

The present study yielded insight into holistic and configural face processing in ASD and neurotypical adolescents by examining behavioral performance (detection rate, response time) and neural correlates (P1, N170, gamma-band activity) with a Mooney stimuli inversion task. The behavioral responses suggest that mechanisms for holistic face processing are in place for both groups. Higher face detection rates for Mooney stimuli in upright orientation compared to inverted were found for both controls and the ASD group. The finding is consistent with previous studies, which also found an intact face inversion effect for individuals with ASD [15, 20–22]. While we cannot eliminate the potential that a part-based processing style influenced face detection rates in the ASD group for prior reports utilizing upright and inverted stimuli [18], our high rates of face identification are unlikely to

be due to any type of parts-based system given the nature of the Mooney stimuli. Despite a similar impact of orientation on behavioral decisions of "face-ness" for both groups, adolescents with ASD were less likely to perceive Mooney stimuli as faces than controls and displayed longer reaction times to make a face decision, which is in line with another study that employed Mooney stimuli [19]. Besides intact holistic face processing, the finding also supports a quantitative instead of a qualitative face perception difference in ASD [22, 24].

The ERP results also implicate group differences in the early neural circuitry within the visual processing system thought to reflect attentional (e.g., P1), rather than perceptual (e.g., N170) processes specific to faces. Within the comparison of face responses contrasting upright and inverted Mooney stimuli, controls displayed faster P1 latencies compared to the ASD group, whereas no differences for N170 amplitude or latency could be detected between groups and by orientation. This finding is in contrast to delayed N170 latencies to realistic faces for individuals with ASD [42]. Within the contrast of face and no face responses for inverted stimuli, controls also showed faster P1 latencies compared to the ASD group. Similarly, to the first comparison, no group differences were detected for N170 amplitude or latencies, which is also in contrast to previous findings [23, 42]. Consistent with other studies utilizing facial stimuli, we did find larger N170 amplitudes in the right compared to the left cluster [4].

We investigated the lower gamma-band (25–45 Hz) to examine feature binding processes proposed to underlie deriving a face percept from the black and white Mooney images. No group differences were found in gamma-band activity for groups across clusters, which contrasts previous findings of *more* GBA in occipital areas for controls compared to adolescents with ASD [45] or *more* GBA in ASD compared to controls [19]. Both groups showed similar activity in the early window, overlapping the P1 and the start of the N170 component. Former studies found larger GBA for controls in comparison to the ASD group [19]. However, prolonged gamma-band activity for the ASD group was detected in comparison to the control group. Increased temporal activity was also found in similar time windows for adolescents with ASD [45].

General early stage processing of Mooney stimuli was identified by the P1 component activity within both comparisons. The P1 is typically associated with early visual attention [35, 36] and source-localized to the visual association cortex [59]. In our experiment, the task emphasized attention toward the stimulus to determine "face-ness," while maintaining a 2-button response mapping. Thus, the task protocol required sustained attention and elicited a large P1 component in both groups. It is also possible that our directions provided a strategy that helped to "normalize" engagement of the face processing circuitry, as suggested by consistent morphology of the component across groups and individuals, with quantitative modulation of latency. Thus, the basic attention and processing mechanisms seem to be available in individuals with ASD and can be manipulated to produce greater responses by directing attention [12, 37]. This is in line with another study that found similar face detection rates after directing the attention to parts of the face [10].

Early stage perceptual face processing has been historically assessed by examining response patterns of the N170 component and later GBA (e.g., 150 to 250 ms or 200 to 300 ms) [4, 39]. In contrast to former studies, we did not find any differences in N170 latency or amplitude between adolescents with and without ASD [42].

Although the N170 was right-lateralized in both groups as previously reported [17, 39], it is worthy to note that most studies employ natural faces and previous research suggests that intact natural faces and eyes result in greater and faster N170 responses [60], and schematic face stimuli might induce weaker neural responses [19]. The composition of Mooney stimuli mainly comprises black and white parts that create a 3D shape of a face [26]. As these stimuli did not contain typical first-order face features (e.g., eyes or nose), they may also trigger a weaker or less consistent N170 response [61]. Latinus and Taylor (2005) found that Mooney stimuli elicited a delayed and enhanced N170 component, but only after participants received a training. We also did not find a face inversion for the Mooney images, but this may reflect that our contrast included only those stimuli that were identified as face and the N170 is associated with a general face detection mechanism [4].

Gamma-band activity has been associated with perceptual coherence. In line with the presented behavioral and ERP results, GBA responses were similar for adolescents with ASD and controls over the first 50 to 200 ms. Our groups did differ in later gamma-band activity from 200 to 350 ms, which has been associated with perceptual binding [39].

Besides the association with higher cognitive functions such as memory and attention [43, 45], early GBA has also been associated with the match of bottom-up and top-down information [43]. Within the MUM model, early GBA reflects the matching of bottom-up signals with memory contents and is enhanced when the matching process yields a positive result [62]. Later bursts have been associated with readout processes like action planning, behavioral control, or memory storage [63]. The prolonged GBA for participants with ASD across time might indicate continued activation of the matching processes.

Another explanation of the prolonged activity in ASD could be an imbalance in precision of top-down predictions and bottom-up sensory processing as suggested by the predictive coding framework [64]. Based on Bayesian decision theory, the framework suggests that we perceive our environment by consistently creating inferences. One part of the inference process is prior knowledge which is extracted from earlier sensory events [65]. These priors are consistently updated when presented with sensory evidence (e.g., Mooney stimulus) and these updates are indexed by prediction errors [66]. Individuals with ASD might have hypo-priors, meaning that whenever they saw a Mooney stimulus their system made larger prediction errors [64]. Cortical responses are considered as an index of prediction errors [65]. The prolonged GBA for individuals with ASD across face and no face responses compared to controls might indicate stronger priors in the controls and prolonged updates within the neural network due to larger prediction errors in the ASD group [66]. The lack of differences for GBA might suggest similar bottom-up perceptual binding, assuming that posterior gamma may be more reflective of a posterior-ventral network (e.g., including inferior-occipital gyri; [67]). Additionally, it might indicate an over-reliance on top-down knowledge and less deviation in perceptual areas [8]. The displayed activation patterns of anterior and posterior clusters across time contribute to the idea of different network activations. The significant decrease of GBA levels from the first to the second time window may suggest that perceptual processes are predominant during early perception, whereas networks in anterior areas are constantly active as part of monitoring and decision-making.

Limitations

Due to too few trials, we were unable to analyze the ERP contrasts involving the no face responses for the upright stimuli. Therefore, an enhanced understanding of holistic processing in ASD could be accomplished by a different attentional task. For example, Castelhano et al. (2013) used different perceptual states and presentation angles for the same physical stimulus or Sun et al. (2012) scrambled the Mooney stimuli to make them even less "face-like" [19, 29]. To further delineate effects of face processing from object processing, another option would be to employ Mooney stimuli that are objects or noise as contrasts.

We did not find a face inversion effect in our ERP data. While Mooney stimuli do resemble faces, they are only face-like. The inversion effect for realistic faces not only reflects both a decrement in performance when inverted, but also the efficiency and reliability of processing when upright. Thus, it may be that processing a Mooney stimulus upright compared to inverted (at this age) may require a more similar activation pattern that results in non-significant differences in scalp ERP amplitude and latency.

Adolescent development reflected a research area of less focused attention, given the inclusion of adolescents either in child samples or in adult samples, and a period wherein some qualitative aspects of the face processing system are mature, although potentially quantitatively different. Our results suggest an intact face inversion effect for adolescents with ASD and minor quantitative differences on the neural level.

Longitudinal study designs might be most suitable to detect behavioral changes as well as the time course of P1, N170, and gamma-band abnormalities as Webb, Neuhaus, and Faja [68] have suggested significant improvement and "normalization" of face neural circuitry into adolescence and adulthood in ASD, particularly in relation to first-order processing.

The analysis of binding processes could also be further addressed with phase information and cross-frequency coupling [57, 69, 70]. Understanding connectivity in long-range connections and between sensory areas and attentional systems would be important in understanding how top-down processes related to the task directions influence perceptual responses.

Conclusions

In this paper, we examined behavioral performance, P1, N170, and gamma-band activity in adolescents with ASD and controls during face perception with a carefully selected (IQ-, sex-, and age-matched), narrow range sample. Processing differences may be due to less efficient holistic face processing in ASD, which is required to perceive Mooney stimuli as faces. However, the general similarities between groups suggest that these neural systems are available in individuals with ASD but may be less pronounced or consistently activated. Thus, the fundamental idea of individuals with ASD having an impaired holistic face processing system should be reviewed.

Abbreviations
ADI: Autism Diagnostic Interview; ADOS: Autism Diagnostic Observation Schedule; ASD: Autism spectrum disorder; EEG: Electroencephalography; ERP: Event-related potential; ICA: Independent component analysis; ITI: Inter-trial interval; WISC: Wechsler Intelligence Scale

Acknowledgements
The authors thank the participants and their families for their time and effort in participation in this project. Additional support was provided by Adham Atyabi, Geraldine Dawson, Anna Kresse, Tisa Nalty, and Jessica Shook.

Funding
Funding was provided by the Cure Autism Now (Webb) and NIH (R01 MH10028, Pelphrey).

Authors' contributions
SN directed the data analysis and interpretation of the data and drafted the manuscript. US contributed to the data analysis and interpretation of the data and revised the manuscript. MS contributed to the data analysis and interpretation of the data and revised the manuscript. JM contributed to the coordination and collection of the data and revised the manuscript. SJW conceived of the study; directed in its design, coordination, analysis, and interpretation; and revised the manuscript. All authors read and approved the final manuscript.

Competing interests
The authors declare that they have no competing interests.

Author details
[1]Berlin School of Mind and Brain, Humboldt-Universität zu Berlin, Berlin, Germany. [2]Department of Psychology, Technische Universität Dresden, Dresden, Germany. [3]Seattle Children's Research Institute, Seattle, USA. [4]Yale University, New Haven, USA. [5]University of Washington, Washington D.C., USA.

References

1. Jemel B, Mottron L, Dawson M. Impaired face processing in autism: fact or artifact? J Autism Dev Disord. 2006;36(1):91–106.

2. Webb SJ, Dawson G, Bernier R, Panagiotides H. ERP evidence of atypical face processing in young children with autism. J Autism Dev Disord. 2006; 36(7):881–90.

3. Taubert J, Apthorp D, Aagten-Murphy D, Alais D. The role of holistic processing in face perception: evidence from the face inversion effect. Vis Res. 2011;51(11):1273–8.

4. Zion-Golumbic E, Bentin S. Dissociated neural mechanisms for face detection and configural encoding: evidence from N170 and induced gamma-band oscillation effects. Cereb Cortex. 2007;17(8):1741–9.

5. Freire A, Lee K, Symons LA. The face-inversion effect as a deficit in the encoding of Configural information: direct evidence. Perception. 2000; 29(2):159–70.

6. Kumar SL. Examining the characteristics of Visuospatial information processing in individuals with high-functioning autism. Yale J Biol Med. 2013;86(2):147–56.

7. Piepers DW, Robbins RA. A review and clarification of the terms 'holistic,' 'configural,' and 'relational' in the face perception literature. Front Psychol. 2012;3:559.

8. Steinberg Lowe M, Lewis GA, Poeppel D. Effects of part- and whole-object primes on early MEG responses to Mooney faces and houses. Front Psychol. 2016;7(February):147.

9. American Psychiatric Association, Diagnostic and Statistical Manual of Mental Disorders (DSM-V), no. 1. 2013.

10. Joseph RM, Tanaka J. Holistic and part-based face recognition in children with autism. J Child Psychol Psychiatry Allied Discip. 2003;44(4):529–42.

11. D'Souza D, Booth R, Connolly M, Happé F, Karmiloff-Smith A. Rethinking the concepts of 'local or global processors': evidence from Williams syndrome, Down syndrome, and autism spectrum disorders. Dev Sci. 2016;19(3):452–68.

12. Webb SJ, Neuhaus E, Faja S. Face perception and learning in autism Spectrum disorders. Q J Exp Psychol. 2016;0218(May):1–44.

13. Van der Hallen R, Evers K, Brewaeys K, Van den Noortgate W, Wagemans J. Global processing takes time: a meta-analysis on local–global visual processing in ASD. Psychol Bull. 2015;141(3):549–73.

14. Frith U. Autism and 'theory of mind. In: diagnosis and treatment of autism. New York: Plenum Press; 1989. p. 33–52.

15. Lahaie A, Mottron L, Arguin M, Berthiaume C, Jemel B, Saumier D. Face perception in high-functioning autistic adults: evidence for superior processing of face parts, not for a configural face-processing deficit. Neuropsychology. 2006;20(1):30–41.

16. Latinus M, Taylor MJ. Holistic processing of faces: learning effects with Mooney faces. J Cogn Neurosci. 2005;17(8):1316–27.

17. O'Connor K, Hamm JP, Kirk IJ. The neurophysiological correlates of face processing in adults and children with Asperger's syndrome. Brain Cogn. 2005;59(1):82–95.

18. Rose FE, Lincoln AJ, Lai Z, Ene M, Searcy YM, Bellugi U. Orientation and affective expression effects on face recognition in Williams syndrome and autism. J Autism Dev Disord. 2007;37(3):513–22.

19. Sun L, et al. Impaired gamma-band activity during perceptual Organization in Adults with autism Spectrum disorders: evidence for dysfunctional network activity in frontal-posterior cortices. J Neurosci. 2012;32(28):9563–73.

20. Rutherford MD, Clements KA, Sekuler AB. Differences in discrimination of eye and mouth displacement in autism spectrum disorders. Vis Res. 2007; 47(15):2099–110.

21. Scherf KS, Behrmann M, Minshew N, Luna B. Atypical development of face and greeble recognition in autism. J Child Psychol Psychiatry Allied Discip. 2008;49(8):838–47.

22. Weigelt S, Koldewyn K, Kanwisher N. Face identity recognition in autism spectrum disorders: a review of behavioral studies. Neurosci Biobehav Rev. 2012;36(3):1060–84.

23. McPartland J, Dawson G, Webb SJ, Panagiotides H, Carver LJ. Event-related brain potentials reveal anomalies in temporal processing of faces in autism spectrum disorder. J Child Psychol Psychiatry Allied Discip. 2004;45(7):1235–45.

24. Akechi H, Kikuchi Y, Tojo Y, Osanai H, Hasegawa T. Neural and behavioural responses to face-likeness of objects in adolescents with autism spectrum disorder. Sci Rep. 2014;4:1–7.

25. George N, Jemel B, Fiori N, Chaby L, Renault B. Electrophysiological correlates of facial decision: insights from upright and upside-down Mooney-face perception. Cogn Brain Res. 2005;24(3):663–73.

26. Grützner C, Uhlhaas PJ, Genc E, Kohler A, Singer W, Wibral M. Neuroelectromagnetic correlates of perceptual closure processes. J Neurosci. 2010;30(24):8342–52.

27. Otsuka Y, Hill HCH, Kanazawa S, Yamaguchi MK, Spehar B. Perception of Mooney faces by young infants: the role of local feature visibility, contrast polarity, and motion. J Exp Child Psychol. 2012;111(2):164–79.

28. Verhallen RJ, Bosten JM, Goodbourn PT, Bargary G, Lawrance-Owen AJ, Mollon JD. An online version of the Mooney face test: phenotypic and genetic associations. Neuropsychologia. 2014;63(1):19–25.

29. Castelhano J, Rebola J, Leitão B, Rodriguez E, Castelo-Branco M. To perceive or not perceive: the role of gamma-band activity in signaling object percepts. PLoS One. 2013;8(6):35–7.

30. Gauthier I, Klaiman C, Schultz RT. Face composite effects reveal abnormal face processing in autism Spectrum disorders. Heal (San Fr.). 2010;49(4):470–8.

31. Jeffery L, Taylor L, Rhodes G. Transfer of figural face aftereffects suggests mature orientation selectivity in 8-year-olds' face coding. J Exp Child Psychol. 2014;126:229–44.

32. Taylor MJ, Batty M, Itier RJ. The faces of development: a review of early face processing over childhood. J Cogn Neurosci. 2004;16(8):1426–42.

33. Dawson G, Webb SJ, McPartland J. Understanding the nature of face processing impairment in autism: insights from behavioral and electrophysiological studies. Dev Neuropsychol. 2005;27(3):403–24.

34. Jeste SS, Nelson CA. Event related potentials in the understanding of autism spectrum disorders: an analytical review. J Autism Dev Disord. 2009;39(3): 495–510.

35. Crist RE, Wu C-T, Karp C, Woldorff MG. Face processing is gated by visual spatial attention. Front Hum Neurosci. 2008;1:10.

36. Jacques C, Rossion B. Electrophysiological evidence for temporal dissociation between spatial attention and sensory competition during human face processing. Cereb Cortex. 2007;17(5):1055–65.

37. Neuhaus E, Kresse A, Faja S, Bernier RA, Webb SJ. Face processing among twins with and without autism: social correlates and twin concordance. Soc Cogn Affect Neurosci. 2016;11(1):44–54.

38. Webb SJ, Merkle K, Murias M, Richards T, Aylward E, Dawson G. ERP responses differentiate inverted but not upright face processing in adults with ASD. Soc Cogn Affect Neurosci. 2012;7(5):578–87.

39. Anaki D, Zion-Golumbic E, Bentin S. Electrophysiological neural mechanisms for detection, configural analysis and recognition of faces. Neuroimage. 2007;37(4):1407–16.

40. Itier RJ, Alain C, Sedore K, McIntosh AR. Early face processing specificity: It's in the eyes! J Cogn Neurosci. 2007;19(11):1815–26.

41. S. J. Webb, R. Bernier, M. Paul, and G. Dawson, Further evidence for an abnormality in the temporal processing of faces in autism, 2003.

42. Hileman CM, Henderson H, Mundy P, Newell L, Jaime M. Developmental and individual differences on the P1 and N170 ERP components in children with and without autism. Dev Neuropsychol. 2011;36(2):214–36.

43. Güntekin B, Başar E. A review of brain oscillations in perception of faces and emotional electric pictures. Neuropsychologia. 2014;58(1):33–51.

44. Kaiser J, Lutzenberger W. Induced gamma-band activity and human brain function. Neuroscientist. 2003;9(6):475–84.

45. Wright B, et al. Gamma activation in young people with autism spectrum disorders and typically-developing controls when viewing emotions on faces. PLoS One. 2012;7:7.

46. Herrmann CS, Fründ I, Lenz D. Human gamma-band activity: a review on cognitive and behavioral correlates and network models. Neurosci Biobehav Rev. 2010;34(7):981–92.

47. Rodriguez E, George N, Lachaux JP, Martinerie J, Renault B, Varela FJ. Perception's shadow: long-distance synchronization of human brain activity. Nature. 1999;397(6718):430–3.

48. Grice SJ, et al. Disordered visual processing and oscillatory brain activity in autism and Williams syndrome. Neuroreport. 2001;12(12):2697–700.

49. Lord C, Rutter M, Le Couteur A. Autism diagnostic interview-revised: a revised version of a diagnostic interview for caregivers of individuals with possible pervasive developmental disorders. J Autism Dev Disord. 1994; 24(5):659–85.

50. Lord C, et al. The autism diagnostic observation schedule-generic: a standard measure of social and communication deficits associated with the spectrum of autism. J Autism Dev Disord. 2000;30(3):205–23.

51. APA. Diagnostic and statistical manual of mental disorders, 4th text. Washington, D.C.: Author; 1994.

52. Mooney CM. Age in the development of closure ability in children. Can J Psychol. 1957;11(4):219–26.

53. Chaumon M, Bishop DVM, Busch NA. A practical guide to the selection of independent components of the electroencephalogram for artifact correction. J Neurosci Methods. 2015;250:47–63.

54. Luck SJ. An Introduction to the Event-Related Potential Technique, Second Edition. Cambridge, MA: MIT Press; 2014.

55. D'Hondt F, et al. Electrophysiological correlates of emotional face processing after mild traumatic brain injury in preschool children. Cogn Affect Behav Neurosci. 2017;17(1):124–42.

56. Tallon-Baudry C, Bertrand O, Delpuech C, Permier J. Oscillatory gamma-band (30-70 Hz) activity induced by a visual search task in humans. J Neurosci. 1997;17(2):722–34.

57. Castelhano J, Bernardino I, Rebola J, Rodriguez E, Castelo-Branco M. Oscillations or synchrony? Disruption of neural synchrony despite enhanced gamma oscillations in a model of disrupted perceptual coherence. J Cogn Neurosci. 2015;27(12):2416–26.

58. Wright B, et al. Gamma activation in young people with autism spectrum disorders and typically-developing controls when viewing emotions on faces. PLoS One. 2012;7(7):e41326.

59. Wong TKW, Fung PCW, McAlonan GM, Chua SE. Spatiotemporal dipole source localization of face processing ERPs in adolescents: a preliminary study. Behav Brain Funct. 2009;5(1):16.

60. Cecchini M, Aceto P, Altavilla D, Palumbo L, Lai C. The role of the eyes in processing an intact face and its scrambled image: a dense array ERP and low-resolution electromagnetic tomography (sLORETA) study. Soc Neurosci. 2013;8(4):314–25.

61. Sagiv N, Bentin S. Structural encoding of human and schematic faces: holistic and part-based processes. J Cogn Neurosci. 2001;13(7):937–51.

62. Herrmann CS, Munk MHJ, Engel AK. Cognitive functions of gamma-band activity: memory match and utilization. Trends Cogn Sci. 2004;8(8):347–55.

63. Rojas DC, Wilson LB. Gamma-band abnormalities as markers of autism spectrum disorders. Biomark Med. 2014;8(3):353–68.

64. Pellicano E, Burr D. When the world becomes 'too real': a Bayesian explanation of autistic perception. Trends Cogn Sci. 2012;16(10):504–10.

65. Stefanics G, Kremlacek J, Czigler I. Visual mismatch negativity: a predictive coding view. Front Hum Neurosci. 2014;8(September):1–19.

66. Friston KJ, Lawson R, Frith CD. On hyperpriors and hypopriors: comment on Pellicano and Burr. Trends Cogn Sci. 2013;17(1):1.

67. Gao Z, Goldstein A, Harpaz Y, Hansel M, Zion-Golumbic E, Bentin S. A magnetoencephalographic study of face processing: M170, gamma-band oscillations and source localization. Hum Brain Mapp. 2013;34(8):1783–95.

68. Webb SJ, Neuhaus E, Faja S. Face perception and learning in autism spectrum disorders. Q J Exp Psychol. 2017;70(5):970–86.

69. Kessler K, Seymour RA, Rippon G. Brain oscillations and connectivity in autism spectrum disorders (ASD): new approaches to methodology, measurement and modelling. Neurosci Biobehav Rev. 2016;71:601–20.

70. David N, Schneider TR, Peiker I, Al-Jawahiri R, Engel AK, Milne E. Variability of cortical oscillation patterns: a possible endophenotype in autism spectrum disorders? Neurosci Biobehav Rev. 2016;71:590–600.

Permissions

All chapters in this book were first published in JND, by BioMed Central; hereby published with permission under the Creative Commons Attribution License or equivalent. Every chapter published in this book has been scrutinized by our experts. Their significance has been extensively debated. The topics covered herein carry significant findings which will fuel the growth of the discipline. They may even be implemented as practical applications or may be referred to as a beginning point for another development.

The contributors of this book come from diverse backgrounds, making this book a truly international effort. This book will bring forth new frontiers with its revolutionizing research information and detailed analysis of the nascent developments around the world.

We would like to thank all the contributing authors for lending their expertise to make the book truly unique. They have played a crucial role in the development of this book. Without their invaluable contributions this book wouldn't have been possible. They have made vital efforts to compile up to date information on the varied aspects of this subject to make this book a valuable addition to the collection of many professionals and students.

This book was conceptualized with the vision of imparting up-to-date information and advanced data in this field. To ensure the same, a matchless editorial board was set up. Every individual on the board went through rigorous rounds of assessment to prove their worth. After which they invested a large part of their time researching and compiling the most relevant data for our readers.

The editorial board has been involved in producing this book since its inception. They have spent rigorous hours researching and exploring the diverse topics which have resulted in the successful publishing of this book. They have passed on their knowledge of decades through this book. To expedite this challenging task, the publisher supported the team at every step. A small team of assistant editors was also appointed to further simplify the editing procedure and attain best results for the readers.

Apart from the editorial board, the designing team has also invested a significant amount of their time in understanding the subject and creating the most relevant covers. They scrutinized every image to scout for the most suitable representation of the subject and create an appropriate cover for the book.

The publishing team has been an ardent support to the editorial, designing and production team. Their endless efforts to recruit the best for this project, has resulted in the accomplishment of this book. They are a veteran in the field of academics and their pool of knowledge is as vast as their experience in printing. Their expertise and guidance has proved useful at every step. Their uncompromising quality standards have made this book an exceptional effort. Their encouragement from time to time has been an inspiration for everyone.

The publisher and the editorial board hope that this book will prove to be a valuable piece of knowledge for researchers, students, practitioners and scholars across the globe.

List of Contributors

Hayley Crawford
Centre for Research in Psychology, Behaviour and Achievement, Coventry University, Coventry CV1 5FB, UK
Cerebra Centre for Neurodevelopmental Disorders, School of Psychology, University of Birmingham, Edgbaston B15 2TT, UK

Chris Oliver
Cerebra Centre for Neurodevelopmental Disorders, School of Psychology, University of Birmingham, Edgbaston B15 2TT, UK

Joanna Moss
Cerebra Centre for Neurodevelopmental Disorders, School of Psychology, University of Birmingham, Edgbaston B15 2TT, UK
Institute of Cognitive Neuroscience, University College London, 17 Queen Square, London WC1N 3AR, UK

Deborah Riby
Department of Psychology, Durham University, Durham DH1 3LE, UK

Na He, Bing-Mei Li, Zhao-Xia Li, Jie Wang, Xiao-Rong Liu, Bin Tang, Wen-Jun Bian, Yi-Wu Shi and Wei-Ping Liao
Institute of Neuroscience and Department of Neurology of the Second Affiliated Hospital of Guangzhou Medical University, Chang-gang-dong Road 250, Guangzhou 510260, China
Key Laboratory of Neurogenetics and Channelopathies of Guangdong Province and the Ministry of Education of China, Guangzhou 510260, China

Heng Meng
Institute of Neuroscience and Department of Neurology of the Second Affiliated Hospital of Guangzhou Medical University, Chang-gang-dong Road 250, Guangzhou 510260, China
Key Laboratory of Neurogenetics and Channelopathies of Guangdong Province and the Ministry of Education of China, Guangzhou 510260, China
Department of Neurology, The First Affiliated Hospital of Jinan University, Guangdong 510630, China Clinical Neuroscience Institute of Jinan University, Guangdong 510630, China

Caitlin M. Hudac and Trent D. DesChamps
Department of Psychiatry and Behavioral Sciences, University of Washington, CHDD Seattle, WA 98195, USA

Raphael A. Bernier and Sara Jane Webb
Department of Psychiatry and Behavioral Sciences, University of Washington, CHDD Seattle, WA 98195, USA
Center for Child Health, Behavior, and Disabilities, Seattle Children's Research Institute, Seattle, WA 98145, USA

Holly A. F. Stessman
Department of Genome Sciences, University of Washington School of Medicine, Seattle, WA98195, USA

Evan E. Eichler
Department of Genome Sciences, University of Washington School of Medicine, Seattle, WA98195, USA
Howard Hughes Medical Institute, Seattle, WA 98195, USA

Emily Neuhaus and Anna Kresse
Center for Child Health, Behavior, and Disabilities, Seattle Children's Research Institute, Seattle, WA 98145, USA

Susan Faja
Boston Children's Hospital and Division of Developmental Medicine, Harvard School of Medicine, Boston, MA 02215, USA

Donna Reid and Chris Oliver
Cerebra Centre for Neurodevelopmental Disorders, School of Psychology, University of Birmingham, B15 2TT, Edgbaston, UK
Faculty of Health and Life Sciences, Coventry University, Coventry CV1 5FB, UK

Hayley Crawford
Cerebra Centre for Neurodevelopmental Disorders, School of Psychology, University of Birmingham, B15 2TT, Edgbaston, UK
Faculty of Health and Life Sciences, Coventry University, Coventry CV1 5FB, UK

Joanna Moss
Cerebra Centre for Neurodevelopmental Disorders, School of Psychology, University of Birmingham, B15 2TT, Edgbaston, UK
Institute of Cognitive Neuroscience, University College London, 17 Queen Square, London WC1N 3AR, UK

Lisa Nelson
Cerebra Centre for Neurodevelopmental Disorders, School of Psychology, University of Birmingham, B15 2TT, Edgbaston, UK

Derby Royal Hospital, Uttoxeter Road, Derby DE22 3NE, UK

Inga Sophia Knoth
Neuroscience of Early Development (NED), 90 Avenue Vincent-D'indy, Montreal, QC H2V 2S9, Canada
Research Center of the CHU Sainte-Justine Mother and Child University Hospital Center, 3175 Chemin Côte Ste-Catherine, Montreal, QC H3T 1C5, Canada

Simon Rigoulot and Sarah Lippé
Neuroscience of Early Development (NED), 90 Avenue Vincent-D'indy, Montreal, QC H2V 2S9, Canada
Research Center of the CHU Sainte-Justine Mother and Child University Hospital Center, 3175 Chemin Côte Ste-Catherine, Montreal, QC H3T 1C5, Canada
Department of Psychology, Université de Montréal, 90 Avenue Vincent-D'indy, Montreal, QC H2V 2S9, Canada
Centre de Recherche en Neuropsychologie et Cognition (CERNEC), 90 Avenue Vincent-D'indy, Montreal, QC H2V 2S9, Canada
International Laboratory for Brain, Music and Sound Research (BRAMS), 1430 Boul Mont-Royal, Montreal, QC H2V 2J2, Canada

Sébastien Jacquemont, Philippe Major, Karine Lacourse and Phetsamone Vannasing
Research Center of the CHU Sainte-Justine Mother and Child University Hospital Center, 3175 Chemin Côte Ste-Catherine, Montreal, QC H3T 1C5, Canada

Jacques L. Michaud
Research Center of the CHU Sainte-Justine Mother and Child University Hospital Center, 3175 Chemin Côte Ste-Catherine, Montreal, QC H3T 1C5, Canada
Faculty of Medicine, Université de Montréal, 2900 boulevard Édouard-Montpetit, Montréal, QC H3T 1J4, Canada

Tarek Lajnef
Department of Psychology, Université de Montréal, 90 Avenue Vincent-D'indy, Montreal, QC H2V 2S9, Canada
Centre de Recherche en Neuropsychologie et Cognition (CERNEC), 90 Avenue Vincent-D'indy, Montreal, QC H2V 2S9, Canada

Karim Jerbi
Department of Psychology, Université de Montréal, 90 Avenue Vincent-D'indy, Montreal, QC H2V 2S9, Canada
Centre de Recherche en Neuropsychologie et Cognition (CERNEC), 90 Avenue Vincent-D'indy, Montreal, QC H2V 2S9, Canada
International Laboratory for Brain, Music and Sound Research (BRAMS), 1430 Boul Mont-Royal, Montreal, QC H2V 2J2, Canada

Centre de Recherche de l'Institut Universitaire en Santé Mentale de Montréal (CRIUSMM), 7401 Rue Hochelaga, Montréal, QC H1N 3M5, Canada
Centre de Recherche de l'Institut Universitaire de Gériatrie de Montréal (CRIUGM), 4565, chemin Queen-Mary, Montreal, QC H3W 1W5, Canada

Michael S. Sidorov and Benjamin D. Philpot
Department of Cell Biology and Physiology, University of North Carolina, Chapel Hill, NC 27599, USA
Carolina Institute for Developmental Disabilities, University of North Carolina, Chapel Hill, NC 27599, USA
Neuroscience Center, University of North Carolina, Chapel Hill, NC 27599, USA

Ronald L. Thibert
Department of Neurology, Massachusetts General Hospital, Boston, MA 02114, USA

Marjan Dolatshahi and Catherine J. Chu
Centre de Recherche en Neuropsychologie et Cognition (CERNEC), 90 Avenue Vincent-D'indy, Montreal, QC H2V 2S9, Canada
International Laboratory for Brain, Music and Sound Research (BRAMS), 1430 Boul Mont-Royal, Montreal, QC H2V 2J2, Canada

Gina M. Deck
Centre de Recherche en Neuropsychologie et Cognition (CERNEC), 90 Avenue Vincent-D'indy, Montreal, QC H2V 2S9, Canada
International Laboratory for Brain, Music and Sound Research (BRAMS), 1430 Boul Mont-Royal, Montreal, QC H2V 2J2, Canada
Present Address: The Neurology Foundation, Rhode Island Hospital and Warren Alpert School of Medicine at Brown University, Providence, RI 02903, USA

Lynne M. Bird
Department of Pediatrics, University of California, San Diego, CA, USA
Division of Dysmorphology/Genetics, Rady Children's Hospital, San Diego, CA, USA

Inês Bernardino and Tânia Marques
CNC.IBILI, Institute for Biomedical Imaging and Life Sciences, University of Coimbra, 3000-548 Coimbra, Portugal

Gilberto Silva, Isabel Catarina Duarte and Miguel Castelo-Branco
CNC.IBILI, Institute for Biomedical Imaging and Life Sciences, University of Coimbra, 3000-548 Coimbra, Portugal
ICNAS, CIBIT, Institute for Nuclear Sciences Applied to Health, University of Coimbra, 3000-548 Coimbra, Portugal

Inês R. Violante
School of Psychology, Faculty of Health and Medical Sciences, University of Surrey, Guildford GU2 7XH, UK

Cristan Farmer, Susan E. Swedo and Audrey Thurm
Pediatrics and Developmental Neuroscience Branch, National Institute of Mental Health, National Institutes of Health, Bethesda, MD 20892, USA

Lauren Swineford
Pediatrics and Developmental Neuroscience Branch, National Institute of Mental Health, National Institutes of Health, Bethesda, MD 20892, USA
Department of Speech and Hearing Sciences, Washington State University, Spokane, WA 99202, USA

Boin Choi
Graduate School of Education, Harvard University, Cambridge, MA, USA
Graduate School of Arts and Sciences, Harvard University, Cambridge, MA, USA

Charles A. Nelson
Graduate School of Education, Harvard University, Cambridge, MA, USA
Graduate School of Arts and Sciences, Harvard University, Cambridge, MA, USA
Laboratories of Cognitive Neuroscience, Division of Developmental Medicine, Boston Children's Hospital, Harvard Medical School, Boston, MA, USA

Kathryn A. Leech
Graduate School of Education, Harvard University, Cambridge, MA, USA
Boston University School of Education, Boston, MA, USA

Helen Tager-Flusberg
Department of Psychological and Brain Sciences, Boston University, Boston, MA, USA

Eileen Haebig, Christine Weber, Laurence B. Leonard, Patricia Deevy and J. Bruce Tomblin
Purdue University, West Lafayette, IN, USA
University of Iowa, Iowa City, IA, USA

Jun Wang
Department of Psychology, Zhejiang Normal University, 688 Yingbin Road, Jinhua, Zhejiang, China 321004

Lauren E. Ethridge
Department of Pediatrics, Section of Developmental and Behavioral Pediatrics, University of Oklahoma Health Sciences Center, Oklahoma City, OK, USA

Department of Psychology, University of Oklahoma, Norman, OK, USA

Matthew W. Mosconi
Clinical Child Psychology Program and Schiefelbusch Institute for Life Span Studies, University of Kansas, Lawrence, KS, USA

Stormi P. White
Department of Psychiatry, Center for Autism and Developmental Disabilities, University of Texas Southwestern Medical Center, Dallas, TX, USA

Devin K. Binder
Center for Glial-Neuronal Interactions, Neuroscience Graduate Program, Division of Biomedical Sciences, School of Medicine, University of California, Riverside, CA, USA

Ernest V. Pedapati and Craig A. Erickson
Department of Psychiatry and Behavioral Neuroscience and Division of Psychiatry, Cincinnati Children's Hospital Medical Center, Cincinnati, OH, USA

Matthew J. Byerly
Center for Mental Health Research and Recovery, Montana State University, Bozeman, MT, USA

John A. Sweeney
Department of Psychiatry and Behavioral Neuroscience, University of Cincinnati, Cincinnati, OH, USA

Kaitlyn E. Francis and Benjamin R. Morgan
Diagnostic Imaging and Research Institute, Hospital for Sick Children, 555 University Avenue, Toronto, Ontario M5G 1X8, Canada

Vanessa M. Vogan
Diagnostic Imaging and Research Institute, Hospital for Sick Children, 555 University Avenue, Toronto, Ontario M5G 1X8, Canada
Department of Applied Psychology and Human Development, Ontario Institute for Studies in Education, University of Toronto, 252 Bloor Street West, Toronto, Ontario M56 1V6, Canada

Margot J. Taylor
Diagnostic Imaging and Research Institute, Hospital for Sick Children, 555 University Avenue, Toronto, Ontario M5G 1X8, Canada
Department of Psychology, University of Toronto, 100 St. George St., Toronto, Ontario M5S 3G3, Canada

Mary Lou Smith
Department of Psychology, University of Toronto, 100 St. George St., Toronto, Ontario M5S 3G3, Canada

Sabine E. Mous
Department of Child and Adolescent Psychiatry/Psychology, Sophia Children's Hospital, Erasmus Medical Center, Wytemaweg 80, 3015 CN Rotterdam, The Netherlands
Division of Child Psychiatry, Department of Psychiatry, Washington University School of Medicine, 660 South Euclid Avenue, Campus St Louis, MO 63110, USA

Allan Jiang, Arpana Agrawal and John N. Constantino
Division of Child Psychiatry, Department of Psychiatry, Washington University School of Medicine, 660 South Euclid Avenue, Campus St Louis, MO 63110, USA

Jessica Klusek
Department of Communication Sciences and Disorders, University of South Carolina, Keenan Building, Suite 300, Columbia, SC 29208, USA

Giuseppe LaFauci and Tatyana Adayev
Department of Developmental Biochemistry, New York State Institute for Basic Research in Developmental Disabilities, 1050 Forest Hill Road, Staten Island, NY 10314, USA

W. Ted Brown
Department of Human Genetics, New York State Institute for Basic Research in Developmental Disabilities, 1050 Forest Hill Road, Staten Island, NY 10314, USA

Flora Tassone
UC Davis MIND Institute, University of California Davis, 2825 50th Street, Sacramento, CA 95817, USA

Jane E. Roberts
Department of Psychology, University of South Carolina, 1512 Pendleton Street, Columbia, SC 29208, USA

R. K. Greene and M. G. Mosner
Department of Psychology and Neuroscience, University of North Carolina at Chapel Hill, Chapel Hill, NC 27514, USA

G. S. Dichter
Department of Psychology and Neuroscience, University of North Carolina at Chapel Hill, Chapel Hill, NC 27514, USA
Department of Psychiatry, University of North Carolina at Chapel Hill School of Medicine, Chapel Hill, NC 27514, USA
Carolina Institute for Developmental Disabilities, University of North Carolina at Chapel Hill School of Medicine, Chapel Hill, NC 27514, USA

Department of Psychiatry, University of North Carolina at Chapel Hill School of Medicine, CB 7155, Chapel Hill, NC 27599-7155, USA

M. Spanos
Duke Clinical Research Institute, Duke University, Durham, NC 27705, USA
Duke Center for Autism and Brain Development, Duke University, Durham, NC 27705, USA
Department of Psychiatry, University of North Carolina at Chapel Hill School of Medicine, Chapel Hill, NC 27514, USA
Duke-UNC Brain Imaging and Analysis Center, Duke University Medical Center, Durham, NC 27705, USA
Carolina Institute for Developmental Disabilities, University of North Carolina at Chapel Hill School of Medicine, Chapel Hill, NC 27514, USA
Department of Psychiatry and Behavioral Sciences, Duke University Medical Center, Durham, NC 27705, USA

L. Sikich
Duke Clinical Research Institute, Duke University, Durham, NC 27705, USA
Duke Center for Autism and Brain Development, Duke University, Durham, NC 27705, USA
Department of Psychiatry, University of North Carolina at Chapel Hill School of Medicine, Chapel Hill, NC 27514, USA
Department of Psychiatry and Behavioral Sciences, Duke University Medical Center, Durham, NC 27705, USA

Alderman
Duke Clinical Research Institute, Duke University, Durham, NC 27705, USA
Department of Psychiatry, University of North Carolina at Chapel Hill School of Medicine, Chapel Hill, NC 27514, USA
Carolina Institute for Developmental Disabilities, University of North Carolina at Chapel Hill School of Medicine, Chapel Hill, NC 27514, USA

T. Chandrasekhar
Duke Center for Autism and Brain Development, Duke University, Durham, NC 27705, USA
Department of Psychiatry, University of North Carolina at Chapel Hill School of Medicine, Chapel Hill, NC 27514, USA

C. E. Walsh
Department of Psychiatry, University of North Carolina at Chapel Hill School of Medicine, Chapel Hill, NC 27514, USA

L. C. Politte
Department of Psychiatry, University of North Carolina at Chapel Hill School of Medicine, Chapel Hill, NC 27514, USA
Carolina Institute for Developmental Disabilities, University of North Carolina at Chapel Hill School of Medicine, Chapel Hill, NC 27514, USA

G. D. Stuber
Department of Psychiatry, University of North Carolina at Chapel Hill School of Medicine, Chapel Hill, NC 27514, USA
Department of Cell Biology and Physiology, University of North Carolina at Chapel Hill School of Medicine, Chapel Hill, NC 27514, USA
Neuroscience Center, University of North Carolina at Chapel Hill School of Medicine, Chapel Hill, NC 27514, USA

J. Bizzell
Duke-UNC Brain Imaging and Analysis Center, Duke University Medical Center, Durham, NC 27705, USA
Carolina Institute for Developmental Disabilities, University of North Carolina at Chapel Hill School of Medicine, Chapel Hill, NC 27514, USA

J. L. Kinard
Carolina Institute for Developmental Disabilities, University of North Carolina at Chapel Hill School of Medicine, Chapel Hill, NC 27514, USA

Sanne Bongers and Pieter F. A. de Nijs
Department of Child and Adolescent Psychiatry/ Psychology, ENCORE NF1 Expertise Centre for Neurodevelopmental Disorders, Erasmus Medical Centre–Sophia Children's Hospital, Rotterdam, The Netherlands

André B. Rietman
Department of Child and Adolescent Psychiatry/ Psychology, ENCORE NF1 Expertise Centre for Neurodevelopmental Disorders, Erasmus Medical Centre–Sophia Children's Hospital, Rotterdam, The Netherlands

Department of Child and Adolescent Psychiatry/ Psychology, Sophia Children's Hospital, Room Sp 2478, CB Rotterdam, The Netherlands

Rianne Oostenbrink
Department of General Paediatrics, ENCORE NF1, Erasmus Medical Centre–Sophia Children's Hospital, Rotterdam, The Netherlands

Marie-Claire de Wit
Department of Paediatric Neurology, ENCORE NF1, Erasmus Medical Centre–Sophia Children's Hospital, Rotterdam, The Netherlands

Caspar W. N. Looman
Department of Public Health, Erasmus Medical Centre, Rotterdam, The Netherlands

Eddy Gaukema, Sandra van Abeelen and Jos G. Hendriksen
Kempenhaeghe Centre for neurological learning disabilities, Heeze, The Netherlands

Sandra Naumann
Berlin School of Mind and Brain, Humboldt-Universität zu Berlin, Berlin, Germany

Ulrike Senftleben
Department of Psychology, Technische Universität Dresden, Dresden, Germany

Megha Santhosh
Seattle Children's Research Institute, Seattle, USA

James McPartland
Yale University, New Haven, USA

Sara Jane Webb
University of Washington, Washington D.C., USA

Index

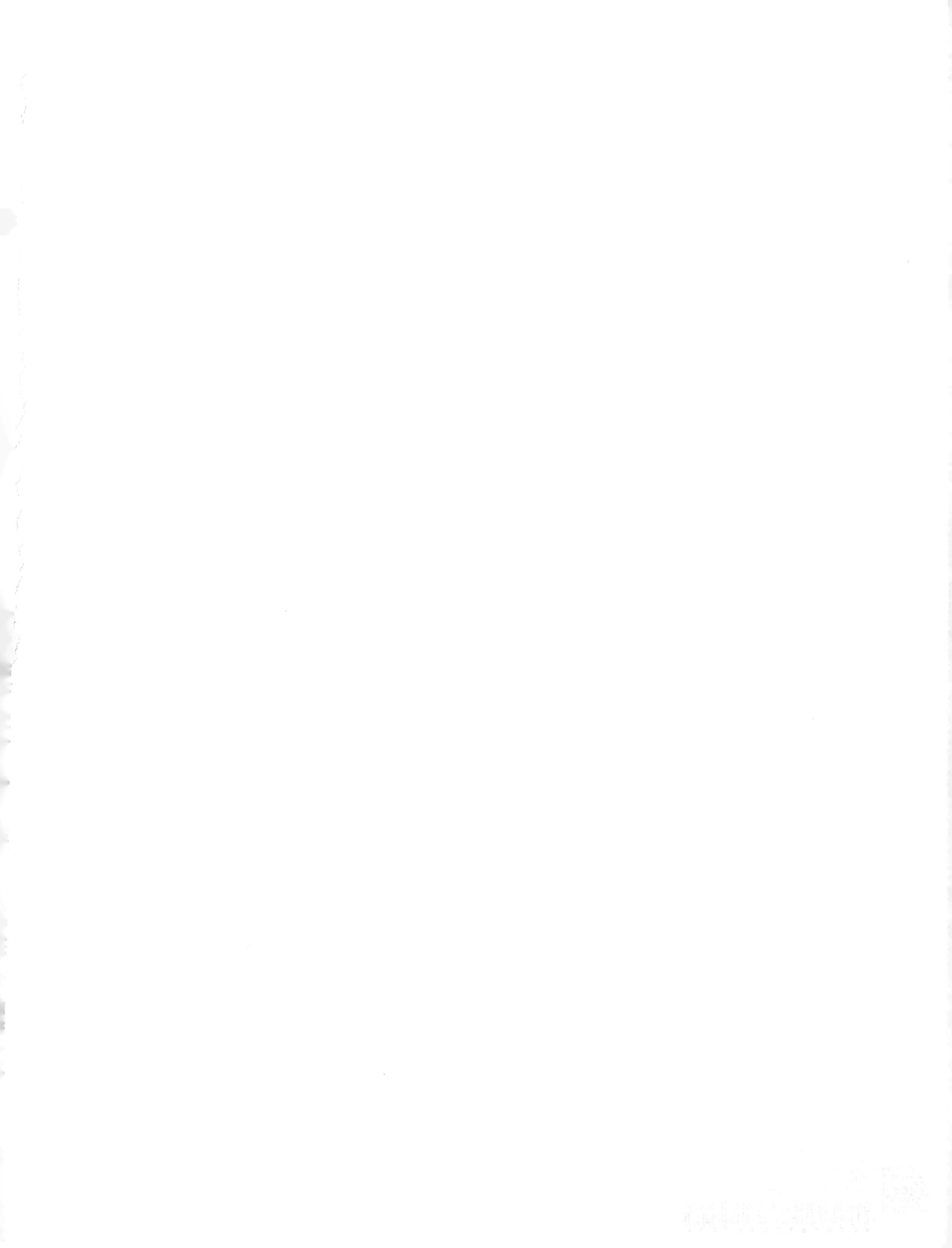